LUNG WATER
AND SOLUTE EXCHANGE

LUNG BIOLOGY IN HEALTH AND DISEASE

Executive Editor: **Claude Lenfant**
Director, Division of Lung Diseases
National Institutes of Health
Bethesda, Maryland

Volume 1   IMMUNOLOGIC AND INFECTIOUS REACTIONS IN THE LUNG, *edited by Charles H. Kirkpatrick and Herbert Y. Reynolds*

Volume 2   THE BIOCHEMICAL BASIS OF PULMONARY FUNCTION, *edited by Ronald G. Crystal*

Volume 3   BIOENGINEERING ASPECTS OF THE LUNG, *edited by John B. West*

Volume 4   METABOLIC FUNCTIONS OF THE LUNG, *edited by Y. S. Bakhle and John R. Vane*

Volume 5   RESPIRATORY DEFENSE MECHANISMS (in two parts), *edited by Joseph D. Brain, Donald F. Proctor, and Lynne M. Reid*

Volume 6   DEVELOPMENT OF THE LUNG, *edited by W. Alan Hodson*

Volume 7   LUNG WATER AND SOLUTE EXCHANGE, *edited by Norman C. Staub*

Other volumes in preparation

PATHOGENESIS AND THERAPY OF LUNG CANCER,
edited by Curtis Harris

GENETIC DETERMINANTS OF PULMONARY DISEASE,
edited by Stephen D. Litwin

CHRONIC OBSTRUCTIVE PULMONARY DISEASE,
edited by Thomas L. Petty

EXTRAPULMONARY MANIFESTATIONS OF RESPIRATORY DISEASE,
edited by Eugene D. Robin

LUNG WATER AND SOLUTE EXCHANGE

Edited by

Norman C. Staub

Cardiovascular Research Institute
University of California, San Francisco
San Francisco, California

MARCEL DEKKER, INC.   New York and Basel

Library of Congress Cataloging in Publication Data

Main entry under title:

Lung water and solute exchange.

    (Lung biology in health and disease; v. 7)
    Includes bibliographies and index.
    1. Pulmonary edema. 2. Lungs. I. Staub, Norman C., 1929–   II. Series.
[DNLM: 1. Pulmonary edema. 2. Lung–Anatomy and histology. 3. Lung–Physiopath-
ology. 4. Microcirculation–Physiopathology. 5. Pulmonary circulation. 6. Body water–
Metabolism. 7. Proteins–Metabolism. Wl LU62 v. 7 / WF600 L965] RC756.L83 vol. 7
[RC776.P8] 616.2'4'008s [616.2'4] ISBN 0-8247-6379-3   77-15047

MARCEL DEKKER, INC.
270 Madison Avenue, New York, New York 10016

Current printing (last digit):
10 9 8 7 6 5 4 3 2 1

PRINTED IN THE UNITED STATES OF AMERICA

CONTRIBUTORS

Lynn H. Blake, Ph.D.   Chief, Interstitial Lung Diseases, Division of Lung Diseases, National Heart, Lung, and Blood Institute, National Institutes of Health, Bethesda, Maryland

Kenneth L. Brigham, B.A., M.D.   Director, Pulmonary Circulation Center and Associate Professor of Medicine, Department of Medicine, Vanderbilt University School of Medicine, Nashville, Tennessee

Richard Casaburi, Ph.D.   Assistant Professor of Medicine, Department of Medicine, Division of Respiratory Physiology and Medicine, Harbor General Hospital Campus, UCLA School of Medicine, Torrance, California

Carroll E. Cross, M.D.   Associate Professor and Director of Pulmonary Laboratories, Department of Internal Medicine and Human Physiology, University of California, Davis, Davis, California

Robert E. Drake, M.D., Ph.D.[1]   Assistant Professor, Department of Anesthesiology, University of Missisippi Medical Center, Jackson, Mississippi

Richard M. Effros, B.A., M.D.   Associate Professor of Medicine, Department of Medicine, Division of Respiratory Physiology and Medicine, Harbor General Hospital Campus, UCLA School of Medicine, Torrance, California

Alfred P. Fishman, M.D.   William Maul Measey Professor of Medicine, and Director, Cardiovascular-Pulmonary Division, Department of Medicine, University of Pennsylvania, Philadelphia, Pennsylvania

Joan Gil, M.D.[2]   Anatomisches Institut der Universität Bern, Bern, Switzerland

Frank E. Gump, M.D.   Professor of Surgery, Department of Surgery, College of Physicians and Surgeons, Columbia University, New York, New York

Present Affiliation

[1] Department of Anesthesiology, University of Texas Medical Branch, Galveston, Texas
[2] Associate Professor of Medicine and Anatomy, Department of Medicine, Cardiovascular-Pulmonary Division, University of Pennsylvania, Philadelphia, Pennsylvania

Denis F. J. Halmagyi, M.D., D.Sc., F.R.A.C.P.[3]   Associate Professor of Physiology in Surgery, Department of Surgery, College of Physicians and Surgeons, Columbia University, New York, New York

James C. Hogg, M.D., Ph.D.   Professor of Pathology, Department of Pathology, McGill University, Montreal, Quebec, Canada

Herbert N. Hultgren, M.D.   Professor of Medicine, Stanford University School of Medicine, Stanford, California, and Cardiology Service, Veterans Administration Hospital, Palo Alto, California

Richard W. Hyde, M.D.   Professor of Medicine and Radiation Biology and Biophysics, University of Rochester School of Medicine and Dentistry, Rochester, New York

Frank N. Low, A.B., Ph.D.   Research Professor in Anatomy, Department of Anatomy, University of North Dakota, Grand Forks, North Dakota

Aldo A. Luisada, M.D.   Distinguished Professor of Medicine and Physiology, The Chicago Medical School, University of Health Sciences, and Chairman, Department of Cardiology, Oak Forest Hospital, Oak Forest, Illinois

Edward C. Meyer, M.D.   Director of Surgery, Department of Surgery, Mercy Catholic Medical Center, Fitzgerald Mercy Division, Darby, Pennsylvania

Giuseppe G. Pietra, M.D.   Associate Professor of Pathology, Departments of Pathology and Medicine, University of Pennsylvania, Philadelphia, Pennsylvania

Norman C. Staub, M.D.   Professor of Physiology, Cardiovascular Research Institute, University of California, San Francisco, San Francisco, California

Aubrey E. Taylor, Ph.D.[4]   Professor of Physiology and Biophysics, Department of Physiology and Biophysics, University of Mississippi Medical Center, Jackson, Mississippi

Karlman Wasserman, M.D., Ph.D.   Professor of Medicine and Chief, Department of Medicine, Division of Respiratory Physiology and Medicine, Harbor General Hospital Campus, UCLA School of Medicine, Torrance, California

Present Affiliation

[3]Chief of Medicine, Penobscot Valley Hospital, Lincoln, Maine
[4]Chairman, Department of Physiology, University of South Alabama Medical School, Mobile, Alabama

FOREWORD

I would be hard put to say whether the expansion of research on the lung and on respiratory disease is a precursor or a result of increasing public awareness of the importance of pulmonary illness. Whatever the case, we have undoubtedly witnessed both phenomena within a relatively short period of time, and with them a rather sobering realization of the limitations in both scientific and general public knowledge of lung disease. New concerns about the impact of environmental and occupational hazards on lung function—impacts that may only manifest themselves in frank disease after decades of seemingly innocuous exposure—serve to remind us all that society pays a heavy price when knowledge lags behind action, and moreover that society looks to science for solutions.

This series of monographs is, therefore, most timely and important. The substantial increase in the number and variety of scientific reports on respiratory and pulmonary topics makes it all the more critical that work in this field be subjected to thorough and comprehensive review as a service to the scientist and the physician who find it virtually impossible to "keep up," let alone to assimilate and evaluate a rapidly growing body of knowledge in an area of human health that is of mounting importance.

Chronic and acute lung diseases are among the major causes of disability and death in all age groups. From a public health standpoint, prevention of these diseases is a goal that amply justifies an increased commitment of research resources. For it is clear that the most effective paths toward prevention will emerge out of disciplined study in many fields, from the physiology and biochemistry of the respiratory system to the pathology and therapy of respiratory disorders.

I feel sure that this series of publications will continue to make a substantial contribution to the science and practice of medicine and to the hopes we have for more effective concepts and methods of preventing a major segment of human disease.

Theodore Cooper, M.D.
Former Assistant Secretary for Health
Department of Health, Education, and Welfare

PREFACE

Considering that more than 7 million ml of blood flow daily through an average man's pulmonary microvessels, it is remarkable that we are not up to our carinas in edema froth most of the time. Clearly, in the course of evolution a major problem was how to overcome fluid leakage into the air spaces of the lung. And it was overcome in a manner so eloquent and simple as to make the most advanced extracorporeal oxygenator look shabby by comparison.

Pulmonary vascular pressure is maintained at a low level by the remarkable infolding of the gas exchange surfaces, which provides a huge cross-sectional area of microvessels, thereby permitting high flow at low resistance. The large endothelial surface area, however, forms an imperfect barrier that leaks water and small molecules and is even somewhat permeable to proteins. Thus, there is normally a slow, steady outward flux of fluid and protein.

The lymph pumping system easily handles this normal fluid leak, as long as passive movements of the lungs with breathing deliver the extra fluid to the initial lymphatics. Once within the lymphatics, fluid is propelled by active contractions of the ducts.

To prevent the filtered fluid from entering the alveoli, there is a second barrier, the *alveolar* epithelium, that is nearly impermeable to the smallest water soluble particles. Thus, excess fluid in the lung's interstitium is removed without encroaching on the air spaces.

This volume is, I believe, the first attempt to systematically treat the fluid and solute exchange of the lung. The first four chapters describe the basic fluid anatomy. The next six chapters deal with quantitative aspects of both normal and abnormal fluid and protein exchange. Since pulmonary edema is a real and life-threatening clinical entity, five chapters are devoted to selected types of edema. The concluding chapter discusses approaches to treatment.

In a rapidly moving field such as this, we run the risk of being out of date before we can get the volume published. Certainly important new information has appeared since the chapter manuscripts were prepared. Nevertheless, the fundamental issues and data do not change. I am sure this volume will usefully serve students and investigators for a long time.

Norman C. Staub
San Francisco, California

vi

INTRODUCTION

This series of monographs was conceived to cover as many aspects as possible of lung biology in health and disease. The previous volumes have, by and large, been concerned with the normal lung and its many functions. This monograph is the first in the series to cover the entire spectrum of approaches and disciplines within a given area—from basic research to clinical considerations, including treatment.

Because the thrust of the volume is pulmonary edema, a clinical entity of great prevalence and severity, some readers, undoubtedly, will think the title *Lung Water and Solute Exchange* is misleading. One should see in this the mark of the basic scientist who edited the volume! I am grateful to Norman Staub for selecting this title because it seems to emphasize the important role that basic science plays in the solution to problems of diseases, a role that is too frequently overlooked.

The first chapter of this volume is written by Dr. Staub, who seems to express regrets, if not apologies, for having left out facets of the subject matter. In response, let me emphasize that this series is not an encyclopedia, but rather an analysis of our state of knowledge and—sometimes indirectly—an identification of our knowledge gaps. The volumes' editors were asked to assemble a list of topics that would be a challenge for present and future researchers. Norman Staub has reached this objective superbly. He has assembled an authorship representing so much expertise and sophistication that the readers, be they students of biology or medicine, researchers or clinicians, will be stimulated.

I am personally grateful to him for having accepted the task and for his outstanding accomplishment.

Claude Lenfant
Bethesda, Maryland

CONTENTS

Part One

ANATOMY OF LUNG WATER
AND SOLUTES

1

Lung Fluid and Solute Exchange

NORMAN C. STAUB

University of California, San Francisco
San Francisco, California

I. Introduction

Although the first measurement of lung fluid exchange occurred less than twenty years ago [1], we have made tremendous progress towards understanding the pathophysiology of edema in an organ that was thought to be relatively inaccessible [2]. In many ways, our knowledge of the lung's microcirculation and the factors governing fluid exchange, particularly in intact animals and man, exceeds similar knowledge about most body organs. It is relatively easy to measure pulmonary blood flow by a variety of techniques, and the recent development of flow-directed catheters has permitted the routine measurement of both upstream (pulmonary artery) and downstream (pulmonary wedge) pressures. In addition, the lung is probably the only organ for which we can determine the capillary blood volume by noninvasive techniques [3].

The impetus for studying fluid exchange is partly due to the clinical importance of pulmonary edema. Edema of peripheral tissues may be unpleasant, unsightly, and certainly undesirable but it is not usually a catastrophic event. In the lung, however, fluid in the alveoli interferes with gas exchange and when mixed with air, forms a stable foam that seriously affects overall ventilation and the distribution of inspired air. There seems to be an increasing number of patients with acute pulmonary edema, the primary etiology of which is not left atrial hypertension. Table 1 summarizes the incidence of acute pulmonary edema in the respiratory intensive care unit of a large county hospital.

Experimentally, progress has occurred along several fronts almost simultaneously, not the least being improved methods for quantifying fluid exchange [4,5]. One important advance is the recognition that clinical pulmonary edema is a late manifestation and that more attention must be focused on the early stage, when excess lung water is entirely interstitial and the process is clinically silent [6].

It is not so surprising, then, that we are now able to devote a volume in this series to lung fluid and solute exchange, whereas at a large international symposium on microvascular fluid exchange in 1969, the lung was scarcely mentioned [7]. Although much is known, there remains much to learn. We still do not have a magic substance to reverse the edema process.

II. Oversights

The work included in this volume represents current research on lung fluid exchange. It is not as all-inclusive as I had originally planned. For any omissions and deficiencies, I accept full responsibility.

There is no separate chapter on lung lymphatics, although Low (Chapter 2) reviews the anatomy of lymphatics in relation to the lung and Halmagyi (Chapter 14) briefly reviews general lymphatic function. Probably the single best review of pulmonary lymphatic anatomy is the work of Lauweryns [8]. Additional material relating to the functional aspects of pulmonary lymphatics can be found in my review [6].

TABLE 1   Noncardiogenic Pulmonary Edema in a Respiratory Intensive Care Unit in 1974

Patients Admitted	
A. Total	927
B. Clinical Edema	65
1. On admission	30
2. As a complication	35

Reproduced courtesy of J. Murray, personal communication

There is no chapter on the radiology of lung edema, particularly new experimental approaches to the qualitative and quantitative estimates of lung water [9].

Although our description of lung fluid distribution in edema, covering gross and histologic aspects, is generally accepted [10], it is by no means complete. The temporal relation between alveolar wall edema and edema in the loose interstitial connective tissue spaces has not been completely clarified and the distribution of lung fluid in high altitude edema, uremic edema, and shock lung remains to be worked out.

Although alveolar flooding [11] is referred to frequently, there is no organized chapter about this phenomenon. What is the trigger mechanism? What are the anatomical sites? This should be a particularly fruitful subject for investigation. Vreim recently showed the identity of interstitial and alveolar fluid in the various kinds of pulmonary edema [12,13]. Gee [14], Egan [15], and Bignon [16,17] are among those currently studying fluid and protein exchange across the alveolar, or airway epithelium. The data appear to be contradictory and the approaches are necessarily indirect. But attention is focused on the problem. There is some discussion in Chapter 10 concerning edema-fluid clearance. But it is probable that alveoli do not flood in the same way as that by which they are cleared.

I particularly regret that there is no organized chapter on cell injury and intracellular edema. Recently, Leaf [18] discussed cell swelling in injury. Effros (Chapter 8) and Brigham (Chapter 9) briefly mention this facet. I must confess to having totally ignored it [6]. My excuse is that we were engrossed with measuring interstitial forces and lymph flow in the early phases of pulmonary edema.

The early studies of pulmonary edema by electron microscopy [19] described intracellular changes, mostly the formation of large blebs. Although some of these changes may have been due to technical difficulties, they have not been completely explained away and are still reported (Chapter 9).

Several specific forms of pulmonary edema could have been included in the section on clinical physiology. Two in particular merit mention. How neurogenic factors function is still unsettled in spite of at least one hundred years of study. Fortunately, Luisada (Chapter 12) discusses one hypothesis concerning neurogenic factors in hemodynamic pulmonary edema. Nevertheless, there is substantial literature invoking neurogenic factors independent of any cardiac effects. Moss [20] claims that denervation of one lung completely prevents the edema of the adult respiratory distress syndrome in that lung. It is his belief that direct neurological influences are responsible for the lung lesions seen in this conglomerate of noncardiogenic edemas. Theodore and

Robin [21] have reviewed the accumulated experience in neurogenic pulmonary edema and have an interesting hypothesis that is subject to experimental
tests.

Microembolization of the lung may be associated with severe edema
clinically and experimentally [22]. Saldeen has reviewed his work in this
field [23]. We are also interested in the mechanisms by which embolization
of the lung may lead to altered fluid and protein exchange [24]. The relative
importance of the physical obstruction and the release of permeability-altering
chemicals that emboli occasion remains to be determined. Some aspects of
this problem are referred to in the final chapter on the treatment of pulmonary edema.

III. Starling and his Hypothesis

I am impressed by how many different interpretations there are of what
Ernest Starling said about transvascular fluid exchange. These different interpretations are evident in various chapters of this treatise. He is credited variously with *enunciating* a law, *giving* an equation, and *stating* a hypothesis.
Whatever one may call it, the real question becomes, Is it true, is it a reasonable approximation, or is it false?

I have reread Starling's main papers of 1894–1896 with the view of
clarifying in my own mind what he wrote. Starling [25] credits Ludwig with
the view that "lymph flow was determined by differences of pressure and
composition between the blood in the vessels and the fluids filling the interstices of the tissues." By the word *composition,* he went on to state, he meant
the chemical composition that set up osmotic interchanges.

He clearly realized that the microvascular endothelium was permeable to
protein. He wrote, "The simplest way of explaining these differences [varia-
tions in lymph protein composition] is to look upon them as due to differences
in the permeability of the filtering medium. The more permeable the medium,
the greater is the effect of changes in the pressure of the filtering fluid and
the greater is the ease with which dissolved proteids pass through it. Thus,
the capillaries of the limbs have only a small permeability. . . . The intestinal
capillaries are more permeable. . . . Highest in the scale of permeability come
the liver capillaries."

Starling never mentioned reflection coefficients. However, he realized
that the effective osmotic pressure was variable because only proteins ($\sigma \sim 1$)
exerted osmotic effects [26] whereas electrolytes ($\sigma \sim 0$) did not. He actually used the word *hindered* ($\sigma < 1$), not the word *impermeable* ($\sigma = 1$), for
proteins. He states it quite clearly: "It must be remembered that the early

workers used animal membranes in their experiments on osmotic interchanges. These membranes permit the passage of water and salts, but *hinder* the passage of coagulable proteid."

As for the actual statement of Starling's hypothesis, we find it in his 1896 paper, a page of which is shown in Figure 1. Nowhere does he enunciate a law nor give an equation. As for the question about the applicability of Starling's hypothesis, it works — and beautifully [27] — although as we shall see in Chapter 8, brief osmotic transients to substances of small molecular weight can be achieved experimentally.

I have tried to trace the first appearances of Starling's hypothesis in equation form as we know it today [27]. Landis [28] made quantitative measurements of capillary hydrostatic pressure and the rate at which fluid passes through the walls of single capillaries. His Figure 10 and the regression equation on page 234 of this reference come close to stating the hypothesis in equation form. His equation considered only the intravascular forces, however.

The complete equation containing the extravascular and intravascular forces appeared in a study of pleural effusions by Iverson and Johansen in 1929 [29]. These investigators were followed in quick succession by Meyer and Holland in 1932 [30], Weech and associates in 1933 [31], and Landis in 1934 [32]. All these equations, however, assumed that the sum of forces equated zero, that is, there was no net fluid filtration.

So far as I can tell, the first filtration equation appears in the paper of Pappenheimer and Soto-Rivera in 1948 [33]!

IV. Plan of the Text

A. Anatomy of Lung Water and Solute Distribution and Exchange

Chapters 2 through 4 deal with some of the basic fluid anatomy and pathology of the lung. In Chapter 2, Low describes the lung's interstitium, emphasizing similarities with other organs and also noting features special to the lung. His interesting conceptual approach to the "total body plan" for interstitium and his scanning electron micrographs lead directly into Chapter 3, wherein Gil reviews in detail anatomical relations within the alveolar walls. Both authors speculate about the functional implications of the structural organization.

These two chapters contain numerous stimulating ideas. For example, I would like to know how it is that Low uses vascular perfusion with aldehyde fixatives to produce severe pulmonary edema in guinea pigs whereas Gil uses a similar procedure to fix normal lung in rats. Further, both authors take the

Feb. 5.   At 4 p.m.
      Height of A = 53 cm. serum.
      Height of B = 40 mm. Hg.
      Height of C = 15 cm. serum.   Experiment stopped.
   At beginning of experiment Δ of serum   = $-$ ·600° C.
          „   „ Δ of outer fluid (1·03 °/₀ NaCl) = $-$ ·630° C.
   At end of experiment Δ of serum   = $-$ ·635° C.
          „   „ Δ of outer fluid = $-$ ·635° C.
   The serum contained 7·56 °/₀ proteids.

The importance of these measurements lies in the fact that, although the osmotic pressure of the proteids of the plasma is so insignificant, it is of an order of magnitude comparable to that of the capillary pressures; and whereas capillary pressure determines transudation, the osmotic pressure of the proteids of the serum determines absorption. Moreover, if we leave the frictional resistance of the capillary wall to the passage of fluid through it out of account, the osmotic attraction of the serum for the extravascular fluid will be proportional to the force expended in the production of this latter, so that, at any given time, there must be a balance between the hydrostatic pressure of the blood in the capillaries and the osmotic attraction of the blood for the surrounding fluids. With increased capillary pressure there must be increased transudation, until equilibrium is established at a somewhat higher point, when there is a more dilute fluid in the tissue-spaces and therefore a higher absorbing force to balance the increased capillary pressure. With diminished capillary pressure there will be an osmotic absorption of salt solution from the extravascular fluid, until this becomes richer in proteids; and the difference between its (proteid) osmotic pressure and that of the intravascular plasma is equal to the diminished capillary pressure.

Here then we have the balance of forces necessary to explain the accurate and speedy regulation of the quantity of circulating fluid. It is evident however that we cannot explain in this way the absorption of serum or other fluids rich in proteids from the serous cavities and connective tissues. I would point out however that we have as yet no sufficient evidence that such fluids are absorbed by the blood vessels. If we inject serum into the pleural cavity we find that it is absorbed very much more slowly than is a similar amount of salt solution. The absorption is indeed so slow that it is impossible to exclude the possibility that the whole of it has taken place through the lymphatics.

from ERNEST H. STARLING
ON THE ABSORPTION OF FLUIDS FROM THE CONNECTIVE TISSUE SPACES
JOURNAL OF PHYSIOLOGY, VOL. 19, PP. 312-326, 1895-96

Starling's early discussion of the importance of proteins to fluid balance and exchange between capillary blood and tissue.

FIGURE 1   Reprinted from Classic Pages, *Circ. Res.*, 21:116, 1967.

view that it is well demonstrated that pinocytotic vesicles in the vascular endothelium and alveolar epithelium participate in transcellular transport. I read the same literature, but I am not convinced. I believe the definitive experiment on the function of vesicles in transvascular transport remains to be done.

Now that an alternative function for endothelial vesicles has been found, however, in rapid substrate conversion [34], perhaps the urgency to find something for vesicles "to do" may abate.

In Chapter 4, Gump brings us up to date on measuring lung-fluid compartments. He clearly identifies what can be done and what ought to be done to standardize and improve the procedures. Studies of human and animal lungs in a variety of edemogenic conditions remain to be done. It would be interesting to determine whether the same amount of interstitial fluid accumulates in lungs during high-pressure edema as opposed to altered vascular permeability edema before the onset of alveolar flooding. Halmagyi implies a difference in his essay on "shock lung," Chapter 14. Even while Gump's chapter was in process, an improved method for lung tissue hemoglobin was published [35] and two groups have been exploring radioisotope methods for separating lung-fluid compartments in intact animals and man [36,37]. Finally, if appropriate methods can be used to preserve lung fluids in edematous lungs, one could use point-counting procedures to determine the distribution of fluid in blood cells, interstitium, and alveoli, as Meyer demonstrates in Chapter 10.

B. Physiology of Transvascular Exchange

In Chapters 5 through 10, the authors develop the physiologic aspects of normal and abnormal lung-fluid and protein exchange. Chapters 5 and 6 deal with mathematical modeling to provide a rational basis for explaining experimental results. Blake states succinctly what the value of mathematical modeling can be. He uses measured data obtained in steady state sheep [27] to develop a consistent multiple-pore model. He explains by equations, graphs, and words (the last, that even ordinary mortals can understand) the complex interaction of solutes and the transport processes (diffusion and convection).

Taylor and Drake review the ways in which the specific coefficients and forces in the fluid and protein flux equations are measured. This is of great value, since theoretical analyses are data-limited, in both reliability and scope. These authors review a wide selection of experimental results and offer several interesting alternative possibilities to explain fluid and protein exchange. The two chapters taken together point out numerous uncertainties that afford fertile ground for future investigations.

In Chapter 7, Hogg reviews blood-flow distribution in the lungs and the changes that occur as pulmonary edema develops. Although his data are indirect, they are interesting, somewhat perplexing, and definitely provocative. Regardless of interpretation, however, they show that extravascular forces, in this case extravascular hydrostatic pressure, are critical to understanding the dynamics of lung-fluid exchange. Strong efforts towards direct pressure measurements are urgently needed.

In Chapter 8, Effros examines the exchange of *small* molecules across the pulmonary vascular endothelium; he makes extensive use of the multiple indicator dilution method and he mentions fluid and solute exchange across the alveolar epithelium. He also considers intracellular edema, a phenomenon we know must exist in toxic lung injury, but about which we know very little.

In Chapter 9, Brigham defines, detects, and discusses altered pulmonary microvascular permeability. He cites several exciting leads from his own work and speculates about mechanisms of increased permeability. This aspect of lung solute and water exchange is moving rapidly.

Although most of our research is directed towards edema formation, we must not neglect the recovery phase after the edemogenic response is over. Thus, Chapter 10 by Meyer is welcome. It is intriguing and stimulating. Here, possibly for the first time, is a thorough review of mechanisms of clearance of the products of edema.

C.   Clinical Physiology of Pulmonary Edema

Chapters 11 through 16 are directed towards clinical research and applications to improved patient care. As always, methods for detecting and measuring edema have been rate-limiting, especially those designed for use in intact animals and man. The authors of Chapter 11 review those methods currently in vogue clinically, and also several methods that are being developed. Their conclusions are that while we are severely restricted now, the future is promising.

Visscher [2] referred to hemodynamic pulmonary edema as the "garden variety," meaning that it is far and away the most common form. In spite of a deluge of research and clinical reports about "noncardiogenic" edema, we must not forget that pulmonary venous hypertension is still the leading cause of pulmonary edema. It is probably the simplest form of edema to study experimentally and will continue to be significant for our understanding of the forces and factors that regulate fluid and protein exchange [27]. Luisada, a pioneer in the study of pulmonary edema, discusses the hemodynamic form from the classical view in Chapter 12. He reviews his hypothesis concerning the role of the central nervous system via the sympathetic vasoconstrictor and cardiac outflow. This is an important point, since neurogenic factors in the genesis of pulmonary edema are being reexamined [21].

In Chapter 13, Pietra and Fishman discuss the possibility of selective injury to the bronchial circulation. Although it is well known that edema of the airway mucosa and submucosa may occur in allergic reactions, little attention has been paid to the bronchial vasculature as a source of significant overall fluid filtration. That is due partly to the fact that anatomically the bronchial vessels appear insignificant compared with the pulmonary blood vessels and that flow through the pulmonary vascular bed is 100 times that through the bronchial circulation. The authors remind us, however, that the size of a vascular bed and the flow through it need not bear any relation to its part in transvascular fluid exchange. Their demonstration of the ultrastructural effects of histamine and bradykinin on bronchial venular "gap" formation with retention of colloidal carbon particles in the gaps is intriguing. However, in Chapter 9, Brigham gives evidence that is directly contradictory — about the action of infused histamine in low doses over much longer periods.

The relative activities of the bronchial and pulmonary circulation in various types of edema are not completely clear. This is another interesting field for investigation.

Halmagyi's Chapter 14 on "shock lung" is not the usual comprehensive review and discussion of the syndrome, but a brief personal essay. He lists several interesting differences between the edema of cardiac failure and that of "acute hypoxic respiratory failure" (the phrase he prefers instead of *shock lung*). His review of lymph function is brief but touches all the main points. He provides a very valuable bibliography, much of it foreign literature. His hypothesis that the lymph pump fails in this syndrome is provocative and dovetails nicely with some of Meyer's discussion in Chapter 10. The clear message is that lymphatics and their function need to be studied so that they may be assigned their proper place in total cardiovascular-interstitial fluid function.

In Chapter 15, Hultgren carefully reviews the clinical entity known as high altitude pulmonary edema. He also reviews the suspected etiologic factors, with emphasis on his own experimental work. Why is this seemingly bizarre form of edema of such interest? First, it is not too uncommon. The incidence at high altitude appears to be increasing, presumably owing, as Hultgren states, to the ready access to high altitude by skiers and mountain climbers. Second, the concept of uneven obstruction of the pulmonary arterial system with overperfusion of the remaining microcirculation, which first Gibbon first described [38] and then Visscher [22], is enjoying increased popularity as the basic injury in several forms of noncardiogenic pulmonary edema [21,24]. Reid [39] has quantitative data in normal adult human lungs on the uneven distribution of smooth muscle in the pulmonary arterioles, thus giving an anatomical basis for uneven vasoconstriction during alveolar hypoxia.

The author makes an important point about the difficulty of studying this problem when no good experimental animal model of high altitude pulmonary edema exists. His plea for vigorous support towards developing a suitable model is most welcome. It has certainly been true for other aspects of fluid and solute exchange that rapid progress followed successful development of an animal paradigm [5].

Chapter 16, the last chapter, covers the treatment of pulmonary edema. Some will no doubt feel that such a chapter is premature. I disagree. Pulmonary edema is a real disease and every effort should be made to apply the improved understanding and awareness of it to patients. Drs. Cross and Hyde have come through with a presentation that ties together many points raised in earlier chapters. It is a fitting conclusion to this treatise because it expresses the rather unsatisfactory status of diagnosis and treatment of clinical pulmonary edema, and at the same time offers numerous hopeful possibilities for eventual mastery of this serious but underrated and misunderstood problem.

V. Terminology

I made an effort in 1971 [40] and again in 1974 [6] to standardize the nomenclature for pulmonary fluid and solute exchange. I hoped to make it consistent with the symbols that pulmonary physiologists already used for gas exchange. Although I have had only a modicum of success in convincing others that they should use the new terminology, you may agree after reading this treatise that I was justified in my desire to regularize the use of terms.

In the lung, there are clearly vessels that are exposed to at least part of the alveolar gas pressure. These are termed *alveolar vessels.* All other vessels, particularly the larger arteries and veins, are said to be *extra-alveolar,* signifying only that they are exposed to an external surface pressure different from that of alveolar vessels. Unfortunately, a mystique has grown that alveolar vessels are capillaries and extra-alveolar vessels are not. This separation has not been demonstrated. One reason I use the murky word *microvascular* is just that we are not entirely clear about which vessels are the sites of fluid and protein exchange.

Likewise, the hydrostatic pressure outside the exchange vessels could be related either to alveolar pressure in the alveolar wall interstitium or to pressure in the extra-alveolar connective tissue in the perivascular, peribronchial, and lobar septal spaces. That is why I use the term *perimicrovascular* interstitial fluid without specifying exactly where this is. The evidence suggests that there are at least two distinct components to the pulmonary vascular bed and its interstitium [41,42,6].

Figure 2 is a model I use when thinking about the hydrostatic forces affecting fluid exchange. It includes two "interstitial" compartments and two or even three "microvascular" pressures.

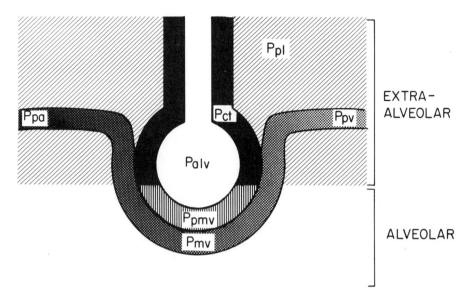

FIGURE 2   Model of fluid-exchange regions of lung. Alveolar compartment is probably the main site of fluid exchange because of its enormous surface area. Perimicrovascular fluid pressure (P_{pmv}) equals alveolar pressure (P_{alv}). For the extra-alveolar vessels, the interstitial connective tissue fluid pressure (P_{ct}) is probably less than (P_{alv}) and related to pleural pressure (P_{pl}). The other abbreviations are for vascular hydrostatic pressures: pulmonary artery (P_{pa}), microvascular (P_{mv}), and venous outflow (P_{pv}).

References

1. A. C. Guyton and A. W. Lindsey, Effect of elevated left atrial pressure and decreased plasma protein concentration on the development of pulmonary edema, *Circ. Res.*, 7:649–657 (1959).
2. M. B. Visscher, F. J. Haddy, and G. Stephens, The physiology and pharmacology of lung edema, *Pharmacol. Rev.*, 8:389–434 (1956).
3. F. J. W. Roughton and R. E. Forster, Relative importance of diffusion and chemical reaction rates in determining rate of exchange of gases in the human lung, with special reference to time diffusing capacity of pulmonary membrane and volume of blood in the lung capillaries, *J. Appl. Physiol.*, 11:290–302 (1957).
4. M. L. Pearce, J. Yamashita, and J. Beazell, Measurement of pulmonary edema, *Circ. Res.*, 16:482–488 (1965).

5. N. C. Staub. Steady state pulmonary transvascular water filtration in un-anesthetized sheep. In *Local Regulation of Blood Flow.* Edited by S. Rodbard, *Circ. Res.,* **28/29** (Suppl. 1):135–139 (1971).

6. N. C. Staub, Pulmonary edema, *Physiol. Rev.,* 54:687–811 (1974).

7. *Capillary Permeability.* Edited by C. Crone and N. A. Lassen. Copenhagen, Munksgaard, 1970.

8. J. M. Lauweryns. The blood and lymphatic microcirculation of the lung. In *Path. Ann.* Edited by S. C. Sommers. New York, Appleton, 1971, pp. 365–415.

9. E. N. C. Milne, Correlation of physiologic findings with chest roentgenology, *Radiologic Clinics of North America,* **11**:17–47 (1973).

10. N. C. Staub, H. Nagano, and M. L. Pearce, Pulmonary edema in dogs, especially the sequence of fluid accumulation in the lungs, *J. Appl. Physiol.,* 22:227–240 (1967).

11. N. C. Staub, M. H. Gee, and C. E. Vreim, Mechanisms of alveolar flooding in acute pulmonary oedema. In *Lung Liquids,* Ciba Foundation Symposium No. 38. Amsterdam, Elsevie, 1976, pp. 255–263.

12. C. E. Vreim and N. C. Staub, Protein composition of lung fluids in acute alloxan edema in dogs, *Amer. J. Physiol.,* **230**:376–379 (1976).

13. C. E. Vreim, P. D. Snashall, and N. C. Staub, Protein composition of lung fluids in anesthetized dogs with acute cardiogenic edema, *Amer. J. Physiol.,* **231**:1466-1469 (1976).

14. M. H. Gee and N. C. Staub, Role of bulk fluid flow in protein permeability of the dog lung alveolar membrane, *J. Appl. Physiol.,* **42**:144-149 (1977).

15. E. A. Egan, Effect of lung inflation on alveolar permeability to solutes. In *Lung Liquids,* Ciba Foundation Symposium No. 38. Amsterdam, Elsevier, 1976, pp. 101–110.

16. J. Bignon, P. Chakinian, G. Feldmann, and C. Sapin, Ultrastructural immunoperoxidase demonstration of autologous albumin in the alveolar capillary membrane and in the alveolar lining material in normal rats, *J. Cell. Biol.,* **64**:503–509 (1975).

17. J. Bignon, M. C. Jaurand, M. C. Pinchon, C. Sapin, and J. M. Warnet, Immunoelectromicroscopic and immunochemical demonstration of serum proteins in the alveolar lining material of the rat lung, *Amer. Rev. Resp. Dis.,* **113**:109–120 (1976).

18. A. Leaf, Cell swelling: A factor in ischemic tissue injury, *Circulation,* **48**: 455–458 (1973).

19. H. Schulz. *The Submicroscopic Anatomy and Pathology of the Lung.* Berlin, Springer, 1959.

20. G. Moss, C. Staunton, and A. A. Stein, Cerebral etiology of the "shock lung syndrome," *J. Trauma,* 12:885–890 (1972).

21. J. Theodore and E. D. Robin, Speculations in neurogenic pulmonary edema, *Amer. Rev. Resp. Dis.,* 113:405–411, 1976.

22. M. B. Visscher, The pathophysiology of lung edema; a physical and physicochemical problem, *Lancet,* 82:43–47 (1962).

23. T. Saldeen, The microembolism syndrome, *Microvasc. Res.*, 11:227–259 (1976).
24. K. Ohkuda, K. Nakahara, and N. C. Staub, Changes in lung fluid and protein balance in sheep after microembolism, *Physiologist*, 19:315 (1976).
25. E. H. Starling, The influence of mechanical factors on lymph production, *J. Physiol.*, 16:224–267 (1894).
26. E. H. Starling, On the absorption of fluids from the connective tissue spaces, *J. Physiol.*, 19:312–326 (1896).
27. A. J., Erdmann, III, T. R. Vaughan, Jr., K. L. Brigham, W. C. Woolverton, and N. C. Staub, Effect of increased vascular pressure on lung fluid balance in unanesthetized sheep, *Circ. Res.*, 37:271–284 (1975).
28. E. M. Landis, The relation between capillary pressure and the rate at which fluid passes through the walls of single capillaries, *Amer. J. Physiol.*, 82:217–238 (1927).
29. P. Iverson and E. H. Johansen, Pathogenese und Resorption von Trans- und Exudaten in der Pleura, *Klin. Wochenschr.*, 8:1311–1312 (1929).
30. F. Meyer and G. Holland, Die Messung des Druckes in Geweben, *Arch. Exp. Path. Pharm.*, 168:580–602 (1932).
31. A. A. Weech, C. E. Snelling, and E. Goettsch, The relation between plasma protein content, plasma specific gravity and edema in dogs maintained on a protein inadequate diet and in dogs rendered edematous by plasmaphoresis, *J. Clin. Invest.*, 12:193–216 (1933).
32. E. M. Landis, Capillary pressure and capillary permeability, *Physiol. Rev.*, 14:404–481 (1934).
33. J. R. Pappenheimer and A. Soto-Rivera, Effective osmotic pressure of the plasma proteins and other quantities associated with the capillary circulation in the hind limbs of cats and dogs, *Amer. J. Physiol.*, 152:471–491 (1948).
34. A. F. Junod, Metabolism, production and release of hormones and mediators in the lung, *Amer. Rev. Resp. Dis.*, 112:93–108 (1975).
35. S. L. Selinger, R. D. Bland, R. H. Demling, and N. C. Staub, Distribution volumes of [^{131}I]albumin, [^{14}C]sucrose and ^{36}Cl in sheep lung, *J. Appl. Physiol.*, 39:773–779 (1975).
36. A. B. Gorin, W. J. Weidner, and N.C. Staub, Noninvasive measurement of altered protein permeability in lungs of sheep, *Amer. Rev. Resp. Dis.*, 111:941 (1975).
37. J. S. Pritchard and G. deJ. Lee, Non-invasive measurement of regional interstitial water spaces, capillary permeabilities and solute fluxes in the lung, using a radioisotope method, *Bull. Physio. Path. Resp.*, 11:137–141 (1975).
38. J. H. Gibbon, Jr., and M. H. Gibbon, Experimental pulmonary edema following lobectomy plasma infusion, *Surgery*, 12:694–704 (1942).
39. L. Reid, Structural and functional reappraisal of the pulmonary artery system, *Scientific Basis of Med. Annual Rev.*, 289–307 (1968).
40. N. C. Staub, Proposed pulmonary space nomenclature. In *Central Hemo-*

dynamics and Gas Exchange, Appendix III. Edited by C. Giuntini. Turin, Minerva Med., 1971, pp. 465–467.

41.   L. D. Iliff, Extra-alveolar vessels and edema development in excised dog lungs, *Circ. Res.,* **28**:524–532 (1971).

42.   G. Bφ, A. Hauge, and G. Nicolaysen, Alveolar pressure and lung volume as determinants of net transvascular fluid filtration, *J. Appl. Physiol.,* **42**:476-482 (1977).

2

Lung Interstitium
Development, Morphology, Fluid Content

FRANK N. LOW

University of North Dakota
Grand Forks, North Dakota

I. Introduction

Pulmonary edema can be interpreted morphologically as "an abnormal accumulation of liquid and solute in the extravascular tissues and spaces of the lung" [1] and physiologically as "a persistent imbalance between the forces that move water into the extravascular spaces and the biologic devices for its removal" [2]. As the removal devices begin to fail, fluid accumulates in abnormal anatomical locations, first in the interstitium far removed from the pleura [3] (or at least in bronchiolar rather than alveolar areas) and only secondarily in the alveolar walls and then the airspaces. This apparent contradiction of a long-established conviction, that capillaries are necessarily the "leaky" portions of the vascular system [4], focuses attention on the interstitium, or tissue (connective tissue) space. A fine structural evaluation of the interstitium with emphasis on its boundaries, its contents, and its position in development is now possible through investigations of recent years. We shall examine these features with some comments on their developmental origin and the formed elements within the area. This essentially morphologic description will be correlated with certain physiologic data, the whole designed as a point of departure for those who want to analyze problems of pulmonary edema.

17

Examining the literature pertinent to fluid and solute exchange at the level of fine structure reveals that relatively little fundamental structural work has been done on the lung itself. Broad analysis therefore necessitates bold extrapolation of basic data derived from areas of the body experimentally more accessible than the lung. Indeed, the greater part of the rationale presented in this chapter relies on data collected about other areas of the body— an unfortunate necessity because of the dearth of primary data derived from experimental observations of the lung itself. This approach naturally proceeds with the assumption that like conditions prevail in lung structures known to be of similar morphologic composition. The reader therefore has to accept the reasoning that basic fine structure is essentially uniform for the entire body. It can then be understood that the lung, although extremely complex in some structural details, is constructed according to a total body plan that does not differ fundamentally for all parts of the organism.

Todd and Bowman [5] in 1845 formulated a body plan that emphasized an epithelium that covered the entire geometric surface of the body.

> This external integument is a part only of a great physiological system, which comprehends also the mucous membranes, and the true or secreting glands; all of which, taken together, and reduced to their most simple expression, are a continuous membrane, more or less involuted, more or less modified in the elementary tissues which compose it or are in connexion with it, and within which all of the rest of the animal is contained. This expanse consists of two elements: a basement tissue composed of simple membrane, uninterrupted, homogeneous and transparent, covered by an epithelium, or pavement, of nucleated particles. Underneath the basement membrane vessels, nerves and areolar tissue are placed.

This complex was understood to include the skin, and the alimentary, respiratory, and genitourinary systems, with the "true" glands that arose from them. The connective tissue underlying the epithelium (*milieu interne* of Claude-Bernard; connective tissue space of morphologists) was recognized to be thicker under certain epithelia and was thus demonstrable as a basement membrane by the basophilic dyes of light microscopy. For somewhat more than a century thereafter, histologists described epithelia as possessing or not possessing a basement membrane, depending on whether or not it was visualized by preparatory techniques then in use. In 1949, Gersh and Catchpole [6], using the newly developed periodic acid–Schiff (PAS) technique, demonstrated a basement membrane beneath *all* epithelia. There were similar, very thin membranes separating muscle, nerve, and fat from the connective tissue space wherever they abutted it. During the next decade, technical improvements in transmission electron microscopy revealed much thinner membranes in the same positions, interposed between the cells of epithelium, muscle, nerve, and fat on the one side and connective tissue space on the other. The designation basement membrane (although now less appropriate descriptively because of newly discovered relations) was carried over without change from light microscopy to these new structures. Visible only with the electron microscope because of small dimensions (~25–50 nm thick, usually separated from their parent cell by a lucid interval of ~20 nm) their somewhat fuzzy outlines became familiar to electron microscopists. Other descriptive terms soon came into use. Fawcett [7] described these structures underneath epithelia and introduced the designation *basal lamina,* reserving the term *membrane* for lipoprotein complexes only. The relation of these laminae to the morphologic plan of the total body was emphasized by Low [8], whose descriptive term *boundary membrane* related them to the connective tissue space (of which they formed external and internal boundaries) rather than the cells with which they were closely associated. This term also identified them with the extracellular connective tissues, of which they are now recognized to be a part. Bennett's term *glycocalyx* [9] was introduced to designate a carbohydrate-rich area separating cells from their surroundings. Although the glycocalyx as described by Bennett was far more widely distributed than its evident coextensiveness with the boundaries of the tissue space, this term has had some general use to designate the structures under consideration. Since relations of tissues with the interstitium are prime to this chapter, the term *boundary membrane* will be used herein. But it should be remembered that it equates with *basement membrane, basal lamina,* and *glycocalyx* as these terms are customarily used in the literature of fine structure. Also, the term *interstitium* is interchangeable with the more descriptive *connective tissue space.*

The scanning electron microscope affords a new and interesting method of three-dimensional visualization of the edematous condition in lungs. This is shown in Figures 1 to 6, of which the three pairs (1 and 2, 3 and 4, 5 and 6) contrast normal and edematous tissue. These preparations were made either by insufflation of aldehyde-fixing fluid into the alveoli via the trachea and bronchial tree, which preserves the normal anatomy of the lung tissues (Figs. 1, 3, and 5), or by pulmonary vascular perfusion with the same fixing fluid at physiologic pressure for 30 min, which causes edema (Figs. 2, 4, 6). In each case the pleural cavity was not disturbed and there was no lung collapse as the tissues were hardened by fixation. Following the initial aldehyde fixation, pieces of lung were postfixed by osmium, dehydrated in ascending grades of acetone, critical-point-dried in liquid CO_2, surface-coated with metal (palladium/gold; 40:60), and finally examined in a scanning electron microscope.

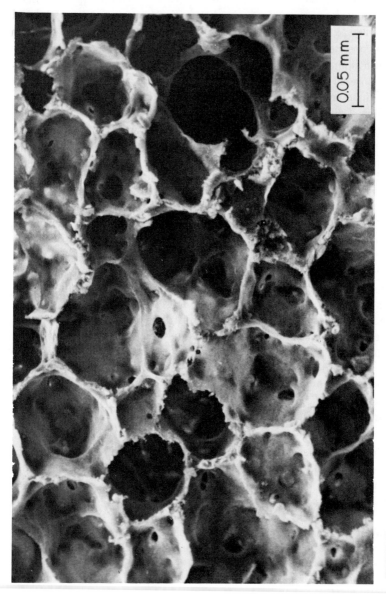

FIGURE 1   Cut surfaces of alveolar walls, guinea pig lung, normal. Note thinness of alveolar walls and relative size of airspaces. Alveolar pores, a normal feature of guinea pig lungs, are numerous.

0.05 mm

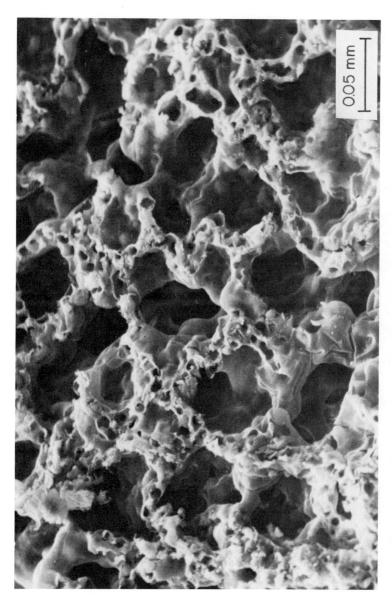

FIGURE 2 Cut surfaces of alveolar walls, guinea pig lung, edematous. Compare with Figure 1. Note the thick, swollen walls, open blood vessels, and distorted airspaces.

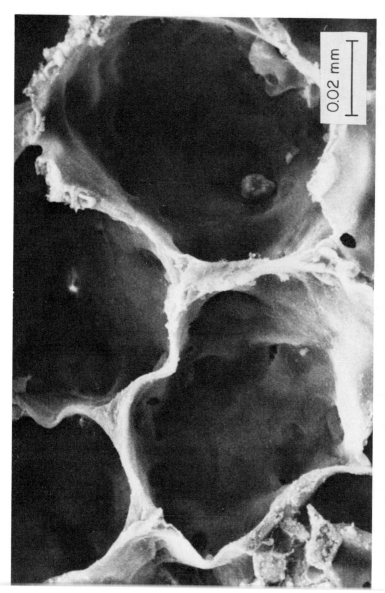

FIGURE 3 Cut surfaces of alveolar walls, guinea pig, normal. Note the thinness of the alveolar walls compared with the size of the airspaces. A free macrophage is in the alveolus at lower right.

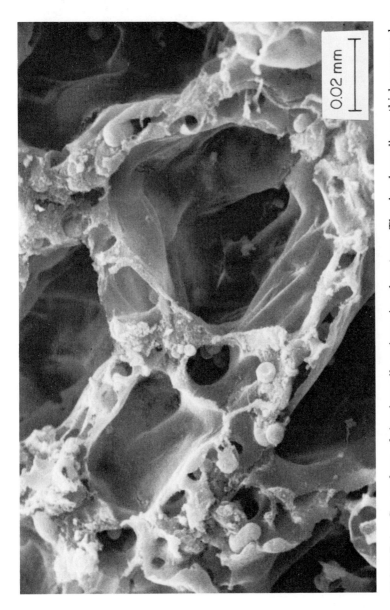

0.02 mm

FIGURE 4 Cut surfaces of alveolar walls, guinea pig, edematous. The alveolar walls are thick compared with those of Figure 3. The airspaces are also considerably reduced.

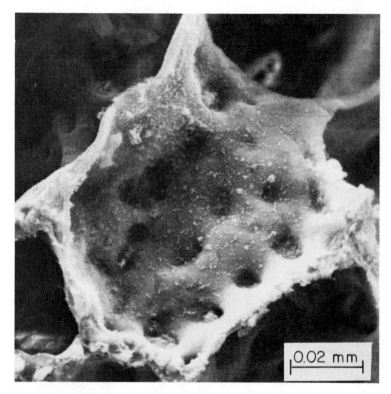

0.02 mm

FIGURE 5 Face-on view of alveolar wall, guinea pig, normal. Note the grid-like pattern produced by the dense capillary network, with individual capillaries projecting into the alveolus.

In each of the fields of Figures 1 to 6, the camera is facing the cut edge of a primarily respiratory portion of the lung parenchyma. The edematous tissue is characterized primarily by thickened alveolar walls, distended and empty blood vessels (due to continued pulmonary perfusion), and airspaces that are reduced and congested. The radical changes in amount of tissue versus airspace in advanced edema is dramatized by these preparations. There is no doubt that considerable fluid escaped into the interstitium of the alveolar walls. Whether or not the alveoli were flooded is not certain since any alveolar fluid would be washed out in the subsequent steps of the technique. Pieces of perfused lung floated when placed in liquid fixer, indicating considerable air content still remaining. Comparable lung pieces that were well insufflated sank in the fixing fluid, indicating that the air passageways had become filled with fixing fluid.

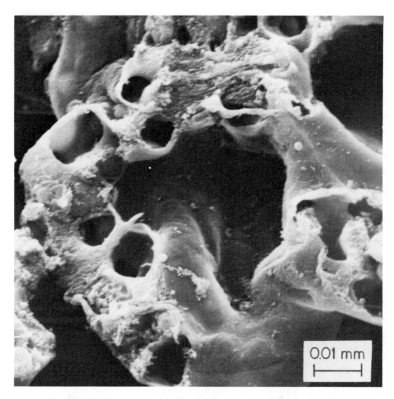

FIGURE 6 Cut surface and face-on view of alveolus, guinea pig, edematous. This micrograph, which should be compared with Figure 5, represents the most extreme edematous condition after long perfusion with buffered aldehydes at physiological pressures observed in our preparations. The interstitial spaces of the alveolar walls are greatly increased and the airspace is drastically reduced.

II. Morphologic Considerations

A. Total Body Plan

The total body of the vertebrate organism can be conceived according to a very simple structural body plan known as the boundary membrane concept [8] (Fig. 7). The external surface of the body is covered by an epithelium, which possesses an external free surface facing the outside world and a basal surface that rests on connective tissue. A boundary membrane (external) separates all epithelium from underlying connective tissue space. Within these

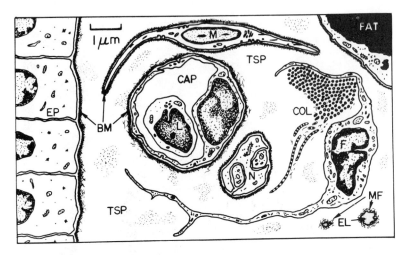

FIGURE 7   A representation of the boundary membrane concept as expressed
in the histologic organization of the total body. A continuous tissue space (TSP)
is separated by boundary membranes (BM) from the cells of epithelium (EP),
endothelium of the capillary (CAP), muscle (M), nerve (N), and fat. The connective tissue, consisting of both cells (F for fibroblast) and fibers (COL for unit
collagen fibers; EL for elastic fibers and MF for microfibrils), are contained in
the tissue space as its true contents. They have no boundary membranes.

external boundaries certain types of cells are similarly separated from the connective tissue space by boundary membranes (internal). These include endothelium, mesothelium (both sometimes included by morphologists with other
epithelia), muscle, nerve, and fat. The only main histologic tissue not yet accounted for is connective tissue. Its structural components, both cells and
extracellular materials, are the "true" contents of the connective tissue space.
They exist within it, without separation from ambient gels and fluids by
boundary membranes. The situation illustrated in Figure 7 is expressed at the
cellular level and persists throughout the body with few exceptions. This
same concept, as applied to the total body, is illustrated in the highly stylized
drawing of Figure 8. This represents the same basic situation as that which
exists early in embryonic life, when the distances between the non-connective-
tissue masses are large and the interstitium is voluminous. This representation
of the body emphasizes the continuity of the connective tissue space. This
continuity, despite the extremely complex geometric manifestations of the
connective tissue space brought about during development (vascularization, innervation, etc.), is maintained, so that the adult organism still possesses one
single, continuously communicating connective tissue space. It is important to

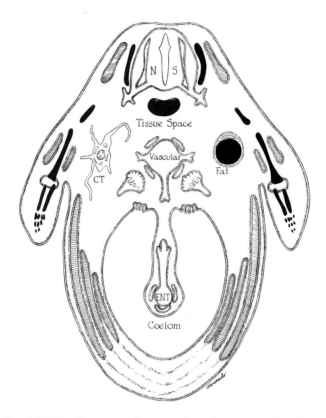

FIGURE 8 A highly diagrammatic expression of the main tissue masses and their relation to the tissue space in the embryo. The epithelium (here represented by the skin, the endoderm of the gut (ENT), the endothelium of the blood vascular system, the mesothelium lining the coelom, and the genitourinary epithelium), the muscular system (here represented chiefly in the body walls), the nervous system (NS), and fat cells are separated from the tissue space. The tissue space contains all the connective tissue cells (CT), fibers, and skeletal elements that have no boundary membranes. The tissue space is clearly single for the entire organism at this stage. Later, its geometric complexity greatly increases but it remains a single space, still expressing the fundamental relations depicted in this figure.

remember that this situation prevails throughout all stages of development and function in the living lung. Exceptions to this "boundary membrane concept" do occur. For example, although at least a small amount of tissue space intervenes between the boundary membranes of capillary endothelium and the membranes of epithelial parenchyma in most parts of the body, the connective tissue space does become obliterated between the two boundary membranes (so that only one membrane is demonstrable) in the renal corpuscles, portions of the alveolar walls of the lung, the central nervous system, the area vasculosa of the cochlear duct, and certain placental areas. Another notable exception to the general rule is the failure of boundary membranes to appear in vascular sinusoids (liver, bone marrow, some lymphoid organs) and around lymphatic capillaries. On close examination, such areas of morphologic exception are found to be accompanied by the special physiologic requirements of that particular area. These dual conditions, exception to a standard morphologic pattern and special physiologic requirements, provide interesting points of departure for the investigator. When thoughtfully used, they strengthen rather than weaken the boundary membrane concept.

B.   Connective Tissues

Cells

Connective tissue cells, which are the true cellular contents of the interstitium, tend to be individual in their relations to their surroundings. They are not usually organized by contact with each other as epithelium, muscle, and nerve cells are. Many move freely about in the extracellular matrix, which is more abundant in the interstitium than anywhere else in the organism. Certain connective tissue cell types, as in bone and cartilage, are trapped by the density of the surrounding matrix. Cell types are numerous and are known by a very complex terminology that often reflects their controversial relations with one another. Only a few connective tissue cells will be mentioned in this account, with emphasis on those most pertinent to considerations of lung structure.

The fiber-forming fibroblasts and the universally phagocytic macrophages are common in all areas of the interstitium. Generally these cells can move about and express their functions according to the environmental conditions about them. Mast cells, with their heparin-rich granules, are also frequent in "areolar" areas of the interstitium. All blood leukocytes can undergo diapedesis and thus can be found in similar areas. Many eosinophils appear to reside permanently in the interstitium. Fat cells, also present in loose connective tissue, merit special mention because they are the only cells of the connective tissue to have boundary membranes. It was formerly thought that a defatted adipose cell reverted to a fibroblast; later evidence [10] has shown that this resemblance is only superficial, since the boundary membrane persists in this condition of stress. A more satisfactory classification of fat cells places them as members of a separate tissue rather than of the connective tissue group.

Fibers

The fibrous tissue of the interstitium (which is extracellular) includes the three fiber types classically recognized in light microscopy: collagen, reticular, and elastic. The range of their dimensions is given in Figure 9. With the advent of electron microscopy, it was discovered that both collagen and reticular

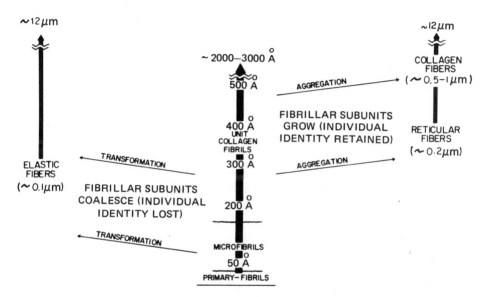

FIGURE 9   This diagram represents the developmental relations among the extracellular fibrous elements of the connective tissues. The main stem of fibrillar growth begins with the primary fibrils; these are the first to appear in ontogeny, and constitute a fine network in the earliest boundary membranes. At the interstitial surface of these membranes, microfibrils soon appear. Microfibrils increase in size and develop into periodically banded unit collagen fibrils. These aggregate to form both the reticular fibers and collagen fibers of light microscopy, in the sequence indicated. It is more difficult to include elastic fibers in a unitary concept of extracellular fibrillar development. The earliest expressions of elastin appear in electron microscopy as if transforming from already formed unit collagen fibrils. Later the homogeneous elastin component becomes surrounded by demonstrably hollow microfibrils, to form the "adult" organization of the elastic fibers of light microscopy. The primary fibrils and microfibrils of the main stem of growth persist in boundary membranes throughout the life of the organism and may provide a permanent fountain source for new fibrillar growth.

fibers are composed of smaller, "unit collagen fibrils," which have an axially repeating periodicity of 50–60 nm (in Epon-embedded thin sections) [11–13]. Elastic fibers were recognized as having a homogeneous core of elastin [14], surrounded by fibrils, which are ~15 nm in diameter and have a demonstrably hollow core. A morphologic set of smaller nonperiodic fibrils, now generally known as microfibrils [15], is routinely demonstrable in electron microscopy. An even smaller fibril type is believed by some to form the framework of boundary membranes [16,17]. These have been referred to as "primary fibrils [17], because of their early formation in ontogenetic development. A contribution by Policard et al. offers considerable detail on the fibrillar contents of the pulmonary interstitium [18]. Developmental sequences are described in a later section; these should clarify the presumptive relations of fibrils and fibers in adult tissue. These relations are expressed in diagrammatic form in Figure 9.

Ground Substance

Throughout the interstitium there is a varying amount of "ground substance." This is unresolvable at the electron-microscopic level with conventional techniques, but is well known through the histochemical techniques of light microscopy. Thus, the PAS technique reveals a concentration of mucopolysaccharides (or glycosaminoglycans) at the site of boundary membranes [6]. High concentrations of acid mucopolysaccharides characterize cartilage, in which, it is known, they stimulate the formation of new fibrils but inhibit individual fibrillar growth [19–21]. In bone, the amorphous matrix does not inhibit fibrillar growth but is heavily supplemented by inorganic crystals of apatite [22]. In most areas of areolar tissue, however, the ground substance is sufficiently hydrated to permit free cells of the connective tissue to move about. Fluid flow is generally not impeded, although most of the interstitium is normally immobile [23]. The general appearance of unit collagen fibrils in the interstitium is shown in Figures 10 and 11, which were obtained from sections 1 μm thick with a high-voltage microscope. These "thick" sections have the advantage of allowing greater thicknesses of tissue to be seen without loss of resolution, than it is possible to see with conventional electron microscopy and its ultrathin sections. In Figure 10, fibrillar elements are sparse and there is no visible impedance to free flow of fluids. Figure 11 represents a moderately heavy population of unit collagen fibrils of such a concentration that they might conceivably interfere with fluid flow. In the interstitium of the lung, the fibrillar concentration is normally between the two concentrations [24] shown, and it is not known to impede free flow of fluids and solutes.

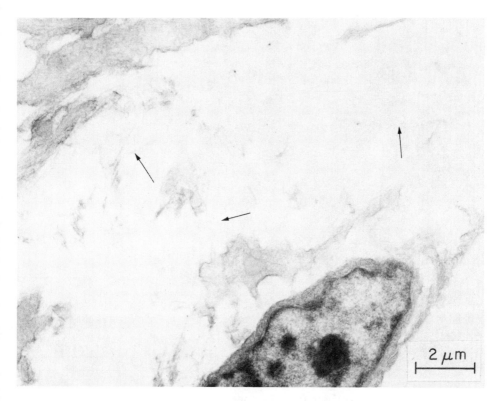

FIGURE 10   Loose connective tissue fibrils viewed in a 1-μm-thick section in a high-voltage electron microscope. This extremely loose arrangement of fibrillar connective tissue (arrows) leaves generous space for tissue fluid and would not be expected to impede free fluid movement. Photomicrograph obtained on the JEM-1000 in the Department of Molecular, Cellular and Developmental Biology, University of Colorado, under the direction of Dr. Keith R. Porter in Boulder, through the courtesy of Dr. Dennis E. Morse.

C.   Blood Vascular System

The blood vascular system is not, properly speaking, one of the contents of the connective tissue space since it is separated from it (with few exceptions) by an endothelial boundary membrane. Its capillary network is, however, so prominently represented in the functional areas of the lung that the fine structure of capillaries merits special attention [25–28]. Endothelial cells encircle the capillary lumen and present to it a predominantly smooth surface,

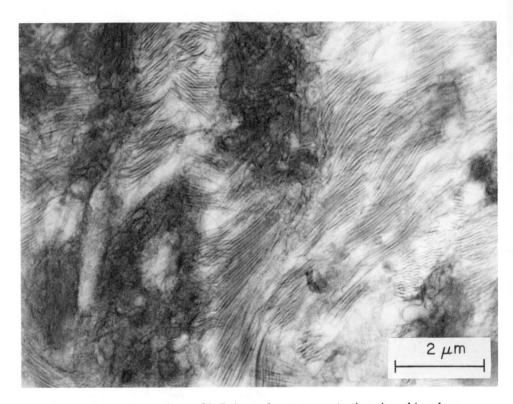

FIGURE 11   Unit collagen fibrils in moderate concentration viewed in a 1-μm-thick section at 1 million volts in a high-voltage electron microscope. The concentration of fibrils in this field, while still moderate compared with concentrations found in tendons and aponeuroses, might be enough to impair the free flow of fluid and solutes through the tissue space. The concentration of fibrils found in normal lung interstitium lies between the concentrations represented in Figures 10 and 11. Same source as Figure 10.

with nuclear position indicated by bulges. There is notable morphometric variation in different areas of the cytoplasm [29]. Wherever endothelial cells come into contact, there are junctions that are continuous along the line of contact. These vary from "tight" junctions to "gap" junctions, which themselves vary from the tight to the "leaky" type, the particular condition depending on the width of the junction. Their permeability is known to vary in sequential segments of the microvasculature [30] and is responsive to physiologic influences [31,32]. Marginal folds occur along areas of endothelial cell contact and tend to project somewhat into the lumen, where they can be seen in the sections of transmission electron microscopy [33]. They are also visible in scanning electron microscopy as they outline cell edges. Their observed relations to diapedesis suggest that they envelop a leukocyte from one or both sides until it is effectively sealed off from the bloodstream and then permit it to enter the space between endothelium and boundary membrane by retraction of the remaining basal portion of the endothelial cytoplasm. Although careful provision seems to exist in this process against incidental escape of serum, the potentiality here for vascular leakage should not be ignored. The site is under study by a group at the Australian National University [34]. Endothelial pinocytosis, or "transport in quanta" at the electron microscopic level, is morphologically demonstrable in capillaries and has been studied in great detail [25]. This process consists of vesicle formation from the plasmalemma of either surface, inclusion of an amount of surrounding substrate, and pinching off to form an independent vesicle that traverses the width of the endothelial cytoplasm. Finally, there is delivery of the vesicular contents to the substrate on the opposite side by fusion of the membrane of the vesicle to the plasmalemma of that side. This source of capillary leakage has been investigated with tracer particles varying from 4.2 to 30 nm in diameter (dextrans, glycogens, and exogenous myoglobin) in experiments that showed approximately 80% of the vesicles containing tracer 60 to 75 sec after injection [35,36]. Pinocytotic vesicles may make up as much as 15% of the volume of the endothelial cytoplasm [25]. It has recently been shown that coalescence of adjacent vesicles may cause patent transendothelial channels with demonstrable transport of small (2-nm) tracer molecules [37]. Pinocytosis is a possible if not readily measurable source of vascular leakage.

The boundary membranes of capillaries apparently have no special features to distinguish them from similar structures elsewhere. Both a fibrous and an amorphous component are recognizable. Small microfibrils about 5 to 10 nm in diameter are found on the surface abutting the tissue space, and somewhat finer fibrils are found deeper in the substance of the membrane [16, 17]. An amorphous material, unresolvable at the electron-microscopic level, decks the fibrillar substrate and produces an overall fuzzy appearance. A lucid interval, usually about 20 nm wide, known as the lamina lucida, separates the boundary membrane from the outer plasmalemma of the endothelium. Boundary membranes are passive rather than active structures, as shown by early work in electron microscopy [38–44]. Tracer materials of colloidal dimensions pass through them only with difficulty, but small molecules and ions are transmitted with essentially unmeasurable rapidity. Most workers using tracers have noticed that tracers are delayed in their passage through these membranes but eventually cross to the other side. Boundary membranes are best interpreted as primarily inert laminae that function as macromolecular filters.

The transition from capillaries to small veins involves no fundamental change in the vascular membrane (endothelium plus boundary membrane) [27] but rather an addition of extracellular connective tissue and fibroblasts to form the walls of the vessel in the connective tissue space outside the vascular membrane.

Lung Epithelium

The transport and tracer studies cited above were performed chiefly on capillary endothelium and associated boundary membranes in various areas of the body. In the alveolar wall of the lung, a similar situation with regard to cell junctions, vesicles of pinocytosis, and boundary membranes applies to the epithelial covering as well as the capillary endothelium. In fact, it is not possible to distinguish between the fine structure of these two complexes on morphologic grounds alone. Their fine structure is identical. Since comparable studies on pulmonary epithelium have not been undertaken, the data applicable to endothelium can be extrapolated to pulmonary epithelium without essential change.

D. Lymphatics

The lymphatics of the lung have long been recognized as extensive and critically important in lung physiology [45–48]. At the gross level, they possess certain interesting morphologic features. It is generally recognized that lung lymphatics exist in two distinct groups. Although they are variously described by different authorities [45–48], the following pattern is generally agreed on. A pleural group drains the visceral surface of the lungs. It follows the lung surface and to some extent the interlobular septa to reach the hilum. The deeper group of lymphatics within the lung parenchyma is divisible into two distinct patterns that are associated with two principal sets of vessels: (1) the set associated with the bronchial tree and pulmonary arterial system, the constituents of which travel deep within the lobules; and (2) the pulmonary venous set, which is primarily interlobular in its course, like the veins that these lymphatics follow. These sets communicate with each other along small veins and with the pleural set near the surface by means of small, capillary lymph ducts. Since numerous anastomoses connect these groups of lymphatics, some writers have been led to minimize their distinctness [49,50]. The presence or absence of valves in pulmonary lymphatics is physiologically significant, especially when edema exists, and valves must be responsible for draining extracellular fluids and solutes efficiently. There appears to be general agreement that lymphatic valves are present in pleural lymphatics and near the hilar nodes. But there is distinct disagreement in the literature about their presence in the lung parenchyma, centrally around the bronchial tree and the pulmonary arteries and veins. Perhaps the original and chief disclaimer of their presence is Miller [45], who emphasizes their paucity or total absence in the parenchyma. Kampmeier [51] supports this view in a developmental study of human lungs. In a more recent developmental study, Tobin [52] concludes that the central part of the lung usually possesses only a few lymphatic valves or is devoid of them. Yoffey and Courtice [53] support this view. An opposite stand is taken by observers who believe that the irregular diameter of injected lymphatics reveals the locations of valves at the points of constriction. On the basis of radiopaque injections of lymphatics, Trapnell [50] writes, "There is clear evidence, therefore, of an abundance of valves in all groups of pulmonary lymphatics." Lauweryns [54,55] tends in this direction (and his analyses involving irreversible flow depend on valves) but states that the valvular structure is "inconsistent in position and competency." The failure of fluid removal in edema suggests an incompetent system of lymphatic valves. But from the purely morphologic standpoint, this matter needs to be resolved by histologic check of serial sections through the central portions of the lung. Determination is especially difficult since identifying a valve in a lymphatic vessel is in itself very uncertain—there is a wide range of structural variation and a lack of clues about the competency of the structures observed [56]. It is generally believed that lymphatic flow proceeds toward the hilum, mostly along bronchial, arterial, and venous lymph vessels. Exception to this "deep to deeper" pattern of flow may occur near the pleural set of vessels. Communications between the deep and pleural sets carry lymph to the pleura. From here it continues along the pleural set either to the hilum or to a point where pleural vessels communicate with the deeper (venous) set. Injection studies yield conflicting results, since thorotrast remains in pleural vessels until the hilum is reached [57] but India ink injections tend to follow communications between pleural vessels and the deeper set [58]. The literature on paths of pleural lymph flow is reviewed by Simer [58]. Especially notable is that those investigators writing on lymphatic flow, which necessarily depends on the topography and efficiency of valves, frequently speak of irregularity and incompetency of the pulmonary lymphatic valves. The extent to which lymphatic channels extend into the interstitium of the terminal or near terminal branches of the bronchial tree is of great interest. All observers agree that lymphatic vessels extend at least into terminal bronchioles but not as far as the alveolar walls (interalveolar septa of Lauweryns [55]). Miller [45] traces lymphatics through respiratory bronchioles and into alveolar ducts, but no farther; that is to say, they are absent in the walls of atria and alveoli. Lauweryns [55], on the other hand, describes them, with convincing illustrations, between the adult "alveolar wall" and the "interlobular, pleural peribronchial or perivascular connective tissue sheets." He defines them by the term *juxta-alveolar lymphatic capillaries.* These vessels constitute the distal end of the bronchial lymphatic tree. The fine structure of lymphatic capillaries presents features of interest, particularly when compared with the fine structural organization of blood vascular capillaries. Lymph capillaries are from two to five times the diameter of blood capillaries [15 to 40 μm) [59]. Notable other differences are (1) the presence of intracellular cytoplasmic filaments [59], which may be presumed to consist of contractile proteins; (2) the presence of loose, or leaky, "junctions" between endothelial cells, which may in places separate as much as 1 to 10 μm, with adhering zonules or gap junctions dispersed irregularly but not continuously along lines of "junction" [59–61]; (3) the absence or marked incompleteness of the boundary membrane that characterizes the vascular membrane of the blood vascular system [59]; and (4) the presence of anchoring filaments of connective tissue that attach to the outer surface of lymph capillaries and effectively attach these surfaces to surrounding connective tissue elements [62].

The classic concept that lymphatics terminate in a system of blind-ended tubules, the lymph capillaries, is well known but was of course formulated at the light-microscopic level of observation. While this idea is not conclusively contradicted in fine-structure findings, there are, as indicated above, modifications of the closed-tubule concept that clearly accommodate the uptake of fluid and large molecules from the surrounding interstitium [60, 62-64]. Both the incompleteness of the boundary membranes that are normally macromolecular filters and the looseness of the endothelial junctions accommodate the idea of such a takeup. By presumption, the cytoplasmic filaments that are capable of contraction and the connective tissue anchors could both, by physical disposition and controlled contracture, accommodate the intake of the lymphatic capillaries. At the level of fine structure, both morphology and physiology could accommodate this important uptake function of lymphatic capillaries. One finds, in examining the lymphatic channels along from the capillaries to larger vessels, that their walls resemble the walls of veins. Although pericytes are absent [65], a boundary membrane becomes complete. The walls increase in thickness, chiefly by addition of connective tissues but also with addition of some isolated smooth muscle cells. Large lymph vessels are difficult to distinguish histologically from veins.

III.   Developmental Background

A.   Total Lung

Development of the lung can conveniently be interpreted in terms of the total body plan. The keynote of the entire process is aggressive growth into the surrounding interstitium by two tubular systems. The epithelium of the bronchial tree and the endothelium of the vascular system both invade the intervening connective tissue space from different directions. A ventral outgrowth of the epithelium of the alimentary canal becomes the trachea, the lung buds, and eventually the entire respiratory tree. The endothelium of the sixth aortic arch is similarly aggressive and eventually accounts for the entire pulmonary circulation, which extends from the right ventricle to the left atrium. In early stages, the tissue space between the epithelial lung bud and the endothelial sixth arch is relatively large compared with these structures. As the size of the embryo increases, there is aggressive growth by both respiratory and vascular components. Effectively the two approach each other but the tissue space is maintained and grows between them as all three systems increase in size. Finally, in the terminal airspaces (the alveoli), the boundary membranes of certain capillary spaces and the alveolar epithelium fuse. Here there is local but partial obliteration of the tissue space, a physical relation that does not occur anywhere else in the lung. The alveolar capillaries receive blood from the right side of the heart via the pulmonary arteries and drain to its left side by the pulmonary veins; this whole system of vessels is separated from the air passageways by varying amounts of tissue space, except in the walls of the alveoli themselves. The epithelium of the airways and the endothelium of the blood vessels all along their respective courses have boundary membranes that face intervening tissue space. The remainder of the walls of both airways and blood vessels develop within this space as expressions of the connective tissues. Connective tissues thus form extracellular fibrils and light-microscopic fibers, and in the larger bronchi, cartilage. Muscle cells develop individual boundary membranes. Peripheral nerve remains separated from other tissues by the boundary membranes of Schwann cells. At least a small amount of tissue space surrounds them except at the functional terminations of individual axons. Lymphatics invade the interstitium from the hilum until a complex network of richly anastomosing vessels finally occupies its characteristic place in the interstitium. Some investigators believe that developing lymphatics originate from veins, whereas others credit their derivation from undifferentiated mesenbhyme [66]. Whatever their origin, it is agreed that their development begins during the second month at the hilum [51,52]. The most vigorous generation of valves occurs during the third and fourth months of gestation. At birth retrograde injection of lymphatics is only limited but becomes impractical in adult lungs. The endothelium of the lymphatics becomes separated from the surrounding interstitium by boundary membranes except at the lymphatic capillary level, where it is deficient, ranging from incomplete to absent. It is important to remember that all through the developmental process, the connective tissue space that surrounds these non-connective tissues persists even down to the alveolar wall, as illustrated in Figures

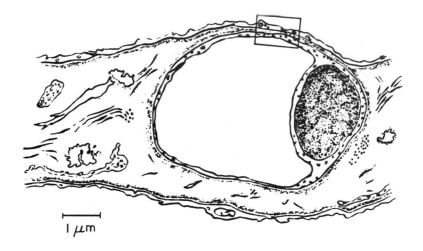

1 μm

FIGURE 12   The essential relations of alveolar air, capillary blood, and interstitium are represented here. The capillary abuts the epithelium above but is
separated from the epithelium below, a situation believed to prevail in the alveolar wall. The tissue space with its various extracellular fibrils is continuous with
the connective tissue space of all the rest of the organism. The area included in
the rectangle is presented in greater detail in Figure 13.

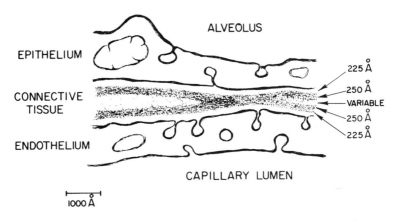

1000 Å

FIGURE 13   The essential physical relations existing at the blood-air barrier
are represented here. At the thinnest expression of the connective tissue space,
epithelium and endothelium with their boundary membranes have pressed it out
of existence. The entire complex here has been observed to be as thin as 500 μm.
Numerous vesicles of pinocytosis are present in both endothelium and epithelium.

12 and 13. It is an unbroken continuation of the same connective tissue
space that exists between externally located epithelium and internally located
endothelium in the relatively simple relations of the embryo in early stages of
development. The continuity of the tissue space is not special to the lung,
since nowhere in the body is this continuity broken. The entire organism
therefore possesses only one tissue space. Epithelial-endothelial relationships
are special in the lung in parts of the alveolar walls only where the tissue
space becomes obliterated (blood-air barrier, illustrated in Figs. 13 and 15) by
fusion of endothelial and epithelial boundary membranes. The fundamental
layers basic to the entire body are retained even here: epithelium, connective
tissues, endothelium—representing the outside covering, the middle tissue, and
the inside lining.

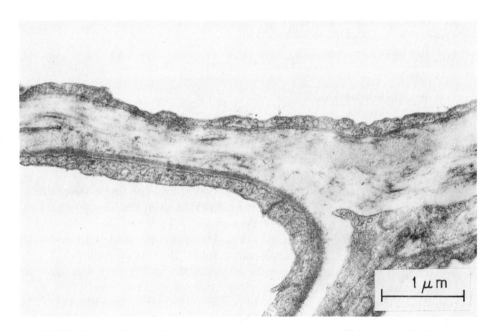

FIGURE 14   Connective tissue intervening between alveoli (above and below
right) and capillary (below left) are represented in this photomicrograph and can
be compared with the lower part of the drawing in Figure 12. The amount of
formed elements (ground substance and fibrils) in the connective tissue space is
typical of the lung and can be compared with the extremes represented in Figures 10 and 11.

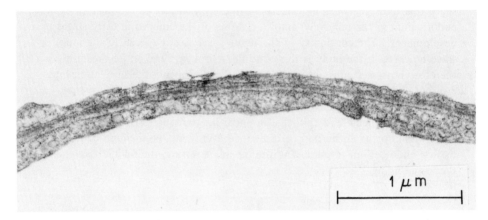

FIGURE 15   The blood-air barrier is expressed by this alveolar wall, in which
the alveolar epithelium and capillary endothelium are separated only by a boundary membrane. Compare with Figure 13.

B.   Connective Tissues

Growth relations among the extracellular connective tissues in the early embryo provide interesting clues to their real and potential relations in the developed organism. A series of studies of developing extracellular connective
tissue in the chick has established a growth continuum involving primary fibrils, microfibrils, and unit collagen fibrils in that order. The first extracellular
connective tissue to appear comprises the primary fibrils of the boundary
membrane of the future ectoderm of the embryo [17]. Within 24 hr this extremely fine fibrillar network becomes decked with amorphous material, and a
boundary membrane of mature appearance results. The first microfibrils
(~4-6 nm) appear upon or close to the surface of the ectodermal boundary
membrane and seem to delaminate into the tissue space. Their growth becomes prolific during the second day of incubation, especially around the
notochord [67,68]. Here masses of them form the fibrillar substrate of the
first cartilaginous vertebral bodies in a substrate rich in acid mucopolysaccharides [69,70]. Their growth here is restricted to a fibril diameter of about
20 to 25 nm. Lateral to this area, comparable inhibition does not operate
and microfibrils increase in diameter, gradually develop the periodicity that
identifies them as unit collagen fibers, and so reach a morphologic end-
point of development [13]. Their further growth and aggregation into the
reticular and collagen fibers of light microscopy is indicated in Figure 9. It is

more difficult to derive elastic fibers from a growth continuum. Their homogeneous component, elastin, appears in the chick, in the aorta, at about one week of incubation, subsequent to the establishment of unit collagenous fibrils [71]. Although the very earliest masses of elastin seem to arise in close physical relation with unit collagenous fibrils, it is difficult to accept a derivation of one from the other because there is thus implied extracellular protein synthesis (the amino acid residues of elastin are distinct from these of tropocollagen)—thought by many to be a biologic impossibility. However, hollow microfibrils (~20 nm) arrange themselves longitudinally around masses of elastin, apparently in such a way that they guide the development of fibril shape [14]. Although these microfibrils are of uncertain origin, it is possible that they are an offshoot of the main stem of microfibril to unit collagen fibril growth, an interpretation that helps a unitary concept of the origin of fibrillar connective tissues (Fig. 9).

IV. Interpretative Remarks

The extremely complex tissue relations observed in the lung, along with its many and varied fine structural characteristics, may well discourage an analyst from trying to rationalize the known events of pulmonary edema. Nevertheless, a reasonable interpretation can be reached if one is willing to interpret the lung in terms of "total-body" structure and function and to assume that bold extrapolation of data originally derived from far-removed parts of the body can be usefully applied to lung problems. Proceeding thus, one can develop along the following lines a rationale of the symptoms of lung edema.

Accumulation of fluid in the interstitium points incontestably to leakage from the vascular system. Quite naturally, the capillary bed, where structural elements intervening between bloodstream and interstitium are at a minimum, has been regarded as the site of leakage. Much work has been devoted to close examination of capillaries with reference to their presumed role in vascular leakage. Three possible sources of leakage are now recognized on both morphologic and physiologic grounds: pinocytosis, leaky junctions, and incidental fluid loss during diapedesis. While all these are true sources of leakage, tracer studies do not bear out the supposition that massive loss of fluid occurs at the capillary level.

As early as 1930, the possibility that both arterioles and venules of near capillary size could leak was investigated [72]. Considerable evidence points to small veins in the systemic circulation as the chief source of leakage [42,43]. Under carefully controlled experimental conditions known to increase vascular leakage, small veins passed tracer substances in large amounts while capillaries in the same area rendered little or no evidence of leakage. Veins as small as

10 μm in diameter and as large as 80 μm were involved, with maximum leakage occurring with the 20-to-30-μm group. Comparable evidence for the lung has been presented by Iliff [73]. When excised lungs had gained 4% to 6% of their original weight, extra-alveolar vessels accounted for 63% of the weight gain. Leakage, as indicated by "cuffing" around the vessels, occurred in veins as large as 750 μm in diameter but in arteries only as large as 200 μm, putting the greater part of the leakage in the veins. A 35% weight gain in the lung was required for production of alveolar edema and the differential between extra-alveolar (venule and arteriole) leakage and alveolar (capillary) leakage was 11 to 1. Iliff believed that pulmonary venules and veins might leak more than comparable vessels of the systemic circulation, and suggested that this warranted investigation.

In considering the evidence cited above, one might reasonably believe that the damaging leakage in lung edema occurs not from the capillary network of the alveolar walls but from leakage into the interstitium, where small veins are present. This would account for the early appearance of abnormal interstitial fluid in the deeper areas of the lung rather than in the primarily respiratory portions. The exact location of veins responsible for massive leakage on the basis of size is interesting to speculate about. All veins immediately draining the alveolar capillaries could be involved, up to those as large as 750 μm in diameter. These would be located not only in the interlobular interstitium but also nearer the hilum. The venous drainage of the bronchiolar tree itself must also be considered. In the larger bronchioles, in which there is a distinct muscular coat, one set of veins occupies the adventitia and another the submucosa. Numerous anastomosing communications connect these two sets and all are of such size as to be suspected of leakage. Since it is known that bronchiolar veins leak in the presence of histamine [74], this rich network may be a significant source of fluid escape and may indeed exceed any other source in cases of pulmonary edema [2].

The secondary appearance of fluid in the alveolar walls, after its first appearance in deeper areas where small veins abound, focuses attention on the unbroken continuity of the connective tissue space. Here fluid flow could be determined by local mechanical forces and perhaps significantly by incidental impedance caused by the formed elements in the interstitium. At the level of the alveolar walls this would consist principally of loosely aligned unit collagen fibrils (some aggregated into reticular fibers) and small elastic fibers. It is also possible that the constriction of fibrillar elements in various parts of the interstitium might change, particularly under stress caused by abnormal conditions. The embryonic developmental pattern, primary fibril to microfibril to unit collagen fibril, may continue its competence into the adult condition, so that the population of unit collagen fibrils might change. However, there is no morphological evidence for a "membrane" separating the connective tissue space deep in the lung from the connective tissue normally existing in the alveolar walls.

It seems very likely that both mechanical and morphologic factors must operate to some extent to prevent immediate draining of interstitial fluid from nonalveolar areas of the tissue space into the alveolar walls themselves. A counterinterpretation, still assuming massive leakage from venules, is that the drainage suggested above is effectively impeded by whatever concentrations of fibrils are present in the connective tissue space and that the secondary flooding of alveolar interstitium is indeed traceable to capillary leakage. This would occur principally via pinocytosis and leaky junctions but at a much lower rate. However, edema normally spreads generally throughout other areas of the entire body by gradual seepage, being stopped only by intense concentrations of connective tissue, such as aponeuroses and their attachments to bone. There is no comparable concentration of connective tissue in the areas of the lung under consideration. It therefore seems reasonable to assume that seepage into alveolar walls from flooded perivenular areas of the interstitium is blocked, or significantly delayed, by local mechanical factors that are rapidly changing and necessarily very difficult to determine.

How the voluminous lymphatics function in removing excess interstitial fluid poses a difficult question. Lymphatic capillaries extend into the interstitium as far as the veins suspected of serious leakage, and farther. They are, moreover, believed to be constructed in the manner of lymphatic capillaries elsewhere in the body. Designed as they are for fluid and large molecule reception, they furnish a puzzle in that their drainage function is not more efficient. The paucity or questionable competence of valves along the greater part of the lymphatic pathways of the lung must necessarily be significant in the mechanics of drainage. If enough competent valves were present, the ever changing mechanical forces of respiration would seem to be an ideal way of propelling any fluid trapped within the lymphatics—always towards the hilum, with eventual return to the bloodstream. It seems that the simple act of coughing or thoracic contraction in the presence of voluntary muscular closure of the larynx would effectively propel lymph in the direction of the thoracic duct. Subsequently its return would be prevented if the valves of the parenchymal lymphatics were numerous enough and competent enough. That this simple mechanical device is not effective in relieving edema suggests valvular incompetency or scarcity. The only other evident cause of failure to clear edematous fluid under pressure would be initial failure of the lymphatic capillaries to take up the excess fluid as edema developed. If this were the case, pressure would only compress the lymphatics and tend to disperse the excess fluid throughout the continuous connective tissue space.

In summary, a notable feature in the search of literature undertaken in preparing this chapter is the frequency with which one finds elaborate analyses of the edematous condition that are based on the conviction that the capillary bed is the only source of vascular leakage. This belief is so strongly entrenched in the literature, reinforced as it is by more than a century of published conviction. Although acceptance of the findings of Majno, Palade, and Schoefl [43] and extrapolation of these principles to the lung as described by Iliff [73] constitute a radical departure from the general opinion on this subject, it might stimulate significant advances in our understanding and approach to the vexatious questions posed by pulmonary edema.

References

1. E. D. Robin, C. E. Cross, and R. Zelis, Pulmonary Edema, *N. E. J. Med.*, **288**:239–246, 293–304 (1972).
2. A. P. Fishman, Pulmonary edema—the water-exchanging function of the lung, *Circulation*, **46**:390–408 (1972).
3. N. C. Staub, H. Nagano, and M. L. Pearce, Pulmonary edema in dogs, especially the sequence of fluid accumulation in lungs, *J. Appl. Physiol.*, **22**:227–240 (1967).
4. M. B. Visscher, F. J. Haddy, and G. Stephens, The physiology and pharmacology of lung edema, *Pharmacol. Rev.*, **8**:389–434 (1956).
5. R. B. Todd and W. Bowman. *The Physiological Anatomy and Physiology of Man.* Vol. 1. London, John W. Parker, 1845, p. 404.
6. I. Gersh and H. R. Catchpole, The organization of ground substance and basement membrane and its significance in tissue injury, disease and growth, *Amer. J. Anat.*, **85**:457–521 (1949).
7. D. W. Fawcett, Physiologically significant specializations of the cell surface, *Circulation*, **26**:1105–1125 (1962).
8. F. N. Low, A boundary membrane concept of ultrastructure applicable to the total organism. In *Proceedings of the third European Regional Conference on EM.* Prague, Publishing House of the Czechoslovak Academy of Sciences, **B**:115–116 (1964).
9. H. S. Bennett, Morphological aspects of extracellular polysaccharide, *J. Histochem. Cytochem.*, **11**:14–23 (1963).
10. L. Napolitano, The differentiation of white adipose cells—An electron microscope study, *J. Cell Biol.*, **18**:663–679 (1963).
11. K. R. Porter and G. D. Pappas, Collagen formation by fibroblasts of the chick embryo dermis, *J. Biophys. Biochem. Cytol.*, **5**:153–166 (1959).
12. E. D. Hay and J. W. Dodson, Secretion of collagen by corneal epithelium. I. Morphology of the collagenous products produced by isolated epithelia grown on frozen-killed lens, *J. Cell Biol.*, **57**:190–213 (1973).

13. D. E. Morse and F. N. Low, The fine structure of developing unit collagenous fibrils in the chick, *Amer. J. Anat.*, **140**:237–262 (1974).

14. R. Ross and P. Bornstein, The elastic fiber. I. The separation and partial characterization of its macromolecular components, *J. Cell Biol.*, **40**:366–381 (1969).

15. F. N. Low, Microfibrils: Fine filamentous components of the tissue space, *Anat. Rec.*, **142**:131–138 (1962).

16. G. E. Palade, Blood capillaries of the heart and other organs, *Circulation*, **24**:368–384 (1961).

17. F. N. Low, Extracellular connective tissue fibrils in the chick embryo, *Anat. Rec.*, **160**:93–108 (1968).

18. A. Policard, A. Collet, and J. C. Martin, L'interstitium pulmonaire. Etude Physiopatholigique, *La Presse Medicale*, **74**:1455–1460 (1966).

19. D. A. Lowther, Chemical aspects of collagen fibrillogenesis. In *Int. Rev. of Connective Tissue Res.* Edited by D. A. Hall. New York, Academic Press, 1963, pp. 63–119.

20. M. K. Keech, The formation of fibrils from collagen solution. IV. Effect of mucopolysaccharides and nucleic acids: An electron microscopic study, *J. Biophys. Biochem. Cytol.*, **9**:193–209 (1961).

21. D. S. Jackson and J. R. Bentley, Collagen glycosaminoglycan interactions. In *Treatise on Collagen.* Vol. 2. Edited by G. N. Ramachandran and B. S. Bould. New York, Academic Press, 1968, pp. 189–214.

22. R. S. Crissman and F. N. Low, A study of fine structural changes in the cartilage-to-bone transition within the developing chick vertebra, *Amer. J. Anat.*, **140**:451–470 (1974).

23. A. C. Guyton, K. Scheel, and D. Murphree, Interstitial fluid pressure. III. Its effect on resistance to tissue fluid mobility, *Circ. Res.*, **19**:412–419 (1966).

24. H. Schultz. *The Submicroscopic Anatomy and Pathology of the Lung.* Berlin, Springer-Verlag, 1959, pp. 32–37.

25. R. R. Bruns and G. E. Palade, Studies on blood capillaries. I. General organization of blood capillaries in muscle, *J. Cell Biol.*, **37**:244–276 (1968).

26. D. W. Fawcett, Comparative observations on fine structure of blood capillaries. In *The Peripheral Blood Vessels, Acad. of Path. Monograph No. 4.* Baltimore, Williams and Wilkins, 1963, pp. 17–44.

27. G. Majno, Ultrastructure of the vascular membrane, *Handbook of Physiology*, Section 2, *Circulation*, **3**:2293–2375 (1965).

28. M. Fillenz, Innervation of pulmonary capillaries, *Experientia*, **25**:842 (1969).

29. M. Simionescu, N. Simionescu, and G. E. Palade, Morphometric data on the endothelium of blood capillaries, *J. Cell Biol.*, **60**:128–152 (1974).

30. M. Simionescu, N. Simionescu, and G. E. Palade, Characteristic endothelial junctions in sequential segments of the microvasculature, *J. Cell Biol.*, **63**:316a (1974).

31. P. Constantinides, Opening of intercellular junctions in arterial endothelium by a chelating agent, *Anat. Rec.*, **172**:295 (1972).

32. M. W. Brightman, M. Hori, S. I. Rapport, T. S Reese, and E. Westergaard, Osmotic opening of tight junctions in cerebral endothelium, *J. Comp. Neur.*, **152**:317–326 (1973).

33. W. Bloom and D. W. Fawcett. *A Textbook of Histology.* 10th ed. Philadelphia, W. B. Saunders, pp. 386–396 (1975).

34. J. W. Quin, J. K. Beh, and A. K. Lascelles, Origin of the various immunoglobulins in lymph from the popliteal lymph node of sheep before and after antigenic stimulation, *Aust. J. Exp. Biol. Med. Sci.*, **52**:887–896 (1974).

35. N. Simionescu and G. E. Palade, Dextrans and glycogens as particulate tracers for studying capillary permeability, *J. Cell Biol.*, **50**:616–624 (1971).

36. N. Simionescu, M. Simionescu, and G. E. Palade, Permeability of muscle capillaries to exogenous myoglobin, *J. Cell Biol.*, **57**:424–452 (1973).

37. N. Simionescu, M. Simionescu, and G.E. Palade, Permeability of muscle capillaries to small heme-peptides—Evidence for the existence of patent transendothelial channels, *J. Cell Biol.*, **64**:586–607 (1975).

38. E. W. Dempsey and G. B. Wislocki, The use of silver nitrate as a vital stain, and its distribution in several mammalian tissues as studied with the electron microscope, *J. Biophys. Biochem. Cytol.*, **1**:111–118 (1955).

39. G. B. Wislocki and A. J. Ladman, The demonstration of a blood-ocular barrier in the albino rat by means of the intravitam deposition of silver, *J. Biophys. Biochem. Cytol.*, **1**:501–510 (1955).

40. M. G. Farquhar, S. L. Wissig, and G. E. Palade, Glomerular permeability. I. Ferritin transfer across the normal glomerular capillary wall, *J. Exp. Med.*, **113**:47–66 (1961).

41. M. G. Farquhar and G. E. Palade, Glomerular permeability. II. Ferritin transfer across the glomerular capillary wall in nephrotic rats, *J. Exp. Med.*, **114**:699–716 (1961).

42. G. Majno and G. E. Palade, Studies on inflammation. I. The effect of histamine and serotonin on vascular permeability: An electron microscopic study, *J. Biophys. Biochem. Cytol.*, **11**:571–605 (1961).

43. G. Majno, G. E. Palade, and G. I. Schoefl, Studies on inflammation. II. The site of action of histamine and serotonin along the vascular tree: A topographic study, *J. Biophys. Biochem. Cytol.*, **11**:607–626 (1961).

44. G. D. Pappas and V. M. Tennepon, An electron microscopic study of the passage of colloidal particles from the blood vessels of the ciliary processes and choroid plexus of the rabbit, *J. Cell Biol.*, **15**:227–239 (1962).

45. W. S. Miller. *The Lung,* 3d ed. Springfield, Ill., Charles C Thomas, 1947, pp. 89–118.

46. H. V. Hayek, *Die Menschlichen Lunge,* Berlin, Springer-Verlag, 1953, pp. 241–246.

47. C. D. Haagensen, C. R. Feind, F. P. Herter, C. A. Slanetz, and J. A. Weinberg. *The Lymphatics in Cancer.* Philadelphia, W. B. Saunders, 1972, pp. 231–245.

48. C. Nagaishi, N. Nagasawa, Y. Okada, M. Yamashita, and N. Inaba. *Functional Anatomy and Histology of the Lung.* Baltimore, University Park Press, 1972, pp. 102-179.

49. A. Karpf, Das innere Lymphgefässsystem der Lunge, *Anat. Anz.,* **116:** 442-451 (1965).

50. D. H. Trapnell, The peripheral lymphatics of the lung, *Brit. J. Radiol.,* **36:** 660-672 (1963).

51. O. F. Kampmeier, The distribution of valves and the first appearance of definite direction in the drainage of lymph in the human lung, *Amer. Rev. Tuberculosis,* **18:**360-372 (1928).

52. C. E. Tobin, Human pulmonic lymphatics, *Anat. Rec.,* **127:**611-633 (1957).

53. J. M. Yoffey and F. C. Courtice. *Lymphatics, Lymph and Lymphoid Tissue.* Cambridge, Mass., Harvard University Press, 1956, p. 161.

54. J. M. Lauweryns, The juxta-alveolar lymphatics in the human adult lung. Histologic studies in 15 cases of drowning, *Amer. Rev. Resp. Dis.,* **102:** 877-885 (1970).

55. J. M. Lauweryns, The blood and lymphatic microcirulation of the lung. In *Pathology Annual.* Edited by S. C. Sommers. New York, Appleton, 1971, pp. 3645-415.

56. L. Boussauw and J. M. Lauweryns, Reconstructions graphiques des valvules lymphatiques pulmonaires, *Comptes Rendus Assoc. des Anat.,* **54:**104-117 (1969).

57. J. J. Singer, The lymphatic drainage of the pleura as demonstrated by thorotrast, *California and West. Med.,* **57:**28-29 (1942).

58. P. H. Simer, Drainage of pleural lymphatics, *Anat. Rec.,* **113:**269-283 (1952).

59. L. V. Leak, Electron microscopic observations on lymphatic capillaires and the structural components of the connective tissue-lymph interface, *Microvasc. Res.,* 2:361-391 (1970).

60. W. J. Cliff and P. A. Nicoll, Structure and function of lymphatic vessels of the bat's wing, *Quart. J. Exp. Physiol.,* **55:**112-121 (1970).

61. L. V. Leak and J. F. Burke, Fine structure of the lymphatic capillary and the adjoining connective tissue area, *Amer. J. Anat.,* **118:**785-809 (1966).

62. L. V. Leak and J. F. Burke, Ultrastructural studies on the lymphatic anchoring filaments, *J. Cell Biol.,* **36:**129-151 (1968).

63. L. V. Leak and J. F. Burke, The removal of particulate material from the connective tissue area by the lymphatic capillaries, *J. Cell Biol.,* **31:**149A (1966).

64. J. R. Casley-Smith, An electron microscopic study of injured and abnormally permeable lymphatics, *Ann. N. Y. Acad. Sci.,* **116:**803-830 (1964).

65. E. E. Fraley and L. Weiss, An electron microscopic study of the lymphatic vessels in the penile skin of the rat, *Amer. J. Anat.,* **109:**85-101 (1961).

66. S. C. J. van der Putte, The development of the lymphatic system in man, *Adv. in Anat., Embryol. and Cell Biol.,* **51**(1):1-60 (1975).

67. E. C. Carlson and F. N. Low, The effect of hydrocortisone on extracellular connective tissue fibrils in the early chick embryo, *Amer. J. Anat.,* **130**: 331–346 (1971).

68. R. G. Frederickson and F. N. Low, The fine structure of perinotochordal microfibrils in control and enzyme-treated chick embryos, *Amer. J. Anat.,* **130**:347–376 (1971).

69. M. D. Olson and F. N. Low, The fine structure of developing cartilage in the chick embryo, *Amer. J. Anat.,* **131**:197–216 (1971).

70. J. J. O'Connell and F. N. Low, A histochemical and fine structural study of early extracellular connective tissue in the chick embryo, *Anat. Rec.,* **167**:425–438 (1970).

71. C. R. Basom, Fine structure of the elastic fiber in the developing chick aorta, *Anat. Rec.,* **160**:506 (1968).

72. P. Rous, H. P. Gilding, and F. Smith, The gradient of vascular permeability, *J. Exp. Med.,* **51**:807–830 (1930).

73. I. D. Iliff, Extra-alveolar vessels and edema development in excised dog lungs, *Circ. Res.,* **28**:524–532 (1971).

74. G. G. Pietra, J. P. Szidon, M. M. Leventhal, and A. P. Fishman, Histamine and interstitial pulmonary edema in the dog, *Circ. Res.,* **29**:323–337 (1971).

3

Lung Interstitium, Vascular and Alveolar Membranes

JOAN GIL

Anatomisches Institut der Universität Bern
Bern, Switzerland

I. Introduction

The contributions that electron microscopists have so far made to our understanding of water and solute exchanges in the lung have not been overwhelmingly significant. In such research, it is often useful to delimit the frame of structures in which events take place. And so we do here. This chapter deals with the structures involved. First, normal morphology of the endothelial and epithelial membranes and of the interstitium is presented. The description is completed by a review of the possible dynamics of these structures during respiratory movements. The second part concerns the electron-microscopic contributions to the field.

II. Relevant Morphologic Notions

In all essential points, the histologic description of the alveolar wall was completed when Low [1] described the epithelial lining membrane of the alveolar

The experimental work of the author was supported by the Swiss National Foundation grant no. 3.034.73.

septa as continuous. A long period of discussion was thus ended. Air-blood barrier is the name given to the tissue elements separating alveolar air from capillary blood. This barrier has been reviewed several times [2,3] and consists of three elements: epithelium, interstitium, and endothelium.

For our purposes it will be more useful to regard the alveolar septum as a whole. The septum includes areas that are primarily for gas exchange, others that are more concerned with the mechanical functions necessary to ensure ventilation of the airspaces, and finally others that probably facilitate fluid drainage and circulation. The two last-mentioned regions, responsible for mechanical movements and fluid drainage, are practically identical and occur within the connective tissue compartment, the interstitium.

A. Epithelial Membrane of Alveolar Septa

Figure 1 is a representative photomicrograph of a lung fixed by instilling the fixatives into the airways; it shows the two main types of pneumocytes that form the epithelial lining. Recent reviews furnish the details of their structure [2,3,4]. Essentially the type I cell is a squamous cell with a nucleus and a pericaryon; it is situated in a crevice of the tissue wall, and sends out thin cytoplasmic extensions. Morphometric data show [5] that type I cells line up to 95% of the total alveolar surface. In performing quantitative studies on epithelial populations of the lung, one must consider different sides of the problem: percentage of septal surface lined by them, volume of the cell, and number of cells compared with other cell types. Our unpublished studies [6] show that the type I cells are the largest of all the epithelial cells in the normal rat lung, taking up 13% of the total parenchymal lung tissue, although they are less numerous than the type II epithelial cells, roughly by 8 to 11.

The type II cell is cuboidal; and in contrast to the type I, it can undergo mitotic division. It seems to accomplish sophisticated biochemical functions, the chief one being the synthesis of part or all of the surface-active material and its secretion into the alveolar space [7]. This cell is typically located in pits and crevices of the alveolar wall, surrounded by neighboring capillary segments. Electron micrographs of lungs fixed by vascular perfusion, where the original tissue-air interface has been preserved, consistently show fluid

---

FIGURE 1   Dog lung fixed by instilling glutaraldehyde into the trachea. The type II alveolar cell contains numerous osmophilic lamellar bodies. A = alveolar space. C = capillary. L = leukocyte inside a capillary. Arrows point at cytoplasmic extensions of type I cells. (From Ref. 4.)

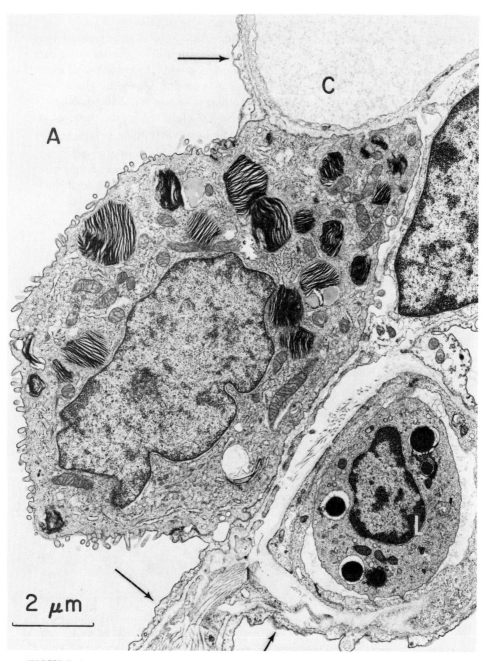

FIGURE 1

pools of variable size lining part of the alveoli. Figure 2 shows a type II cell apparently delivering its secretion product into one of these fluid pools. Figure 3 is a scheme of the situation prevailing in life. The total amount of type II cells is often grossly underestimated. If it is permissible to extrapolate data obtained on rats [8] to humans, then a human would be provided with some 5×10^9 to 7×10^9 type II cells. They constitute a diffuse exocrine gland of considerable size, and very little or nothing is known about the quantity of their output, except that with a radioactive half-life of 14 hr, the turnover of saturated phosphatidyl cholines in the whole lung is very rapid [9].

In connection with fluid exchange in the lung, one must always remember the intra-alveolar lining layer of surface-active material. From electron-microscopic studies, it is evident that we have a fluid pool of considerable size as a part of the intra-alveolar lining layer. The amount of surface-active

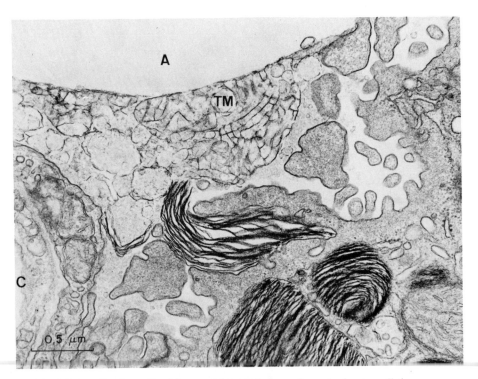

FIGURE 2   Rat lung fixed by vascular perfusion. A pool of extracellular-lining layer, containing tubular myelin (TM), a liquid crystal, is seen over a type II cell. A lamellar body is being delivered into the pool. Compare with Figure 3. A = alveolar space.   C = capillary.   (From Ref. 4.)

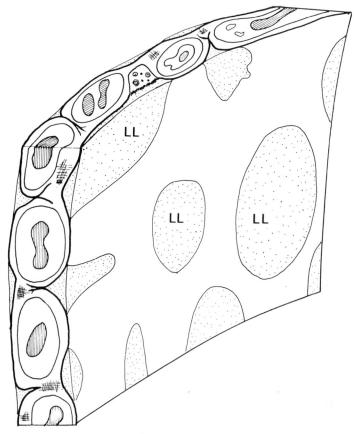

FIGURE 3   Scheme of alveolar septum as seen in lungs fixed by vascular per-fusion. Smoothing of the alveolar surface is achieved by tissue plasticity and by pools of intra-alveolar, extracellular-lining layer (LL). Type II cells are mostly covered by fluid pools.

material or of fluid-lining layer present in a lung is not known; nor are the exact secretion and breakdown pathways known nor the mechanism that reg-ulates these pathways. It is easy to demonstrate incorporation of extraneous material into the lining layer (see Figs. 9 and 10 in Sections III.A and III.B).

Type I cells are generally supposed [10] to derive from the type II cells. Their extensions, as suggested by the scheme of Figures 3 and 4a, achieve a considerable degree of plasticity, which helps to keep the free surface energy low. In connection with fluid balance, however, it is more important to note that they contain, like the endothelial cells, numerous pinocytotic or

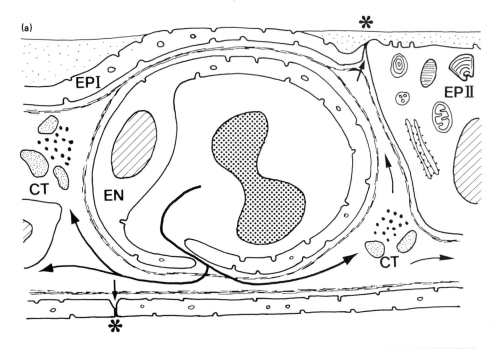

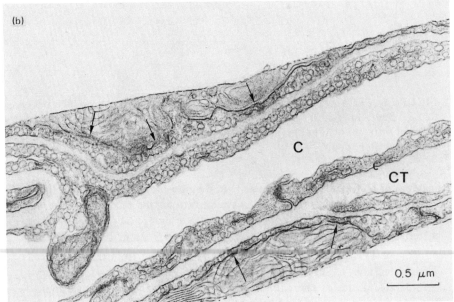

FIGURE 4

plasmalemmal vesicles (Figs. 4a and b). In general, pinocytosis, (cytopempis) serves the purpose of material uptake by the cell. In endothelia, however, pinocytotic vesicles apparently accomplish a shuttle transport function across the cell [11, 12]. There is some evidence that in the alveolar type I cell, pinocytosis is also a transport function [13-15]. This is probably because the type I cell has undergone a special differentiation called "topological" [16]. This means that the cell enlarges its surface to form a sophisticated and thin cytoplasmic shell in the three-dimensional space. Then the vesicle moves across the cell rather than toward the pericaryon.

The epithelial membrane is tightly closed by means of regular zonulae occludentes, cell junctions characterized by a variable number of ridges connecting two cell membranes of neighboring cells. Staehelin [17] has recently published a detailed review of the structure of tight junctions. These complexes occur between all the epithelial cells. Some information on the permeability of tight junctions for water or ions is available (see Ref. 17). It has been established that epithelial tight junctions never can be permeated by macromolecules, in contrast to the endothelial intracellular complexes, which can be leaky (to be discussed later). Hence the plasmalemmal, or pinocytotic, vesicles are the only means of bypassing intercellular junctions in the alveolar epithelium, as indicated by the scheme of Figure 4a.

B. Endothelial Membrane and Capillary Arrangement

Weibel [18] first recognized that in the fully inflated lung the two-dimensional network of capillaries can be regarded as hexagonal. We shall not discuss here the more recent notion of pulmonary sheet flow [19], which in the context of

---

FIGURE 4   (a) Scheme of asymmetrical alveolar septum. The designation EP I indicates extensions of type I cells; EP II, a type II cell; EN, an endothelial cell; and CT, connective tissue elements. Pools of intra-alveolar, extracellular-lining layer are shown to even out the alveolar surface. The epithelial zonulae occludentes (asterisks) are impermeable to macromolecules, whereas the endothelial intercellular junctions (long arrow) are supposedly in part permeable. The thick side of the septum (where the basal laminae are not fused) and the connective tissue between capillary segments are open for macromolecule and water circulation. (Compare with Fig. 8.) (b) Septum of dog lung fixed by vascular perfusion. Arrows point to the outer surface of the alveolar epithelial lining layer, covered by pools of tubular myelin figures, a form of intraalveolar surfactant. On the upper side, both basal laminae are fused; one can see on the lower side some connective tissue (CT) between epithelium and endothelium

the present topic is probably of little significance. Figure 5 shows a realistic schematic representation of the arrangement of capillary segments in the fully distended alveolar septum. One feature is especially notable: the alveolar septum contains a loose framework of connective tissue fibers, which appear in a straight plane when the alveolar septum is completely distended. It follows that the capillary segments must continuously cross the midplane of the septum. This facilitates the folding of the alveolar wall.

The pulmonary capillaries do not differ significantly from other closed, nonfenestrated capillaries. Forty-five percent of the tissue cells in the rat lung are endothelial although they account only for 27% of the total tissue volume [6].

Like type I cells, endothelial cells contain numerous pinocytotic vesicles that may function as a shuttle system [11,13,14]. To the best of our knowledge, nothing is known about nervous or humoral influences on pinocytosis. The membrane of these vesicles seems to be identical with the cell membrane.

The cell junctions are at first glance identical with the junctions seen in other tissues: Cell margins can overlap or interdigitate or end bluntly. In all cases one observes junctional complexes that can be regarded, if we follow conventional nomenclature, as tight junctions, or zonulae occludentes [13–15,20]. There has been much discussion on the existence of oval slits or open channels in the junctional complexes of endothelia. Karnovsky described them [21] as having a diameter of 4 nm. According to him, these slits would be the morphological equivalent of the "small" pores, while pinocytotic vesicles would correspond to the "large" pores of the physiologists. This view can no longer be sustained in this form. It will be discussed again in the section dealing with tracer studies.

Very recent studies of the endothelial junctions with the freeze-fracture technique published simultaneously by two different laboratories [22,23] shed new light on the substructure of the endothelial junctions. Both articles describe epithelial junctions as classical tight zonulae occludentes made up of several rows of interconnecting ridges on the protoplasmic fracture face and complementary interconnecting grooves on the exoplasmic face. The endothelial junction is, in contrast, poorly developed with fewer and less frequently interconnected rows that show occasional discontinuities. Inoue et al. [23] indicate that the mean depth of an epithelial zonula occludens is 0.26 ± 0.02 mμ while the corresponding figure for the endothelium is 0.17 ± 0.01 mμ. Schneeberger and Karnovsky [22] tentatively estimate the occasional areas of discontinuity of the junctional rows in the endothelium to be between 13.6 to 48.0 nm long with a mean of 25.8 ± 2.6 nm. Therefore, the endothelial junctions can be regarded as comparatively "leaky," similar to those described for renal tubular cells. These findings appear to lend strong support to the contention [24] that only the alveolar epithelium is a tight membrane, whereas the capillaries are permeable, although they do not clarify the size of particles that can freely cross the vascular membrane.

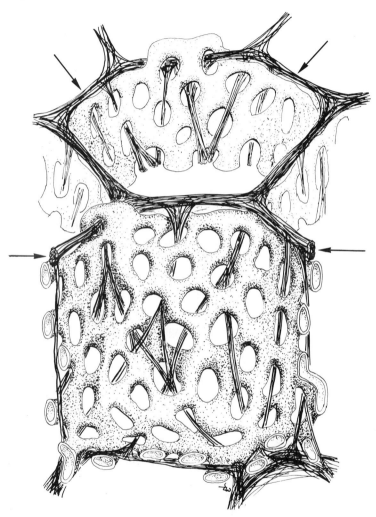

FIGURE 5 Scheme of fully distended alveolar walls. The epithelial membrane has been omitted. Connective tissue fibers form in the midplane a loose network that is continuously crossed by capillary segments. In vivo, this fibrous skeleton undergoes plastic adaptations. Arrows point at the reinforced entrance rings of the alveoli, which are the most peripheral elements of the axial connective tissue. (From Ref. 4.)

The pericytes are usually regarded as a part of the wall of capillaries. A detailed study on the occurrence of pericytes in the alveolar wall has been recently published [25]. This finding is important because pericytes may be contractile cells. They have the same appearance in the lung as in other organs: the nucleus and the pericaryon run parallel to the axis of the vessels and send out perpendicular short cytoplasmic extensions that embrace the capillary. In electron micrographs they can be recognized because they are embedded in the basal lamina of the endothelial cell. The side of the pericyte closest to the endothelium is smooth and contains filaments, while the opposite side shows numerous pinocytotic vesicles. The function of the pericytes is not known. They are more numerous in the lungs of large animals than in smaller ones; thus in the common laboratory rodents they are rare.

C.   Interstitium

There are three different constituents of the fibrous continuum of the lung [4]:

1.   Axial connective tissue, which comes from the hilum and in which all the airways and pulmonary arteries are embedded. These connective tissue sheaths are the places in which, according to Staub et al. [26], edema fluid accumulation would begin.

2.   Peripheral connective tissue, which is identical with the connective tissue of the visceral pleura.

3.   Parenchymatous connective tissue, situated inside the alveolar walls (shown in Figs. 4 and 5).

This classification serves only didactic purposes; all three constituents are a functional unit. They are primarily for ventilating the lung. Secondarily they are involved in fluid circulation. All three elements are locked inside a space lined on both sides by alveolar epithelium (Fig. 4)—the lung interstitium. The axial and peripheral connective tissue contains lymphatic vessels; the parenchymatous does not, although it constitutes the largest and most leaky region of the interstitium.

Parenchymatous connective tissue consists of elastic and collagen fibers that form a loose basket around every single alveolus (Fig. 5). It has been suggested (see Refs. 3,27) that these fibers are a drainage pathway for fluid pools inside the alveolar wall. The fluid, following these fibers, would rapidly reach the axial and peripheral regions, where lymphatic vessels occur. The findings by Staub [26] strongly suggest that quantitatively the main direction of drainage is towards the axial connective tissue. Even if this is so, however, the formation of periarterial cuffs around small pulmonary arteries described by other authors [28] could hardly be explained by this mechanism.

Capillaries can be regarded as tunnels embedded in the parenchymatous interstitium. We have already discussed the occurrence of potentially contractile cells, the pericytes, in their wall. Kapanci et al. [29] have shown on the other hand that stripes of lung parenchyma are actively contractile and that actin can be demonstrated inside many interstitial cells, which are probably different from the pericytes. Thus we have two elements that can undergo active contraction. One can speculate that they may influence the local perfusion level, which in turn would secondarily bear on quantitative permeability.

Little information on quantitative composition of the interstitium is available. In the rat lung parenchyma [6] interstitium makes up 47% of the total tissue. Of this, 35% is cellular and 12% noncellular (fibers and fluid). Interstitial cells, largely fibrocytes, account for 33% of the total amount of lung cells and are, after the endothelial cells, the most numerous. One must remember that the rat lung is not particularly rich in connective tissue! In judging their significance, it would be important to know how many of these interstitial cells contain actin and are contractile [29].

Until recently, problems posed by the organization of the "amorphous" ground substance of the interstitium have been neglected. Recent studies by Wiederhielm et al. [30] show that the partition of fluid between two phases, a gel-like mucopolysaccharide compartment and a free-fluid phase containing plasma proteins, probably is very important to capillary water balance. According to these authors, the osmotic pressures exerted by the two-phase system are higher than the algebraic sum of the two components. This notion implies a considerable volume exclusion, resulting in unexpectedly high local protein concentrations. The two-phase system produces also an "osmotic buffering" effect. The fluid in the so-called amorphous ground substance probably flows in rivulets toward the lymphatics along connective tissue fibers. Disruption of the gel mucopolysaccharide phase will profoundly affect local osmotic equilibrium.

The alveolar septum is asymmetrical with regard to the capillary segments as shown in Figure 4. The significance of this fact for fluid circulation was probably first recognized by Cottrell et al. [31] and has been stressed several times [32]. The endothelial and the epithelial cells are continuously underlined by a basal lamina, which is known to be a form of collagen [33].*

*The term *basement membrane* should be reserved for membranes visible in light microscopy that give a positive reaction with certain histochemical stains. A typical example is the basement membrane of the ciliated epithelium of trachea and bronchi. The *basal lamina* can be visualized only with the electron microscope and has a different composition.

Basal laminae are 50–100 nn thick and constitute the universal frontier of the interstitium. Although no attachments between the lamina and the cell membranes of epithelial and endothelial cells can be visualized in ordinary specimens, they undoubtedly exist. The anchorage points can be shown for certain endothelia partially detached after a severe experimental vasoconstriction [34].

As others have pointed out [15, 31, 32], the basal laminae of endothelium and epithelium are fused on one side but not on the opposite side (Fig. 4). This means that the air-blood barrier is thin on one side and relatively thick on the other. Areas in which the basal laminae are fused appear to be sealed for fluid circulation. They cannot be widened even in severe edematous conditions (Fig. 7). The other side, however, is open for fluid drainage.

D. Dynamic Implications

We recently discussed anatomical factors that account for the mechanical properties of the lung [4]. Consideration of this subject is simplified if we keep in mind the classification of connective tissue just presented. The axial connective tissue, whose final extensions are the reinforced entrance rings of the alveolar mouths, is connected with the hilum; it represents therefore a relatively fixed element of the fibrous continuum. Not so the subpleural peripheral connective tissue, which is closely associated with the chest wall and the diaphragm and participates in the respiratory movements. The parenchymal connective tissue of the septum (Fig. 5) is caught between the two other systems, with which it is continuous, and is submitted to stress changes more or less like a bellows. Activity in this fibrous backbone of the alveoli leads to a folding and unfolding of the alveolar wall, or in other words, to recruitment and derecruitment of gas exchange area [35,36]. This may include alveolar recruitment, especially when volume changes are extensive [35,37], but probably in most cases within the tidal volume, the changes affect smaller areas of the alveolar wall. Electron micrographs of derecruited septa [35] show that the gaps between folds are filled with fluid. Figure 6 shows an extensive zigzag reversible folding in a perfused isolated rabbit lung; other areas of the same lung were very well expanded and this derecruitment must be

FIGURE 6   Isolated rabbit lung fixed by vascular perfusion. Extensive foldings in zigzag partly identified by arrows. Some of the derecruited air spaces are marked by asterisks. Lining layer (LL) is seen on the free surface and partly inside derecruited air spaces. A = alveolar space; C = capillary. Similar areas are circled in Figure 7.

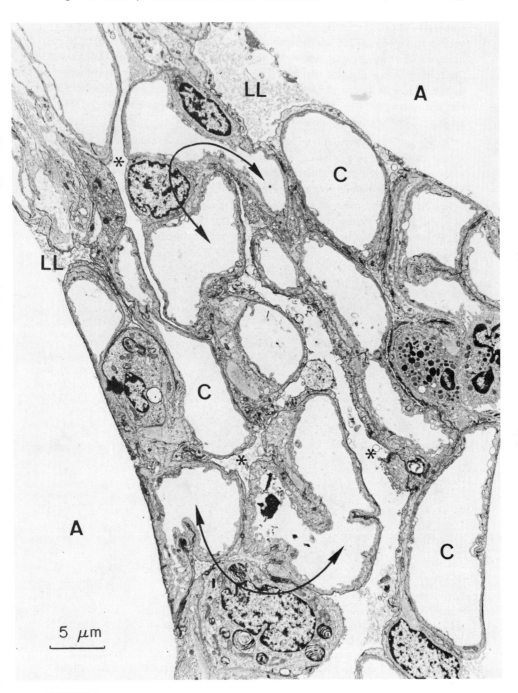

FIGURE 6

considered focal. One suspects that the exact geometry of the fold lines is subject to rapid changes during breathing movements. Available evidence [36] indicates that capillary segments also undergo deep changes in connection with the folding of the alveolar surface. The question arises whether these local dynamic changes affect some of the factors involved in the equations for passive transport [27,38]. We can offer only a speculative answer, but chances are high that they do.

Figure 7 shows a light micrograph of an isolated, excised rabbit lung similar to the one in Figure 6. Several areas of local collapse are circled. Arrows point at intraseptal capillaries that appear to be closed in spite of the wide lumen seen in the derecruited area. Physiologic literature [39] indicates that even when alveolar pressure exceeds vascular pressures by 10 cm H_2O, amounts of blood move between arteries and veins. The derecruited areas seen in Figure 7, seemingly "corner" or "edge" vessels, are likely candidates for staying open.

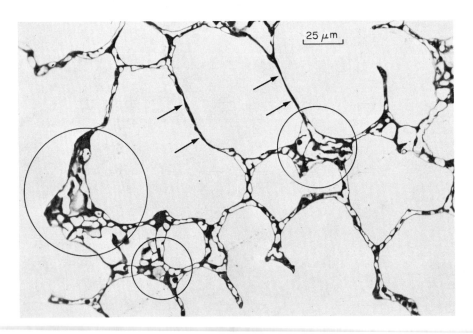

FIGURE 7   Isolated rabbit lung fixed by vascular perfusion inside a subatmospheric-pressure chamber at intermediate inflation (60%) of its total lung capacity (TLC). Small areas of derecruitment of the gas-exchange surface are circled (compare with Fig. 6). Note the near collapse of capillary segments in well-distended areas of the septum. This picture suggests that physical forces driving fluid exchange may differ locally.

In a derecruited area (Figs. 6 and 7) there is no recoil force inside the alveolar space, which is filled with fluid. This by itself could change the interstitial pressure. Additionally, nothing is known about the osmotic properties of the intra-alveolar fluid. There is also a realistic chance that as a consequence of the folding, fluid drainage pathways are obstructed. And finally, folding of the capillaries can also affect the level of blood perfusion and thus the hydrostatic pressure in the vascular compartment. Summarizing, it is difficult to overlook the situation prevailing inside the derecruited areas, and there is a possibility that under certain circumstances, these areas become leaky and give rise to focal fluid accumulation. The existence of active contractile cells in the interstitium complicates this picture still more.

III. Water Circulation and Macromolecule Passage in the Alveolar Septum

The findings of electron microscopists have contributed to the study of fluid and macromolecule exchange. Our review of their work comprises three aspects: (1) fluids that can be seen directly; (2) tracer studies; and (3) possibilities of morphometry.

A. Fluids: Electron-Microscopic Aspects

Water can exist in increased amounts in three different places.

1. In the interstitium in the wide sense. There is a possibility of seeing fluid in this particular site since it produces a widening of the space. As clearly shown in Figure 8, of a rat lung perfused at excess pressure, fluid tends to accumulate in thicker parts of the barrier [31] or in connective tissue strands connecting neighboring capillaries. Morphometric estimates of the water volume present between epithelial membranes and endothelium are possible and have been made [40], although we are unable to distinguish between the gel-like and the free-fluid phase previously described. In our own studies on normal rat lungs fixed at moderate of inflation by vascular perfusion [6], the volume of noncellular "interstitium" was estimated at 12%, but this included connective tissue fibers.

2. There is a definite possibility that the water content of cells partly changes. Pathological studies show that the epithelial or endothelial membranes can also undergo swelling [40,41,42]. This problem could be clarified by comparative quantitative studies between edematous and carefully controlled normal lungs.

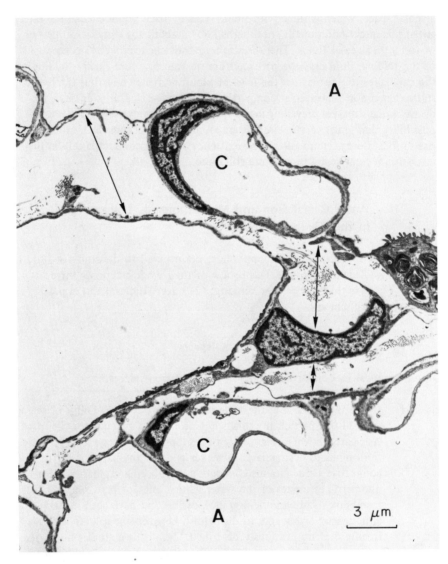

FIGURE 8   Rat lung perfused with glutaraldehyde at excess pressure (about 50 mmHg) to reveal water circulation spaces. While one of the capillary sides is intact (compare with Figs. 4a and 4b), the other has undergone very extensive dilatation (arrows). The lining layer has been washed out and the alveolar tissue surface is very irregular, possibly indicating filling of the alveolar space (A) with non-electron-dense fluid.

3.   Alveoli may be filled with non-electron-dense, i.e. invisible, fluid. The possibility that alveoli are filled with an ultrafiltrate has been discussed but is generally rejected [27]. Electron microscopy will not settle the problem. If alveoli are to have intrinsic stability, however, the normal fluid-air or tissue-air interface must be smooth; in other words, the interface must possess the lowest possible free energy. This is indicated in Figs. 2 and 4 and has been discussed elsewhere [43]. In electron micrographs of lungs that have alveoli filled with an artificial electron-dense edema fluid like hemoglobin (Fig. 9), two different interfaces can be recognized: a fluid-air interface, which is smooth, and a tissue-fluid interface, which is irregular. In our experiments with lungs fixed by vascular perfusion to preserve the lining layer, we have often observed that the lack of any visible fluid-lining layer parallels the presence of a very irregular alveolar surface [43,44]. Our interpretation of this situation is that water has crossed the tissue barrier and washed out the lining layer— that it now fills the alveolar space, abolishing the tissue-air interface and thus causing the epithelial membrane to have an irregular surface. This formulation seems to be reliable but it is difficult to make a practical use of it.

During studies on isolated, ventilated, and perfused rabbit lungs (unpublished results), we have repeatedly observed under different conditions sudden weight increases paralleled by apparent volume increases of the lungs. Since light- and electron-microscopic investigation of these specimens failed to show a commensurate interstitial edema, we suspected that the alveoli might be filled with fluid, but we could never obtain any direct evidence other than the presence of a very irregular alveolar surface.

To end this section, it is necessary to consider two technical problems.

1.   How realistic are the chances of fixing fluids for electron microscopy in situ? Chemical fixatives for electron microscopy are effective only on substrates able to undergo some cross-linkage. Specifically, it is impossible to preserve plain water. We have shown that by a perfusion technique, it is possible to preserve intra-alveolar edema from oxygen poisoning [44,45]; the fluid is rich in albumin. In the same work, however, edema fluid following acute circulatory overload could not be seen.

2.   One must remember the problem of the osmotic and oncotic pressure of the fixatives [46]. There is always a possibility that fixatives

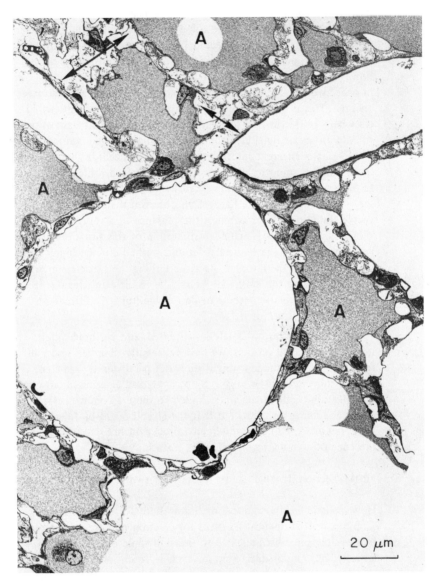

FIGURE 9   Rat lung perfused with aqueous hemoglobin at 50 mmHg and subsequently fixed by vascular perfusion. Hemoglobin, which is electron-dense, is irregularly distributed in different alveoli (A). While the tissue-air interface is smooth, the tissue-hemoglobin interface is irregular. In some areas (arrows) the interstitium is widened without containing electron-dense material. Capillaries are empty.

induce measurable changes in the amount of fluid or in the volume of the cells. It is very important to use standard solutions of known osmolarity to obtain reproducible results.

B. Tracer Studies at the Electron Microscope Level

The structures relevant for macromolecule transport in the lung, then, are the intercellular junctions of the endothelium and the pinocytotic vesicles, formerly thought to be the anatomical counterpart of the small and large pores, respectively. The most important studies on tracer passage in the lung are those by Schneeberger and Karnovsky [13,14] and by Pietra et al. [15].

Schneeberger-Keeley and Karnovsky [13] concluded from experiments making use of horseradish peroxidase (molecular weight 40,000 daltons; diameter 3 nm) administered intravenously and instilled into the nose, that the cell junctions are the morphologic equivalent of the small pores and that the vesicles represent the large pores. The epithelial tight junctions could not be permeated. Later Pietra et al. [15] put forward the theory of the "stretchable" pores, in describing the endothelial cell junctions of dog lungs perfused with hemoglobin (molecular weight 64,000 daltons; diameter 6 nm) at different pressures. The slits are opened only under conditions of hypervolemia—as these conditions could be simulated by perfusing the hemoglobin solutions (7 g/100 ml) at a pressure of 50 mmHg.

The experiments of Pietra, which we have reproduced (Fig. 9), clearly show that the intercellular junctions of the vascular membrane can leak. It is not clear whether they are important in macromolecular exchange under normal conditions or only under pathological conditions, i.e., when hemodynamic edema exists.

In a subsequent work, using horseradish peroxidase and larger tracers, Schneeberger and Karnovsky [14] confirmed that tracer passage through the endothelial clefts depended on the injection of large volumes of fluid; this finding lent further support to the theory of the stretchable pores of Pietra et al. The investigators insisted, however, that pinocytotic vesicles are important under normal conditions.

Recently, Nicolaysen and Staub [47] investigated, at the light-microscopic level, the passage of albumin with Evans blue labeled in rapidly frozen mouse lungs. They found apparent equilibration 3 to 5 hr after injection. Available ultrastructural studies do not explain how this equilibration comes about.

Very recently two independent groups published accounts on the permeability of muscle capillaries to small hemepeptides [11] and horseradish peroxidase [12]. Both articles support the view that pinocytotic vesicles are the most important shuttle system across the endothelial cell. Endothelial junctions either are impermeable [11] or allow passage of very limited amounts of the tracer [12]. Simionescu et al. [11] suggest the existence of transendothelial channels, visible in the form of plasmalemmal vesicles. If the lung capillaries are comparable to the muscle capillaries, we shall have to conclude that shuttle vesicles are the key transport feature for macromolecules. As previously pointed out, little is known about control, activation, or inhibition of pinocytosis.

We have performed some experiments with horseradish peroxidase and hemoglobin and fixed the lungs by vascular perfusion to try to see the possible incorporation of these tracers into the alveolar lining layer (Figs. 9 and 10). By using conditions that did not produce hypervolemia, we could find horseradish peroxidase incorporated into the intra-alveolar-lining layer in a few places (Fig. 10); this finding usually involved some search. The interstitium close to these intra-alveolar deposits was mostly free, but sometimes it contained traced deposits. One should note, in examining pictures in which the tracer appears in the interstitium of the thin part of the barrier, that if this area does not participate in fluid circulation [31], the tracer can have arrived only by pinocytosis. Very recently Bignon et al. [48] showed with immunochemical methods the presence of plasma albumin in the normal lining layer; this finding is additional proof that macromolecules pass across the barrier into the airspaces.

C. Morphometry: Conditions and Possibilities

There appears to be a consensus on the need for carrying out quantitative studies on histologic specimens. Morphometry is a system of practical procedures based on stereological principles that establish the quantitative relation between original structures in three-dimensional space and their traces seen in random two-dimensional sections. As a general tool for histopathologic work, these procedures have been reviewed several times [49,50]. Essentially, random pictures are compared with a test system consisting of points, lines, and a test frame, and in many cases, the task of the investigator is reduced to a simple point counting.

Morphometry is being used so extensively in pulmonary studies that even a brief review would be too complex here. It is surprising, however, to notice that morphometric studies on pulmonary edema or fluid exchange in the lung in general are rare or nonexistent and it is worth while discussing why. If we examine some examples of recent papers on lung morphometry, we distinguish several groups to which it is applied.

1. Structural changes produced under pathologic conditions, such as oxygen poisoning [40,51], controlled exposure to environmental pollutants [41], respiratory distress syndrome in adult humans [52], and emphysema development [53].

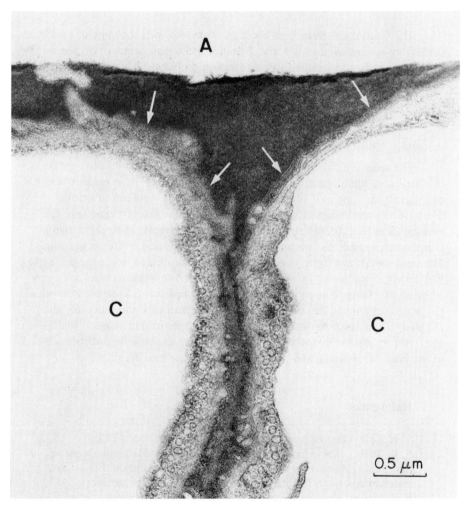

FIGURE 10 Incorporation of horseradish peroxidase into the extracellular-lining layer of a normal rat lung. Arrows point at the interface tissue lining layer. In other places of the specimen, some pinocytotic vesicles with the tracer could be seen.

2. Structural studies in normal lungs aimed at obtaining baseline data for comparing structure and function in phenomena such as diffusing capacity [54] or adaptation of alveolar surface to environmental conditions [55] or for studying normal growth and cell differentiation [56].

3. Studies aimed at investigating functional changes of structures such as alveolar surface or capillary network [35,37].

The fixation problem here becomes acute. In fact, the type of problems commonly studied in groups 1 and 2 do not make high demands on the investigator's ability to handle difficult fixation problems. This is different for group 3, or for the electron-microscopic investigation of the fluid content of the lung. In these cases, we must resort to what is called a physiological fixation [46], i.e., fixation of the organ after adjusting and monitoring its physiologic condition by an administration unlikely to interfere with the feature under study. This means in most cases either rapid freezing or vascular perfusion.

The second difficulty met in quantitative sutides on fluid distribution is the focal and inhomogeneous distribution of fluid pools. It is evident that if one regards the lung as a whole, one must distinguish between interstitial edema in the axial connective tissue surrounding the airways, especially the periarterial cuffs [26,28], and interstitium in the alveolar wall. Essentially, morphometric methods require randomly distributed and isotropic structures. The axial connective tissue is neither randomly distributed nor isotropic, since it is clearly convergent. In such cases, morphometric work requires some adaptations. Often it is enough to adapt the sample size to the point at which the structures studied can be regarded as homogeneously and randomly distributed, for instance by working at different magnification stages. The limiting factor at present in applying morphometry to studying fluid distribution in the lung lies in fixing and preserving free extracellular fluid.

References

1. F. N. Low, Electron microscopy of rat lung, *Anat. Rec.*, 113:241 (1953).
2. E. R. Weibel, The ultrastructure of the alveolar-capillary membrane or barrier. In *The Pulmonary Circulation and Interstitial Space*. Edited by A. P. Fishman and H. H. Hecht. Chicago, University of Chicago Press, 1969.
3. E. R. Weibel, Morphological basis of alveolar-capillary gas exchange, *Physiol. Rev.*, 53:419 (1973).
4. E. R. Weibel and J. Gil, Structure-function relationships at the alveolar level. In *Bioengineering Aspects of the Lung*. Edited by J. B. West. New York, Marcel Dekker, 1977, pp. 1–81.

5. Y. Kapanci, E. R. Weibel, H. P. Kaplan, and F. R. Robinson, Pathogenesis and reversibility of the pulmonary lesions of oxygen toxicity in monkeys. II. Ultrastructure and morphometric studies, *Lab. Invest.*, **20**:101 (1969).

6. D. Haies, J. Gil, and E. R. Weibel, Morphometry of lung cells. I. Cell populations of rat lung parenchyma, to be published.

7. J. Gil and O. K. Reiss, Isolation and characterization of lamellar bodies and tubular myelin from rat lung homogenates, *J. Cell Biol.*, **58**:152 (1973).

8. S. L. Kauffman, P. H. Burri, and E. R. Weibel, The postnatal growth of the rat lung. II. Autoradiography, *Anat. Rec.*, **180**:63 (1974).

9. D. F. Tierney, J. A. Clements, and H. J. Trahan, Rates of replacement of lecithins and alveolar instability in rat lungs, *Amer. J. Physiol.*, **213**:671 (1967).

10. M. J. Evans, L. J. Cabral, R. J. Stephens, and G. Freeman, Renewal of alveolar epithelium in the rat following exposure to NO_2, *Amer. J. Pathol.*, **70**:175 (1973).

11. N. Simionescu, M. Simionescu, and G. L. Palade, Permeability of muscle capillaries to small heme-peptides. Evidence for the existence of patent transendothelial channels, *J. Cell Biol.*, **64**:586 (1975).

12. M. C. Williams and S. L. Wissig, The permeability of muscle capillaries to horseradish peroxidase, *J. Cell Biol.*, **66**:531 (1975).

13. E. E. Schneeberger-Keeley and M. J. Karnovsky, The ultrastructural basis of alveolar-capillary membrane permeability to peroxidase used as a tracer, *J. Cell Biol.*, **37**:781 (1968).

14. E. E. Schneeberger and M. J. Karnovsky, The influence of intravascular fluid volume on the permeability of newborn and adult mouse lungs to ultrastructural protein tracers, *J. Cell Biol.*, **49**:319 (1971).

15. G. G. Pietra, J. P. Szidon, M. M. Leventhal, and A. P. Fishman, Hemoglobin as a tracer in hemodynamic pulmonary edema, *Science*, **166**:1643 (1969).

16. E. R. Weibel, A note on differentiation and divisibility of alveolar epithelial cells, *Chest*, **65**:195 (1974).

17. L. A. Staehelin, Structure and function of intercellular junctions, *Intern. Rev. Cytol.*, **39**:191 (1974).

18. E. R. Weibel. *Morphometry of the Human Lung*. Heidelberg, Springer, 1963.

19. S. S. Sobin, H. M. Tremer, and Y. C. Fung, Morphometric basis of the sheet-flow concept of the pulmonary alveolar microcirculation in the cat, *Circ. Res.*, **26**:397 (1970).

20. R. R. Bruns and G. E. Palade, Studies on blood capillaries. I. General organization of blood capillaries in muscle, *J. Cell Biol.*, **37**:244 (1968).

21. M. J. Karnovsky, The ultrastructural basis of capillary permeability studied with peroxidase as a tracer, *J. Cell Biol.*, **35**:213 (1967).

22. E. E. Schneeberger and M. J. Karnovsky, Substructure of intercellular junctions in freeze-fractured alveolar-capillary membranes of mouse lung, *Circ. Res.*, **38**:404–411 (1976).

23. S. Inoue, R. P. Michel, and J. C. Hogg, Zonulae occludentes in alveolar epi-thelium and capillary endothelium of dog lungs studied with the freeze-fracture technique, *J. Ultrastr. Res.*, **56**:215–225 (1976).

24. A. E. Taylor and K. A. Gaar, Estimation of equivalent pore radii of pul-monary capillary and alveolar membranes, *Amer. J. Physiol.*, **218**:1133–1140 (1970).

25. E. R. Weibel, On pericytes, particularly their existence in lung capillaries, *Microvasc. Res.*, **8**:218 (1974).

26. N. C. Staub, H. Nagano, and M. L. Pearce, Pulmonary edema in dogs, es-pecially the sequence of fluid accumulation in the lungs, *J. Appl. Physiol.*, **22**:227 (1967).

27. N. C. Staub, Pulmonary edema, *Physiol. Rev.*, **54**:678 (1974).

28. J. B. West, Pulmonary hemodynamics and edema. In *Central Hemodynam-ics and Gas Exchange*. Edited by C. Giuntini. Turin, Minerva Medica, 1971.

29. Y. Kapanci, A. Assimacopoulos, C. Irle, A. Zwahlen, and G. Gabbiani. "Contractile interstitial cells" in pulmonary alveolar septa: A possible reg-ulator of ventilation/perfusion ratio? Ultrastructural, immunofluorescence and in vitro studies, *J. Cell Biol.*, **60**:375 (1974).

30. C. A. Wiederhielm, J. R. Fox, and D. R. Lee, Ground substance mucopoly-saccharides and plasma proteins: Their role in capillary water balance, *Amer. J. Physiol.*, **230**:1121–1125 (1976).

31. T. S. Cottrell, O. R. Levine, R. M. Senior, J. Wiener, D. Spiro, and A. P. Fishman, Electron microscopic alterations at the alveolar level in pulmon-ary edema, *Circ. Res.*, **21**:783 (1967).

32. J. P. Szidon, G. G. Pietra, and A. P. Fishman, The alveolar-capillary mem-brane and pulmonary edema, *N. E. J. Med.*, **286**:1200 (1972).

33. M. J. Cowan and R. G. Crystal, Lung growth after unilateral pneumonec-tomy: Quantitation of collagen synthesis and content, *Amer. Rev. Resp. Dis.*, **111**:267 (1975).

34. P. H. Burri and E. R. Weibel, Beeinflussung einer spezifischen cytoplasma-tischen Organelle von Endothelzellen durch Adrenalin, *Z. Zellforsch.*, **88**:426 (1968).

35. J. Gil and E. R. Weibel, Morphological study of pressure-volume hysteresis in rat lungs fixed by vascular perfusion, *Respir. Physiol.*, **15**:190 (1972).

36. E. R. Weibel, P. Untersee, J. Gil, and M. Zulauf, Morphometric estimation of pulmonary diffusion capacity. VI. Effect of varying positive pressure inflation of air spaces, *Respir. Physiol.*, **18**:285 (1973).

37. T. G. Klingele and N. C. Staub, Alveolar shape changes with volume in iso-lated, air-filled lobes of cat lung, *J. Appl. Physiol.*, **28**:411 (1970).

38. N. C. Staub, Pathogenesis of pulmonary edema, *Amer. Rev. Resp. Dis.*, **109**:358 (1974).

39. D. Y. Rosenzweig, J. M. B. Hughes, and J. B. Glazier, Effects of transpul-monary and vascular pressures on pulmonary blood volume in isolated lung, *J. Appl. Physiol.*, **28**:553–560 (1970).

40. G. S. Kistler, P. R. B. Caldwell, and E. R. Weibel, Development of fine structural damage to alveolar and capillary lining cells in oxygen-poisoned rat lungs, *J. Cell Biol.*, **32**:605 (1967).
41. C. G. Plopper, D. L. Dungworth, and W. S. Tyler, Morphometric evaluation of pulmonary lesions in rats exposed to ozone, *Amer. J. Pathol.*, **71**:395 (1973).
42. R. E. Brooks, Ultrastructure of lung lesions produced by ingested chemicals. I. Effect of the herbicide paraquat on mouse lung, *Lab. Invest.*, **25**: 536 (1971).
43. J. Gil and E. R. Weibel, Improvements in demonstration of lining layer of lung alveoli by electron microscopy, *Respir. Physiol.*, **8**:13 (1969/70).
44. J. Gil, Edema formation in the lung: Quantitative morphological methods, *Bull. Physio-pathol. Resp.*, **7**:1077 (1971).
45. J. Gil, Methods for demonstration of interstitial and alveolar edema by electron microscopy. In *Central Hemodynamics and Gas Exchange.* Edited by C. Giuntini. Turin, Minerva Medica, 1971.
46. J. Gil, Preservation of tissues for electron microscopy under physiological criteria. In *Technique of Biochemical and Biophysical Morphology.* Edited by D. Glick and R. M. Rosenbaum. New York, Wiley-Interscience, 1977.
47. G. Nicolaysen and N. C. Staub, Time course of albumin equilibration in interstitium and lymph of normal mouse lungs, *Microvasc. Res.*, **9**:29 (1975).
48. J. Bignon, P. Chahinian, G. Feldmann, and C. Sapin, Ultrastructural immunoperoxidase demonstration of antologous albumin in the alveolar capillary membrane and in the alveolar lining material in normal rats, *J. Cell Biol.*, **64**:503 (1975).
49. E. R. Weibel, Stereological principles for morphometry in electron microscopic cytology, *Intern. Rev. Cytol.*, **26**:235 (1969).
50. E. R. Weibel, Stereological techniques for electron microscopic morphology. In *Principles and Techniques of Electron Microscopy.* Vol. 3. Edited by M. A. Hayat. New York, Van Nostrand Reinhold, 1972.
51. Y. Kapanci, R. Tosco, J. Eggermann, and V. E. Gould, Oxygen pneumonitis in man. Light and electron microscopic morphometric studies, *Chest*, **62**:162 (1972).
52. M. Bachofen and E. R. Weibel, Basic pattern of tissue repair in human lungs following unspecific injury, *Chest*, **65**:145 (1974).
53. W. M. Thurlbeck, Internal surface area and other measurements in emphysema, *Thorax*, **22**:483 (1967).
54. E. R. Weibel, Morphometric estimation of pulmonary diffusion capacity. I. Model and method, *Respir. Physiol.*, **11**:54 (1970/71).
55. P. H. Burri and E. R. Weibel, Morphometric estimation of pulmonary diffusion capacity. II. Effect of environmental PO_2 on the growing lung, *Respir. Physiol.*, **11**:247 (1971).
56. P. H. Burri, J. Dbaly, and E. R. Weibel, The postnatal growth of the rat lung. I. Morphometry, *Anat. Rec.*, **178**:711 (1974).

4

Lung Fluid and Solute Compartments

FRANK E. GUMP

College of Physicians and Surgeons
Columbia University
New York, New York

I. Introduction

Certain assumptions about the distribution of water, sodium, hemoglobin, and albumin in the lung make it possible to calculate virtual volumes of distribution for these substances. They are normal constituents of the body and are in dynamic equilibrium in the lung. Their use as distribution indicators represents a departure from more widely applied techniques using exogenous indicators with limited times for equilibration. Although techniques for calculating virtual distribution volumes for physiologic indicators are limited to biopsy or postmortem specimens, they do provide information about pulmonary vascular, interstitial, and intracellular tissues that cannot be obtained in any other way. Measurements of the various pulmonary compartments are especially important since these determinations frequently serve as the standard for comparison with less invasive in vivo measurements. A clear understanding of the underlying assumptions and also of some of the technical problems involved is important if these measurements are to help our understanding of pulmonary function.

II. Water and Wet Weight of Lungs

A. Human Lung Weight
at Postmortem Examination

Pathologists have long used scales as a way of identifying organs in abnormal condition removed at postmortem and the lung has been no exception. It is generally accepted that both lungs weigh between 800 and 1000 g in patients who die of noncardiorespiratory diseases [1,2].

A recent study is of interest in that a systematic effort was made to explore the relation between weight and normal or abnormal histology [3]. The authors examined records on 1019 patients and found that 350 (17.2% of the 2038 lungs) were thought to be normal following careful microscopic examination. These lungs fell into the weight range previously mentioned, while the lungs of patients who had died of pulmonary edema or pneumonia had marked increases in weight. The increased lung weight noted in these conditions has generally been attributed to an increase in lung water, and a variety of methods have been used in an effort to measure such increases.

B. Wet Weight To Dry Weight Ratio

A very straightforward approach is simply to weigh the lung wet after removal and then to repeat this measurement after the lung has been dried to a constant weight. There is no argument that this provides a completely accurate determination of the water content of the specimen. Unfortunately, it neglects the contribution of blood trapped in the lung. Previous studies frequently assumed that almost all the blood was successfully removed by opening the large pulmonary vessels and draining the lung by gravity [4]. When homogenates of such drained lungs are analyzed for hemoglobin, it becomes evident that significant amounts of blood still remain. If the blood contribution is taken into account, ratios of wet weight to dry weight show the lung to have a very high water content. In careful studies on five normal human lungs removed at postmortem we found the extravascular water content to average 78%. In nine patients who died of posttraumatic pulmonary insufficiency and who had had marked increases in lung weight, the percentage of extravascular water had increased to 86% (Table 1). This marked increase in wet- to dry-weight ratio is the result of the dramatic weight gain seen in lungs removed from patients who died of posttraumatic pulmonary insufficiency. Threefold increases have been reported, and doubling of the usual postmortem weight is not unusual [5].

TABLE 1 Postmortem Lung Compartments in Normal Humans and Those Dying of Posttraumatic Pulmonary Failure

Patient no.	Weight (g)	Blood volume (ml)	Nonblood solids (g)	Extravascular water (ml)	Extravascular sodium (ml)	Extravascular albumin (g)
Normal Lungs						
1	363	52	61	249	180	4.2
2	257	57	49	149	77	1.5
3	318	84	55	179	107	1.5
4	357	87	56	215	120	3.9
5	328	67	55	200	127	2.8
Mean ± 1.0 SD	325 ± 42	67 ± 19	55 ± 4	198 ± 38	122 ± 38	2.8 ± 1.3
Posttraumatic Pulmonary Failure						
1	867	321	87	440	282	11.6
2	766	188	100	467	358	9.4
3	1028	275	86	649	645	19.7
4	810	236	120	440	290	13.1
5	1270	357	97	795	586	15.1
6	745	230	118	384	363	6.9
7	1014	281	104	612	507	15.8
8	841	218	74	536	366	11.6
9	989	185	89	704	500	12.0
Mean ± 1.0 SD	925 ± 167	255 ± 59	97 ± 15	585 ± 139	433 ± 131	12.8 ± 3.7

Note: All data normalized to /m^2 BSA.

When fluid accumulation is less marked, the wet- to dry-weight ratio (especially when uncorrected for retained blood) may be misleading. Pulmonary fluid that accumulates interstitially or in the alveoli obviously contains a variety of solutes and determination of pulmonary edema should take into account absolute increases in water as well as the wet- to dry-weight ratio (or percentage of water) [6].

C.   Extravascular Lung Water

Unfortunately it is not easy to normalize absolute pulmonary water content. As noted, lung weights, which primarily depend on water, vary widely even in the "normal" postmortem lung. Whimster found these normals to range from 680 to 725 g, with a standard derivation close to 100 g. Body weight, sex, and race had no effect on the lung weight but there was a possible correlation with height [3]. In our own studies involving human lungs, lung water was related to body surface area (BSA), in which height is a factor. In 5 so-called normal postmortem lungs—of young adults who died suddenly without time for hospitalization or therapy—extravascular lung water averaged 198 ± 38 ml/m^2 BSA (Table 1). Staub reported on 13 "normals" and found extravascular water to average 383 g, but this value was not normalized for body surface area [7]. Assuming a BSA of 1.7 m^2 to be typical, the two values are obviously quite comparable. In the same review, Staub reported marked increases in extravascular water in pulmonary edema (1145 g), whereas we found similar increases in 9 surgical patients who died of posttraumatic pulmonary insufficiency (585 ± 139/m^2 BSA) [8]. It may be that normalization using the patient's stature would be preferable to using BSA, the calculation of which includes body weight. Fresh lung weight as a fraction of body weight was recommended by Visscher but the large variations in human body composition make this ratio of little value in clinical studies [9]. This would be especially true in situations in which abnormal water accumulation in the lungs is associated with generalized edema and its associated weight changes.

The foregoing discussion makes it clear that the water compartment of the lung is large and can be approximated simply by weighing the excised lung. The water percentage of excised lungs can be precisely quantified by drying the lung to a constant weight and comparing wet to dry weight, but this neglects the contribution of blood, which can be drained out only to a very limited extent. Quantification of pulmonary blood volume by approaches now to be outlined makes it possible to determine extravascular lung water gravimetrically. This volume can best be normalized by relating it to the subject's height and provides a sensitive index of abnormal gain or loss of pulmonary water.

III. Hemoglobin (Blood Compartment)

A. Preparation of the Lung

Human pulmonary tissue must be obtained either by biopsy in the course of thoracotomy or from postmortem tissues. The biopsy techniques introduce the problem of sampling that may not be representative. Furthermore, the operation and possibly the underlying condition that led to surgery may also disturb the baseline conditions that are being sought. When lungs are obtained at postmortem, the entire lung can be used, but postmortem changes that take place between the time of death and autopsy represent a serious problem. It is now well established that blood and fluid content of the lung increases with time after death [10]. Numerous animal studies with a variety of species all show that not only is the method of sacrifice important in determining the amount of blood in the lungs but the time delay between death and examination is also critical [11-13]. Whereas most organs lose weight after death, lungs gain both fluid and blood. Rapid exsanguination will limit postmortem changes [12] and this process may have been helpful in our studies of normal lungs. These tissues were obtained from the New York Medical Examiner's office and consisted of young adults who died traumatically without opportunity for therapy. Hemorrhage was a factor in all five deaths although only one patient was specifically said to have become exsanguinated. Our postmortem studies in hospitalized patients who died with acute respiratory failure undoubtedly reflect artifacts related to the inevitable delay between death and autopsy. Since postmortem changes are inevitable, studies with postmortem tissues must make every effort to control this variable by minimizing the time delay or at least trying to make it a constant.

Studies in vitro have also varied, using homogenization of the entire lung, a lobe, or an even smaller segment. The effects of gravity on regional pulmonary blood distribution are well documented for both ante- and postmortem conditions and unless these factors can be controlled it is almost mandatory to homogenize the entire lung to evaluate the pulmonary blood compartment properly [14,15].

B. Extracting and Measuring Hemoglobin

Many methods designed to extract and measure hemoglobin from biologic tissues have been described. The ability to separate and quantify blood, free of lung tissue, continues to represent a challenge for the biochemist. The usual technique consists of converting blood to acid hematin, which is then quantified by spectrophotometric analysis. When this method is directly applied to untreated lung homogenates, difficulties may ensue. Despite thorough homogenization, separating the blood and lung tissues is difficult. Even if all the hemoglobin is converted to acid hematin, it may not be evenly distributed in the lung [16]. More vigorous separation or homogenization will result in better distribution but the resulting mixture is cloudy even after filtration and centrifugation. Under these circumstances optical density is increased in comparison with standards prepared from blood without pulmonary tissue.

Complete homogenization of the lung tissue is essential and if this is done, some technique designed to eliminate spectrophotometric interference is necessary. Our own studies were done using ether-alcohol extraction, since repeated extraction with a 4:1 mixture of ether and 95% alcohol will extract the acid hematin from the water-lung mixture. A recent study has examined five different techniques for estimating the blood content of excised lung tissue including those just mentioned [16]. The author concluded that even ether-alcohol extraction failed to yield consistently satisfactory results, probably because of lipid compounds that continued to interfere with spectrophotometric analysis. Pretreatment with acetone was advocated, and it was reported that this procedure improved the acid hematin ether-alcohol extraction method. Hemoglobin levels in pulmonary tissue have also been determined by measuring the peroxidase activity of free heme pigments under specially buffered conditions. The method is reported to be reproducible and sensitive to hemoglobin concentrations of 5 mg% [17].

It is also possible to determine hemoglobin by transforming it into cyanohemoglobin. A solution of potassium ferricyanide can be added, and after hemolysis of all the blood in the homogenized pulmonary tissue the cyanohemoglobin concentration of the clear red supernatant liquid can be determined spectrophotometrically [18].

Staub and his associates have reported on the use of the cyanmethemoglobin method to measure residual lung blood [19]. These workers homogenized the entire lung and felt that satisfactory identification of hemoglobin in pulmonary tissue was possible by this technique.

Simplification of these somewhat exacting techniques is possible when isotopes can be used. The method requires injecting [^{131}I] albumin as a plasma marker before excision of the lung and thus applies better to experimental studies than to postmortem. Homogenization, centrifugation, and filtration are still necessary before gamma counting but the calculations are straightforward [20].

The foregoing discussion is important since it emphasizes that separating hemoglobin from pulmonary tissue and measuring it is not without pitfalls. Careful attention to detail is necessary, but current methods do make it possible to determine accurately the residual hemoglobin in the lung.

C. Calculating Blood Volume

Once the amount of hemoglobin in the lung is known, it becomes possible to calculate the pulmonary blood volume. In postmortem studies, one can assume a normal value for hemoglobin for men or for women, and that is how we calculated a blood volume for the five normal young adults who died suddenly without hospitalization. For the patients who died with posttraumatic pulmonary insufficiency, we were able to use the last hemoglobin recorded in the hospital record. These patients had been in critical condition, and daily hemoglobin determinations were available.

Other investigators have used postmortem blood samples, since blood in many of the large veins remains unclotted for hours following death. Bachmann withdrew samples bilaterally from subclavian and femoral veins and reported that there was very little difference in the hemoglobin concentration from these four sites [21]. Backmann also relied on work done by Schleyer, who found that the escape of serum from capillaries with a resultant increase in hemoglobin concentration did not become significant until 24 hr after death took place [22]. We did not find good agreement between the four postmortem sampling sites as reported by Backmann and felt that an antemortem value for large-vessel hemoglobin concentration was far more reliable. When this is not available, average normal values can be used but the chance of serious error does exist.

Even when an accurate estimate of large-vessel hemoglobin concentration is available, there is concern about the relation between large-vessel hematocrit (LVH) and pulmonary hematocrit. Rapaport and his coworkers found the correction to be somewhat less than 5% [23]. Dow, Hahn, and Hamilton, and also Lawson and his associates, arrived at a similar figure [24,25]. However, these studies were all carried out using Evans blue for plasma volume and ^{51}Cr-labeled red cells for the red cell mass. Blood volume determinations using Evans blue and radioactive red cells are always larger than when some other plasma tag is used [26-29]. When RISA is used in place of Evans blue, it becomes apparent that the difference between the hematocrit in the pulmonary vessels and the LVH is not very great [30]. This is partly because in the living organism most of the blood in the central or pulmonary circuit is in large vessels. After death, when the lung is passively drained, the hematocrit of the blood remaining in the smaller pulmonary vessels may vary from hematocrit in the large vessels. This suggests that an effort should be made to measure plasma volume by a tracer whenever this is possible, to avoid the errors inherent with an assumed hematocrit value.

When residual blood volume is determined from the total hemoglobin in the lung, it must also include the blood contained in the bronchial circulation.

Although this blood is intrapulmonary, it is not actually part of the lesser circulation. However, bronchial blood flow is only 1% to 2% of the cardiac output [31], and probably less than half of this is actually in the lung at any time. It is included in the calculation of the pulmonary blood compartment.

Other approaches to calculating pulmonary blood volume have been described and are somewhat more accurate because the specific gravity of blood and homogenate are not the same. Furthermore, LVH or hemoglobin concentration is related to volume, usually 100 ml of blood, while aliquots of the homogenate are usually weighed. Formulas have been designed to take these factors into account and require a blood specimen before excision of the lungs. Hemoglobin concentration and blood density and wet and dry weights must be determined from this systemic blood sample. Similarly, hemoglobin concentration in the homogenate, specific gravity, and the wet weight of the lungs are needed to determine the weight of blood in the lungs [32].

Isotopic techniques have also been used in estimating the pulmonary blood compartment. This requires labeling red cells and injecting these cells with [^{125}I] albumin. A period of mixing, usually 10 to 15 min, is necessary and then the lung is removed. A systemic blood sample is also necessary, and after it is taken differential counting can be used to calculate both the erythrocyte and plasma volume of the excised lung [33]. Holcroft and Trunkey [34] have recently described a similar technique.

D. Comparison of Gravimetrically Determined Pulmonary Blood Volume to Other Methods

The average total weight of the lung (meaning both right and left lobes) is approximately 700 g, despite slightly higher values given by some pathologists. In the five healthy young adults who died suddenly without hospitalization or treatment, the mean lung weight was 325 ± 42 g/m^2 body surface area; the mean lung weight for the usual adult is about 600 g. The blood content of the lung has been reported to be approximately 30% of the total wet weight. It should be noted that blood was drained from the large pulmonary vessels in these subjects before homogenization. Other investigators [21,35] have reported higher values for the undrained lung.

Gravimetric values can be compared with values determined in several other ways. The most common technique for estimating pulmonary blood volume in vivo is the "needle-to-needle" volume obtained from the indicator dilution technique. This value, more often referred to as the central blood volume, usually includes blood in the heart chambers; if the indicator bolus is injected into the pulmonary artery and the sampling is done in the left atrium, however, these blood reservoirs are eliminated. Unfortunately, there is evidence that the failure to include a mixing chamber (right or left ventricle) in the circuit may lead to inaccuracies. Techniques involving double injection or double sampling have been used, however, to obviate this problem. Careful studies by Dock [36] and Milnor and their coworkers [37], using the double-injection single sampling technique, reported mean values of 246 and 365 ml/m² BSA, respectively. These values include blood that would be lost on draining postmortem lungs, so the higher values are consistent with the postmortem studies already mentioned.

When pulmonary *capillary* blood volume is measured by the method of Roughton and Forster, the value obtained is more closely related to blood remaining in the drained lung. Values of 65 ml (or 38 ml/m² BSA) have been reported [38] and are close to the values that we found in the five normal postmortem lungs (67 ± 19 ml/m² BSA).

Pulmonary capillary blood volume values have also been reported by Weibel, who used careful anatomical measurements in human lungs [39]. This investigator reported a pulmonary capillary blood volume of approximately 2 ml/kg body weight, which would be 82 ml/m² BSA for a 70 kg/1.7 m² adult. This is very close to the postmortem values that we have reported for drained lungs.

Vreim and Staub compared pulmonary capillary blood volume measured by the method of Roughton and Forster with an ingenious technique of direct measurement that is also based on direct histologic examination [40]. These investigators studied cat lungs that were frozen with liquid propane minutes after the indirect measurement of pulmonary capillary blood volume. Alveolar surface area, alveolar wall thickness, and alveolar wall volume were then determined histologically. The point count method was used to establish the fraction of alveolar wall volume occupied by red blood cells; then pulmonary capillary blood volume was calculated directly with the peripheral hematocrit value. In 18 cats, the direct measurement was 22% larger than the average indirect determination of capillary blood volume, but it was evident that both methods were reliable.

Once the pulmonary blood compartment has been identified, it becomes possible to divide the lung into three well-defined compartments. The total wet weight of the lung represents the starting point and the pulmonary blood weight constitutes the first compartment. Extravascular water can be measured by drying an aliquot of the homogenized lung to a constant weight, but the contribution of blood to this solid residue must be subtracted. This can be done after the blood weight is determined. Once the blood contribution to the lung solids has been subtracted, this compartment and the blood compartment can be added. The difference between this sum and the original wet weight of the lung constitutes the extravascular water compartment, which includes both interstitial and intracellular water.

It is possible to extend this three-compartment lung, consisting of blood, extravascular water, and nonblood solids, by further dividing extravascular water. Sodium has often been used for this purpose since its distribution is primarily extracellular.

IV. Pulmonary Sodium Space

Sodium represents a physiologic test substance normally in dynamic equilibrium in the body. It has an advantage when the virtual volume of distribution is being estimated in that no equilibration time is needed.

Sodium determination in biologic tissue is far less complex than measuring hemoglobin. Most investigators have ashed the tissue samples [41,8,42, 43]. A flame photometer can then be used for the final determination of the sodium content of the sample.

The original reports by Fishman and his coworkers used the ratio of total sodium per gram of wet lung to sodium concentration in microequivalents per millitter of protein-free plasma water to define the volume distribution of this electrolyte. The distribution volume of sodium was not corrected for the contribution from red blood cells since corrected volumes, calculated from the volume of blood in the lungs, the hematocrit, and the sodium content of red blood cells, differed from the uncorrected by only 2.4% [41].

In our studies, we calculated the extravascular distribution of sodium in an effort to define the interstitial space. Such calculations require that the total sodium in the lung homogenate be reduced by the amount accounted for in the blood compartment. This can readily be accomplished once the blood or plasma volume is known provided that a systemic plasma sample is available for determining sodium concentration. As noted previously, the small amount of sodium in red cells is not large enough to require special treatment. The remaining sodium is extravascular and to calculate the distribution volume, it is necessary to know the extravascular concentration. In our studies, we assumed that the extravascular or interstitial concentration was equal to the concentration in plasma. This neglects the Donnan equilibrium and the fact that interstitial electrolyte concentrations are somewhat lower than simultaneously determined plasma levels. The two values are closely related, however, and if extravascular sodium is to be used as an indicator of interstitial fluid volume, uncertainties regarding its extravascular concentration are actually of less concern than our inability to define precisely its distribution boundaries. Sodium penetrates the cells to some degree so it is clear that the sodium space represents an overestimate of interstitial volume.

When an exogenous indicator such as sucrose is used to define the extravascular, extracellular space, a far smaller volume results. When sucrose and chloride spaces were compared simultaneously in the sheep lung, the chloride space was found to be at least one and a half times the space measured by sucrose [44]. This illustrates the limitations inherent in using chloride ion to define interstitial fluid volume. Sodium has no advantages over chloride and may even penetrate cells to a slightly greater degree [45]. Despite these limitations, sodium and chloride are of value in any effort to define interstitial fluid volume. While sucrose is undoubtedly a more precise marker in that it is completely excluded from the cell, it represents an exogenous indicator that needs a period of equilibration. Equilibration times may vary in some of the conditions under study to say nothing of the fact that only endogenous substances can be used in postmortem tissue analysis. A better marker normally present in interstitial fluid would be of real value and might be found by systematic investigation of some of the other ionic substances present in body fluids.

In the lung, sodium undoubtedly communicates with the fluid lining the alveoli and especially with pulmonary edema fluid. The pulmonary interstitial space plus the alveolar gas space combine to make up the extravascular, extracellular compartment of the lung and both these areas have to be considered in the extravascular distribution of sodium, or chloride. Under normal conditions, however, the interstitial space is separated from the alveolar gas by an alveolar epithelial barrier that is considered to be impermeable to nearly every solute.

Efforts have recently been made to separate pulmonary extravascular, extracellular fluid into its interstitial and alveolar components. Since these two spaces cannot readily be separated by the usual tracers that other compartmentalization studies use, electron-microscopic techniques have been called on. Weibel and his associates have used stereological techniques extensively and they can describe changes in interstitial and alveolar tissues volumes in semiquantitative terms [46,47]. Light microscopy has also been used by Staub and his associates to examine the sequence of fluid accumulation in experimental pulmonary edema [48,49]. Fishman and his colleagues have also studied this process. They used the presence of hemoglobin in extravascular sites as a "tracer" in the pathogenesis of experimental hemodynamic edema [50]. A similar technique was reported by Moss and his associates but they modified the sodium ion so it could be identified in interstitial tissues [51]. All such electron-microscopic studies are limited by technical difficulties in preparing the lung and the fact that postmortem studies are not possible. Even human biopsy specimens are not readily converted into satisfactory electron micrographs, so that morphologic approaches will continue to be valuable in experimental rather than clinical studies.

Actual measurements of extravascular pulmonary sodium distribution were first reported by Fishman and his coworkers [41] and Mendenhall and his associates [43]. Both groups were surprised by the extent of this compartment, which was approximately 60% of the wet weight of the lung. Fishman postulated a layer of interstitial fluid inside the gaseous side of the alveolar surface as a possible explanation for the large extravascular sodium space. Our studies in the five postmortem lungs revealed an extravascular distribution volume of 122 ± 38 ml/m^2, or 40% of the wet weight. This represents a somewhat smaller value but is still quite large considering the limited interstitial area that one sees when the lung is viewed through a microscope.

When the interstitial space is measured more precisely by an exogenous tracer that remains completely extracellular, it still occupies a large fraction of the extravascular water. Such a study was carried out in human pulmonary tissue removed at thoracotomy by Vaughan and his coworkers, who injected [^{14}C] sucrose 10 min before lung biopsy. In 10 patients undergoing pulmonary resection the interstitial space measured 0.60 ± 0.28 of extravascular water [52]. Pulmonary edema would obviously increase the interstitial volume, and in 5 patients who died of pulmonary edema we found that the sodium space rose to 0.56 of the wet weight, or 0.76 of the extravascular water in the lung.

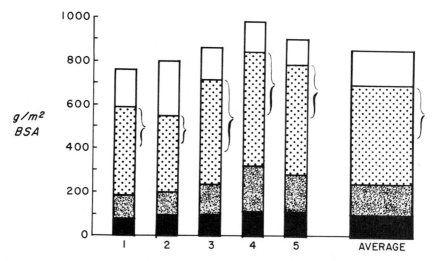

FIGURE 1   Postmortem determinations of virtual distribution volumes in five patients who died in acute pulmonary edema. The compartments starting from the top represent blood, extravascular sodium, nonsodium extravascular water, and nonblood solids. The brace represents extravascular albumin, and the calculations are based on the arbitrary assumption that interstitial albumin concentration is 3 g/100 ml (see text).

Much of the debate in the pathogenesis of pulmonary edema relates to the transition from interstitial edema to alveolar flooding. Schulz postulated early involvement of the alveolar spaces [53] but more recent work suggests that alveolar wall edema is extensive preceding spillover into the alveoli. Sodium space measurements alone cannot answer this question because the alveolar gas space is in series with the interstitial tissue. However, we were able to show large increases in sodium distribution in patients with acute respiratory failure but no clinical evidence of pulmonary edema; these findings implied that at least under these circumstances this compartment can be increased more than 300% before there is clinically detectable overflow into the alveoli (Figs. 1 and 2). Interpreting these findings is complicated because all patients had evidence of some degree of consolidation on chest films taken before they died. Undoubtedly sodium-containing fluid was present in the consolidated areas and the large increase in sodium distribution undoubtedly represents a combination of interstitial and alveolar compartments.

Similar findings were observed in an experimental study in which steam inhalation was used to promote alveolar capillary leakage [54]. In this study, extravascular water was determined instead of sodium distribution. Increases of approximately 200% were associated with well-aerated alveoli as judged by

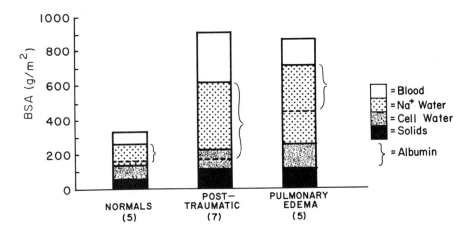

FIGURE 2 Comparison of distribution volumes in 5 "normal" postmortem lungs—7 patients who died of posttraumatic pulmonary insufficiency and 5 patients of pulmonary edema. Even though the posttraumatic and pulmonary edema lungs weighed approximately the same, differences in the individual compartments are evident. The individual values for the pulmonary edema lungs are shown in Figure 1, and the values for the normals and the posttraumatic pulmonary insufficiency patients are recorded in Table 1.

TABLE 2 Postmortem Lung Compartments in Normal Dogs and Those with Burns of the Lung

Dog no.	Body wt. (kg)	Lung wt. (g)	Blood wt. (g)	Extravascular water (g)	Extravascular solids (g)
Control Dogs					
1	15.9	149	46	82	21
2	15.0	155	53	79	23
3	17.3	178	62	84	32
4	14.5	171	48	96	27
5	16.0	161	56	83	22
Mean 1.0 ± SD	15.7 ± 1.07	162.8 ± 11.7	53.0 ± 6.4	84.8 ± 6.5	25.0 ± 4.5
Steam Inhalation					
1	15.2	239	44	152	43
2	13.6	285	17	243	25
3	15.0	248	50	165	33
4	17.0	200	42	136	22
5	19.1	231	46	161	24
6	19.5	242	77	134	31
7	15.9	281	42	201	38
8	20.5	251	45	164	42
9	18.2	240	42	166	32
10	17.1	198	44	123	31
Mean 1.0 ± SD	17.1 ± 2.2	241.5 ± 28.5	44.9 ± 14.4	164.5 ± 35.2	32.1 ± 7.25

normal roentgenographic appearance and the lack of alveolar fluid accumulation histologically. The increased water recorded in this study included both intracellular as well as interstitial water but it supports the concept that a considerable increase in extravascular water accumulation is possible without clinical or x-ray evidence of pulmonary edema (Table 2).

V. Albumin Compartment

When the lung is expanded by edema fluid, the protein in this fluid is soluble and consists of plasma protein. Hemingway was one of the first to quantify soluble protein in a study of guinea pig lungs [55]. In his studies, the lungs were ground to a paste in sand and the ground residue extracted with a 1% NaCl solution. This removed the soluble proteins, which were contrasted to the insoluble pulmonary nitrogen taken as a measure of the structural tissue of the lung.

A serious problem with the technique was that the soluble protein fraction included hemoglobin, which had to be determined separately, and also numerous other proteins that were not characterized. It is probably better to determine the albumin content of pulmonary tissue since albumin constitutes the principal component of soluble protein.

The extent of the albumin compartment in normal or diseased lungs is not readily determined, even after measurements of total pulmonary albumin concentration by electrophoresis of the soluble protein fraction. In our studies we homogenized entire lungs and centrifuged an aliquot at 10,000 rpm for 10 min. Total soluble protein content of the supernatant solution was determined with an AO refractometer. The albumin fraction was then determined by electrophoresis. The position of the albumin peak was established by comparison with a plasma sample. Normally the supernatant solution showed only two large peaks, albumin and hemoglobin. The intravascular albumin fraction was readily calculated from the large-vessel plasma albumin concentration and the previously determined pulmonary blood volume. However, calculation of extravascular albumin distribution volume necessitates a value for extravascular or interstitial albumin concentration. Some workers feel that lung lymph protein is identical in composition to the protein in the interstitial fluid. The volume of the extravascular, extracellular space and the total extravascular albumin content of the lung can be measured from the volume of distribution of a suitable indicator in excess of intravascular volume. Such measurements make it possible to calculate interstitial albumin concentration if it is assumed that the albumin is uniformly distributed throughout interstitial fluid. When albumin concentration in interstitial fluid is calculated in this fashion it ranges between 0.3 and 0.7 of the plasma concentration [6].

Albumin concentration in pulmonary interstitial fluid is also well below the albumin concentration in pulmonary lymph. This was reported in a recent study by Vaughan, Erdmann, and Staub, who measured total extravascular water, albumin content, and the $[^{14}C]$ sucrose extravascular space in sheep lungs [57]. RISA was given before the study, and after three to seven days to to allow for equilibration with body albumin, $[^{14}C]$ sucrose was administered intravenously. After sacrifice, the lungs were weighed wet, analyzed for residual blood, total extravascular water $[^{14}C]$ sucrose, and ^{125}RISA. Calculations showed the albumin concentration in interstitial water to be low in contrast to levels in pulmonary lymph as determined in previous studies. The authors concluded that either there is a large interstitial excluded volume for albumin or albumin is concentrated in lymph. These possibilities have been further explored in Staub's recent review article [6].

A recent study using different methods also postulated concentration of pulmonary interstitial fluid before it was collected as thoracic duct lymph [58]. Northrup and Humphrey used an intravenous injection of RISA dogs that had been cannulated in the right thoracic duct. Timed collections of lymph provided flow and mean transit time, which they multiplied to derive "apparent" pulmonary lymph volume. This volume was only about 15% of the space (extravascular) measured by the double indicator dilution method. They postulated that the discrepancy might be caused by a resorption of water from lymph to blood that occurred in the lymph nodes traversed by pulmonary lymph before it reached the right thoracic duct.

Difficulties of this sort will continue until it becomes possible to analyze pulmonary interstitial fluid directly in order to determine its albumin concentration. In our studies we calculated an extravascular albumin compartment based on the completely arbitrary assumption that the interstitial concentration was 3 g/100 ml [8]. While a virtual volume can be calculated using this assumption, the finding doesn't mean very much, and probably a better method would be to report the findings in terms of the *amount* or *content* of extravascular albumin.

VI. Evaluation and Future Applications of Compartmentalization

Investigations of the pathogenesis of pulmonary edema and the acute respiratory insufficiency syndrome have focused attention on the increased lung weight associated with these conditions. Compartmentalization of the lung into individual virtual volumes of distribution has been of help in understanding what compartments or spaces contribute to the marked increase in total lung weight.

Furthermore, comparison of intravascular and extravascular composition and volume provides a new insight into how pulmonary capillaries partition electrolytes and albumin.

Much of our previous understanding of abnormal pulmonary capillary function has been based on histologic examination of pulmonary tissue, but a variety of artifacts and also variation between sampling sites has made interpretation difficult. The homogenization of entire lungs and then their reconstitution following chemical analysis provides a new dimension in the study of pulmonary pathology.

Certain limitations are obvious and must be recognized. Pulmonary hemoglobin must be determined carefully but even when this has been accomplished, calculating its volume of distribution requires knowledge of the pulmonary blood hemoglobin concentration. The large-vessel hematocrit is a reasonable approximation but it is possible to improve the precision of this determination by using radioisotopes. Provided that the blood compartment can be determined with precision, its contribution to solids can be subtracted from an aliquot of the pulmonary homogenate dried to a constant weight. In this fashion the blood compartment and a "solid" compartment can be identified and the remainder of the wet weight of the original lung is extravascular water. These three compartments can be determined with excellent precision but further compartmentalization has limitations. In our studies we used sodium as a marker for interstitial fluid, since the interstitial space is of great interest in pulmonary edema and also posttraumatic pulmonary insufficiency. The ability of sodium, or any other electrolyte marker, to define this space is limited because of intracellular penetration and the fact that the sodium-containing interstitial fluid is continuous with intra-alveolar fluid. For this reason the sodium space is only an approximation of the interstitial space of the lung.

The final compartment or virtual volume examined in this report is albumin. Although the quantity, or lung content, of extravascular albumin can be determined reasonably well, its distribution volume will remain uncertain until it becomes possible to examine pulmonary interstitial fluid and measure its albumin concentration.

Most compartmentalization studies have dealt with entire lungs excised at postmortem or when the experimental preparation was sacrificed. Future application of these techniques will probably rely more on biopsy specimens; thus postmortem artifacts would be avoided and sequential determinations made possible. Much has already been done in this area from skeletal muscle biopsies. A detailed description of the needle biopsy technique was provided by Bergstrom, who used 20–80-mg samples from the lateral aspect of the quadriceps femoris [59]. Neutron activation analysis made it possible to do multiple analysis for sodium, potassium, chloride, and phosphorus on these small samples. Skeletal muscle, like the lung, can be divided into extracellular and intracellular phases. To determine the concentration of a single ionic species in the intracellular space, one must subtract the extracellular ionic content from the total tissue ion content. This requires estimating the extracellular fluid volume; and this was done by the chloride method, assuming minimal intracellular penetration by this ion. These authors were interested in muscle electrolytes and made no effort to identify a separate blood compartment in these muscle biopsies. There is no reason, however, why virtual volumes of distribution for blood, interstitial fluid (extravascular chloride or sodium distribution), and intracellular fluid cannot be determined. The ability to analyze small samples of any tissue, whether it is muscle, lung, or liver, means that compartmentalization studies can now be far more widely applied in clinical research.

References

1. D. M. Pryce and E. F. Ross. *Ross' Postmortem Appearances.* London, Oxford University Press, 1963, p. 283.
2. F. W. Sunderman and F. Boerner. *Normal Values in Clinical Medicine.* Philadelphia, W. B. Saunders, 1949, p. 641.
3. W. F. Whimster, Normal lung weights in Jamaicans, *Amer. Rev. Resp. Dis.,* **103**:85 (1971).
4. O. R. Levine, R. B. Mellins, R. M. Senior, and A. P. Fishman, The application of Starling's law of capillary exchange to the lungs, *J. Clin. Invest.,* **46**:934 (1967).
5. R. L. Simmons, A. M. Martin, Jr., C. A. Heisterkamp, III, and T. B. Duchen, Respiratory insufficiency in combat casualties. II. Pulmonary edema following head injury, *Ann. Surg.,* **170**:39 (1969).
6. N. C. Staub, Pulmonary edema, *Physiol. Rev.,* **54**:678 (1974).
7. N. C. Staub, Pathogenesis of pulmonary edema, *Amer. Rev. Resp. Dis.,* **109**:358 (1974).
8. F. E. Gump, Y. Mashima, A. Ferenczy, and J. M. Kinney, Pre- and postmortem studies of lung fluids and electrolytes, *J. Trauma,* **11**:474 (1971).
9. M. B. Visscher, F. J. Haddy, and G. Stephens, The physiology and pharmacology of lung edema, *Pharmacol. Rev.,* **8**:389 (1956).
10. T. Sjostrand, On the principles for the distribution of the blood in the peripheral vascular system, *Skand. Arch. Physiol. Suppl.,* **71**:1 (1935).
11. F. M. Boyd and L. M. Knight, Postmortem shifts in the weight and water levels of body organs, *Toxicol. Appl. Pharmacol.,* **15**:119 (1963).
12. S. H. Durlacher, W. G. Banfield, and A. D. Bergnes, Postmortem pulmonary edema, *Yale J. Biol. Med.,* **22**:565 (1950).
13. J. M. Lauweryns and N. Bourgeois, Neonatal hyaline membrane disease: Light and electron microscopical studies. In *Current Research in Chronic*

Respiratory Disease. Washington, U. S. Department of Health, Education, and Welfare Publication 1879, 1969, p. 3.

14. W. S. Miller. *The Lung.* Springfield, Illinois, Charles C Thomas, 1943, p. 3.

15. J. B. West. *Ventilation Blood Flow and Gas Exchange.* Oxford, Blackwell, 1965.

16. B. E. Marshall, Determination of the blood content of lungs in vitro, *J. Appl. Physiol.,* **31**:643 (1971).

17. J. W. Holcroft and D. D. Trunkey, Extravascular lung water following hemorrhagic shock in the baboon, *Ann. Surg.,* **180**:408–417 (1974).

18. R. Backmann. *Blutvolumen, Gefässbett und Blutverteilung in der Lunge.* Stuttgart, Gustav Fischer Verlag, 1969, p. 2.

19. K. L. Brigham, W. C. Woolverton, L. Blake, and N. C. Staub, Increased sheep lung vascular permeability caused by *Pseudomonas bacteremia, J. Clin. Invest.,* **54**:792 (1974).

20. B. E. Marshall and M. Q. Wyche, Pulmonary extravascular water volume during halothane-oxygen anesthesia in dogs, *Anesthesiology,* **32**:530–536 (1970).

21. R. Backmann, Blutgehalt and Blutverteilung in den Lungen gesunder und kranker Menschen, *Beitr. Path. Anat.,* **125**:222 (1961).

22. F. Schleyer. *Postmortale klinisch-chemische Diagnostik und Todzeitbestimmung.* Stuttgart, Thieme, 1958.

23. E. Rapaport, H. Kuida, F. W. Haynes, and L. Dexter, Pulmonary red cell and plasma volumes and pulmonary haematocrit in the normal dog, *Amer. J. Physiol.,* **185**:127 (1956).

24. P. Dow, P. F. Hahn, and W. F. Hamilton, The simultaneous transport of T 1824 and radioactive red cells through the heart and lungs, *Amer. J. Physiol.,* **147**:493 (1946).

25. H. C. Lawson, W. F. Cantrell, J. E. Shaw, D. L. Blackburn, and S. Adams, Measurement of cardiac output in the dog by the simultaneous injection of dye and radioactive red cells, *Amer. J. Physiol.,* **170**:277 (1952).

26. A. E. Lewis, Estimation of plasma volume of the heart, *Amer. J. Physiol.,* **172**:203 (1953).

27. J. W. Pearce, On the regulation of blood volume. In *Cardiology,* Part 6, 1961.

28. L. Y. Senn and K. E. Karlson, Methodologic and actual error of plasma volume determination, *Surgery,* **44**:1095 (1958).

29. D. G. Vidt and L. A. Sapirstein, Distribution volume of T 1824 and chromium labelled red cells immediately following intravenous injection, *Circ. Res.,* **5**:129 (1957).

30. D. Parrish, D. E. Strandess, Jr., and J. W. Bell, Differences between plasma and red cell flow characteristics of the pulmonary vascular bed, *Amer. J. Physiol.,* **200**:619 (1961).

31. H. D. Bruner and C. F. Smidt, Blood flow in the bronchial artery of the anesthetized dog, *Amer. J. Physiol.,* **148**:648 (1947).

32. M. L. Pearce, J. Yamashita, and J. Beazell, Measurement of pulmonary edema, *Circ. Res.,* **16**:482 (1965).

33. P. Aarseth and G. Bo, Content of blood and of extravascular water in cat lungs during changes in total blood volume, *Acta Physiol. Scand.,* **85**:343 (1972).

34. J. W. Holcroft and D. D. Trunkey, Pulmonary extravasation of albumin during and after hemorrhagic shock in baboons, *J. Surg. Res.,* **18**:91 (1975).

35. L. Dexter and G. T. Smith, Quantitative studies of pulmonary embolism, *Amer. J. Med. Sci.,* **247**:37 (1964).

36. D. S. Dock, W. L. Kraus, E. Woodward, L. Dexter, and F. Haynes, Observations on pulmonary blood volume in man, *Fed. Proc.,* **18**:37 (1959).

37. W. R. Milnor, A. D. Jose, and C. J. McGaff, Pulmonary vascular volume, resistance and compliance in man, *Circulation,* **12**:130 (1960).

38. F. J. W. Roughton and R. E. Forster, Relative importance of diffusion and chemical reaction rates in determining the rate of exchange of gases in the human lung, *J. Appl. Physiol.,* **11**:290 (1957).

39. E. R. Weibel. *Morphometry of the human lung.* New York, Academic Press, 1963.

40. C. E. Vreim and N. C. Staub, Indirect and direct pulmonary capillary blood volume in anesthetized open thorax cats, *J. Appl. Physiol.,* **34**:452 (1973).

41. A. P. Fishman, E. L. Becker, and H. W. Fritts, Jr., et al., Apparent volumes of distribution of water electrolytes and hemoglobin within the lung, *Amer. J. Physiol.,* **188**:95 (1957).

42. F. N. Low, Extracellular components of the pulmonary alveolar wall, *Arch. Int. Med.,* **127**:847 (1971).

43. R. M. Mendenhall, P. M. Ramorino, and B. Gerstl, Water, sodium and potassium content of human, guinea pig and rabbit lung, *Proc. Soc. Exp. Biol. Med.,* **82**:318 (1953).

44. N. C. Staub, personal communication.

45. M. B. Cleland, J. R. Pluth, W. Tauxe, and J. W. Kirklin, Blood volume and body fluid compartment changes soon after closed and open intracardiac surgery, *J. Thor. Surg.,* **52**:698 (1960).

46. E. R. Weibel, Structure in space and its appearance on sections. In *Proceedings of the Internal Congress on Stereology* 2nd Chicago. Edited by H. Elias. New York, Springer, 1967.

47. E. R. Weibel, Morphological basis of alveolar capillary gas exchange, *Physiol. Rev.,* **53**:419 (1973).

48. N. C. Staub, The pathophysiology of pulmonary edema, *Human Pathol.,* **1**:419 (1970).

49. N. C. Staub, H. Nagano, and M. L. Pearce, Pulmonary edema in dogs, especially the sequence of fluid accumulation in the lungs, *J. Appl. Physiol.,* **22**:227 (1967).

50. G. G. Pietra, J. P. Szidon, M. M. Leventhal, and A. P. Fishman, Hemoglobin as a tracer in hemodynamic pulmonary edema, *Science,* **166**:1643 (1969).

51. G. S. Moss, T. das Gupta, B. Newson, and L. M. Nyhus, Effect of hemorrhagic shock on pulmonary interstitial sodium distribution in the primate lung, *Ann. Surg.,* **177**:211 (1973).
52. T. R. Vaughan, Jr., D. J. Ullyot, and N. C. Staub, Interstitial albumin concentration in the lung, *Clin. Res.,* **21**:673 (1973).
53. H. Schulz. *The Submicroscopic Anatomy and Pathology of the Lung.* Berlin, Springer-Verlag, 1959, p. 87.
54. F. E. Gump, B. A. Zikria, and Y. Mashima, The effect of interstitial edema on pulmonary function in the dog, *J. Trauma,* **12**:764 (1972).
55. A. Hemingway, A method of chemical analysis of guinea pig lung for the factors involved in pulmonary edema, *J. Lab. Clin. Med.,* **35**:817 (1950).
56. R. D. H. Boyd, J. R. Hill, and R. W. Humphreys et al., Permeability of lung capillary macromolecules in fetal and newborn lambs and sheep, *J. Physiol.,* **201**:567 (1969).
57. T. R. Vaughan, Jr., A. J. Erdmann, III, and N. C. Staub, Subdivisions of lung extravascular water space and calculated interstitial albumin concentration in sheep, *Fed. Proc.,* **30**:379 (1971).
58. W. F. Northrup, III, and E. W. Humphrey, Albumin permeability in the pulmonary capillaries, *Surg. Forum,* **25**:224 (1974).
59. J. Bergstrom, Muscle electrolytes in man, *Scand. J. Clin. Lab. Invest.,* Vol. 14, Suppl. 68. 1962.

Part Two

TRANSVASCULAR EXCHANGE

5

Mathematical Modeling of Steady State Fluid and Protein Exchange in Lung

LYNN H. BLAKE

National Heart, Lung, and Blood Institute
National Institutes of Health
Bethesda, Maryland

I. Introduction

Mathematical models have become important tools in biologic investigations. If such models are properly developed and used, they can provide insight into the relations between the physical variables and processes influencing the system being studied. The resulting interplay of experimental investigation and theoretical model can be an essential factor in developing the experimental design and interpreting the data.

The purpose of this chapter is to review briefly the application of mathematical models to solute and fluid transport across neutral membranes; to investigate the influence of membrane structure (pore sizes and numbers), hydrostatic pressure, and solute concentrations on the steady state membrane exchange; and to describe the application of an "equivalent" pore model to the lung.

II. Mathematical Models and Membrane Transport

A. General

Mathematical models now reach into almost every field of biologic research. In many cases, they are no longer a luxury but an indispensable tool for the design, execution, and interpretation of experimental investigations. Like any research tool, the mathematical model has a utility that is directly related to its intelligent application.

There are many kinds of mathematical modeling. Since many biologic systems are complex, mathematical formulations have been developed to reproduce experimental data without regard to underlying processes or mechanisms. Such models can be extremely useful in considering the performance of biologic systems, although the components of the model are not always identifiable with the components and mechanisms of the physiologic system. Nevertheless, without such specificity, the models can be arbitrarily adjusted to reproduce experimental data and so used to explore the relations between various systems. For complex biologic systems, the insight such models provide has proved useful.

If a mathematical model is properly developed, it can reveal not only what is happening within a system but why it is happening. If the molecular processes of a system can be described by mathematical equations that can be written in terms of the physiologic parameters, the mechanisms of the process can be investigated. This kind of model provides mathematical equations to describe the change of mass, momentum, energy, charge, and the like within a specified volume as a function of the exchange occurring across the boundaries of the volume under consideration. Therefore, a well-defined volume must be identifiable and the processes that control the exchange across the boundaries of this volume must be described in mathematical terms embracing the physiologic parameters involved.

Such a model can provide us with two benefits. It can first provide an improved understanding of the physical parameters and processes that influence the variables we experimentally measure. Agreement between the results from a model and experimental data supports the validity of the experiment and also helps us to understand better how the system functions.

The second advantage of a model is that it allows for a theoretical investigation of the sensitivity of the variables being measured to changes in the experimental conditions. If we find from the model that the variable being measured is insensitive to the processes of interest, we may be directed to select a new variable to measure. In contrast, we may find that the variable being measured is so sensitive to an uncontrollable condition that it will be very difficult to interpret the experimental results. Such difficulty can lead to an improved experimental design. Consequently, the interplay between the experimental design and the theoretical model becomes an essential step in developing and interpreting experimental research.

Any mathematical model should be validated by comparing it with experimental data covering a wide range of conditions. This parametric investigation may demonstrate the inadequacies of the model and could lead to a more complete understanding of the physical processes involved.

For the pulmonary exchange considered here, the primary process is the passive transport of fluid and protein across the pulmonary vascular (endothelial) membrane of the lung. A simple model of this exchange is shown in Figure 1. A large volume of fluid and protein enters the lung, as shown. Under normal conditions, a net flow of approximately 0.003% of this fluid occurs across the endothelial membrane. This filtrate leaves the lung through the lymphatic system, as shown. When the lymphatic system cannot handle the net fluid exchange across the endothelial membrane, the lung becomes edematous, and as an extreme, flooding of the alveoli occurs.

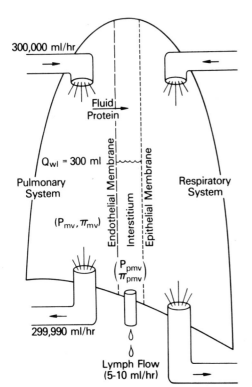

FIGURE 1 Simple lung model of pulmonary vascular exchange (total lung model).

Since the fluid and protein transport across the endothelial membrane is the key process, a significant effort has been made to understand this exchange more fully. Studies of steady state transvascular exchange in the lung have recently been reviewed by Staub [1, 2] and Taylor [3].* Therefore, the pathophysiology of the mechanisms involved will not be discussed here. We shall examine how the mathematical model can be applied to these processes and interpreted relative thereto.

B. Total Lung Model

One approach to understanding steady state fluid and protein exchange in the lung is to consider the lung a total unit. This model of the total lung has been used for isolated and perfused lung preparations [4, 5] as well as for intact sheep [6]. In this approach, the general Starling equation is applied to the total lung, for which the characteristics of the endothelial membrane are described by the transfer coefficients.

The general Starling equation describes the net flux of fluid across a membrane under steady state conditions:

$$\dot{Q}_f = K_f \, [(P_{mv} - P_{pmv}) - \sigma(\Pi_{mv} - \Pi_{pmv})] \tag{1}$$

where $\dot{Q}_f$ is the next transvascular fluid flow; K_f is the fluid conductance (filtration coefficient); P_{mv} and P_{pmv} are the hydrostatic pressures on each side of the membrane; σ is the "effective" reflection coefficient of the membrane; and Π_{mv} and Π_{pmv} are the protein osmotic pressures on each side of the membrane. If it is assumed that the endothelial membrane separates two well-mixed chambers with a hydrostatic and an osmotic pressure, as shown in Figure 1, then the filtration coefficient for the total lung can be calculated by measuring the net transvascular fluid flow, the microvascular hydrostatic pressure, and the osmotic pressure difference, and assuming a value for the reflection coefficient. A summary of experimental filtration coefficient data and the techniques and assumptions used to obtain them are presented by Staub [2].

To provide an improved understanding of pulmonary exchange and to elaborate on the sensitivity of the processes involved to the physiologic parameters and membrane structure, an "equivalent" pore model has been developed. This model provides the opportunity for investigating the influence of an equivalent membrane structure and of each of the physiologic conditions that may be associated with the transport upon the total exchange by each of the transport mechanisms involved.

*See Chapter 6 of this volume.

C. Equivalent-Pore Model

The second approach to characterizing the transvascular exchange has been to describe the exchange barrier as an equivalent membrane with pores through which the transport can occur. Pappenheimer and his coworkers [7] introduced a pore theory based on the concept of equivalent pores through which the solute and fluid would be exchanged by diffusion and convection. Transport, it was assumed, would take place through uniform cylindrical pores that occupied a small fraction of the membrane surface. This model was formalized by Renkin [8] with several subsequent refinements. The physics of transport through neutral porous membranes has received considerable attention in recent years [9, 10]. The theoretical model here considered includes the fundamentals of the equivalent-pore theory, with the Onsager reciprocity hypothesis assumed.

The net fluid J_v and solute J_s transport through an equivalent pore of radius R_p in a neutral membrane can be written [11]

$$J_v = L_p \left[(P_{mv} - P_{pmv}) - \sum_{s=1}^{n} \sigma_s (\Pi_{mv_s} - \Pi_{pmv_s}) \right] \tag{2}$$

$$J_s = \omega_s (\Pi_{mv_s} - \Pi_{pmv_s}) + (1 - \sigma_s) \overline{C}_s J_v \tag{3}$$

where P_{mv} and P_{pmv} are the hydrostatic pressures; Π_{mv_s} and Π_{pmv_s} are the osmotic pressure due to solute s; $\overline{C}_s$ is the average concentration of solute s across the membrane; and σ_s, ω_s and L_p are three transport coefficients (reflection, diffusional permeability, and fluid conductivity). The total fluid Q_f and solute $\dot{Q}_s$ fluxes across a membrane with uniform pores can therefore be written as the product of the transport per pore and the number of pores per membrane area f integrated over the total membrane area A_m:

$$Q_f = \int_{A_m} f J_v \, dA_m \tag{4}$$

$$\dot{Q}_s = \int_{A_m} f J_s \, dA_m. \tag{5}$$

Under the assumptions already noted, the conservation of mass of protein s and the fluid within the interstitial region of Figure 1 can be written as follows:

$$Fluid \quad \frac{\partial}{\partial t} (V_I) = \dot{Q}_f - q_w \tag{6}$$

$$Solute\ s \quad \frac{\partial}{\partial t} (V_I C_{Is}) = \dot{Q}_s - q_w C_{Is} \tag{7}$$

where V_I is the volume of the interstitial region; q_w is the egress from the region through the lymph system; and C_{Is} is the concentration of solute s in the interstitial fluid. Since it is assumed for this development that the transmembrane water and solute exchange is at a steady state,* Equation (7) becomes

$$\dot{Q}_s - \dot{Q}_f \, C_{Is} = 0 \tag{8}$$

since the egress flux is equal to the transmembrane flux from Equation (6). Therefore, for steady state conditions, the interstitial fluid solute concentration is

$$C_{Is} = \frac{\dot{Q}_s}{\dot{Q}_f} \tag{9}$$

and a solute concentration ratio between the interstitial fluid and plasma is given as

$$\frac{C_{Is}}{C_{Ps}} = \frac{\dot{Q}_s}{C_{Ps} \, \dot{Q}_f} \tag{10}$$

When a uniform pore membrane separates dilute solutions of a single solute s, Equation (10) can be written as a ratio of the interstitial-plasma concentration ratios C_{Is}/C_{Ps}.

$$\frac{C_{Is}}{C_{Ps}} = \frac{\omega_s \, RT + [(1 - \sigma_s)/2] \, J_v}{\omega_s \, RT + [(1 + \sigma_s)/2] \, J_v} \tag{11}$$

Perl [12] has recently used this concentration ratio in investigating albumin exchange between plasma and interstitium in nonliver capillary beds of the body and dog-paw muscle. The theoretical values for the transport coefficients can be calculated for water and solute s in transport through a pore of radius R_p [13, 14]

$$\omega_s = \frac{A_{sd} \, D_s}{\Delta X \, RT} \qquad \sigma_s = 1 - \frac{A_{sf}}{A_{wf}} \qquad L_p = \frac{A_{wf} \, R_p^2}{\Delta X \, 8\eta} \tag{12}$$

where A_{sd} is the solute diffusion area; D_s is the solute free-diffusion coefficient; ΔX is the membrane thickness (assumed uniform); R is the gas constant; T is temperature; η is the viscosity coefficient; and A_{sf}/A_{wf} is the ratio of the pore area for solute filtration to the area available for water filtration. The empirical

---

*Equations (6) and (7) are currently being solved with the multiple-pore membrane model in a theoretical investigation of the transient conditions that are associated with experimental preparations of osmotic shock and tracer washouts.

equations for A_{sf}/A_p, A_{wf}/A_p, and A_{sd}/A_p are given in the Appendix to this chapter. Therefore, for given values for pore radius, length, and solute (molecular radius and free-diffusion coefficient), the three transport coefficients can be calculated for a given temperature T and viscosity coefficient η.*

A simplified form of the concentration ratio (Eq. 11) can be developed by assuming the mean concentration $\overline{C}_s$ to be equal to the plasma concentration C_{Ps}, and describing the transport coefficients σ_s and ω_s by analytical approximations that are valid for solute radii significantly smaller than the pore radii. This simplified concentration ratio equation, referred to as the Renkin equation [8], is given as

$$\frac{C_{Is}}{C_{Ps}} = \frac{1 + (A_{wf} D_s/\Delta X J_v)}{(A_{wf}/A_{sf}) + (A_{wf} D_s/\Delta X J_v)} \tag{13}$$

This relation was shown to describe the transport across artificial membranes [8]. The Renkin equation has also been solved implicitly to determine an equivalent-pore system in biologic membranes that would produce the measured concentration ratio and fluid flux [15, 16]. Effective pore radii of 40 to 50 Å were found. It was recognized, however, that the membrane structure predicted by the implicit solution of the Renkin equation did not provide a complete description of the experimental results with biologic membranes [17-19].

Two other approximations of Equation (11) are regularly made, although the inherent assumptions are seldom enunciated. If a membrane is considered with a reflection coefficient of unity for the specific solute ($\sigma_s = 1.0$), the concentration ratio simplifies to

$$\frac{C_{Is}}{C_{Ps}} = \frac{\omega_s RT}{\omega_s RT + J_v} \tag{14}$$

which is referred to as the diffusional approximation [20]. On the other hand, if the fluid flux J_v is sufficiently large that

$$\frac{1 + \sigma_s}{2} J_v \gg \omega_s RT$$

a second simplification to the concentration ratio can be written,

$$\frac{C_{Is}}{C_{Ps}} = \frac{1 - \sigma_s}{1 + \sigma_s} \tag{15}$$

*In these studies, the following were assumed constant: T = 32°C; η = 1.0 centipoise; ΔX = 5000 Å; D_a = 9.3 × 10^{-7} cm^2/sec; D_g = 6.7 × 10^{-7} cm^2/sec.

which is known as the convection approximation. A comparison of the results of these approximations with the general solution of Equation (11) will be made for specific examples of concentration gradients and membrane structures.

It is important to note that the general concentration ratio of Equation (11) is for dilute solutions. For dilute solutions, the osmotic pressure for a solute is a linear function of the solute concentration (van't Hoff approximation),

$$\Pi_s = C_s RT. \tag{16}$$

Experimental data have shown, however, that the relation between the osmotic pressure and the normal human plasma protein concentrations is not linear. The osmotic pressure-concentration relation for plasma protein concentrations (including those of sheep used in our experimental studies) can be described by a cubic fit [21]:

$$\Pi_s = AC_s + BC_s^2 + DC_s^3 \tag{17}$$

where A, B, and D are constants. When this nonlinearlity is introduced into Equation (3), the general solute interstitial-plasma concentration ratio for one solute s can be written

$$\frac{C_{Is}}{C_{Ps}} = \frac{\omega_s \, (RT + \hat{F}_s) + [(1 - \sigma_s)/2] \, J_v}{\omega_s \, RT + [(1 + \sigma_s)/2] \, J_v} \tag{18}$$

where $\hat{F}_s$ is a correction term that is a function of higher-order terms of the concentration ratio C_{Is}/C_{Ps}. For dilute solutions, this correction term is zero; however, for the protein concentrations considered, the correction term has a significant effect on the calculated concentration ratio.

Therefore, for assumed pore size, plasma protein concentration, and difference in hydrostatic pressure, the solute concentration ratio across a homogeneous membrane can be determined by an iterative solution of Equation (18).

III. Characteristics of Membrane Transport

The results from Equation (18) are presented for a variety of membrane and solute characteristics. These results show the influence of membrane pore structure, solute concentrations, and hydrostatic pressure on the solute transfer as indicated by the concentration ratio. The calculations are as follows: the pore size is assumed and the transfer coefficients—that is, reflection coefficient σ_s, diffusional permeability ω_s, and fluid conductivity L_p—are calculated for each solute by Equation (12). For a given solute plasma concentration, a given hydrostatic pressure difference, and an assumed interstitial protein concentration, the fluid transport can be calculated for each set of pores by Equation (2). The concentration ratio for each solute can then be calculated from Equation (18); and the new values for the interstitial solute concentrations thus determined are used to recalculate the fluid flux. This iteration is repeated until the solutions for the interstitial concentrations are found.

A. Single-Pore Membrane Separating Mixtures of One Solute

The theoretical concentration ratios for albumin are shown in Figure 2 as a function of membrane-pore radii from 36 to 1500 Å for hydrostatic pressure differences from 1 to 40 cm H_2O. A plasma concentration of albumin of 0.58 mM (4 g/100 ml) was considered, for which the albumin molecule was assumed to be spherical and have a radius of 34 Å.

The results show that at small differences of hydrostatic pressure, the concentration ratio is insensitive to pore size. Only at higher pressure differences (greater than 5 cm H_2O) does the concentration ratio for a single-solute mixture become sensitive to membrane-pore size and then only at the small values of pore size.

As Equation (3) shows, the solute flux is composed of two transport mechanisms, diffusion and convection. Since the model assumes well-mixed

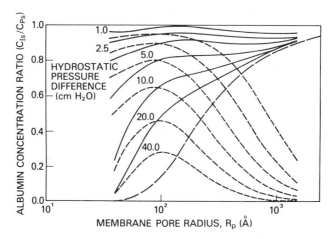

FIGURE 2 Albumin concentration ratios across a single-pore membrane as a function of hydrostatic pressure difference and membrane pore radius. [——— General solution (Eq. 18), ———— Diffusion approximation (Eq. 14), — — — Convection approximation (Eq. 15)]

chambers on both sides of the membrane, the relative transport through pores of different sizes becomes a function of the relative effects of pore radius on the three transport coefficients. As Equation (12) shows, the hydraulic coefficient is a function of the fourth power of pore radius, compared with a second-power effect in solute permeability. For a pore size much larger than the solute, the reflection coefficient approaches zero and the primary mechanism of solute transport is convection. For this pore-solute relation, the solute has very little interaction with the membrane and the concentration ratio across the membrane approaches unity and is independent of hydrostatic pressure, as shown by Figure 2, at large values of pore size.

In contrast, as the membrane-pore size approaches the size of the solute, the reflection coefficient σ_s approaches unity; therefore, the convective sieving becomes very restrictive to the total convective solute transport. The solute permeability ω_s also approaches zero but the relative effect is less restrictive than on the convective flow; therefore, for regions of pore size near solute size, solute diffusion is the primary source of solute transport. A combination of these two transport mechanisms accounts for the exchange in the intermediate-pore-size region.

Even though diffusion is the principle source of solute transport in the small-pore region, convective fluid flow has a significant influence on the concentration ratio across the membrane. If no convective flow exists, the diffusional flux will bring two chambers into equilibrium, as shown in Figure 2 for the small values of hydrostatic pressure. As the hydrostatic pressure difference increases, a "washout" effect is experienced in the interstitium, with consequent decrease in the concentration level of the interstitial fluid and a resulting lowering of the concentration ratio. This lowering of the concentration in the interstitial fluid brings about an osmotic potential buildup to counteract the convective flow. The resulting concentration ratios are shown in Figure 2.

Also shown in Figure 2 are the two common simplifications of the concentration ratio, the diffusional and convective approximations. In comparison with the more complete solution, the convective approximation, Equation (15), is valid only for very high pressure differences or very-large-pore-solute geometry, for which convective flow is the primary mode of solute transport. On the contrary, the diffusional approximation, Equation (14), is applicable when the pore size is comparable with the size of the solute and when there are small pressure differences, for which the diffusional flux predominates. It is noted, however, that even for the small pore-size and pressure difference region, the diffusional approximation does not provide an asymptote to the complete solution, since the van't Hoff assumption is required in the diffusional approximation. These illustrative results suggest that even for a single-solute mixture, care must be used in applying these two simplifying approximations.

As Figure 2 shows, one of the problems of using the albumin concentration ratio as an indicator of pore size is the insensitivity of pore size to the concentration ratio. This is especially true at the lower pressure differences and at higher pore sizes. To improve the utility of concentration ratios as indicators of equivalent-pore structure of membranes, a multiple-solute mixture was considered.

B. Single-Pore Membrane Separating Mixtures of Two Solutes

Equation (18) was solved by numerical iteration for two solutes, albumin and globulin; in this model, the influence of the two solutes affects the osmotic pressure terms of the fluid transport. For illustration, a plasma albumin concentration of 0.58 mM (4 g/100 ml) and a globulin concentration of 0.18 mM (3 g/100 ml) were considered with water in the two-chamber system of Figure 1. The results of the concentration ratios of each are presented as a function of uniform pore size and hydrostatic pressure difference. The results of Figure 3 show that the concentration ratio of globulin is more sensitive to pore size than to albumin, so that a set of concentration ratios of albumin *and* globulin is sufficient to characterize the equivalent membrane pore size. These results show the benefit of measuring at least two solutes when characterizing membrane pore structure by concentration ratios.

It is important to note the difference between the protein concentration ratios in Figure 2 and the ratios in Figure 3 for the same hydrostatic pressure differences and the same plasma concentration. This is illustrated in Figure 4

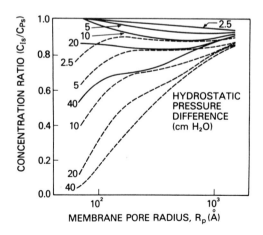

FIGURE 3 Concentration ratios of albumin (————) and globulin (– – – – –) across a single-pore membrane as a function of hydrostatic pressure difference and membrane pore radius for plasma concentrations of albumin (0.58 mM) and globulin (0.18 mM).

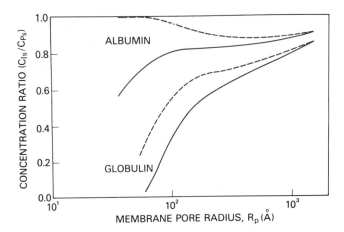

FIGURE 4 Concentration ratios of albumin and globulin across a single-pore membrane for each solute alone (———) and for two-solute mixtures (—————) as a function of membrane-pore radius and a constant hydrostatic pressure difference (10 cm H_2O) for plasma concentrations of albumin (0.58 mM) and globulin (0.18 mM).

by the plot of both albumin and globulin concentration ratios for a hydrostatic pressure difference of 10 cm H_2O. These results are for a membrane having pores of uniform size. The plasma concentrations for each protein are the same as the results given in Figure 2 and 3. The marked increase in the concentration ratios of each of the solutes when considered in a mixture shows the strong coupling between two solutes in membrane transport. This coupling occurs through the influence of the osmotic potential of each solute in a mixture.

This example illustrates the need for careful modeling in interpreting experimental concentration ratios, especially when the mixtures considered become as complex as blood plasma and interstitial fluids.

C. Multiple-Pore Membrane Separating Mixtures of Two Solutes

In a multiple-pore model, an equation for the concentration ratio analogous to Equation (18) can be written [22]

$$\frac{C_{Is}}{C_{Ps}} = \frac{\sum\limits_{i=1}^{m} f_i \left\{ \omega_{si} (RT + \hat{F}_{si}) + [(1 - \sigma_{si})/2] J_{vi} \right\}}{\sum\limits_{i=1}^{m} f_i \left\{ \omega_{si} RT + [(1 + \sigma_{si})/2] J_{vi} \right\}} \tag{19}$$

where f_i is the number of pores of radius i per unit membrane area. This more general concentration ratio will be used to investigate the influence of a membrane of multiple pore sizes and numbers of pores that separates a two-solute, nondilute mixture at various levels of hydrostatic pressure.

The sensitivity of the concentration ratio for a membrane with two pore sizes is shown in Figure 5. For a plasma solute mixture of albumin (0.58 mM) and globulin (0.18 mM), concentration ratios are plotted as a function of the pore number ratio—the number of pores with a given radius to one pore of a radius of 1000 Å. Results are presented for three different values of the hydrostatic pressure difference.

The effect of each set of pores on the total solute transport is shown to be a function of the pore number ratio, the hydrostatic pressure difference, the pore size, and the protein (albumin or globulin). At small values of pore sizes, the concentration ratios are very sensitive to the pore number ratio. As the pore size is larger, the two sizes becomes more nearly equal and the influence of the second pore system becomes negligible.

At small values of hydrostatic pressure difference, where diffusional transport represents the primary mode of solute exchange, the pore number ratio has only a modest effect on the total concentration ratio. As the value of pressure difference increases, the influence of convective transport significantly increases, resulting in more dramatic effects of the pore number ratio. Therefore, the results show that a second-pore-size system becomes important when the difference in pore sizes is large and when convection is significant in the total exchange.

IV. Pulmonary Model

A. Pulmonary Vascular Membrane

The characteristic vascular structure of the pulmonary bed is illustrated in Figure 6. The exchange considered here is between the plasma and the interstitium across the vascular membrane. Electron-microscopic investigation of the vascular membrane have suggested two morphological characteristics that could influence the fluid and solute exchange across it. First, intercellular junctions between the endothelial cells produce a direct pathway. It has been suggested that these junctions may vary in radius from approximately 20 Å, referred to as small pores, to approximately 1000 Å, referred to as large pores; uniform diameter is assumed. In our equivalent-pore model of the vascular membrane, cylindrical pores of three different radii will be considered. *Small pore* will refer to those pores with radii less than 34 Å, which allow complete protein sieving (albumin, $r_a = 34$ Å; globulin, $r_g = 54$ Å). *Intermediate pore* will refer to pores with radii

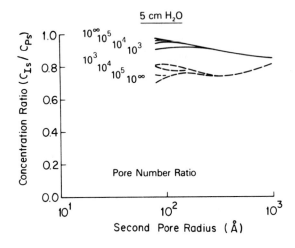

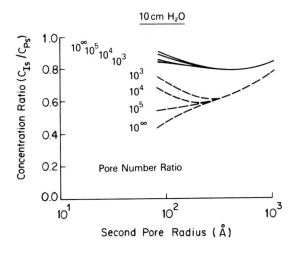

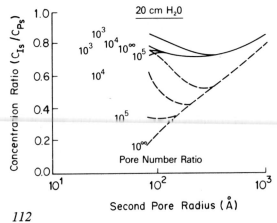

FIGURE 5 *(see facing page for legend)*

112

greater than 34 Å and less than approximately 300 Å, which allow partial sieving of the solutes considered. Pores of approximately 1000 Å, designated *large pores,* allow no protein sieving.

Second, cytoplasmic vesicles may transport solute from the plasma into the interstitium. Although what vesicles do in the pulmonary vascular exchange is unclear [23], vesicular transport has been represented by an equivalent diffusional flux [24, 25].*

In addition to the transport associated with pores and vesicles, the endothelial cell membrane may allow water flow through the cell cytoplasm [25]. This transport, as characterized by Solomon [14] for red cells, can be described by equivalent intercellular pores. These equivalent intercellular pores have been calculated to be of the order of 5 Å for the red cell [14].

It was our intent to develop a methematical description of the fluid and protein exchange across the endothelial membrane by using the equivalent-pore model. Applying the equivalent-pore model to biologic membranes has shown that a membrane with uniform-sized pores may not completely account for the experimental results [18]. Several modifications of the uniform pore model have been suggested. Perl has suggested that the pores may be made up of a wide portion, 200 Å, and a narrow portion, 40 Å [19]. To account for the experimental observations on large-molecule transport, Renkin [20] suggested a membrane with pores of two different radii. A two-pore model was also used by Boyd [17] to interpret the results on the permeability of the sheep lung. Boyd found that a uniform-pore system (radius of 150 Å as calculated from the Renkin equation) would predict the measured transport of the large molecules. To accommodate the total protein transport, a second pore system with pores of 1000 Å radius was required. In the theoretical description of the two-pore model Boyd used, the second pore system was not allowed to interact with the transport of the first. A correction term was simply added to the results of the Renkin equation that allowed for solute transport by convection only.

We have therefore developed a general multiple-transport model that

---

*Although a diffusional model of vesicular transport was included in our theoretical model, the results presented in the studies referred to do not consider this form of transport. Preliminary results suggest, however, that vesicular exchange does not significantly influence the diffusional and convective transport.

FIGURE 5 Concentration ratios for albumin (————) and globulin (— — — —) across a two-pore membrane as a function of hydrostatic pressure (5 cm H_2O, 10 cm H_2O, and 20 cm H_2O), second pore radius, and pore number ratio (number of pores with the second pore radius to one pore of 1000-Å radius) for plasma concentrations of albumin (0.58 mM) and globulin in (0.18 mM).

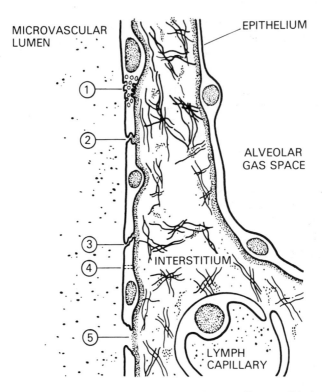

FIGURE 6 Characteristic vascular structure showing five possible transport pathways: (1) vesicules, (2) intermediate pores, (3) small pores, (4) intracellular pores, and (5) large pores.

calculates the transport of water and two solutes across an equivalent membrane having pores of three different radii. In this increased generality, our theoretical model is more akin to the two-pore model of Winne [26] as used by Arturson [27].

The model describes the diffusive and convective transport through three sets of pores for a membrane of unit area. We can therefore investigate the sensitivity of membrane structure (pore sizes and numbers) and physiological variables (hydrostatic and osmotic pressures) on the endogenous albumin, globulin, and fluid exchange processes in the pulmonary vascular bed.

It is important to note that the total lung model implies that the total protein and fluid exchange in the lung occurs between two well-mixed chambers, as shown in Figure 1. It was our intent, with our model, to investigate the

TABLE 1   Assumptions for Mathematical Model of Pulmonary Microvascular Exchange

VASCULAR MEMBRANE
   Passive transport
   Cylindrical pores (small, intermediate, and large)
   Uniform thickness
   Permeability constant per unit area

INTERSTITIAL FLUID
   Well-mixed (at local level)
   Constant pressure
   Drained only by nonsieving lymph duct

PLASMA
   Well-mixed (no unstirred layers)
   Constant pressure along microvessel
   Linear vertical pressure distribution in the lung

effects of distribution in the lung on the total exchange. The transport was therefore calculated for a membrane of unit area and the exchange then integrated over the total lung, to compare the theoretical results with the experimental results.

The assumptions made in the theoretical model are summarized in Table 1. For the conditions considered, the alveolar membrane is impermeable to both protein and fluid [1, 2] and it is assumed that the interstitial region is drained by a nonsieving lymph duct [28, 3]. The transport is calculated for a membrane of unit area, and the unit membrane is assumed to contain a set of the three-pore system the model embraces. The plasma and interstitial regions near this unit membrane are assumed to be locally well mixed and at steady state [27, 28].

B. Distributed Lung Model

Since both the distribution of the total vascular membrane area and the pore size distribution in the lung are unknown, the model assumes the following: (1) the pore size and number are constant throughout the lung and can be represented by a three-pore system; and (2) the vascular membrane area is a linear function of the mass of the lung.

To calculate this total fluid transport, it is required that the mass distribution of the lung be a function of lung height.* This lung mass distribution has

---

*This represents one of the earliest results of this modeling approach. That is, we could not proceed with the distributed model without some basic information about the lung mass distribution.

been determined [29] by slowly freezing dead sheep suspended in the prone position, sectioning the thorax perpendicular to the horizontal plane with a band saw, and weighing the lung slices cut at 2-cm intervals up the lung. Mass distributions have been obtained from four sheep by this procedure.

We defined the lung mass fraction M_f:

$$M_f \equiv \frac{\rho_L \overline{\Delta A_L} (h) \Delta h_L}{M_L} \tag{20}$$

where $\overline{\Delta A_L}$ is the average area over the 2-cm height Δh_L; ρ_L is the average lung density; and M_L is the total mass of the lung. The experimental mass fraction distribution was determined for four sheep, and the average is shown in Figure 7 as a function of lung height. If the apex of the left atrium is used as a reference point, as it was in the sheep experiments [30], the center of mass of the lung is shown to be approximately 2 cm above this point.

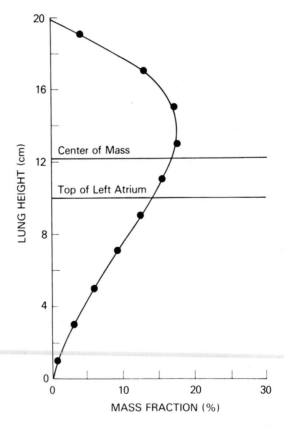

FIGURE 7   Measured lung mass fraction distribution (sheep).

The transvascular fluid exchange for any section of the lung (h_1 to h_2) is therefore given [22]

$$\dot{Q}_f(h) = M_L a_m \sum_{h_1}^{h_2} M_f(h) \, f \, J_v \tag{21}$$

where the lung mass fraction and filtration per pore remain a function of lung height, and it is assumed that the vascular membrane area per unit mass of the lung a_m is a constant. Similarly, the solute transport over any section of the lung is

$$\dot{Q}_s(h) = M_L a_m \sum_{h_1}^{h_2} M_f(h) \, f \, J_s. \tag{22}$$

By substituting Equations (21) and (22) into Equation (10), one can find the average lymph-to-plasma ratio for any section of the lung, $(L/P)_{sh}$:

$$\left(\frac{L}{P}\right)_{sh} = \frac{\displaystyle\sum_{h_1}^{h_2} M_f(h) \, f \, J_s}{C_{ps} \displaystyle\sum_{h_1}^{h_2} M_f(h) \, f \, J_v} \tag{23}$$

By summing Equations (21) and (23) over all sections of the lung, we can obtain the total fluid exchange and the average lymph-to-plasma ratio for the total lung and compare these findings with the experimental results. For the three-pore model, these totals can be written

$$\dot{Q}_{fT} = M_L a_m \sum_{i=1}^{3} \sum_{0}^{h_L} M_f(h) \, f_i \, J_{vi} \tag{24}$$

$$\left(\frac{L}{P}\right)_S = \frac{\displaystyle\sum_{i=1}^{3} \sum_{0}^{h_L} M_f(h) \, f_i \, J_{vi}}{C_{ps} \displaystyle\sum_{i=1}^{3} \sum_{0}^{h_L} M_f(h) \, f_i \, J_{vi}}. \tag{25}$$

With the assumption of lung homogeneity and with the measured values of plasma solute concentration, mass fraction distribution, and a three-pore vascular model, the total fluid exchange and the average lymph-to-plasma ratio (Eqs. 24, 25) can be solved if the hydrostatic pressure difference across the vascular membrane is known as a function of lung height.*

The most straightforward approach is to assume that the hydrostatic pressure in the microvasculature at the level of the left atrium is the mean between the pulmonary artery pressure and the pressure in the left atrium. Some theoretical and experimental evidence, however, suggests that under normal lung conditions the precapillary resistance loss is greater than the postcapillary resistance. A simple linear model for microvascular pressure has therefore been used by numerous investigators [31, 32]. This microvascular hydrostatic pressure is written

$$P'_{mv} = P_{la} + K(P_{pa} - P_{la}) \tag{26}$$

where the microvascular pressure P_{mv} at the level of the left atrium is given as a function of the pulmonary artery pressure P_{pa}, the left atrium pressure P_{la}, and the linearity constant K. In this study, Equation (26) will be used as a description of the microvascular pressure at the lung height equal to the apex of the left atrium with a constant K value of 0.4.

Because of the graviational effect on the lung, a hydrostatic microvascular pressure head is experienced over the vertical height of the lung. West has suggested a hydrostatic-pressure-distribution model for the lung that contains the possibility of three distinct pressure zones [33]. In the data presented here, however, the pressure distribution over the lung P_{mv} was assumed to be a linear function of lung height. This means that even at the apex of the lung, the microvascular pressure is greater than the alveolar pressure. This is equivalent to the zone III model of West.**

To illustrate the distributed fluid and protein transport in the sheep lung, Equations (24) and (25) were solved for the lung-mass fraction shown in Figure 7 [29], a microvascular pressure of 12 cm H_2O at the left atrium, plasma contrations of 0.58 mM for albumin and 0.18 mM for globulin (normal values for sheep), and a vascular membrane with an assumed uniform pore size of 100 Å. For these assumptions, the distribution of the lymph fraction (fluid exchange at height h divided by the total fluid exchange) as a function of lung height is shown in Figure 8. Although the center of mass for the lung is approximately 3 cm above the level of the left atrium, the centroid of fluid transport is approximately 2 cm below the left atrium. This shows the strong influence of hydro-

*In practice, we avoided measuring, or calculating, the vascular membrane area per unit mass of the lung a_m; instead, we compare changes in the fluid exchange to a baseline condition. This assumes that a_m is always a constant.
**A more complete model for microvascular-pressure distribution associated with the three zones defined by West is being incorporated into the theoretical model.

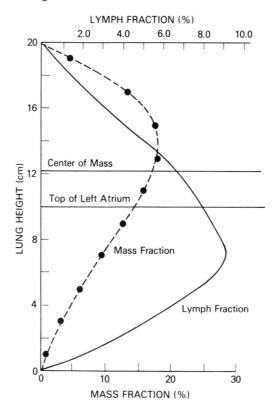

FIGURE 8 Distribution of lymph fraction (top axis) and mass fraction (bottom axis) as a function of lung height (sheep).

static pressure on the fluid-exchange distribution in the lung. These results support the recognized fact that fluid accumulation first occurs in the dependent regions of the lung.

Experimental evidence suggests that under "normal" conditions the distribution of lung fluid is essentially uniform [6]; therefore, the lymphatic system must provide an effective drain for the dependent regions of the lung. If interstitial fluid accumulation occurs, the interstitial pressure would increase, thus decreasing the net hydrostatic pressure difference across the membrane. This would provide a natural control to the magnitude of the net fluid exchange that occurs.

The distributed lymph-to-plasma ratios for albumin and globulin are shown in Figure 9. These results show that the lymph-to-plasma protein ratios are a direct function of lung height, suggesting an interstitial "washout" effect due to the higher fluid exchange in the dependent regions of the lung. As the

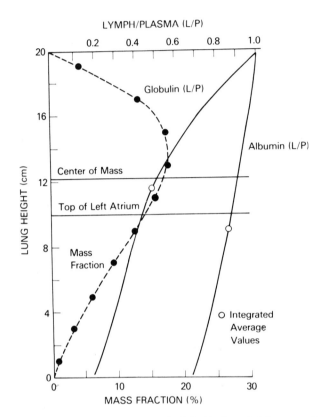

FIGURE 9 Distribution of albumin and globulin lymph/plasma ratios as a function of lung height. The open circles are average lymph/plasma ratios for albumin and globulin.

hydrostatic pressure difference is less, the fluid exchange due to convection is also less, and the diffusion transport brings the solute concentrations into near equilibrium at the apex of the lung.

The lower lymph-to-plasma ratios in the dependent region of the lung also act to decrease the net fluid exchange in this region. As shown by the fluid flux equation (Equation 2), the osmotic difference tends to counteract the increase in hydrostatic pressure. Therefore, even though the hydrostatic-pressure distribution within a lung affects the distribution for the fluid and solute exchange experienced, there are mechanisms within the lung that provide natural regulation of this distributed exchange. Further investigation of this distributed exchange and of the influence of the physiological and structural conditions is needed.

C. Results

The integrated results from this distributed theoretical model have been compared with experimental results from a steady state sheep preparation [22]. For illustration, the experimental and theoretical lymph-to-plasma ratios from four unanesthetized sheep are shown in Figure 10. The experimental ratios of the albumin and globulin concentrations measured in the lymph to the concentrations in the plasma over a range of microvascular pressures referenced to the left atrium are shown by the dots and triangles. The curves represent the solutions from the theoretical model using a three-pore model (Table 2). As shown, the comparison of theory and experimental results are good over the microvascular pressure range 10 to 35 cm H_2O.

The theoretical and experimental values of net lung-fluid filtration are presented in Figure 11. The filtration results presented correspond directly to the solute transport results of Figure 10. The results are presented as a

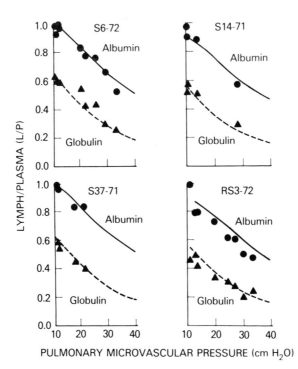

FIGURE 10 Comparison of multiple-pore theoretical model and experimental sheep lymph/plasma ratios for albumin and globulin over a range of microvascular pressures (referred to the left atrium) in four sheep.

TABLE 2   Vascular Membrane Model

Cylindrical pores	Relative number	Equivalent radius (Å)
Small	1300	20
Intermediate	1	125
Large	$<10^{-5}$	1000

percentage of baseline flow, where a baseline pressure of 12 cm H_2O was selected. This represents an average "normal" baseline microvascular pressure for the sheep when referred to the left atrium.

   The results of Figure 11 show a reasonable correlation between the theoretical model and experimental results for two of the four sheep. For the other two, the theoretical results predicted higher values of fluid filtration than what was experimentally measured. This difference tends to become more

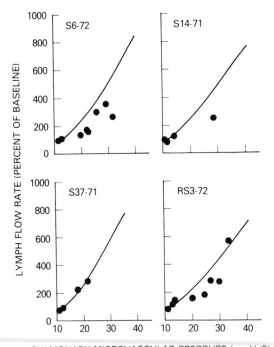

FIGURE 11 Comparison of multiple-pore theoretical model and experimental sheep fluid exchange (lymph flow) over a range of microvascular pressures (referred to the left atrium) in four sheep.

pronounced at higher levels of microvascular pressure. A further investigation of this apparent filtration problem is required to be able to understand more fully the discrepancy between the theoretical and experimental results at higher levels of microvascular pressure.

The theoretical distribution of the albumin, globulin, and water transported across the vascular membrane of the sheep lung is illustrated by Figure 12. The results of the theoretical model showed the intermediate pore to be the key site for protein transport, with approximately 70% of the exchange occurring by diffusion and 20% by convection. The solutes transported by convective flow through the large pores represented the remaining 10% of solute transport. Diffusion through the large pores represented an insignificant fraction of the total protein exchange. As seen in Figure 12, in a comparison of albumin and

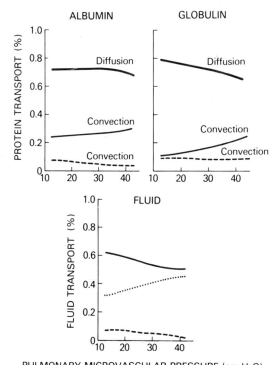

FIGURE 12 Comparison of the fraction of solute and fluid exchange for each transport mechanism and pore size as a function of the microvascular pressure (referred to the left atrium). [. . . . . . . Small pore, ———— Intermediate pore, − − − − − Large pore.]

globulin, the transport of the larger, globulin molecule is more sensitive to the mode of transport.

The fluid exchange was found to be essentially divided between the intermediate and small pores, with the contribution of the large pores less than 5% since there were so few in this model. Although a significant increase occurs in the fluid transport through the intermediate and small pores with an increase in microvascular pressure, the influence of the osmotic potential tends to decrease the relative amount transported through the intermediate pores at the increased pressure levels. These two modes of water transport become approximately equal at higher values of vascular pressure. These results emphasize the importance of the small-pore system in our model and the need for additional investigation into its structural characteristics.

A basic model of pulmonary vascular exchange has been developed that includes the characteristic transport mechanisms of the vascular membrane. For a single-membrane structure, the integrated protein transport results from the model compared well with experimental results from four unanesthetized sheep over a wide range of pulmonary microvascular pressure valves. The relative magnitude of each transport mechanism was evaluated and the key modes of transport identified.

The model has also been applied to a sheep preparation in which increased lung vascular permeability was produced by *Pseudomonas* bacteremia [34]. It was found that a slow intravenous infusion of *Pseudomonas aeruginosa* bacteria into unanesthetized sheep caused a dramatic, prolonged, but reversible increase in pulmonary transvascular fluid and protein flow.

The three-to-tenfold increase in lymph flow that was observed after the infusion was significantly higher than results from increases in hydrostatic pressure alone. The equivalent-pore model was used to investigate the possible mechanisms by which the bacteria could be influencing transvascular exchange in the sheep lung.

We found that our three-pore model would predict the protein and lymph flow for the baseline conditions of this preparation; however, the steady state lymph flow and lymph-to-plasma ratios after *Pseudomonas* was introduced could not be predicted from the model except by an effective change in the membrane permeability. The experimental data after *Pseudomonas* was introduced could be correlated reasonably well with the theoretical model when the intermediate-pore radius was increased from 125 Å to 150 Å and the small-pore area was approximately doubled. Therefore, the large changes in fluid and protein filtration experienced by the bacteria were shown as possibly corresponding with small changes in the endothelial membrane structure.

The concept that large changes in filtration can result from small changes in the exchanging membrane structure is important and is consistent with the observations that the lesion caused by *Pseudomonas* was found to be entirely reversible in most sheep [34]. This suggests that severe edema in humans occurring in the absence of heart failure may not necessarily be the result of extensive, irreversible damage to the lung's vascular endothelium.

The model is now being modified to include additional solute molecules, membrane "slits" as well as pores, and nonlinear hydrostatic pressure gradients as a function of lung height and non-steady-state conditions. The influence of these additional variables on the pulmonary exchange can thus be investigated.

V. Conclusion

We have been concerned here with applying mathematical models to the transmembrane exchange of fluids and proteins in the lung. Certain assumptions can be made by the mathematical model, and work with the models leads to the potential for further experimental and theoretical work. A model was used to investigate the influence of the vascular membrane structure on the transvascular exchange of fluid and protein in two sheep preparations. The results of the studies show that for endogeneous plasma protein concentrations of the sheep, the interactions of the transport mechanisms across the vascular membrane of the lung are sufficiently complex that simple approximations of this exchange may not be valid. Theoretical calculations should include nondilute effects of the osmotic pressures, at least two protein concentrations, a multiple-pore-size equivalent membrane, and a well-distributed hydrostatic pressure.

The results from the theoretical model suggest three important characteristics of the vascular membrane structure. First, a multiple-pore-size model is required that includes a one pore system having pores smaller than the albumin molecule; second a few large equivalent pores can exist in the membrane; and third, small changes in the equivalent-pore sizes of the vascular membrane can result in big changes in the fluid exchange. In the sheep preparation of permeability change, these membrane structure changes were found to be reversible.

These studies have outlined the need for further theoretical and experimental investigations of these exchange processes. The influence of additional structural and physiologic changes on these processes and the application of these results to the human lung should be continued.

VI. Appendix

The restrictive pore areas for solute diffusion A_{sd}, for solute filtration A_{sf}, and for water filtration A_{wf} are given by the following empirical equations:

$$\frac{A_{sf}}{A_p} = \left[2\left(1 - \frac{a_s}{R_p}\right)^2 - \left(1 - \frac{a_s}{R_p}\right)^4 \right]$$

$$\times \left[1.0 - 2.104\left(\frac{a_s}{R_p}\right) + 2.09\left(\frac{a_s}{R_p}\right)^3 - 0.95\left(\frac{a_s}{R_p}\right)^5 \right]$$

$$\frac{A_{wf}}{A_p} = \left[2\left(1 - \frac{a_w}{R_p}\right)^2 - 1\left(\frac{a_w}{R_p}\right)^4 \right]$$

$$\times \left[1.0 - 2.104\left(\frac{a_w}{R_p}\right) + 2.09\left(\frac{a_w}{R_p}\right)^3 - 0.95\left(\frac{a_w}{R_p}\right)^5 \right]$$

$$\frac{A_{sd}}{A_p} = \left(1 - \frac{a_s}{R_p}\right)^2 \times \left[1 - 2.104\left(\frac{a_s}{R_p}\right) + 2.09\left(\frac{a_s}{R_p}\right)^3 - 0.95\left(\frac{a_s}{R_p}\right)^5 \right]$$

where a_s is the radius of the solute molecule, a_w is the radius of the water molecule, and A_p is the pore area. In these studies, the following were assumed constant: $a_w = 1.5$ Å; $r_a = 34$ Å; and $r_g = 54$ Å.

References

1. N. C. Staub, "State of the art" review, Pathogenesis of pulmonary edema, *Amer. Rev. Resp. Dis.*, **109**:358-372 (1974).
2. N. C. Staub, Pulmonary Edema, *Physiol. Rev.*, **54**, 678-811 (1974).
3. A. E. Taylor, W. J. Gibson, H. J. Granger and A. C. Guyton, The interaction between intracapillary and tissue forces in the overall regulations of interstitial fluid volume, *Lymphology*, **6**:192-208 (1973).
4. K. A. Garr, A. E. Taylor and L. J. Owens, Effects of capillary pressure and plasma protein on development of pulmonary edema, *Amer. J. Physiol.*, 213:79-82 (1967).
5. R. L. Goodale, B. Goetzman and M. B. Visscher, Hypoxia and iodoacetic acid and alveolocapillary barrier permeability to albumin, *Amer. J. Physiol.*, 219:126-1230 (1970).

6. A. J. Erdmann, T. R. Vaughan, W. C. Woolverton, K. L. Brigham and N. C. Staub, Effects of increased vascular pressure on lung fluid balance in unanesthetized sheep, *Circ. Res.,* **37**:271 (1975).

7. J. R. Pappenheimer, Passage of molecules through capillary walls, *Physiol. Rev.,* **33**:387-423 (1953).

8. E. M. Renkin, Filtration, diffusion and molecular sieving through porous cellulose membrane, *J. Gen. Phys.,* **38**:225-243 (1954).

9. C. P. Bean, The physics of porous membranes—neutral pores. In *Membranes.* Vol. 1. Edited by G. Eisenman, Marcel Dekker, New York, pp. 1-54 (1972).

10. W. Perl, A friction coefficient, series-parallel channel model for trans-capillary flux on non-electrolytes and water, *Microvasc. Res.,* **6**:169-193 (1973).

11. A. Katchalsky and P. F. Curran, *Nonequilibrium Thermodynamics in Biophysics,* Cambridge, Mass., Harvard University Press, 1967.

12. W. Perl, Convective and permeation of albumin between plasma and inter-stitium, *Microvasc. Res.,* **10**:83-94 (1975).

13. O. Kedem and A. Katchalsky, A physical interpretation of the phenomen-ological coefficients of membrane permeability, *J. Gen. Physiol.,* **45**: 143-179 (1961).

14. A. K. Solomon, Characterization of biological membranes by equivalent pores, *J. Gen. Physiol.,* **51**:335s-364s (1968).

15. J. R. Pappenheimer, E. M. Renkin and L. M. Borrero, Filtration, diffusion and molecular sieving through peripheral capillary permeability, *Amer. J. Physiol.,* **167**:13-46 (1951).

16. E. M. Landis and J. R. Pappenheimer, Exchange of substances through capillary walls. In *Handbook of Physiology.* Section 2, Vol. 2. *Circulation.* Edited by W. F. Hamilton and P. Dow. Washington: American Physiology Society, 1963, Chap. 29.

17. R. D. H. Boyd, J. R. Hill, P. W. Humphreys, I. C. S. Normand, E. O. R. Reynolds and L. B. Strang, Permeability of lung capillaries to macro-molecules in foetal and new-born lambs and sheep. *J. Physiol.,* **201**: 567-588 (1969).

18. J. R. Pappenheimer, Osmotic reflection coefficients in capillary mem-branes. In *Capillary Permeability.* Edited by C. Crone and N. A. Lassen. New York, Academic Press, 1970, pp. 278-290.

19. W. Perl, Modified filtration-permeability model of transcapillary trans-port—A solution to the Pappenheimer pore puzzle? *Microvasc. Res.,* **3**: 233 (1971).

20. E. M. Renkin, Transport of large molecules across capillary walls, *Physiologist,* **7**:13-28 (1964).

21. H. Ott, Die Errechnung des kolloidosmotischen Serumdruckes aus dem Eiweiss-Spektrum, *Klin. Wochenschr.,* **34**:1079-1083 (1956).

22. L. H. Blake and N. C. Staub, Pulmonary vascular transport in sheep: A mathematical model, *Microvasc. Res.,* **12**:197-220 (1976).

23. R. R. Bruns and G. E. Palade, Studies on blood capillaries, *J. Cell Biol.*,
     37:244-276 (1968).
24. S. M. Shea and M. J. Karnowsky, Brownian motion: A theoretical explana-
     tion for the movement of vesicles across the endothelium, *Nature,* **212**:
     353-355 (1966).
25. S. M. Shea and M. J. Karnowsky, Vesicular transport across endothelium:
     Simulation of a diffusion model, *J. Theor. Biol.,* **24**:30-42 (1969).
26. D. Winne, Die Capillarpermeabilitat hochmolekularer substanzen, Pfluger
     Arch. Ges. Physiol., **283**:119-136 (1965).
27. G. Arturson, T. Groth and G. Grotte, The functional ultrastructure of the
     blood-lymph barrier, *Acta Physiol. Scand. Suppl.,* **347**:1-30 (1972).
28. D. G. Garlick and E. M. Renkin, Transport of large molecules from plasma
     to interstitial fluid and lymph in dogs, *Amer. J. Physiol.,* **219**:1595-1605
     (1970).
29. R. Sobel and N. C. Staub, Effect of lung mass distribution on micro-
     vascular filtration coefficient, *Fed. Proc.,* **33**:412 (1974).
30. N. C. Staub, Steady state pulmonary transvascular water filtration in
     unanesthetized sheep, *Circ. Res.,* **28/29** (Suppl.):135-139 (1971).
31. K. A. Garr, A. E. Taylor, L. J. Owens and A. C. Guyton, Pulmonary
     capillary pressure and filtration coefficient in the isolated perfused lung,
     Amer. J. Physiol., **213**:910-914 (1967).
32. P. Uter, U. Kotzerke, R. Rufer and W. Schodel, Kolloidosmotischer
     durch die Alveolar-Capillar-Schranke in der Hundelunge, *Pfluger's Arch.,*
     294:1-16 (1967).
33. J. B. West, *Ventillation of Blood Flow and Gas Exchange,* Oxford, Black-
     well Scientific Publications, 1967.
34. K. L. Brigham, W. C. Woolverton, L. H. Blake and N. C. Staub, Increased
     sheep lung vascular permeability caused by *Pseudomonas* bacteremia,
     J. Clin. Invest., **54**:792-804 (1974).

6

Fluid and Protein Movement Across the Pulmonary Microcirculation

AUBREY E. TAYLOR AND ROBERT E. DRAKE

University of Mississippi Medical Center
Jackson, Mississippi

I. Introduction

Since the development of pulmonary edema is associated with many pathological disorders, physiologists and clinicians have used a variety of experimental models to investigate the movement of water and solutes out of the pulmonary capillary system. Only a few experiments, however, have been designed to measure the movement of fluid and plasma proteins out of the pulmonary capillaries into the interstitium. In most studies, the movement of fluid into the airspaces was measured, not the movement across the capillary membrane. In addition, due to the extreme complexity of the pulmonary circulation in the upright human lung, very little information is available concerning transvascular fluxes of fluid and protein in human lungs. The purpose of this chapter is to develop the basic transport equations relative to volume and protein movement across the pulmonary exchange vessels and to evaluate available experimental data relative to a basic model of fluid and protein transport. No model is any

The work reported in this manuscript from our laboratory was supported by a National Institutes of Health grant, HL 11477.

better than the basic assumptions from which it is made, and as this chapter develops it will become quite apparent to the reader that many of the parameters necessary to describe the protein and fluid movements have simply not been measured in the pulmonary capillary bed. We hope that this chapter will stimulate thought towards developing adequate methods for measuring these parameters and evaluating their effect on fluid and protein movement across the pulmonary microcirculation.

II. Volume Movement Across the Pulmonary Vascular System

A. General

The mathematical notation for tissue forces and flows defined by Staub [1] is used throughout this chapter. Many workers in the field of capillary transport use the notation of Kedem and Katchalsky [2], which is completely developed in the textbook by Katchalsky and Curran entitled *Nonequilibrium Thermodynamics in Biophysics* [3]. However, others may use notations that are not consistent with what Kedem and Katchalsky or Staub use. Staub has defined a notation for flows and forces in the pulmonary vascular system that will avoid any ambiguity among notations used by different investigators. Any kind of mathematical approach to a biologic or a physiologic system is more readable if all investigators studying that system agree to use the same symbols for important parameters. As respiratory physiologists have learned, a well-defined set of symbols and parameters is an important tool in transmitting information within any given field.

The movement of volume across the pulmonary microvascular system can be described by a simple equation relating volume flow per 100 g of tissue, $\dot{Q}_F$, to conductance (a term that has been defined in physiology as the filtration coefficient, $K_{F_{MV}}$) times the difference in hydrostatic and osmotic heads across the membrane. The equation is written in the following fashion:

$$\dot{Q}_F = K_{F_{MV}} [(P_{MV} - P_{PMV}) - \sum_{i=1}^{k} [\sigma_{MV_i} (\pi_{MV_i} - \pi_{PMV_i})]. \qquad (1)$$

where P_{MV}, P_{PMV}, π_{MV_i}, π_{PMV_i} and σ_{MV_i} refer to microvascular hydrostatic pressure, perimicrovascular hydrostatic pressure, microvascular colloid osmotic pressure of the ith protein species, perimicrovascular colloid osmotic pressure of the ith species and the reflection coefficient of the ith species respectively. A very simple analysis involving the movement of fluid out of the pulmonary microvascular system into the alveoli was developed in our laboratory several years ago, with the assumption that the microvascular and alveolar membranes behaved as a double membrane series system. This analysis revealed that filtration into the alveoli will not occur until the microvascular pressure is raised to values that very nearly equal the colloid osmotic pressure of the plasma that perfuses the lung. This model prediction agrees well with many experimental observations [4-7]. The model also predicted that any filtration coefficient calculated during the formation of pulmonary edema, KF_{ED}, will be less than the filtration coefficient of the pulmonary capillary, KF_{MV}, or of the alveolar membrane, KF_A, as seen in the following equation:

$$KF_{ED} = \frac{KF_{MV} \, KF_A}{KF_{MV} + KF_A} \tag{2}$$

With flows across two membranes in series, the magnitude of total flow will more closely represent that membrane with the lesser volume conductance. In addition, during the formation of pulmonary edema, the alveolar membrane is most likely disrupted, and if the disruption does not occur in all alveoli at the same time, then the rate of edema formation cannot be analyzed to get information about the filtration coefficient of the microvascular membrane [8, 9].

Using the notation P_{MV} for microvascular pressure instead of a notation for capillary pressure is very important, we believe. It may well be that there are different beds within the pulmonary circulation and even different filtering characteristics along the length of any individual pulmonary capillary; and to imply that only one capillary pressure describes the effective microvascular pressure may be seriously in error. Designating pressure surrounding the microvasculature P_{PMV} is also a better functional notation than simply describing tissue pressure, because several areas in lung tissue may contribute to an average pressure calculated in any given experimental model. The last term in Equation (1) contains colloid osmotic pressure of plasma and tissue for the ith species, and another very important membrane parameter, the reflection coefficient σ_{MV_i}. The reflection coefficient was defined by Staverman [10] as equal to 1 for membrane that is impermeable to a given solute; that is, solutes would reflect 100% of the calculated Van't Hoff osmotic pressure across the membrane. The value of σ_{MV_i} equals zero for a membrane to which the solute is freely permeable. Again, we think it is extremely important to realize that we shall be discussing the reflection coefficient of the microvascular system, which may be not only alveolar septal capillaries but also small arteries and veins.

B. Basic Forces

Microvascular Pressure

Equation (1) is derived assuming that solute and volume movement occurs through the same channels. Obviously, this is not true in any capillary bed. What the equation describes in a heterogenous membrane system is some average

KF_{MV}, P_{MV}, P_{PMV}, σ_{MV_i}, π_{MV_i} and π_{PMV_i} that will fit a particular experimental model. There are no direct measurements of pulmonary microvascular pressure similar to those measured for several peripheral beds [11-14]. Pappenheimer and Soto-Rivera [15] have developed an indirect method of estimating micro-vascular pressure in isolated organs and Gaar et al. [16, 17] have used this technique to measure P_{MV} in isolated dog lung. The basic assumption made in determining an isogravimetric microvascular pressure is that the organ is in an isogravimetric state, neither gaining nor losing weight. Flow is then reduced and venous pressure is elevated to maintain the isogravimetric state (PV_i). This same procedure is repeated in successive steps, and the isogravimetric blood flow $\dot{Q}B_i$ is linearly related to the isogravimetric venous or arterial pressures by their respective resistances:

$$P_{PM_i} = PA_i - RA\,\dot{Q}B_i$$

$$P_{PM_i} = PV_i + RV\,\dot{Q}B_i$$

(3)

The midpoint of the filtering bed is considered to be P_{PM_i} and is not an anatomi-cal midpoint but a filtration midpoint of the microvascular bed. Figure 1 is a representation of data from which the isogravimetric microvascular pressure has been obtained by this procedure. The upper left panel is from the work of Johnson and Hanson [18] on isolated dog intestine, the upper right panel is a determination of isogravimetric microvascular pressure by Pappenheimer and Soto-Rivera [15] in the dog hind limb, and the lower curve is a determination of the isogravimetric microvascular pressure by Gaar et al. [16] in dog lung. There are several possible problems associated with determining microvascular pressure by this procedure. One possible problem is that we are dealing with an isolated system. If the capillary-tissue system has changed during removal from the animal, then the isogravimetric microvascular pressure may not reflect the normal microvascular pressure in the intact lung.

A recent study by Diana will illustrate this point [19]. Diana measured the isogravimetric microvascular pressure in an isolated hind limb preparation. He also measured tissue pressure by the capsular technique Guyton developed [20]. The pressures measured from these implanted capsules were either posi-tive or only slightly negative, which is quite different from the pressure meas-ured in intact hind limb (averaging –7 mmHg in several hundred determinations). It appears that the isolated hind limb is edematous, which would lead to over-estimation of the intact microvascular pressure.

The important parameters measured by the isogravimetric pressure tech-nique are the arterial and the venous resistance. If these two resistances are known, then one should be able to calculate an average microvascular pressure for any intact lung preparation for which the arterial and venous pressures are

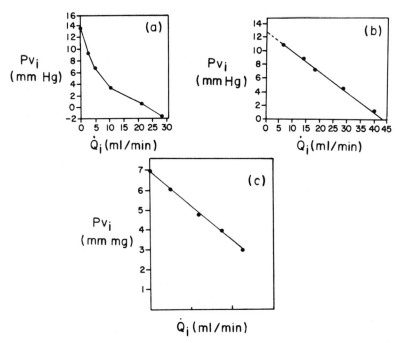

FIGURE 1 Isogravimetric pressure measurements in intestine (a), in hind leg (b) and lung (c). PV_i refers to the isogravimetric venous pressure and $\dot{Q}_i$ refers to the isogravimetric blood flow. Under these conditions, the organ gains no weight. The isogravimetric capillary pressure (PC_i) is determined by extrapolation of the pressure-flow relationship until it intercepts the Y-axis at $Q = 0$. The venous resistance appears to be constant in the hind limb (a) and lung (c), but becomes nonlinear at low flows in the intestine (b). Diagram (a) is reprinted from P. C. Johnson and K. M. Hanson, *Circ. Res.*, **19**:766 (1966), by courtesy of the publisher. Diagram (b) is reprinted from J. R. Pappenheimer and A. Soto-Rivera, *Amer. J. Physiol.*, **152**:471-491 (1948), by courtesy of the publisher. Diagram (c) is reprinted from K. A. Garr, Jr., A. E. Taylor, L. J. Owens, and A. C. Guyton, *Amer. J. Physiol.*, **216**:1370-1373 (1969), by courtesy of the publisher.

known. The microvascular pressure, since it is obtained in an isogravimetric state, is calculated by assuming $\dot{Q}F = 0$ in Equation (1), and it equals the sum of all other forces in the equation. If all the forces are defined by this equation and the organ is at a stationary state, then the microvascular pressure has been measured at that time. For tissues with high tissue protein concentration, such as intestine and lung, $P_{MV} < \pi_{MV}$; for skeletal muscle capillaries, $P_{MV} \cong \pi_{MV}$ [15, 16, 21].

Another microvascular characteristic that is revealed during the measurement of isogravimetric capillary pressure is that in some beds, elevation of venous pressure results in a change of venous resistance. This is quite apparent in Johnson and Hansen's work (see Fig. 1a) but it does not appear to be a significant problem with the venous resistance calculations for the hind limb or lung tissue [15, 16, 22].

Isogravimetric microvascular pressure measurements have been much lower than the values determined by direct micropuncture techniques in several capillary beds [15, 19, 23]. Intaglietta has recently pointed out that since the interstitial volume was increased due to tissue edema, the capillary pressure measured by this technique would not be the same as a direct measurement. However, the argument presented by Intaglietta suggests a measurement error in the wrong direction; i.e., the isogravimetric capillary pressure equals the sum of all other forces in Equation (1) and if the perimicrovascular colloid osmotic pressure has decreased or perimicrovascular pressure has increased, then the measured microvascular pressure will actually be higher than normal. If proteins leak into the tissues during the isolation procedure, then P_{MV} would be underestimated. Miller has recent evidence that indicates no significant protein leakage when blood flow is interrupted for two hours in a hind limb preparation [24]. And Nicoloff et al. [25] have observed that the pulmonary microvascular membrane does not appear to be damaged following fairly severe hypoxia. Protein leakage could certainly cause a problem with PMV_i measurements, but available data do not support the hypothesis that it does occur [26].

There are currently many arguments about why there is a difference between the isogravimetric microvascular pressures and pressures obtained by direct puncture techniques. The most probable cause for this discrepancy is that pressure is usually measured in a flowing capillary, whereas in reality, there may only be a small number of open capillaries in a given capillary bed at any given time. The isogravimetric microvascular pressure measurement would also, in most instances, overestimate the functional and true capillary pressure, since one would expect to have slight tissue edema because of isolation procedures and lack of an intact and functional lymphatic system.

We had believed that the determination of P_{MV} for isolated lungs was basically correct. However, we recently investigated the effects of elevated venous pressure on the calculation of P_{MV}, as shown in Figure 2, and realized that the venous resistance decreased with increasing pressure. As the venous system of the lung becomes distended owing to the increased pressure, the venous resistance decreases. This has been determined in many instances experimentally, but it has usually been discussed in terms of the total resistance to flow through the lung [17, 27]. It appears that most of the decreased total resistance is caused by changes in venous resistance. The change in venous

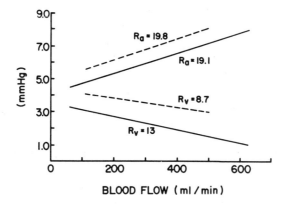

FIGURE 2 A plot of isogravimetric venous pressure (lower two curves) and isogravimetric arterial pressure (upper two curves) at two different isogravimetric states in isolated dog lung. Note the change in venous resistance (dotted lines) at the higher initial venous pressure. Unpublished observations.

resistance in Figure 2 is modest, but other experiments demonstrate that larger increases in venous pressure decrease venous resistance to very small values. Figure 2 demonstrates that the microvascular pressure responsible for fluid movements in intact lungs may almost equal the left atrial pressure, and only a very small drop is required to move the blood from the average filtration midpoint into the left atrium. This same result is also apparent in the data of Agostoni and Piiper [28]. Therefore, any estimation of capillary pressure in an intact animal, especially when venous pressure is elevated, must be reevaluated using correct values for pulmonary arterial and venous resistances.

Since pulmonary arterial pressure in dogs averages between 12 and 32 mmHg and the left atrial pressure averages between 2 and 12 mmHg [29], the normal microvascular pressure would likely be between 7 and 9 mmHg as measured by Gaar [16] and Agostoni [28]. For the remainder of this section, we shall discuss microvascular pressure as though it were some average pressure and use the value 4 mmHg for normal left atrial pressure. It is quite apparent, however, that if one models accurately the pulmonary microcirculation, one must include the systolic and diastolic pressures in both the pulmonary arteries and the left atrium in order to describe adequately the perfusion that exists at different lung levels. (The last section of this chapter will deal with this particular problem when a more complete model of pulmonary fluid movement is considered.)

Colloid Osmotic Pressure of the Plasma

The colloid osmotic pressure of the plasma can be determined by several techniques. The osmometer recently developed by Prather et al. [30] can be used to measure the plasma protein osmotic pressure, or the plasma osmotic pressure can be calculated by the equation derived both empirically and theoretically by Landis and Pappenheimer [12]. However, the actual osmotic pressure caused by the colloids at the microvascular tissue interface may be quite different from the value determined by an osmometer, which has a membrane more limiting than the microvasculature, or by an equation that is derived from normal albumin and globulin ratios. The effect is probably not important in a simple model that uses average values for the parameters, like Equation (1). However, when one tries to model the osmotic pressure at a pore that may be small enough to restrict passage of globulin although it allows albumin to pass through, the method of defining osmotic pressure presents a real problem. A later section, which develops the permeability characteristics of plasma proteins across the pulmonary microvasculature, indicates that all protein fractions must be considered— not simply the albumin and globulin—in assessing colloid osmotic pressure.

   In most instances, the plasma colloid osmotic pressure in dogs averages 20 mmHg and the plasma albumin-to-globulin ratios are relatively low, the average being very close to 1. Intaglietta [31] has recently measured plasma colloid osmotic pressure for many different species, and these measurements should prove helpful in estimating capillary dynamics in a very divergent group of animals. The plasma colloid osmotic pressure must be determined for each laboratory model. For instance, when animals are bled to obtain blood for extracorporeal perfusing circuits, plasma colloid osmotic pressures of 14 to 15 mmHg are not unusual for these animals.

   Although an accurate measurment of colloid osmotic pressure is desirable in each experiment model, the Landis and Pappenheimer equation, we have found, agrees well with osmometer measurements. Table 1 is a computer print-out of this equation, which you may find helpful in estimating colloid osmotic pressure of either lymph or plasma. It must be realized, however, that this represents only some average estimate of colloid osmotic pressure.

Perimicrovascular Pressure

One of the most controversial topics in physiology today is, What is the hydro-static pressure surrounding pulmonary exchange vessels? Subcutaneous tissue fluid pressure has been measured and is subatmospheric, averaging about –7 mmHg [20, 32-36], by the implanted capsule method of Guyton, and – 4 mmHg by Scholander's wick method [35, 37-40]. But some methods of estimating perimicrovascular pressures yield positive values [41]. Pressure determinations

TABLE 1 Colloid Osmotic Pressure Calculated from Landis and Pappenheimer's Equation

C_p	0.0	0.1	0.2	0.3	0.4	0.5	0.6	0.7	0.8	0.9
0	0.000	0.212	0.426	0.645	0.866	1.091	1.320	1.551	1.787	2.026
1	2.269	2.516	2.766	3.020	3.278	3.540	3.806	4.077	4.351	4.629
2	4.912	5.199	5.490	5.786	6.086	6.391	6.700	7.014	7.332	7.655
3	7.983	8.316	8.653	8.996	9.343	9.696	10.054	10.416	10.784	11.157
4	11.536	11.920	12.309	12.704	13.104	13.510	13.922	14.339	14.762	15.190
5	15.625	16.065	16.512	16.964	17.423	17.887	18.358	18.835	19.318	19.808
6	20.304	20.806	21.315	21.831	22.353	22.882	23.417	23.959	24.508	25.064
7	25.627	26.197	26.774	27.358	27.949	28.547	29.152	29.765	30.385	31.013
8	31.648	32.291	32.941	33.598	34.264	34.937	35.618	36.307	37.004	37.708
9	38.421	39.142	39.871	40.608	41.353	42.106	42.868	43.638	44.417	45.204

Source: Courtesy of Dr. Robert Brace.
Note: The equation is $\pi = 2.1C_p + 0.16C_p^2 + 0.009C^3$, where C_p is the total protein concentration in g/100 ml.

made in dog lungs by Guyton's experimental procedures have yielded pressures that are subatmospheric, averaging -6 mmHg [42]. Other investigators feel, however, that the pressure surrounding the exchange vessels of the lung need not be subatmospheric and may indeed be very close to alveolar pressures [43]. Several factors must be considered in order to arrive at some proper understanding of the pressure that surrounds the pulmonary exchange vessels.

Simply because alveolar pressure is zero, it does not require that the fluid pressures surrounding the exchange vessels be zero, since at least three types of pressures exist within tissues. Agostoni, in discussing pleural pressure, has defined these pressures: (1) a fluid pressure, which is present in the very thin fluid layer that separates visceral pleura from parietal pleura; (2) a surface-averaged pressure, which represents the force tending to collapse the lung; and (3) a deformation or contact pressure [44]. The sum of the fluid and deformation pressures equals the surface-averaged pressure of the lung.

Guyton has extended this same concept of different pressures to explain how a negative pressure can exist in interstitial fluids. He postulates (1) a fluid pressure that provides the force that moves fluid across membranes; and (2) a solid tissue pressure that is exerted by contact points throughout the interstitium. The solid pressure does not require that fibers must transfer pressures to only attachment planes, but merely that the pressure is transmitted in ways other than through fluid elements. He also holds that (3) total pressure equals the sum of fluid and solid pressures and is the pressure that tends to collapse vessels [45-48].

The alveoli have a collapse factor of about 4 mmHg. Obviously, if there were not a counterbalancing pressure in the opposite direction, then the alveoli would collapse. The counterbalancing pressure could simply be provided by contact points such that the solid tissue pressure is negative, referred to the tissue. Or perimicrovascular pressure could have a minimal value of -4 mmHg, which is equal to the collapse tendency of the alveoli. A very concise review of pulmonary tissue pressures has been recently written by Hughes [49], and you will find in that work a more complete analysis of pulmonary tissue pressures.

Another indication that interstitial fluid pressure is negative is that pulmonary microvascular pressure is quite low relative to other vascular beds. Some other tissue force must counterbalance capillary pressure or fluid will be pulled out of the interstitium continuously. This force could be either interstitial colloid osmotic pressure or interstitial fluid pressure. Most physiologists now agree that a combination of both forces are responsible for the differences between microvascular hydrostatic and colloid pressures.

Levine and associates have provided data that indicate a negative perimicrovascular pressure in dog lung; they have not, however, considered the perimicrovascular protein concentration a significant tissue factor [5, 6, 50].

As this chapter develops, the concept of a subatmospheric perimicrovascular pressure will emphasize pressures measured in dog lung. There are convincing arguments, however, against subatmospheric pressures especially in sheep lung (Section IV of this chapter).

Tissue Colloid Osmotic Pressure

The tissue colloid osmotic pressure has never been measured directly in lung tissue, and lymphatic protein has been used to estimate this parameter. Figure 3 shows a typical experiment from our laboratory using an isolated dog lung in which we have measured lymph flow and lymph protein content after elevating pulmonary venous pressure. It can be seen from this plot that the control lymphatic protein concentration is about 5.5 g/100 ml. The lymph protein concentration in numerous experimental animals have averaged 70% of plasma levels [1, 51]. Recent investigations by Levine [52], however, have demonstrated that if albumin and chloride are confined to the same spaces within the lung, then the extravascular protein content cannot be as high as that determined for pulmonary lymph. Dog lung tissue may be entirely different from sheep lung tissue, since Vaughan et al. have surmised that proteins have a volume of distribution different from that for sucrose [53]. Also, a recent study

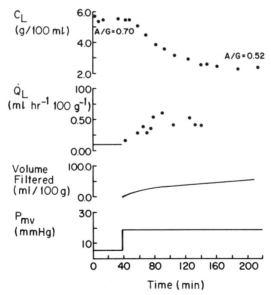

FIGURE 3 Changes in lymph-protein concentration (C_L), lymph flow ($\dot{Q}_L$), and volume filtered as P_{MV} is increased from 6 to 15 mmHg. Reprinted from Drake and Taylor, unpublished observations.

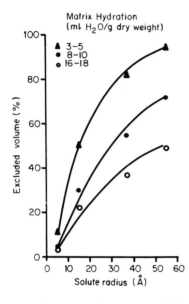

FIGURE 4 Plot of exclusion phenomena for an umbilical gel tissue model from Granger. The closed circles represent normal gel hydration; the open circles represent overhydration; and the triangles represent dehydration. Note that albumin is excluded at each hydration state. Reprinted from H. J. Granger et al. [56].

by Johnson and Richardson [54] indicates that intestinal lymphatics may also have a higher protein concentration than that within the intestinal interstitium. How can this apparent difference be resolved? There is no doubt that lymphatic proteins could be quite different from the protein surrounding any individual capillary, owing to some concentrating mechanism within the lymphatics [55]. However, the lymphatic draining any particular region should at least reflect some average protein content of that region, as Taylor and Gibson have determined for subcutaneous lymphatics [36].

Figure 4 demonstrates the exclusion principle for a Wharton's jelly model which Granger et al. [56] developed. These data were obtained using Wharton's jelly at three different hydrations: normal, dehydrated, and overhydrated. Albumin is excluded at all three hydration states and even when the umbilical gel is highly swollen, the albumin molecule is still excluded by 35%. It must be emphasized that Wharton's jelly has a very high concentration of hyaluronic acid and the concentration of gel in pulmonary tissues is not known. For peripheral tissues, Garlick and Renkin [57] have calculated a 25% exclusion for large molecules; and for proteins in sheep pulmonary tissue, Staub has calculated a 50% exclusion. However, Levine's data indicate almost no exclusion of albumin relative to that of choride in dog lung.* Therefore, either some of the estimates

---

*An argument can be made against using Cl⁻ as a marker for extravascular space, since the mucopolysaccharides have a negative change. However, the agreement between Levine's Cl spaces and the Na spaces measured by other investigators is quite good. Comparison of a sucrose space with the albumin space would be most helpful in evaluating this argument.

are inaccurate or dog lung is very different from sheep lung or umbilical tissue in concentration of gel and protein exclusion phenomena within the interstitium.

Obviously, it is very difficult to assess a functional tissue colloid osmotic pressure, since the colloid osmotic pressure may be quite different at different points in the interstitium, or even along the length of the capillary. One of the main questions that must be answered is, How is lymph protein related to tissue protein? Until this question is resolved, we simply wil have to use lymph to approximate tissue fluid.

Capillary Membrane Filtration Coefficient

So far we have discussed four parameters. Only three are known to any degree of accuracy, even in an isolated perfused system, much less for the very complex intact pulmonary microcirculation. The same situation is true with the microvascular filtration coefficient. A brief review of filtration coefficient measurements in other beds is necessary in order to point out the difficulties of measuring this parameter. The first measurements of filtration coefficients were made by Landis, in which he directly measured filtration from a single capillary [11]. Later, Pappenheimer [15, 58] developed an indirect method for obtaining the filtration coefficient of an isolated hind limb preparation. The filtration coefficient was obtained by elevating venous pressure and determining the weight transient. Since a very constant rate of weight gain was observed following venous pressure elevations in isolated limbs, the slope of the weight-grain curve can be determined, and when divided by the initial pressure head yields the fluid filtration coefficient (usually expressed as $g\ min^{-1}\ mmHg^{-1}\ 100\ g^{-1}$ tissue). There is one important point to consider concerning this type of measurement; if we try the same procedure for lung tissue, that is, elevate pulmonary venous pressure until a constant weight gain is attained by the lungs, then fluid will be filtering not only into the interstitium but also into the alveoli. Most estimates of the pulmonary filtration coefficient have been made by measuring wet- and dry-weight ratios of lungs at different left atrial pressures [21, 59]. The filtration coefficients determined by this procedure at low left atrial pressures are about one-tenth the filtration coefficient measured in hind limb. However, one can simply not use the total weight gain to calculate a filtration coefficient. For instance, with left atrial pressure elevation, if the fluid leaves the pulmonary circulation very rapidly, then the tissue forces will change—i.e., tissue pressure will increase, tissue colloid osmotic pressure will decrease. If the total weight gain is then divided by the initial pressure head, a small filtration coefficient will be found. Since the filtration coefficient is a rate, then the total weight gain could be small but filtration could occur very rapidly.

Figure 5 is a plot of the data from several lungs from our laboratory; in these procedures, we elevated pulmonary venous and arterial pressure by exactly the same amount and determined the weight gain of an isolated lung [60, 61].

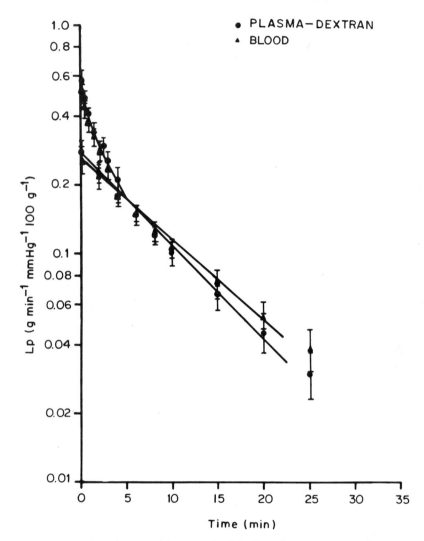

FIGURE 5 A plot of KF_{MV} (designated LP in figure) as a function of time as determined in dog lung by Taylor and Garr. Plasma dextran was used as a perfusing fluid ($\bullet$) and compared with whole blood ($\blacktriangle$). Note that both fluids yield similar values and that KF_{MV} is large for dog lungs. Reprinted from A. E. Taylor and K. A. Garr, Jr., *Revista Argent. Angio.*, **3**:26-40 (1969), by courtesy of the publishers.

The slopes of the weight gain curve were then plotted as a function of time on semilogarithmic, as shown in Figure 5. There are two distinct components of this curve, the fast component as the lung blood vessels fill (capacitance effect) and a slower component, which represents filtration of fluid into the lung interstitium. When the slower component is extrapolated to zero time, the calculated filtration coefficient is 0.25 g(min $\times$ mmHg $\times$ 100 g)$^{-1}$, which is a large filtration coefficient. There are other experiments in the literature from which one can obtain a KF_{MV} of similar magnitude. The work of Lunde and Waaler [62] and Bø and Waaler [63] on rabbit lungs yields filtration coefficients of the same order of magnitude. Also, Uter has determined a capillary filtration coefficient much higher than that for the alveolar membrane [64]. Perl and associates [65] have recently measured a KF_{MV} of about one-half the magnitude of ours; however, their measurement was made at a given time and does not represent the extrapolated filtration coefficient. Finally, the data of Weiser and Grande [66] also yield a large initial filtration coefficient.

The calculated filtration coefficient could be too large if the capacitive elements are still changing during the slow component of the weight-gain curve. We have recently reevaluated this measurement by comparing the weight gain curve to hematocrit changes over the entire experimental procedure. The weighing procedure and volume changes calculated by hematocrit changes yield similar total volume changes. This agreement indicates that lung weight gains following the initial blood volume shift reflect transvascular flux of fluid out of the pulmonary circulation. The KF_{MV} estimated from Lunde's data can be calculated independent of blood volume changes, since the blood volume shift was measured simultaneously with weight changes by radioisotope procedures. Also, Weiser and Grande measured both blood volume and tissue volume changes during the first 5 min following elevation of pulmonary venous pressure. Their results allow yet another calculation of KF_{MV} independent of blood volume shifts.

Another method by which the filtration coefficient can be obtained is measuring or calculating all the tissue and microvascular forces, i.e., the hydrostatic pressures in the microvasculature and interstitium, the colloid osmotic pressure in the interstitium and in the capillaries, and total lymph flow from an organ. The total lymph flow can then be divided by the force imbalance to yield KF_{MV}:

$$\dot{Q}L = \dot{Q}F = KF_{MV} [\Delta P_{drop}] \quad \text{or} \quad KF_{MV} = \frac{\dot{Q}L}{\Delta P_{drop}} \tag{4}$$

This is the method of choice for measuring the filtration coefficient if all the forces and flows are known very accurately. At present we do not know all the forces or flows very accurately for dog pulmonary tissue. For instance, if the pulmonary lymphatic protein does not reflect tissue protein, then the imbalance across the capillary would be difficult to assess and the filtration coefficient may be overestimated using Equation 4. There are several other determinations of pulmonary filtration coefficients in the literature for dog lungs, but these are either measurements of the filtration coefficient of the combined pulmonary microvasculature and alveolar membrane (most likely dirupsted alveolar membranes) [4, 6] or measurements of the accumulated tissue volume divided by the change in left atrial pressure instead of the initial slope of the weight gain curve [5, 6, 50, 59].

Erdmann et al. [67] have used Equation (4) to estimate KF_{MV} for intact sheep lungs. Their value of KF_{MV} is very small, approximately 0.01 to 0.02 ml/ (min $\times$ mmHg $\times$ 100 g). As you can see from Figure 6, the pressure drop is considerable, especially at the lower filtration coefficients, averaging 5 mmHg at normal lymph flows and 20 mmHg at a fivefold increase in lymph flow. If these filtration coefficients are correct, then sheep lungs should be able to withstand considerable increases in left atrial pressure before intra-alveolar edema develops [67].

Finally, a very important observation concerning fluid movement out of the pulmonary microvascular system has been made by Iliff [68]. She has found by differentially studying lungs in perfusion zones I, II, and III that different segments of the filtration surface, called arterial extra-alveolar, alveolar, and venous extra-alveolar vessels, had differing filtration characteristics. The extra-alveolar arterial vessels accounted for 16% of the filtration in a static zone III lung, and the alveolar 38%, and extra-alveolar venous vessels 46%. Whether this difference is due to either different porosities or greater surface areas or both

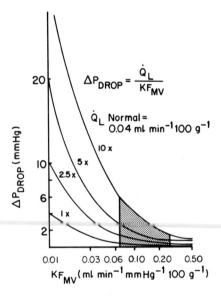

FIGURE 6 A plot of net filtration pressure (ΔP_{drop}) as a function KF_{MV}, at different lymph flows. The normal lymph flow was assumed to equal that determined from dog studies using right duct lymph flow. The shaded area represents calculated KF_{MV} for dog lungs. Note that ΔP_{drop} is very small even for tenfold differences in lymph flow. Staub's filtration coefficient for sheep lung would be represented by a KF_{MV} of 0.01, which would yield a very large ΔP_{drop} both for normal lymph flow (4 mmHg) and for a fivefold increase in lymph flow (20 mmHg).

is not clear. Any model of fluid movement across the pulmonary exchange vessels must incorporate this feature of the microvascular membrane. An anatomical investigation of this phenomenon like the one of Majno and Palade [69] for skeletal muscle would be most beneficial.

Reflection Coefficient

The reflection coefficient was defined by Staverman [10] and is related to molecular sieving in the following way. Consider a fluid that is being filtered through a membrane. The concentration of a substance in the filtrand (C_F) is found to have a concentration in the filtrate of C_S. Now if C_S/C_F equals 1, then the molecule is not sieved at the membrane. If $C_S/C_F = 0$, then the membrane is impereamble to the molecule. The ratio C_S/C_F is the sieving coefficient and is related to σ in the following way:

$$\sigma = 1 - \frac{C_S}{C_F}. \tag{5}$$

Pappenheimer investigated the molecular sieving of several molecules in an isolated hind limb and calculated an effective or equivalent pore of 40-Å radius for these capillaries. Kedem and Katchalsky, using nonequilibrium thermodynamics, developed the basic equations describing sieving in biological membranes and derived the following equation to relate σ to the area available for solute (A_S) and the area available for water (A_W) [2]:

$$\sigma = 1 - \frac{A_S}{A_W} \tag{6}$$

Durbin used the Kedem and Katchalsky equations and measured σ for several molecules in three different membrane systems [70]. Figure 7 demonstrates the theoretical relation between σ and the ratio of the radius of the probing molecule, a, to an effective pore radius of the membrane with cylindrical pores assumed). The data obtained for a dialysis membrane are also shown on this plot. The functional relation between σ and a/r can be used for any membrane pore system for which the size of the molecule is known.

No estimates of σ_{MV} for plasma proteins are available for dog lung but Staub's group has calculated σ_{MV_p} from a model approach. One cannot simply use plasma protein concentrations in lymph relative to plasma to determine σ_{MV_i}. That this would cause serious error can be seen when peripheral lymph is used. The albumin concentration of peripheral lymph is about 1 g/100 ml and of plasma about 4 g/ml. If σ_{MV} were calculated from these data, we should obtain

$$\sigma_{MV} = 1 - \frac{1}{4} = 1 - 0.25 = 0.75. \tag{7}$$

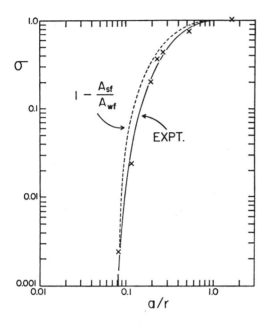

FIGURE 7 A plot of 1 – A_{sf}/A_{wf}, or σ, as a function of molecular radius of probing molecule a divided by pore radius r, from Durbin. The experimental points are for σ's measured across a dialysis membrane. This curve is extremely useful for estimating σ for any pore-molecule systems. Reprinted from R. P. Durbin, *J. Gen. Physiol.*, **44**:315-326 (1960), by courtesy of the publishers.

The reflection coefficient could not possibly be this small for the total capillary surface area. If lung lymph is used, then the apparent σ would be found of the order of 0.1 to 0.2, which is impossible. Obviously, a single σ cannot describe the lymphatic protein concentrations observed in diffusion studies and a distribution of pores is necessary to explain the observed values.

Staub and associates [1] have recently constructed a model that predicts a σ_{MV} for albumin of 0.8 and of globulin 0.9, for the sheep pulmonary microvascular membrane. In Chapter 8, Effros discusses the measurements of σ in more detail and this is also discussed in Section II of this chapter. The value of σ_{MV} for several large molecules should be measured in some experimental lung model, but if they are of the order of magnitude Staub has calculated, then it would be difficult to detect any difference among the plasma proteins in their sieving characteristics in lung tissue.

Chinard's group (personal communication [71]) has recently shown that osmotic transients pull fluid both from the interstitium and from endothelial cells. A complete discussion of this problem is presented by Lifson and Tosteson in a recent symposium on capillary dynamics [72, 73]. Basically, the observed σ's should be much larger if the endothelial cells have total filtration areas that are equivalent to the larger endothelial gaps. In fact, the observed σ for all molecules would be 0.50 unless the endothelial gaps restrict the molecules. It may be impossible, however, because of other factors, to adequately measure σ in lung tissue. Grabowski has recently suggested that fluid is pulled from the interstitium, decreasing tissue pressure to a very low value and resulting in a diminished net volume flow for a given initial osmotic head [74]. Also, Perl [65] has proposed that native tissue solutes are sieved as the osmotic transient occurs and that the actual osmotic head across the capillary is much lower than the initial perfusate concentration.

Despite the many problems in measuring σ_{MV} in lung, much more work must be done in an attempt to assess this parameter before the effective porosity of the pulmonary microvascular membranes can be described. Until some average σ_{MV} is measured for at least albumin and globulin, we must assume some value that is not greatly different from the one used by Starling, i.e., $\sigma_{MV} \cong 1$.

Imbalance in Forces, Net Filtration Heat (ΔP_{drop})

Normally, the forces previously discussed do not sum to zero since a small amount of filtrate is continually entering the lymphatics. This imbalance in the Starling forces must also be considered when one tries to analyze volume movement across any capillary system. Figure 6 shows the principle of net filtration pressure. For high filtration coefficients, the drop is not large even for a tenfold increase in lymph flow, but for low filtration coefficients the net filtration pressure can be quite significant. Figure 6 shows filtration coefficients that have been measured in dog lungs (shaded area) for normal and 2.5, 5, and 10 times normal lymph flows. Since right-duct lymph flow increases only 2.5-fold when left atrial pressures are elevated in intact animals, the net filtration drop cannot be very large in these preparations. If lymph flow is underestimated, however, then the true filtration drop could be significant.

From our experiments with dog lungs, the pressure drop is not a significant factor, since the filtration coefficient is large and lymph flow is extremely small. Staub and associates, however, calculate a considerable filtration head in sheep lungs, because lymph flow is large relative to the calculated filtration coefficient [67]. Mortillaro has recently measured the net filtration pressure for isolated dog intestine [75]. The net filtration pressure in this system was 5 mmHg for a venous pressure of 30 mmHg but very small at normal venous pressures. The maximum drop that we have observed in several dog lungs has been about 0.5 mmHg and this pressure drop was measured at 30 mmHg venous pressure. If lung lymph flow in dog lungs is only 4 ml/hr (lower curve of Figure 6), then it is difficult to calculate any large-force imbalance unless KF_{MV} is underestimated by almost an order of magnitude. There is always the distinct possibility that all lymph from the lungs cannot be collected—perhaps it will be only a very small portion. If this is the case, then a large pressure drop could exist across the pulmonary capillary.

Lymph Flow

Figure 3 shows lymph flow from a large lymphatic that joins the right lymph duct; from an isolated dog lung experiment. The flow is very low relative to measurements made for intact right lymph duct preparations [51, 76]. Furthermore, we see no lymph flow unless the lung is ventilated, indicating that respiratory movements are necessary to propel lymph in an isolated lung. This has also been observed in isolated human cadaver lungs [77, 78]. Since sodium pentobarbital was used to anesthetize the animal, the intrinsic pumping ability of the lymphatics might be altered, and respiratory movements are the only lymphatic pump available [79, 80].

The lymph flow is increased to values six times normal following elevation of venous pressure. This is a larger increase than what has been observed in intact animals (2.5 times) following large elevations of left atrial pressure. Our lymphatic preparation certainly does not measure all lung lymph flow, but should at least reflect changes representative of the behavior of the entire lung [81]. We feel that the intact right lymph duct preparation may primarily reflect lymph from other extra pulmonary sites, and such large increases of pulmonary lymph flow could be masked.

Some investigators consider lymph flow an unimportant factor in preventing the formation of pulmonary edema [82], mainly because lymph flow is so small. But, ΔP_{drop} is the important parameter of lymph flow, not total flow as discussed in Section II, 7.

Staub's group has developed an excellent preparation for studying sheep-lymph flow and most of the pertinent new data have been obtained in this model. A recent review article by Staub [1] discussed lymph flow and tissue protein removal, and we shall discuss this important tissue factor in Section III.

Obviously much more work must be done along these lines in order to understand the mechanisms of lung-lymph flow and protein composition. Two excellent books on the lymphatic system, Rusznyák, Földi, and Szabó [79] and Yoffey and Courtice [80] can furnish the reader with a more complete description of lymph flows in several capillary beds.

Compliance of the Pulmonary Interstitium

Figure 8 is a plot of lung compliance [ml/(mmHg $\times$ 100 g)] as a function of calculated perimicrovascular fluid pressure from dog lungs. This curve was calculated in an isogravimetric dog-lung system. The lung was allowed to obtain an isogravimetric condition and venous pressure was elevated by a known amount. The lung gained weight until it reached a new isogravimetric state. The compliance was calculated as the difference in weight gain between the two

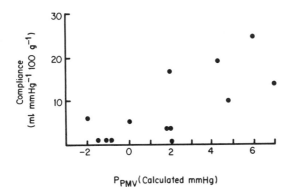

PPMV(Calculated mmHg)

FIGURE 8 Plot of interstitial compliance of isolated dog lung at a different calculated P_{PMV}. The compliance is small at low values of P_{PMV} and increases tenfold at values of $P_{PMV} > 2$ mmHg. Reprinted from Drake and Taylor, unpublished observations.

isogravimetric points divided by the change in calculated microvascular pressure, using values for venous and arterial resistances as measured by Gaar et al. [16]. As you can see from this plot, at pressures below 2 mmHg the compliance of the lung tissue averaged 3 ml/(mmHg × 100 g). At higher capillary pressures, the lung tissues expand dramatically for small changes in perimicrovascular pressures. The compliance averaged 20 ml/(mmHg × 100 g) for calculated pressures greater than +2 mmHg. To our knowledge, this is the only attempt to measure some type of tissue-volume curve for pulmonary tissue. This compliance curve indicates that dog lungs change weight by about 30% to 50% before intra-alveolar edema develops, as measured by histologic means. This is a very important function curve and much more work needs to be done along these lines to understand how tissue pressure changes with increases in pulmonary tissue volumes. The curve shown in Figure 8 incorporates a degree of uncertainty, since the perimicrovascular pressure was calculated by measuring all other forces in Equation (1), and assuming that lymphatic protein was equal to tissue protein.

Edema Safety Factor

The pulmonary extravascular water volume does not expand greatly until P_{MV} is equivalent to π_{MV}. Guyton and coworkers have developed the concept of tissue safety factors to describe the changes in tissue forces which oppose the filtration pressure [45, 83-85]. When P_{MV} is increased, P_{PMV} will increase, π_{PMV} will decrease, and ΔP_{drop} will increase. The sum of these three changes in the tissue forces is the edema safety factor. We can compute the total safety factor for pulmonary tissue, but the contribution of each factor is currently still uncertain [47, 48, 86].

The value P_{PMV} could increase from -7 to +2 mmHg before the compliance of the tissue changes and π_{PMV} could decrease from the average values of 14 mmHg to about 5 mmHg (Figure 3, and Staub [43, 87]). These two forces would yield a total safety factor of 22 mmHg. There is still some argument about whether lymphatic protein concentration reflects tissue protein concentration. If it does not, then the total safety factor would not be this large. As can be seen from this computation, the remaining force ΔP_{drop} cannot be very large since the total measured safety factor is only about 18 to 20 mmHg [4].

A very interesting observation was made by Uhley et al. about changes in the safety factor observed with chronic elevations of left atrial pressure. They observed a large increase in lymph flow in their chronic animals. The size of ΔP_{drop} must become important under these conditions and perhaps π_{PMV} decreases to low values, as is seen in intestinal lymph with chronic portal hypertension by Witte [88]. KF_{MV} may also decrease in these preparations, which would make ΔP_{drop} even more important. The changes in tissue safety factors prevent pulmonary edema formation in patients with chronically elevated left atrial pressures, but more experimental work is necessary to determine the exact contribution of each of the safety factors [89, 90].

III.   Protein Movement Across
the Microvascular Exchange Vessels

A.   General

The equation describing protein movement ($\dot{Q}_P$) for a single homogeneous membrane is as follows:

$$\dot{Q}_P = \dot{Q}_F (1 - \sigma_P) \, \overline{C}_P + P_P A \, \Delta C \tag{8}$$

where $\overline{C}_P$ is the average protein concentration across the capillary [$(CP_{MV} + CP_{PMV})/2$], P_P is the permeability coefficient, A is the surface area of membrane, and ΔC is the concentration difference across the membrane.

This equation is for a single protein species across a homogeneous barrier where the solute and solvent cross the membrane through the same aqueous channels. This equation states simply that the molecules can cross a membrane by two different physical processes. One process is bulk flow, as described by the first term in Equation (8). If σ equals zero, then a pressure head across this system pushes fluid through the membrane at the existing concentration of the plasma. At values of $\sigma_P > 0$, evaluation of the term becomes more difficult.

Proteins can also cross membranes by diffusion, which is represented by the second term of Equation (8). This diffusional term is usually measured with isotopes for membrane systems with zero volume flow. There is another possible mechanism by which proteins may cross a living membrane and that is vesicular transport (cytopempsis [91, 92]). Schneeberger-Keeley and Karnovsky [93, 94] have demonstrated that horseradish peroxidase does not appear to leave pulmonary capillaries by endothelial vesicles. The peroxidase molecules appear to cross the pulmonary microvasculature through the interspaces between the overlapping endothelial cells. These findings were confirmed by Szidion et al. using horseradish peroxidase and hemoglobin as the tracer molecule [9]. However, Simionescu et al. [95] and Themann et al. [96] have shown in both diaphragm and heart muscle that vesicular transport is very important in the movement of large molecules across these capillaries.* Perhaps a more careful investigation of pulmonary endothelial vesicles can identify a contribution of vesicular transport to protein transvascular fluxes.

Pappenheimer [58] was the first to describe an equivalent-pore model and you will find in the classical review by Landis and Pappenheimer [12] a complete development of this concept. Basically, it is assumed that the pores have an equivalent radius that describes the diffusion and filtration processes that occur in a given experimental model. Both cylindrical and slit equivalent pores have been used to describe the diffusion processes and Renkin has developed a mathematical model to calculate A_S/A_W [97]. The relation in Figure 7 was calculated from Renkin's equation, and indicates a good fit of the data obtained from a dialysis membrane. We can obtain the parameters in Equation (8)– KF_{MV}, P_P, and σMV_P–from three different experimental approaches. The measurement of KF_{MV} has been discussed at length in Section II. The value P_P can be calculated from either diffusion data or an analysis of lymphatic protein fluxes. The value σMV_P can be calculated using the osmotic transient analysis as described in Section IIIC of this chapter.

Obviously, we cannot describe any capillary in terms of a single diffusional barrier for protein leakage. But we must consider the membrane as having several types of pores. A simple calculation will demonstrate this problem. The endothelial cells are not permeable to protein, so that their contribution to movement of protein through pores need not be considered. If the lung lymph albumin concentration is 2.5 g/100 ml and lymph flow is 4 ml/hr, then 0.10 g

---

*One of the main objections to crediting vesicular transport is that the process is too slow to describe the normal protein leakage. The work of Simionescu shows that the vesicular turnover is very rapid, only 5 to 20 sec, indicating sufficient time for this process to transport protein across the microvascular wall. Another possible way that large dextran molecules could cross the capillary is by being aligned in a direction perpendicular to the pore. Since there is net filtration in the microvascular bed, then this possibility certainly exists.

albumin moves across the lung capillaries per hour. Assume that there are holes or slits in the pulmonary circulation that allow the exact concentration of protein in the plasma to be transferred into the lymphatics by bulk flow. Since 0.10 g/hr of protein is removed by the lymphatics, then lymph flow could be only 2.5 ml for a total plasma filtrate. This is a very oversimplified calculation, but it easily demonstrates the need for more than one pore size at the microvascular membrane to describe protein flux.

B. Calculation of Pore Dimensions Using Lymphatic Data

Most investigators would agree that the peripheral capillaries have two types of effective pores—a small-pore system (40-Å radius) and a large-pore system (200 to 350 Å radius) [12, 31, 91, 98-104]. Boyd [105, 106] and Staub [1] also observed the presence of a large-pore system in sheep lung. Figure 9 schematically represents Grotte's data from dog hind limb and Boyd's data from sheep lung. For Grotte's work [99], the permeability of the small-pore system predominates with probing molecules whose radii are below 40 Å. However, at molecular radii above 40 Å the lymph-to-plasma ratios of the probing molecules are almost equal. A similar finding can be seen from Boyd's data (see Fig. 4 in Ref. 106). At molecular radii below 80 Å, the L/P ratios fall very dramatically with increasing molecular size. The data of P. M. Taylor [107] from dog lung lymph yields L/P ratios of 0.72 for albumin and 0.43 for globulins, an observation that agrees well with Boyd's data for smaller molecules. Mayerson also observed constant L/P ratios for large-molecular-weight substances for cervical lymph [91].

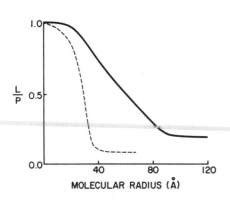

MOLECULAR RADIUS (Å)

FIGURE 9 Plot of lymph/plasma ratios of large molecules from Grotte's work on hind limb (———) and Boyd's on sheep lung (———). Note the extreme difference between the leakage of large molecules into the interstitium for the two beds; however, both beds demonstrate a constant value at increasing molecular radii of the probing molecules. Based on G. Grotte, *Acta Chem. Scand. Suppl.*, **211**:1-84 (1971), and R. D. Boyd et al., *J. Physiol.*, **201**:567-588 (1969).

There is no agreement on what constitutes this large-pore system. The large-pore system can be described by either large "leaks" or vesicular transport. Mayerson et al. [91] showed that large leaks could explain the large-pore system in intestinal and liver lymph by the reasoning that L/P ratio did not approach a constant value at large molecular sizes but decreased slowly with increasing molecular size.

Renkin [92] developed the first quantitative approach to protein movement across peripheral capillaries by analyzing the lymph-to-plasma ratios of large dextrans from Grotte's [99] and Mayerson's [91] earlier studies. Renkin (Ref. 91, equation 7) derived the following equation to analyze protein movement across the capillary:

$$\frac{C_L}{C_P} = \frac{\dot{Q}_F + D_S A_W / \Delta X}{\dot{Q}_L (A_W / A_S) - 1 + \dot{Q}_F + D_S A_W / \Delta X} \tag{9}$$

where A_W is pore area available for water, A_S the restricted pore area for solute, D_S the free-diffusion coefficient of solute as measured in water, C_L the concentration of protein in lymph, C_P the plasma concentration of protein, and ΔX the membrane thickness. Furthermore, C_L / C_P must be measured in a steady state and lymph must be identical to tissue fluid. If $\dot{Q}_F = \dot{Q}_L$, the equation can be reduced to

$$\frac{\dot{Q}_L \, C_L / C_P}{1 - C_L / C_P} = \frac{\dot{Q}_F + D_S \, A_W / \Delta X}{A_W / A_S - 1}. \tag{10}$$

If $\dot{Q}_F$ is small, the equation reduces to

$$PA = \frac{\dot{Q}_L \, C_L / C_P}{1 - C_L / C_P} = \frac{D_S \, A_W / \Delta X}{A_W / A_S - 1}. \tag{11}$$

If $\dot{Q}_F \gg D_S \, A_W / \Delta X$, Equation (10) reduces to

$$\frac{\dot{Q}_L \, C_L / C_P}{1 - C_L / C_P} = \frac{\dot{Q}_F}{A_W / A_S - 1}. \tag{12}$$

Equation (8) can also be used to arrive at a similar equation:

$$PA = \frac{\dot{Q}_L \, C_L - (1 - \sigma_{MV_P}) \, \overline{C}_S}{(C_P - C_L)}. \tag{13}$$

Renkin used these equations and the data from Landis and Pappenheimer to estimate the effects of diffusion and bulk flow in the small-pore system of peripheral capillaries. The value $D_S A_W/\Delta X$ was equal to 5×10^{-2} cm^3/(sec × 100 g) and lymph flow was only 6×10^{-4} ml/(sec × 100 g) in Renkin's experiments. Since there was a difference of 10 between diffusional and bulk flow terms (assuming that the volume flow occurred through small holes), then diffusion predominates in the small-pore system (40 Å). When large pores predominate, the lymphatic removal of both albumin and globulin will be increased in proportion to the filtration through the larger pores [92, 103].

If the PA product or L/P ratio remain constant for large molecules, then the protein movement is not occurring through large leaks, since some sieving should be observed. Renkin feels that the large-pore system is actually endothelial vesicular transport [57, 92, 103].

Garlick and Renkin [57] increased filtration in a hind limb preparation and observed that the PA product (left term in Equation 11) remained constant. Protein flux $(\dot{Q}_L \cdot C_L)$ can increase, because the tissue protein concentration decreases and increases ΔC across the capillary membrane. Filtration through large pores or slits should increase the protein flux over and above the increase in ΔC. Renkin explained his experimental findings on vesicular transport. Lassen has recently challenged this concept [102]; however, Lassen uses total body lymph for his argument. It may be safely assumed that this represents predominantly liver and intestinal protein flows, and Mayerson has shown these to have large-pore systems [91].

The use of L/P ratios or PA products is helpful if the experimental model can be investigated in a variety of conditions, such as increased filtration pressure or conditions that should only change pore dimensions. However, L/P ratios could be quite erroneous if lymph does not reflect tissue fluid. The protein flux calculated from the product of lymph flow and lymph concentration is not affected by any concentrating mechanism of the lymphatics and can be used to estimate permeability coefficients (P_P).

An equivalent pore model calculated from L/P ratios can be quite misleading. Boyd's original data were described as two distinct sets of large pores for lung tissue. Of course this is true. But how many of these large pores are necessary to give the experimental results? Only a very small amount of protein enters the lymph per hour. The most logical interpretation of these data is that the lung has two large-pore distributions, but also a small-pore system. But since the lung has such a tremendous capillary surface area, then the number of large pores relative to the small-pore system is great enough to account for lymphatic protein although their total area is still very small.

For $\dot{Q}_P$ or L/P ratios to be calculated, the system must be in a steady state and this had led to controversy about peripheral tissues (see Haddy [100] and Renkin [103]). The isolated lung requires about 1.5 to 2 hr to reach a new steady state for lymph protein concentration following elevation of venous pressure. Staub has found that 1 to 2 hr is required for sheep lung to arrive at a steady state following any given transient. Figure 3 demonstrates that lymph flow reaches a new steady state much more rapidly than protein concentration, so both of these parameters must be at a steady state following a transient so that lymphatic data, not just lymph flow, can be interpreted. Renkin has found that 40 min is the time needed to reach a new steady state [57] in a paw preparation; and Mortillaro [75] has found that 30 to 40 min is needed for the intestine to reach a new steady state.

Finally, if surface area instead of P_P increases during some experimental maneuver, then other indicators of surface-area changes are necessary for separating the effect, such as measurements of KF_{MV}. A recent article by Diana shows what is necessary for calculating changes in surface area relative to P_P changes [19, 23].

C. "Stretched Pores"?

Renkin, in a recent article [103], has pointed out that in some capillary beds intercellular gap widening, or "stretched pores" [108], is a distinct possibility. This reveals another subject on which experimental findings for different experimental lung models do not agree.

Pietra et al. [109] demonstrated that hemoglobin and horseradish peroxidase did not easily enter pulmonary interstitial spaces at normal pulmonary arterial pressure. As arterial pressure was increased, the horseradish peroxidase and hemoglobin tracer easily crossed the membrane through the slits between endothelial cells. Pietra's observations were made on dog lung and there are few data about this animal relative to P products of albumin or large globulins following increases of microvascular pressure.

Figure 3 shows some data obtained in our laboratory. The initial A/G ratio for lymph fluid was 0.70; as the filtration proceeded and the protein content of the lymph decreased to 2.5 g/100 ml the A/G ratio decreased to 0.52. In six other experiments, similar results were obtained, indicating that globulin flows increased with elevated P_{MV}, a finding consistent with "pore stretching." Parving et al. [110] have recently provided results for "pore stretching" of systemic capillaries following acute volume expansion.

Erdmann and associates [67] found no increases in the flux of globulin fractions relative to albumin after elevations of left atrial pressure in sheep lung; in fact, they still observed selectivity among the various protein fractions at elevated left atrial pressures. Thus it appears that a large-pore system exists in sheep lung without "pore stretching," although the data of Boyd [106] as recently analyzed by Michel [111] appear also to be consistent with some vesicular transport.

Again, the data on protein flows collected from dog and sheep lungs are quite different. The data from dog lungs are very scant, however, whereas there are considerable data for intact sheep lung. The data accumulated for isolated dog lungs indicate that proteins can cross the microvascular barrier via a population of small and large pores, and that a "stretched-pore" effect can be seen with elevations of P_{MV}. Before this problem can be adequately resolved, the removal by the lymphatics of several molecular species must be studied in dog lungs for a variety of experimental conditions.

D. Equivalent-Pore Models

The data of Staub and associates are the most complete on transvascular flux of proteins across the pulmonary microvascular membrane in any species. They have calculated that three distributions of pores exist in sheep pulmonary microvascular membrane: 1300 20-Å-radius small pores per one intermediate pore of 125 Å radius and one pore of 1000-Å radius per 100,000 intermediate pores. Staub [1] states that these findings also agree substantially with the findings of Boyd et al. [105, 106] and of Humphreys et al. [112].

In a previous study, we tried to determine the equivalent or effective pore radius of the pulmonary exchange vessels in isolated dog lung [60]. The approach of Kedem and Katchalsky [2] and Vargas and Johnson [113] was used to analyze the osmotic transients produced by small lipid insoluble substances.

First, KF_{MV} was determined in each isogravimetric lung. Then the lung was perfused with a known concentration of the test molecule ($\Delta\pi$). The initial slope of the osmotic weight transient $(\Delta W/dt)_0$ was then analyzed to obtain σMV_i from the following relations:

$$\left(\frac{\Delta W}{\Delta t}\right)_0 = KF_{MV}\sigma MV_i\Delta\pi_i$$

or

$$\sigma MV_i = \frac{(\Delta W/\Delta t)_0}{KF_{MV}\Delta\pi_i}. \tag{14}$$

The calculated σ_{MV} for three small molecules was very small, and the effective pore was estimated to have a radius of 50 to 60 Å. Chapter 8 in this text provides new data from the work of Effros, Perl, and Chinard. They were able to obtain a much larger value for $(\Delta W/\Delta t)_0$ in their preparation. Our osmotic transients have always demonstrated a perfusion artifact, and it may well be that many events occurred at the pulmonary exchange vessels before we measured $(\Delta W/\Delta t)_0$. The new findings are more compatible with a larger contribution of water flow through endothelial cells, as well as between them. It is evident from this discussion that we do not know the dimensions of the small-pore system, and any particular model of pore sizes is in no way a clear-cut solution. More data must be collected, especially for large molecules, so that the effective dimensions of the small-pore system can be established.

The indicator dilution techniques have not proved useful in estimating the permeability coefficients of the pulmonary capillary membrane for small solutes since the extraction is very small. The concentration of protein in lymph can be used to calculate $P_P A$, but we do not know the surface area of the exchange vessels.

Staub and associates have calculated a permeability coefficient for albumin and globulin of 0.046×10^{-7} cm/sec and 0.01×10^{-7} cm/sec. The data of Taylor et al. [107] and Boonyaprakob et al. [114] can be used to estimate permeability coefficients for albumin of 0.15×10^{-7} cm/sec for the lung of adult dogs and 0.33×10^{-7} cm/sec for puppy lung.

IV. General Model of Protein and Fluid Movement

We have so far assumed that P_{MV}, P_{PMV}, and π_{PMV} are uniform in lung. This assumption would be valid if the lung were perfused at the same arterial and venous pressure at each level. The work of West and associates [115] demonstrates that this is not the case; there are different perfusing pressures in the dependent zones of the lung relative to apical regions.

West has defined three different zones for an upright lung: (1) zone III, for which the pulmonary venous pressure is greater than the alveolar pressure and in which flow is determined by the difference between pulmonary venous and arterial pressures; (2) zone II, for which alveolar pressure is greater than venous pressure and in which flow is determined by the difference between arterial and alveolar pressures; and (3) zone I, for which alveolar pressure exceeds the arterial pressure at that level and no flow occurs.

The average distance from the bottom to the top of the lung is about 15 cm in the standing dog. The left atrium is located one-third the distance up the chest wall as measured from the sternum in the standing dog. Since pulmonary arterial pressure averages 20 mmHg in dogs (27 cm H_2O) and left atrial pressures averages 8 mmHg (11 cm H_2O) (relative to the left atrium), then the dog lung is in a zone III condition.

At different lung levels, even a zone III condition, the arterial pressure will change. At the bottom of the lung, the pulmonary arterial pressure will be 31 cm H_2O and at the apex only 17 cm H_2O. The pulmonary venous pressure will be 15 cm H_2O at the base of the lung and decrease to 1 cm H_2O at the top of the lung. Since the pressures vary at each lung level, then microvascular pressure will be different at each lung level. Using the resistance of the arteries and veins as measured by Gaar [16], P_{MV} is calculated as 21.4 at the base of the dog lung and 7.4 at the apex. Our latest work indicates that P_{MV} at the base of the lung may be very close to venous pressure rather than an estimate of P_{MV} using:

$$P_{MV} = P_{LA} + 0.4 (P_{PA} - P_{LA}). \tag{15}$$

Staub has recently presented a model that incorporates pressure changes at various lung heights in order to interpret lymph data. Obviously the more dependent zones of the lung should filter more than the upper regions of the lung; but to calculate the amount of filtration at each lung level, one must know P_{PMV} and π_{PMV}. Staub assumes that P_{PMV} is zero, which we feel may not be correct. We believe that P_{PMV} will become more negative at upper lung levels. The value P_{PMV} obtained is -4 cm H_2O at the bottom of the lung, contrasted with -18 cm H_2O at the uppermost portion of the lung.

One major objection to our contention is that the septal P_{PMV} does not have to be subatmospheric, since flow continually occurs from the septal to the junctional tissues. A pressure drop associated with this flow can be calculated and is small; however, many assumptions must be made to make this calculation and the assumptions used in the calculation have not been experimentally tested.

Since Staub's model assumes no difference in P_{PMV} at different lung levels, he has made the assumption that π_{PMV} increases in the apical regions of the lungs. This could certainly be so; but if it is so, how much do the apical regions of the lungs filter? How much protein leaks into the tissue spaces in this region? These are variables that we do not understand at present. Our simple model would yield a π_{PMV} of about 9 cm H_2O at each lung level; if less filtration occurs at the top of the lung, then P_{PMV} would be less negative and π_{PMV} would increase.

The total lymph flow from the lung could be partitioned into each lung level if ΔP_{drop} and the capillary surface area were known for each level. But with the uncertainties of P_{PMV} and π_{PMV}, only a very biased model can be constructed.

The different capillary pressures at each lung level indicate that most lymph is probably formed in the dependent zones of the lung and that only during systole are the upper zones filtering. If total lymph flow is divided by some average drop, using an average capillary pressure to calculate ΔP_{drop}, then KF_{MV} calculated by this procedure will be underestimated. If it is also assumed that the entire lung is filtering, then another serious error is introduced into the calculation of KF_{MV}. If the lymph from the upper regions of the lung is high in protein and combines with lymph of a lower concentration from the lower regions of the lung, then π_{PMV} will be overestimated.

If lymph protein is used to calculate the permeability coefficient of lung, then P_P may be seriously underestimated, since the protein may not be uniformly crossing the capillary membranes in each lung zone. Since the filtration characteristics of arterial and venous extra-alveolar vessels and septal capillaries are quite different, then the arterial and venous protein fluxes would be quite different at each lung level.

The problems associated with the uneven blood flow distribution in different zones become even more acute when one is dealing with the human lung. For what is the capillary pressure in zone I and in zone II conditions? Obviously, we must depend on some average computation and only a model approach such as Staub used will allow us to gain any insight into this very difficult and interesting physiologic problem.

V. Conclusion

We have tried to show the basic approaches used in physiology to study fluid and protein movement across the microvascular system. Problems exist with each approach, both physically and physiologically. Our review is intended not as a negative criticism of permeability work conducted on the lung, but as an indicator of areas for which new or more rigorous experimental approaches are necessary.

Three basic questions remain to be answered by some experimental approach: (1) How is lymph fluid related to tissue fluid? (2) What is the perimicrovascular pressure in the septal regions of lung? (3) What are the dimensions of the small-pore system in lung? Question 1 can best be answered by an anatomical approach coupled with physiologic measurements. Perhaps applying fluorescent antibody techniques for albumin or globulin will allow an interpretation of lymph protein concentration relative to tissue protein concentration. Question 2 is even more difficult to answer; but if we can relate lymph fluid to tissue fluid, then a force balance study similar to investigations in Staub's laboratory and ours can at least establish some average perimicrovascular pressure.

The dimensions of the small-pore system are beginning to emerge from the recent work of Effros (Chapter 8), Chinard [71], and Perl [65], but larger molecules must be investigated in lung to measure adequately the restriction characteristics of the small pores. The approach using lymph data coupled with isogravimetric procedures should yield results that can be interpreted more concisely.

The computer approach of Staub is the only way that experimental findings can be coupled to events that occur in the intact lung, because of the extreme difficulty in assessing pulmonary blood flow, pressures, and microvascular forces. Until these parameters are estimated to a better degree, then we must rely on some simple model to relate tissue colloid osmotic pressure, perimicrovascular pressure, and lymph flow to interstitial volume changes seen following elevation of left atrial pressure.

Finally, I feel that an experimental preparation using different lung zones must be developed in order that data obtained in vitro can be extrapolated to intact animal and human lungs.

Acknowledgments

We should like to thank Ms. Pamela Collins for her preparation of this manuscript and Dr. B. Cook for his many helpful discussions.

References

1. N. C. Staub, Pulmonary edema, *Physiol. Rev.*, **54**:678 (1974).
2. O. Kedem and A. Katchalsky, Thermodynamic analysis of the permeability of biological membranes to nonelectrolytes, *Biochim. Biophys. Acta*, **27**:229-246 (1958).
3. A. Katchalsky and P. F. Curran. *Nonequilibrium Thermodynamics in Biophysics.* Cambridge, Mass.: Harvard University Press, 1965.
4. C. C. Guyton and A. W. Lindsey, Effect of elevated left atrial pressure and decreased plasma protein concentration of the development of pulmonary edema, *Circ. Res.*, **7**:649-657 (1959).
5. O. R. Levine, R. B. Mellins, and A. P. Fishman, Quantitative assessment of pulmonary edema, *Circ. Res.*, **17**:414-426 (1965).
6. O. R. Levine, R. B. Mellins, R. M. Senior, and A. P. Fishman, The application of Starling's law of capillary exchange to the lungs, *J. Clin. Invest.*, **46**:934-944 (1967).
7. N. C. Staub, H. Nagano, and M. L. Pearce, Pulmonary edema in dogs, especially the sequence of fluid accumulation in the lungs, *J. Appl. Physiol.*, **22**:227-240 (1967).
8. A. E. Taylor and K. A. Gaar, Jr., Measurement of the hydraulic conductivity of the pulmonary capillary membrane in the isolated lung, *Proceedings of the International Union of Physiological Sciences*, **7**:43A (1968).
9. J. P. Szidon, G. G. Pietra, and A. P. Fishman, The alveolar-capillary membrane and pulmonary edema, *N. E. J. Med.*, **286**:1200-1204 (1972).
10. A. J. Staverman, The theory of measurement of osmotic pressure, *Rec. Trans. Chim.*, **70**:344-352 (1951).

11. E. M. Landis, Microinjection studies of capillary blood pressure in human skin, *Heart,* **15**:209-228 (1930).

12. E. M. Landis and J. R. Pappenheimer, Exchange of substances through the capillary walls. In *Handbook of Physiology,* Vol. 2, Section 2. Baltimore, Waverly Press, 1963, pp. 961-1034.

13. M. Intaglietta and B. W. Zweifach, Microcirculatory basis of fluid exchange. In *Advances in Biological and Medicine Physics,* Vol. 15. New York and London, Academic Press, 1974, pp. 111-155.

14. B. W. Zweifach, Microcirculation, *Annu. Rev. Physiol.,* **35**:117-150 (1973).

15. J. R. Pappenheimer and A. Soto-Rivera, Effective osmotic pressure of the plasma proteins and other quantities associated with the capillary circulation in the hind limb of cats and dogs, *Amer. J. Physiol.,* **152**:471-491 (1948).

16. K. A. Gaar, Jr., A. E. Taylor, L. J. Owens, and A. C. Guyton, Pulmonary capillary pressure and filtration coefficient in the isolated perfused lung, *Amer. J. Physiol.,* **213**:910-914 (1967).

17. K. A. Gaar, Jr., A. E. Taylor, And A. C. Guyton, Effect of lung edema on pulmonary capillary pressure, *Amer. J. Physiol.,* **216**:1370-1373 (1969).

18. P. C. Johnson and K. M. Hanson, Capillary filtration in the small intestine of the dog, *Circ. Res.,* **19**:766 (1966).

19. J. N. Diana and M. H. Laughlin, Effect of ischemia on capillary pressure and equivalent pore radius in capillaries of the isolated dog hind limb, *Circ. Res.,* **35**:77-101 (1974).

20. A. C. Guyton, A concept of negative interstitial pressure based on pressures in implanted perforated capsules, *Circ. Res.,* **12**:399-414 (1963).

21. P. C. Johnson, Effect of venous pressure on mean capillary pressure and vascular resistance in the intestine, *Circ. Res.,* **16**:294-300 (1965).

22. G. J. Grega, R. M. Daugherty, Jr., J. B. Scott, D. P. Radawski, and F. J. Haddy, Effect of pressure, flow, and vasoactive agents on vascular resistance and capillary filtration in the canine fetal, newborn, and adult lung, *Microvasc. Res.,* **3**:297-307 (1971).

23. J. N. Diana, S. C. Long, and H. Yao, Effect of histamine on equivalent pore radius in capillaries of isolated dog hind limb, *Microvasc. Res.,* **4**: 413-437 (1972).

24. G. L. Miller, R. L. Kline, J. B. Scott, E. J. Haddy, and G. J. Grega, Canine forelimb lymph flow and protein concentration following the relief of prolonged ischemia, *Physiologist,* **16**:397 (1973).

25. D. M. Nicoloff, H. M. Ballin, and M. B. Visscher, Hypoxia and edema of the perfused canine lung, *Proc. Soc. Exp. Biol. Med.,* **131**:22-26 (1969).

26. A. B. Fisher, R. W. Hyde, and J. S. Reif, Insensitivity of the alveolar septum to local hypoxia, *Amer. J. Physiol.,* **223**:770-776 (1972).

27. S. Permutt, P. Caldini, A. Maseri, W. H. Palmer, T. Sasamori, and K. Zierler, Recruitment versus distensibility in the pulmonary vascular bed. In *The Pulmonary Circulation and Interstitial Space.* Chicago, University of Chicago Press, 1969, pp. 375-390.

28. E. Agostoni and J. Piiper, Capillary pressure and distribution of vascular resistance in isolated lung. *Amer. J. Physiol.,* **22**:1033-1036 (1962).
29. W. F. Hamilton, R. A. Woodbury, and E. Vogt, Differential pressures in the lesser circulation of the unanesthetized dog, *Amer. J. Physiol.,* **125**: 130-141 (1939).
30. J. W. Prather, K. A. Gaar, Jr., and A. C. Guyton, Direct continuous recording of plasma colloid osmotic pressure of whole blood, *J. Appl. Physiol.,* **24**:602-605 (1968).
31. M. Intaglietta and B. W. Zweifach, Measurement of blood plasma colloid osmotic pressure. I. Technical aspects, *Microvasc. Res.,* **3**:72-82 (1971).
32. K. Aukland, Autoregulation of interstitial fluid volume: Edema-preventing mechanisms, *Scand. J. Clin. Lab. Invest.,* **31**:247-254 (1973).
33. J. S. Calnan, P. M. Ford, P. J. L. Holt, and J. J. Pflug, Implanted tissue cages—A study in rabbits, *Brit. J. Plast. Surg.,* **23**:164-174 (1972).
34. K. Kirsch, W. Rafflenbeul, and H. Roedel, Untersuchungen zur Ursache des negativen interstitiellen Gewebsdruckes (Gyton-Kapsel). *Pflug. Arch.,* **328**:193-204 (1971).
35. J. W. Prather, D. N. Bowes, D. A. Warrell, and B. W. Zweifach, Comparison of capsule and wick techniques for measurement of interstitial fluid pressure, *J. Appl. Physiol.,* **31**:942-945 (1971).
36. A. E. Taylor, W. H. Gibson, H. J. Granger, and A. C. Guyton, The interaction between intracapillary and tissue forces in the overall regulation of interstitial fluid volume, *Lymphology,* **6**:192-208 (1973).
37. J. J. Ladegaard-Pederson, Measurement of the interstitial pressure in subcutaneous tissue in dogs, *Circ. Res.,* **26**:765-770 (1970).
38. P. F. Scholander, A. R. Hargens, and S. L. Miller, Negative pressure in the interstitial fluid of animals, *Science,* **161**:321-328 (1968).
39. P. D. Snashall, J. Lucas, A. Guz, and M. A. Floyer, Measurements of interstitial "fluid" pressure by means of a cotton wick in man and animals, *Clin. Sci.,* **41**:35-53 (1971).
40. S. B. Stromme, J. E. Maggert, and P. F. Scholander, Interstitial fluid pressure in terrestrial and semiterrestrial animals, *J. Appl. Physiol.,* **27**: 123-126 (1969).
41. C. A. Wiederhielm and Burt V. Weston, Microvascular, lymphatic, and tissue pressures in the unanesthetized mammal, *Amer. J. Physiol.,* **225**: 992-996 (1973).
42. B. J. Meyer, A. Meyer, and A. C. Guyton, Interstitial fluid pressure. V. Negative pressure in the lungs, *Circ. Res.,* **22**:263-271 (1968).
43. N. C. Staub, The pathophysiology of pulmonary edema, *Human Path.,* **1**: 419-432 (1970).
44. E. Agostoni, Mechanics of the pleural space, *Physiol. Rev.,* **52**:57-128 (1972).
45. A. C. Guyton and T. G. Coleman, Regulation of interstitial fluid volume and pressure, *Ann. N. Y. Acad. Sci.,* **150**:537-547 (1968).
46. A. C. Guyton, H. J. Granger, and A. E. Taylor, Interstial fluid pressure, *Physiol. Rev.,* **51**:527-563 (1971).

47. A. C. Guyton, A. E. Taylor, H. J. Granger, and W. H. Gibson, Regulation of interstitial fluid volume and pressure. In *Neurohumoral and Metabolic Aspects of Injury.* New York, Plenum Publishing Corp., 1973, pp. 111-118.

48. A. E. Guyton, A. E. Taylor, and H. J. Granger, Analysis of types of pressure in the pulmonary spaces: Interstitial fluid pressure, solid tissue pressure and total tissue pressure. In *Central Hemodynamics and Gas Exchange.* Turin, Minerva Medica, 1971, pp. 41-55.

49. J. M. B. Hughes, Pulmonary interstitial pressure, *Bull. Physio-Path. Resp.,* 7:1095-1123 (1971).

50. R. B. Mellins, O. R. Levine, R. Skalak, and A. P. Fishman, Interstitial pressure of the lung, *Circ. Res.,* 24:197-212 (1969).

51. M. F. Warren and C. K. Drinker, The flow of lymph from the lungs of the dog, *Amer. J. Physiol.,* **136**:207-221 (1942).

52. O. R. Levine, R. B. Dell, E. Bowe, and A. I. Hyman, Pulmonary extravascular chloride space and albumin content in adult dogs and puppies, *Ped. Res.,* 8:270-274 (1974).

53. T. R. Vaughan, Jr., A. J. Erdmann, and N. C. Staub, Subdivisions of lung extravascular water space and calculated interstitial albumin concentration in sheep, *Fed. Proc.,* **30**:379 (1971).

54. P. C. Johnson and D. R. Richardson, The influence of venous pressure on filtration forces in the intestine, *Microvasc. Res.,* 7:296-306 (1974).

55. A. E. Taylor and H. Gibson, Model of the concentrating ability of the lymphatic vessels, *Lymphology* 8:43-49 (1975).

56. H. J. Granger, J. Dhar, and H. I. Chen. Structure and function of interstitium. In *Proceedings of the Albumin Workshop.* J. T. Sgouris and A. René, eds., Division of Blood Resources N.H.L. Institute, Bethesda, Maryland, pp. 114-125, 1975.

57. D. G. Garlick and E. M. Renkin, Transport of large molecules from plasma to interstitial fluid and lymph in dogs, *Amer. J. Physiol.,* **219**:1595-1065 (1970).

58. J. R. Pappenheimer, E. M. Renkin, and L. M. Borrero, Filtration, diffusion and molecular sieving through peripheral capillary membranes, *Amer. J. Physiol.,* **167**:13-46 (1951).

59. O. R. Levine, F. Rodriguez-Martinez, and R. B. Mellins, Fluid filtration in the lung of the intact puppy, *J. Appl. Physiol.,* 34:683-686 (1973).

60. A. E. Taylor and K. A. Gaar, Jr., Calculation of equivalent pore radii of the pulmonary capillary and alveolar membranes, *Revista Argent. Angio.,* 3:26-40 (1969).

61. A. E. Taylor and K. A. Gaar, Jr., Estimation of equivalent pore radii of pulmonary capillary and alveolar membranes, *Amer. J. Physiol.,* **218**:1133-1140 (1970).

62. P. K. M. Lunde and B. A. Waaler, Transvascular fluid balance in the lung, *J. Physiol.,* **205**:1-18 (1969).

63. G. Bφ, A. Hauge, G. Nicolaysen, and B. A. Waaler, Does interstitial lung edema cause changes in lung compliance? *N. E. J. Med.,* **289**:218-219 (1973).

64.   P. Uter, U. Kotzerke, and W. Schoedel, Filtration von Flussigheit durch die Alveolar-Capillar-Schranke in der isolierten Hundenlunge, *Pflug. Arch.*, 289:174-179 (1966).

65.   W. Perl, P. Chowdhury, and F. P. Chinard, Reflection coefficients of dog lung and endothelium to small hydrophilic solutes, *Am. J. Physiol.*, 228: 797-809 (1975).

66.   P. C. Weiser and F. Grande, Estimation of fluid shifts and protein permeability during pulmonary edemagenesis, *Amer. J. Physiol.*, 225:1028-1034 (1974).

67.   A. J. Erdmann, III, T. R. Vaughn, W. C. Wolverton, K. L. Brigham, and N. C. Staub, Effect of increased vascular pressure on lung fluid balance in unanesthetized sheep, *Circ. Res.*, 37:271-284 (1975).

68.   L. D. Iliff, Extra-alveolar vessels and oedema development in excised dog lungs, *J. Physiol.*, 207:85P-86P (1970).

69.   G. Majno and G. E. Palade, Studies on inflammation. I. Effect of histamine and serotonin on vascular permeability: An electron microscopic study, *J. Biophys. Biochem. Cytol.*, 11:571-606 (1961).

70.   R. P. Durbin, Osmotic flow of water across permeable cellulose membranes, *J. Gen. Physiol.*, 44:315-326 (1960).

71.   F. P. Chinard, W. Perl, and R. M. Effros, Pulmonary endothelial membrane characteristics: Temperature effects, *Fed. Proc.*, 33:412 (1974).

72.   N. Lifson, Revised equations for the osmotic transient method. In *Capillary Permeability*. New York, Academic Press, 1970, pp. 302-305.

73.   D. C. Tosteson, *Discussion*. In *Capillary Permeability*. New York, Academic Press, 1970, pp. 658-664.

74.   E. F. Grabowski, Osmotic weight transients in myocardium: A convective diffusion model. In *Proceedings of the 1974 Summer Computer Simulation Conference*, 1974, pp. 618-688.

75.   N. A. Mortillaro and A. E. Taylor, Edema safety factor in intesting, *Fed. Proc.*, 33:411 (1974).

76.   H. H. Uhley, S. E. Leeds, J. J. Sampson, and M. Friedman, Right duct lymph flow in dogs measured by a new method, *Dis. Chest*, 37:532-534 (1960).

77.   A. S. Hendin, Postmortem demonstration of inspiratory constriction of deep lymphatic vessels of the human lung, *Invest. Radio.*, 9:1-6 (1974).

78.   A. S. Hendin and R. H. Greenspan, Ventilatory pumping of human pulmonary lymphatic vessels, *Radiology*, 108:553-557 (1973).

79.   J. Rusznyák, M. Földi, and G. Szabó, Lymphatics and lymph circulation. In *Physiology and Pathology*. 2nd ed. Oxford, Pergamon Press, 1967.

80.   J. M. Yoffey and F. C. Courtice. *Lymphatics, Lymph and the Lymphomyeloid Complex*. London, Academic Press, 1970.

81.   E. C. Meyer and R. Ottaviano, Right lymphatic duct distribution volume in dogs. Relationship to pulmonary interstitial volume, *Circ. Res.*, 35: 197-203 (1974).

82.   K. Oka, Experimental studies on the pulmonary edema investigation with special reference to permeability of the pulmonary capillary from the standpoint of pulmonary lymphatic return, *Jap. Cir. J.*, 37:1343-1354 (1973).

83. A. C. Guyton, Interstitial fluid pressure. II. Pressure-volume curves of interstitial space, *Circ. Res.,* **16**:452-460 (1965).

84. A. C. Guyton, Interstitial fluid pressure-volume relationships and their regulation. In *Ciba Foundation Symposium on Circulatory and Respiratory Mass Transport.* London, A. J. Churchill, 1969, pp. 4-20.

85. A. C. Guyton, I. Compliance of the interstitial space and the measurement of tissue pressure, *Pflug. Arch. Suppl.,* **336**:S1-S20 (1972).

86. A. C. Guyton, Pulmonary alveolar-capillary interface and interstitium. Introduction to Part I. In *The Pulmonary Circulation and Interstitial Space.* Chicago, University of Chicago Press, 1969, pp. 3-7.

87. N. C. Staub, T. R. Vaughan, Jr., A. J. Erdmann, III, K. L. Brigham, and W. C. Wolverton, Evidence for high efficiency and sensitivity of the lung's lymph pump in unanesthetized sheep, *Microvasc. Res.,* **4**:331 (1972).

88. C. L. Witte, Y. C. Chung, M. H. Witte, O. F. Sterle, and W. R. Cole, Observations on the origin of ascites from experimental extrahepatic portal congestion, *Ann. Surg.,* **170**:1002-1015 (1969).

89. H. N. Uhley, S. E. Leeds, J. J. Sampson, and M. Friedman, Role of pulmonary lymphatics in chronic pulmonary edema, *Circ. Res.,* **11**:966-970 (1962).

90. H. N. Uhley, S. E. Leeds, J. J. Sampson, N. Rudo, and M. Friedman, The temporal sequence of lymph flow in the right lymphatic duct in experimental chronic pulmonary edema, *Amer. Heart J.,* **72**:214-217 (1966).

91. H. S. Mayerson, C. G. Wolfram, H. H. Shirley, Jr., and K. Wasserman, Regional differences in capillary permeability, *Amer. J. Physiol.,* **198**: 155-160 (1960).

92. E. M. Renkin, Transport of large molecules across capillary walls, *Physiologist,* **7**:13-28 (1964).

93. E. E. Schneeberger-Keeley and M. J. Karnovsky, The ultrastructural basis of alveolar-capillary membrane permeability to peroxidase used as a tracer, *J. Cell Biol.,* **37**:781-793 (1968).

94. E. E. Schneeberger-Keeley and M. J. Karnovsky, The influence of intravascular fluid volume on the permeability of newborn and adult mouse lungs to ultrastructural protein tracers, *J. Cell Biol.,* **49**:319-334 (1971).

95. N. Simionescu, M. Simionescu, and G. E. Palade, Permeability of muscle capillaries to exogenous myoglobin, *J. Cell Biol.,* **57**:424-452 (1973).

96. H. Themann, G. Keuker, and V. Westphal, Elektronenmikroscopische Untersuchungen zuer Permeation exogerer Peroxidase durch das Endothel der herzmuskel Kapillaren, *Cytobiologie,* **3**:13 (1971).

97. E. M. Renkin, Filtration, diffusion and molecular sieving through porous cellulose membranes, *J. Gen. Physiol.,* **38**:225-243 (1954).

98. R. D. Carter, W. L. Joyner, and E. M. Renkin, Effects of histamine and some other substances on molecular selectivity of the capillary wall to plasma proteins and dextran, *Microvasc. Res.,* **7**:31-48 (1974).

99. G. Grotte, Passage of dextran molecules across the blood-lymph barrier, *Acta Chir. Scand. Suppl.,* **211**:1-84 (1956).

100. F. J. Haddy, J. B. Scott, and G. J. Grega, Effects of histamine on lymph protein concentration and flow in the dog forelimb, *Amer. J. Physiol.,* 223:1172-1177 (1972).

101. W. L. Joyner, R. D. Carter, G. S. Raizes, and E. M. Renkin, Influence of histamine and some other substances on blood lymph transport of plasma protein and dextran in the dog paw, *Microvasc. Res.,* 7:19-30 (1974).

102. N. A. Lassen, H. H. Parving, and N. Rossing, Filtration as the main mechanism of overall transcapillary protein escape from the plasma, *Microvasc. Res.,* 7:i-iv (1974).

103. E. M. Renkin, R. D. Carter, and W. L. Joyner, Mechanism of the sustained action of histamine and bradykinin on transport of large molecules across capillary walls in the dog paw, *Microvasc. Res.,* 7:49-60 (1974).

104. K. Wasserman, L. Loeb, and H. S. Mayerson, Capillary permeability to macromolecules, *Circ. Res.,* 3:549-603 (1955).

105. R. D. H. Boyd, J. R. Hill, P. W. Humphreys, I. C. S. Normand, E. O. R. Reynolds, and L. B. Strang, Permeability of lung capillaries to macro-molecules in foetal and newborn lambs and sheep, *J. Physiol.,* 201: 567-588 (1969).

106. R. D. H. Boyd, J. R. Hill, P. W. Humphreys, I. C. S. Normand, E. O. R. Reynolds and L. B. Strang, Passage of large molecules from lung capil-laries to lymph in fetal and newborn lambs and sheep. In *The Pulmonary Circulation and Interstitial Space.* Chicago, University of Chicago Press, 1969.

107. P. M. Taylor, U. Boonyaprakov, V. Waterman, D. Watson, and E. Lopata, Clearances of plasma proteins from pulmonary vascular beds of adult dogs and pups, *Amer. J. Physiol.,* 213:441-449 (1967).

108. H. H. Shirley, C. G. Wolfram, K. Wasserman, and H. S. Mayerson, Capil-lary permeability to macromolecules: Stretched pore phenomenon, *Amer. J. Physiol.,* 190:189-193 (1957).

109. G. G. Pietra, J. P. Szidon, M. M. Leventhal, and J. P. Fishman, Hemo-globin as a tracer in hemodynamic pulmonary edema, *Science,* 166: 1643-1646 (1969).

110. H. H. Parving, S. L. Nielsen, and N. A. Lassen, Increased transcapillary escape rate of albumin, IgG and IgM after acute volume expansion in man, *Amer. J. Physiol.,* in press.

111. C. C. Michel, Flows across the capillary wall. In *Cardiovascular Fluid Dynamics.* Vol. 2. New York, Academic Press, 1972, pp. 241-298.

112. P. W. Humphreys, I. C. S. Normand, E. O. R. Reynolds, and L. B. Strang, Pulmonary lymph flow and the uptake of liquid from the lungs of the lamb at the start of breathing, *J. Physiol.,* 193:1-29 (1967).

113. F. Vargas and J. A. Johnson, An estimate of reflection coefficients for rabbit heart capillaries, *J. Gen. Physiol.,* 47:667-677 (1964).

114. U. Boonyaprakob, P. M. Taylor, D. W. Watson, V. Waterman, and E. Lopata, Hypoxia and protein clearance from the pulmonary vascular beds of adult dogs and pups, *Amer. J. Physiol.,* 216:1013-1019 (1969).

115. J. B. West, C. T. Dollery, and A. Naimark, Distribution of blood flow in isolated lung; relation to vascular and alveolar pressures, *J. Appl. Physiol.,* 19:713-724 (1964).

7

Effect of Pulmonary Edema
on Distribution of Blood Flow in the Lung

JAMES C. HOGG

McGill University
Montreal, Quebec, Canada

I. Introduction

In a classic study on the effect of noxious gases on the lung, Sir Joseph Barcroft [3] stated, "The pathology of gas poisoning has been full of surprises but never was I more surprised than when I discovered that it was possible for a goat to live with its arterial blood fully, or almost fully, oxygenated, but with its lung four times its ordinary weight." He went on to speculate in what must have been one of the earliest statements of the ventilation-perfusion concept, that this could only be so if the blood flow to the edematous regions of the lung was markedly reduced (Fig. 1). Although gas poisoning probably causes pulmonary edema by increasing capillary permeability, in high-pressure pulmonary edema gas exchange is equally maintained until gross edema occurs, so that interference with gas exchange by edema is an abrupt terminal event [2, 3]. Just how blood flow is shifted away from edematous lung regions is the topic for consideration in this chapter and to discuss it effectively the mechanical factors thought to control blood flow must be considered.

The quantity of blood flowing through a given region of the lung is determined by the resistance of the vessels in that region and the driving pressure

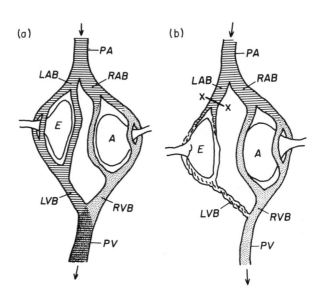

FIGURE 1 PA = pulmonary artery. PV = pulmonary vein. LAB and RAB = right and left arterial branches. LVB and RVB = right and left venous branches. E = edema. A = air. Barcroft noted that if blood flow were not decreased through the edematous regions, marked unsaturation of the pulmonary venous blood should occur (a). He observed no such desaturation in his experiments, and concluded that blood flow was reduced in the edematous areas, with most of the flow going to air-containing tissue (b). Reprinted from J. Barcroft, *J. Royal Army Med. Corps,* **34**:155-173 (1920), by courtesy of the publishers.

causing blood to flow through them. Therefore, if pulmonary edema were to affect the blood flow received by a particular lung region, it must do so either by changing the resistance of the vessels in that region or by changing the pressure driving blood through them. Before considering the possible mechanisms by which pulmonary edema might change the factors responsible for delivering regional blood flow, it may be helpful to review some basic knowledge of flow through tubes. Flow through rigid tubes is governed by the Poiseuille equation, which can be written

$$\text{flow} = \Delta P \times \frac{\Pi}{8} \times \frac{1}{\eta} \times \frac{r^4}{1}$$

where ΔP is the pressure difference between two intramural points, $1/\eta$ is a factor relating to the viscosity of the fluid, and $r^4/1$ is a geometric factor relating to the radius of the vessel r and its length l. This equation is not strictly applicable to distensible tubes such as blood vessels because an increase in driving pressure will increase the intraluminal pressure so that the vessel will dilate and lengthen. The geometric factor of the Poiseuille equation $r^4/1$ indicates that the effect of small changes in radius of the vessel will markedly change flow because the effect is related to the fourth power of the radius. Length changes, on the other hand, will have a much smaller effect in the other direction so that the overall effect of increasing the transmural pressure of the vessel will be to decrease vascular resistance and increase flow.

II. Resistance of the Alveolar and Extra-alveolar Vessels

A. General

As the transmural pressure of the pulmonary blood vessels is of primary importance in determining their resistance, it is important to consider the magnitude and nature of pressure surrounding the pulmonary blood vessels. In most organs, the variation in transmural pressure of blood vessels is related chiefly to changes in intravascular pressure, since interstitial pressure is nearly constant. In the lung, on the other hand, the pressure outside the vessels is quite variable because the vessels in alveolar walls are for practical purpose surrounded by alveolar gas pressure, whereas the extra-alveolar vessels are surrounded by lung interstitial pressure. Indeed, experimental work from several laboratories [4, 5] suggests that from a mechanical point of view the pulmonary blood vessels can be usefully separated into alveolar and extra-alveolar compartments—because the vessels in these compartments behave differently. For example, it has been shown that vessels in the alveoli decrease as the lung is inflated with positive pressure, and that when alveolar pressure exceeds pulmonary arterial pressure, blood flow ceases because these vessels collapse. The larger vessels in the extra-alveolar compartment, on the other hand, behave differently in that they increase with lung inflation [4, 5]; and this change takes place even when a constant relation is maintained between vascular and alveolar pressure. This change occurs because the appropriate pressure outside the extra-alveolar vessels is lung interstitial pressure, which becomes more negative with lung inflation, so that the transmural pressure of these vessels increases with lung inflation, and they dilate.

In considering the resistance to the blood flow in any lung region, it follows that the extra-alveolar and alveolar vessels will act as two resistances in series and that the resistance of each set of vessels will vary depending on their transmural pressure. As the intravascular pressures are closely similar in both sets of vessels, this difference in behavior occurs because the appropriate surrounding pressure is alveolar gas pressure in the case of the alveolar vessels and lung interstitial pressure in the case of the extra-alveolar vessels.

B.   Alveolar Vessels

Since the pressure surrounding the alveolar vessels is alveolar gas pressure, it can be easily measured and is uniform throughout the lung. These vessels are also easily collapsible and therefore analagous to a sluice [6] or a Starling resistor [7]. West and his colleagues [8] realized that because all the vascular pressures increase from lung top to bottom due to gravity, while alveolar pressure remains constant, the lung could be divided into zones with different resistances. Using as a model the Starling resistor, which behaves as though the driving pressure is the difference between inlet (pulmonary artery pressure) and surrounding pressure (alveolar pressure), they showed that blood flow could be predicted for different lung regions. Obviously, when the alveolar pressure was greater than the pulmonary artery pressure, no flow occurred (zone 1). Blood flow increased rapidly with distance down the lung as long as alveolar pressure was less than arterial pressure but greater than venous pressure (zone II), because gravity steadily increased the driving pressure—the difference between arterial and alveolar pressures in this region. Once venous pressure becomes greater than alveolar pressure (zone III), the driving pressure becomes the difference between arterial and venous pressure, and gravity no longer has the effect of increasing the driving pressure down the lung, since the arterial pressure and the venous pressure increase at the same rate. However, they thought that blood flow continued to increase in zone III because the continually increasing mean vascular pressure caused the blood vessels to dilate and decrease their resistance. Whether or not blood flow continuously increases in zone III will be considered after the extra-alveolar vascular resistance has been discussed.

C.   Extra-alveolar Vessels

The exact pressure acting on the outer surface of an extra-alveolar vessel, in contrast to an alveolar vessel is very difficult to measure but must be an average of the pressures that the solid and liquid components in and around the interstitial space exert on it [9]. The existence of both solid and liquid pressures in the same space can perhaps be best illustrated considering the pressure in the pleural space. The pleural surface pressures is the pressure that prevents the lung from collapsing by its own recoil. The existence of a pleural liquid pressure different from the surface pressure was first appreciated clearly by Setnikar et al. [10, 11], who found that the pressure in the pleural liquid was very much more negative than the pressure required to overcome the elastic recoil of the lung. Agostoni and his colleagues [12] suggested that this very negative liquid pressure was due to the excess of fluid absorption on the visceral pleura over fluid filtration in the parietal pleura. The absorption of liquid pulls the pleural membranes into close apposition, generating solid tissue pressure at the points of contact between visceral pleura and parietal pleura. The pleural surface pressure, therefore, is the sum of the pleural liquid pressure and the pleural solid pressure, and under static conditions this sum is equal and opposite in sign to the elastic recoil of the lung. The pressure surrounding the extra-alveolar vessels can similarly be influenced by the solid and liquid pressures within the extra-alveolar interstitial space. The solid pressures are those transmitted to this space by the surrounding alveolar attachments and the liquid pressures are those related to the liquid that the space contains. An increase in the amount of liquid in the extra-alveolar interstitial space tends to make the pressure in this space more positive and thereby decrease the transmural pressure of the extra-alveolar vessels. West and his colleagues [13, 14] defined a zone at the lung base where flow decreased, and they believed that this region, which they called zone IV, might have an increased resistance because of the collection of fluid around the larger extra-alveolar vessels in the peribronchovascular space. It is possible that fluid might collect preferentially in the interstitial space at the lung base either because of greater transcapillary exchange in this region or because of poorer lymphatic drainage out of the lung base. The crude methods of measuring lung water by wet/dry ratios do not indicate any increase down the lung in normal upright dogs [2], but if small amounts of liquid can change interstitial pressure, this method may not be sensitive enough to detect such a change.

A recent observation in our own laboratory (Fig. 2) showed that the reduction in flow at the lung base began near the top of zone III (i.e., at about the height above the lung base equal to left atrial pressure) in seven out of eight experiments. This suggests that in intact animals flow is *decreasing* in zone III, where the driving pressure ($P_a - P_v$) is constant, so that the decreased flow must be due to an increase in resistance. This increased resistance must be associated with a decreased transmural pressure, and as the mean vascular pressure is increasing down the lung, the extravascular pressure of either the alveolar or extra-alveolar vessels must be increasing at a rate faster than the intravascular pressure.

Staub [15] calculated that the bulk of the capillary filtrate comes from zone III since it is primarily in this region that the balance of forces in the Starling equation operates in favor of filtration rather than absorption. It is possible that the pressure surrounding the alveolar vessels is greatest in zone III if a relatively small increase in fluid in the pericapillary interstitial space caused a rise in the pericapillary pressure. This rise in pericapillary pressure could result in a decrease in the transcapillary distending pressure and an increase in resistance of the alveolar vessels. It is also possible that any excess interstitial fluid in zone III collects around the extra-alveolar vessels, where it could lower the transmural pressure and increase the resistance of the extra-alveolar vessels.

These considerations make it obvious that the precise nature of the pressure in the interstitial space surrounding both the alveolar and extra-alveolar vessels must be known before it is possible to determine which resistance is

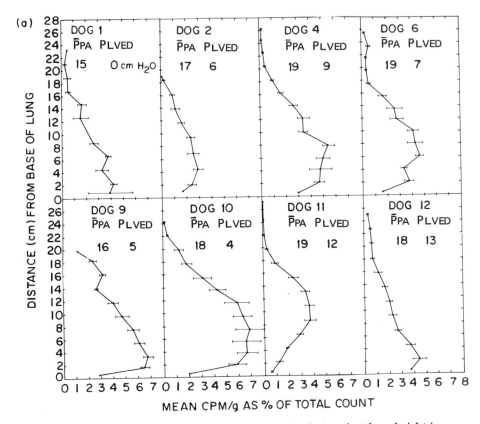

FIGURE 2 (a) Data showing blood flow on the abscissa against lung height in eight experiments. Reprinted from A. L. Muir et al., *J. Appl. Physiol.*, **33**:763-769 (1972), by courtesy of the publishers. *(Continued on facing page)*

important in calculating pulmonary blood flow. This knowledge is not now available, but some isolated facts make it seem likely that the increased resistance is zone III is in the alveolar vessels. One piece of evidence against the extra-alveolar vessels as the site of increased resistance in zone III is that fluid is known to collect in the perivascular space early in edema, when there is little if any effect on blood flow. Secondly, the factor responsible for the reduction in flow in alveolar edema is interstitial fluid (to be described), so that it is conceivable that pericapillary pressure increases and transmural pressure of the alveolar vessels decreases under these circumstances.

It is of interest that when left atrial pressure is raised, the point of flow reversal moves only a short distance up the lung (Fig. 3) and appear to occur at the level at which the wet/dry ratio shows the sharpest increase (dog IV, 12 cm).

(b)

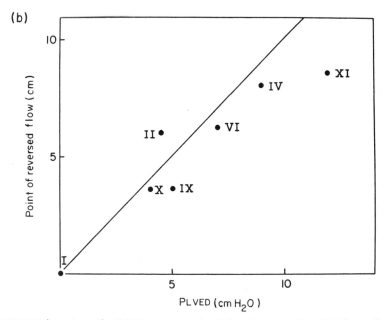

FIGURE 2 *(continued)* (b) Shows a good relation between lung height at the point of flow reversal and PLVED referred to the lung base. Data such as this suggest that the blood flow may decrease throughout zone III. See text for discussion.

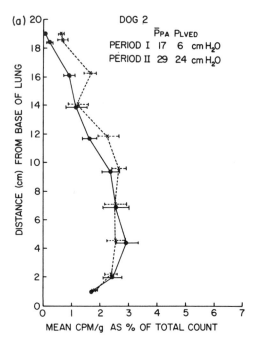

FIGURE 3 (a) Data show relative distribution of total blood flow per gram of lung in control conditions (———) and after the induction of interstitial pulmonary edema (———). Although the relative blood flow at the base has decreased slightly, the absolute flow must have increased, since cardiac output increased. (See text and Table 1). Reprinted from A. L. Muir et al., *J. Appl. Physiol.*, **33**:763-769 (1972), by courtesy of the publishers. *(continued on next page)*

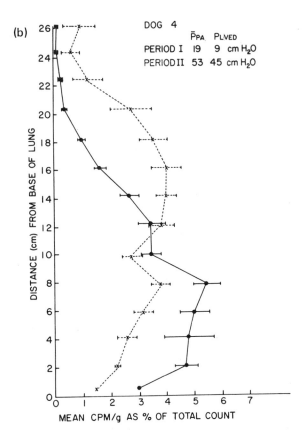

FIGURE 3 *(continued)* (b) Similar data from an experiment in which alveolar edema was produced, showing that this caused a marked change in relative blood flow to the base and also in absolute flow, since the cardiac output (see Table 1) was nearly the same under both control and edematous conditions. *(Continued on facing page)*

TABLE 1 Summary of Measured Parameters for dog II and dog IV (Figure 3)

Dog	$\bar{P}_{PA}$ (cm H_2O)		PLVED (cm H_2O)		Cardiac output (liters/min.)		Plasma Osmotic Pressure (mmHg)		Pa_{O_2} (mmHg)		Pa_{CO_2} (mmHg)		pH_a	
	1	2	1	2	1	2	1	2	1	2	1	2	1	2
II	17	29	6	24	2.70	6.98	12.0	6.7	91	108	45	34	7.28	7.21
IV	19	53	9	45	1.20	1.54	18.4	4.2	100	102	35	25	7.31	7.20

SOURCE: Based on Muir et al., *J. Appl. Physiol.*, **39**:885-890 (1975), by courtesy of the publishers.
NOTE: Interstitial edema was produced in dog II and alveolar edema in dog IV. Period 1 = Control. Period 2 follows cardiopulmonary overload produced by inflation by an aortic balloon and infusion of 4 to 5 liters of saline.

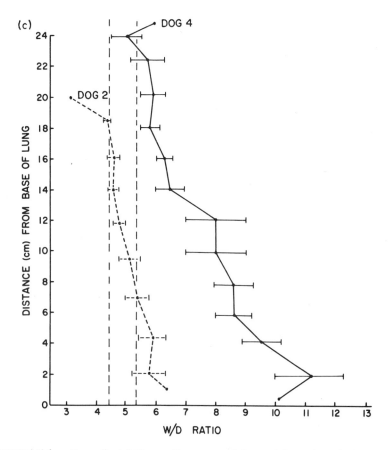

FIGURE 3 *(continued)* (c) Shows the wet- and dry-weight ratios of the lung at different lung heights for the two experiments shown in (a) and (b) compared with the W/D ratios from normal lungs studied under the same conditions. Vertical dashed lines equal ±SD from the mean.

As the entire lung is under zone III conditions in the edematous period, it could be that the pericapillary pressure increases in the lung regions only where the lymphatics are unable to clear the fluid out of the perimicrovascular space.

III. Effects of Edema on Pulmonary Vascular Resistance

A. General

The sequence of changes in the lung as pulmonary edema develops has been described in detail elsewhere [16]. Briefly, the fluid appears to collect in the bronchovascular interstitial space, then in the alveolar wall, and at the corners of the alveoli in the airspace, and finally rapidly fills the airspace, reducing the volume of the filled alveoli. Interestingly, the airspace filling is patchy—the alveoli either become completely full or remain empty of fluid. Theoretically, pulmonary vascular resistance could be altered by pulmonary edema in several ways. First, as noted above, the collection of fluid in the bronchovascular interstitial space could raise the interstitial pressure and decrease the transmural pressure of the extra-alveolar pulmonary vessels so that their resistance increases. Second, if the widening of the alveolar walls indicates fluid collecting in the alveolar wall interstitial space, this could decrease the transmural pressure of the capillaries and increase their resistance. Third, when fluid collects in the alveolar space so that alveolar gas pressure is replaced by the liquid pressure of the edema fluid, this could compress capillaries and increase their resistance. Fourth, as alveolar edema also produces partial collapse of the fluid-filled alveoli, this reduction in lung volume could affect the resistance of the extra-alveolar vessels—with the reduced volume the perivascular interstitial pressure would become more positive so that the transmural pressure of the extra-alveolar vessels would decrease. It is also possible that several of these mechanisms might operate simultaneously, so that the local change in pulmonary vascular resistance in edema may be a result of a complex combination of mechanisms. With these possibilities in mind, we now review the experimental results to determine if possible what relative importance these various factors have in regulating blood flow in pulmonary edema.

B. Effect of Increased Bronchovascular Interstitial Fluid on Blood Flow

One expects that as fluid collects in the bronchovascular interstitial space in the early stages of edema, the increased volume of fluid would make the pressure in this space more positive—so that the transmural pressure of the extra-alveolar vessels would decrease and their resistance would increase. Since this fluid collects first at the lung base [2], one might expect that the resistance of the extra-alveolar vessels in this region would rise so that flow at the base would decrease and there would be a compensatory increase in flow to the upper lung regions. As we have seen, West and his colleagues [13, 14] observed a zone of reduced blood flow at the lung base that occurred normally and they attributed this to a cuff of edema fluid around the vessels at the lung base. Subsequently [14], they showed that in isolated perfused lungs this cuff of fluid would increase in the early stages of pulmonary edema and further reduce the blood flow at the lung base. Their hypothesis that perivascular edema was responsible for local increase in vascular resistance remained extremely attractive until

Ritchie, Shauberger, and Staub [17] repeated West's experiments and showed that they got only a reduction in flow at the lung base under the specific conditions of low flow and low driving pressures. A little later, Naimark and his colleagues [18] showed that gross edema was required before there was a significant shift in blood flow away from the dependent lung regions, and Muir and his associates [2] confirmed this finding; the second group provided both histologic and physiologic data that showed that gross alveolar edema had to exist before there was a significant shift in blood flow away from the lung base. Data from the experiments of Muir et al., shown in Figure 3, compare the effects of interstitial and alveolar edema. This comparison shows that when interstitial edema was present (dog II), there was relatively little effect on blood flow to the lung base. Indeed, as the measure induced to create edema raised cardiac output in this experiment (Table 1), the absolute flow to the edematous lung region was increased. However, when alveolar edema was produced (dog IV), both the relative and the absolute blood flow decreased to the lung base. These studies suggest that the collection of fluid in the bronchovascular interstitial space has little effect on blood flow and that gross alveolar edema is required before the vascular resistance at the lung base increases appreciably. Just how alveolar edema causes the vascular resistance to increase is considered next.

C. Effect of Alveolar Edema on Pulmonary Blood Flow

The study of Staub and his colleagues [16] showed that the earliest change at the alveolar level during the development of edema was a widening of the alveolar wall. If this were to represent a collection of fluid outside capillaries, it is conceivable that the alveolar interstitial pressure might rise and cause a decrease in the capillary transmural pressure. This would depend on the ability of the type I cell to maintain a pressure drop across it so that fluid pressure in the pericapillary space could rise above alveolar gas pressure. As the capillaries and type I cells share the same basement membrane, one would like to know if fluid could really collect in the substance of the basement membrane and what effect this collection might have on the pressure surrounding the capillary. Direct information relating to this point, is, unfortunately, very difficult to get. A second possible mechanism whereby events at the alveolar level might influence regional blood flow is the collection of fluid in the air space. The substitution of fluid pressure for gas pressure in the alveolus could decrease the transmural pressure of the alveolar vessels and thereby increase their resistance. Finally, as filling the alveoli seems to reduce the volume of the filled alveoli, it is also possible that this local reduction in lung volume [19, 20] could increase the interstitial pressure so that the transmural pressure of both alveolar and extra-alveolar vessels might decrease so that there resistance would increase.

Two laboratories have recently collaborated [21] in an attempt to investigate the relative importance of these three mechanisms (i.e., reduced volume, alveolar fluid, interstitial fluid). The general approach has been to use a double isotope technique, which allows comparing blood flow in small regions of the lung first in control conditions and again after a specific manipulation. In this way, it has been possible to study the effects of filling the alveolar space with fluid that under some circumstances remains in the airspace and under other circumstances fills both the air and interstitial spaces. In addition, since both edema and artificially introduced alveolar fluid cause a decrease in alveolar volume, the effect of lung volume change was examined independently. Blood flow was measured by tagging the pulmonary circulation under control conditions, by injecting macroaggregates of albumin labeled with 99^m technetium. Following the experimental manipulation, the pulmonary circulation was tagged with a second macroaggregate labeled with ^{131}I. The animal was then killed and frozen in the position of study, and after freezing, the thorax was sliced and lung samples obtained with a cork borer. It was assumed that the macroaggregates were removed in one pass through the lung and lodged in the pulmonary circulation in proprotion to the blood flow, so that the total amount of an isotope present in the lung Q_t was proportional to the total pulmonary blood flow. It therefore follows that the amount of isotope in each sample is proportional to the blood flow received by that sample at the time that particular macroaggregate was injected, Q_r. If the amount of isotope in each sample Q_r is expressed as a percentage of the total amount of that isotope present in the entire lung Q_t, the fraction of the total pulmonary flood flow received by the sample at the time of injection of the macroaggregate can be computed (Q_r/Q_t). The influence of the experimental manipulation on the distribution of blood flow can then be studied by comparing the percentage of the cardiac output the sample received in the experimental period with the percentage of the blood flow that the sample received in the control period. This ratio, which can be abbreviated to ΔQ, indicates the change in the percentage of the total blood flow that each lung sample received.

$$\Delta Q = \frac{(Q_r/Q_t)_{expt}}{(Q_r/Q_t)_{ctrl}}$$

An increase in ΔQ indicates that the manipulation caused an increase in flow to the lung region and a decreased ΔQ indicates that the region received a reduction in blood flow following the manipulation.

To test the relative effects of filling the alveolar spaces with fluid and filling both the alveolar and the interstitial spaces, two experiments were done. In one group, the effect of filling the alveolar space was measured by introducing autologous plasma into the alveolar space. Since the plasma in the alveoli was iso-osmotic with the dog's own plasma and since protein is slowly absorbed from the alveolar surface [22], it is reasonable to assume that this fluid will remain in the airspace. In other experiments, autologous plasma was diluted by half with saline so that the protein concentrate in the alveolar fluid would be approximately 50% of the protein concentration in the vascular space; this fluid would then be caused to flood the interstitial space as well as fill the airspace of the lung. Finally, as both naturally occurring lung edema and artificial filling of the alveoli with fluid via the airways causes a reduction in lung volume, the effect of the lung volume reduction was examined in separate experiments. This was done by causing patchy atelectasis to be produced in the animal's lungs as they breathed pure oxygen under negative pressure conditions.

Under the conditions of the first set of experiments where the airspaces were filled with iso-osmotic plasma (Fig. 4a), there was no tendency for blood flow to decrease in the areas receiving the greatest amount of instilled fluid. This result indicates that replacing alveolar gas with liquid does not cause a significant reduction in blood flow. Indeed, in some areas blood flow seemed to increase under these conditions.

In the second set of experiments, when the fluid was diluted with saline so that the osmotic forces would be such that the fluid would enter the interstitial space from the airspace, a significant reduction in blood flow occurred (Fig. 4b). These data suggest that vascular resistance rose under these circumstances because the interstitial space was overloaded with fluid. The increased resistance was presumably owing to the rise in the perivascular pressure, which decreased the transmural pressure of either alveolar or extra-alveolar vessels, or both. Whether the extra-alveolar or the alveolar vessels are primarily responsible for the increased resistance is difficult to determine. As other experiments showed that gross edema around extra-alveolar vessels in the bronchovascular interstitial space had little effect on blood flow, it seems more likely that the effect in these experiments was from increased resistance of the alveolar vessels.

In the third set of experiments, atelectasis was induced by having the animals breath O_2 at low lung volumes, and these experiments showed that reduced lung volume had no separate effect on blood flow. Comparing these three sets of experiments and the results found in airspace edema, it seems reasonable to conclude that it is the alveolar wall component of the airspace edema that increase vascular resistance and reduces blood flow.

Taken together, these results suggest that the mechanism responsible for redistributing blood flow in acute pulmonary edema is associated with alveolar filling and probably due to the alveolar wall component of airspace edema. That blood flow is well maintained so long as the airspace is empty and is reduced sharply when the alveoli becomes edema-filled provides an efficient mechanism whereby blood flow can be reduced to areas of the lungs that can

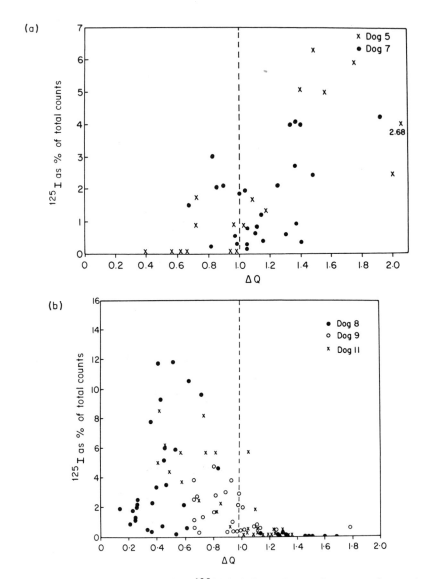

FIGURE 4 Data show that when ^{125}I-labeled autologus plasma was inserted into the alveoli, blood flow tended to increase ($\Delta Q > 1$) in the areas of lung receiving the greatest amount of plasma. Reprinted from A. L. Muir et al., *J. Appl. Physiol.*, **39**:885-890 (1975), by courtesy of the publishers. (b) Shows that when the ^{125}I-labeled plasma was diluted with saline so that the fluid would be absorbed from the alveolar space into the interstitium, blood flow was decreased ($\Delta Q > 1$).

no longer be ventilated. This mechanism allows for good matching of ventilation and perfusion of the lung, and therefore good gas exchange until very late in the edematous process. Indeed, the failure in gas exchange that finally ensues is likely because fluid flows into airways from alveoli so that the airways to the relatively normal open alveoli become occluded.

References

1. J. Barcroft, Severe problems of the circulation during gas poisoning, *J. Royal Army Med. Corps,* **34**:155-173 (1920).
2. A. L. Muir, D. L. Hall, P. Despas, and J. C. Hogg, Distribution of blood flow in the lungs in acute pulmonary edema in dogs, *J. Appl. Physiol.,* **33**:763-769 (1972).
3. S. I. Said, J. W. Longacher, R. K. Davis, C. M. Banejee, W. M. Davis, and W. J. Woodell, Pulmonary gas exchange during the induction of pulmonary edema in anesthetized dogs, *J. Appl. Physiol.,* **19**:403-407 (1964).
4. J. B. L. Howell, S. Permutt, D. F. Proctor, and R. L. Riley, Effect of inflation of the lung on different parts of the vascular bed, *J. Appl. Physiol.,* **16**:71 (1961).
5. C. Macklin, Evidence of increase in the capacity of the pulmonary arteries and veins of dogs, cats and rabbits during inflation of the freshly excised lungs, *Rev. Canad. Biol.,* **5**:199-232 (1946).
6. J. Bannister and R. W. Torrance, The effects of tracheal pressure upon flow: Pressure relations in the vascular bed of isolated lungs. *Quart. J. Exptl. Physiol.,* **45**:362 (1960).
7. S. Permutt, B. Bromberger-Barnea, and H. N. Bane, Alveolar pressure, pulmonary venous pressure, and the vascular waterfall, *Med. Thorac.,* **19**:239-260 (1962).
8. J. B. West, C. T. Dollery, and A. Naimark, Distribution of blood flow in isolated lung; relation to vascular and alveolar pressures, *J. Appl. Physiol.,* **19**:713-724 (1964).
9. J. M. B. Hughes, Pulmonary interstitial pressure, *Bull. Physio-Path. Resp.,* **7**:1095-1123 (1971).
10. I. Setnikar and E. Agostoni, Factors keeping the lung expanded in the chest, *Proceedings of the International Union of Physiological Sciences,* **1**:281-286 (1962).
11. I. Setnikar, E. Agostoni, and A. Taglietti, Entita caratteristiche e origine della depressurie pleurica, *Arch. Sci. Biol.* (Bologna), **41**:312-325 (1957).
12. E. Agostoni, A. Taglietti, and I. Setnikar, Absorption force of the capillaries of the visceral pleura in determination of intrapleural pressure, *Amer. J. Physiol.,* **191**:277-282 (1957).
13. J. B. West, Perivascular oedema: A factor in pulmonary vascular resistance, *Amer. Heart J.,* **70**:570-572 (1965).

14. J. B. West, C. T. Dollery, and B. E. Heard, Increased pulmonary vascular resistance in the dependent zone of the isolated dog lung caused by perivascular edema, *Circ. Res.*, **17**:191-206 (1965).

15. N. C. Staub, Pulmonary edema, *Physiol. Rev.*, **54**:678-811 (1974).

16. N. C. Staub, H. Nagano, and M. L. Pearce, Pulmonary edema in dogs, especially the seuqence of fluid accumulation in the lungs, *J. Appl. Physiol.*, **22**:227-246 (1967).

17. B. C. Ritchie, G. Shauberger, and N. C. Staub, Inadequacy of perivascular edema hypotheses to account for the distribution of pulmonary blood flow in lung edema, *Circ. Res.*, **24**:807-814 (1969).

18. A. Naimark, B. W. Kirk, and W. Chernecki, Regional water volume, blood volume and perfusion in the lung. In *Central aerodynamics and gas exchange*. Turin, Minerva Medica, 1971, p. 139-157.

19. J. C. Hogg, P. Holst, P. Corry, E. Ruff, E. Housely, and E. Norris, Effect of regional lung expansion and body position on pulmonary perfusion in dogs, *J. Appl. Physiol.*, **31**:97-101 (1971).

20. J. M. B. Hughes, J. B. Glazier, J. E. Maloney, and J. B. West, Effect of extra-alveolar vessels on the distribution of blood flow in dog lungs, *J. Appl. Physiol.*, **25**: 701-712 (1968).

21. A. L. Muir, J. C. Hogg, A. Naimark, and W. Chernecki, The effect of alveolar liquid on the distribution of blood flow in dog lung, *J. Appl. Physiol.*, **39**:885-890 (1975).

22. E. C. Meyer, E. A. Dominguez, and K. G. Bensch, Pulmonary lymphatic and blood absorption of albumin from alveoli: A quantitative comparison, *Lab. Invest.*, **20**:1-8 (1969).

8

Small Solutes and Water

RICHARD M. EFFROS

Harbor General Hospital
School of Medicine
University of California, Los Angeles
Torrance, California

I. Introduction

The Starling hypothesis of capillary fluid balance [1-3] has proved to be one of the most useful approximations of modern physiology. The approximation made by Starling was that the capillaries are freely permeable to low-molecular-weight solutes but essentially impermeable to high-molecular-weight solutes. Although concentration gradients of proteins are maintained across capillary walls, similar gradients of electrolytes and sugars cannot be sustained across the same barrier. The value of this premise was that it directed the attention of physiologists to the importance of plasma proteins in preventing the development of interstitial edema.

Starling recognized that while the approximation was appropriate for skeletal muscle vessels, it was not applicable to all organs. He noted that it could not be made for liver sinusoids, which leaked both small and large molecules; and he was probably aware that the cerebral capillaries are relatively impermeable to small and large molecules, a phenomenon observed as early as 1886 that has been attributed to a "blood-brain barrier" [4]. With the development of more sophisticated experimental techniques, it has become clear that even in skeletal muscle, the diffusion of small solutes into the interstitium is by no means instantaneous, and it has been suggested in several studies that changes in vascular concentrations of salts and sugars can transiently dehydrate the interstitial compartment.

It has been the objective of a number of investigators, including the author, to define the role of small solutes in governing fluid balance within the lung. The principal purpose of this chapter is to review the relatively unsatisfactory status of our knowledge in this regard. A significant amount of attention must be given to data obtained from other organs besides the lung, since some of these measurements should be repeated in the lung and since they provide a basis for comparing the permeability of pulmonary and systemic capillaries.

The passage of solutes and water through membranes can be characterized by four parameters: (1) solute permeability P, (2) filtration coefficient P_f, (3) solute reflection coefficient σ_d, and (4) the solvent drag reflection coefficient σ_f. Current information regarding the magnitude of each of these parameters will be reviewed in turn for the passage of small solutes and water across the pulmonary capillaries. The possible effect of small solutes in moderating fluid flow across the capillaries (osmotic buffering) will be considered and the nature of the dehydration that hypertonic solutions of these agents produce will be discussed. Thereafter, a brief survey will be made of the meager but important information that has been obtained for the alveolar epithelial membrane.

II. Morphologic Basis of Capillary Solute and Water Exchange

Although it has been taught that transfer of solutes and blood occurs exclusively through the capillary walls, evidence has been obtained that solute exchange and filtration can also occur across the venules and arterioles in both the lung and systemic vascular beds [5-7]. Under some pathologic circumstances, a considerable amount of fluid can also cross the bronchial vessels, further complicating matters [8]. For the sake of convenience and in the absence of specific information, the exchange site in the lung will be referred to as the pulmonary "capillary bed" and only the nonbronchial vessels will be considered.

The pulmonary capillaries are classified as "continuous" to indicate that the pulmonary endothelial cells are unfenestrated and surrounded by a continuous basement membrane. It is generally believed that the movement of small hydrophilic solutes is limited to the intercellular clefts where the margins of the endothelial cells are joined. These slitlike separations are similar to those in skeletal-muscle capillaries; they are 20 nm wide over most of their length, but narrow to intercellular junctions, or *macuale occludentes,* which are only 4 nm wide and 20 nm long [9]. Morphologic evidence that the narrow portions of the clefts can permit passage of solutes is based on the studies of Schneeberger-Keeley, Karnovsky [10, 11], and Pietra et al. [12, 13], which show that with expansion of the blood volume or increases of arterial pressure, horseradish peroxidase and hemoglobin can traverse the junctions. Data have also been obtained by Michel that both sodium chloride and the dye patent blue V penetrate systemic capillaries at discrete sites that probably represent the intercellular junctions [14]. Morphologically, the area of the junctions represents less than 0.1% of the endothelial surface [9], and it has been estimated that only one-thirtieth of the junctional area is actually open [15].

On the basis of both plant and animal studies, it has been concluded that the cell membrane is itself perforated with very much smaller pores (0.4 nm), which permit passage of both water and small hydrophillic solutes [16-19]. Lipophilic substances readily dissolve in the membrane and diffuse into the cells more quickly than hydrophilic solutes. (Evidence for a similar structure of pulmonary cell membranes will be discussed later.)

The existence of a small population of large defects (12 to 35 nm) has also been inferred from the appearance of some large protein molecules in the lymph [20]. It is not clear to what extent these substances are delivered by pinocytosis. Since we are considering the movement of small solutes and water, and these large pores are probably of lesser importance in this regard, no further consideration is given to them here.

The lung is one of the most vascular organs of the body. The blood volume represents fully one-half of its total weight compared with only 8% of body weight as a whole [21,22]. Using [^{14}C] sucrose as an extracellular indicator, Selinger et al. calculated that the interstitial fluid represented 30% of the extravascular water volume [23]. The corresponding Cl$^-$ space constituted about 40% of the extravascular water volume, suggesting either entry of Cl$^-$ into cells or exclusion of sucrose from part of the interstitium. It is generally assumed that the interstitial electrolyte content is similar to that of plasma. Small differences may be expected due to a Donnan effect; this effect results in a relatively greater number of small cations in the plasma, where protein concentrations are greater, and a correspondingly greater number of anions in the interstitial fluid. The sodium content of the pulmonary tissue is relatively large and there is evidence that some of the pulmonary cells contain higher concentrations of sodium ion than parenchymal cells elsewhere [22,24,25].

III.   Tracer Permeability

A.   Methodology

To determine the permeability P of a membrane to any substance, two basic measurements must be made: the rate at which the substance crosses the membrane and the driving forces responsible for this movement. The driving forces across the vascular bed are primarily gradients of hydrostatic pressure and solute concentration. Measurements of driving forces and flows are easily obtained if the membranes can be isolated and mounted in an appropriate chamber. This procedure is obviously not feasible in studies of capillary permeability; therefore more indirect methods must be used to provide this information. The solute must be injected into the vasculature or tissues and passage into or out of the blood must then be determined.

Before radioisotopes were introduced into biological research, studies of capillary permeability to low-molecular-weight solutes such as sodium and potassium ion were hampered by technical and physiologic problems. Unless large quantities of solute were injected, changes in concentrations could not be measured. Unfortunately, the osmotic and physiologic effects of these injections complicated interpretation of such studies. The advantages of radioisotopes were quickly appreciated after they became available, just before World War II, and during the years that followed an impressive amount of research was conducted on the disappearance of these substances from the circulation [26].

The properties of most tracers resemble the properties of the natural isotopes with sufficient precision that it has been assumed that the former provide adequate information about the latter and this assumption still seems reasonable. It was further assumed however, that the arterial activity of the isotope could be used as an accurate gauge of the concentration differences between blood and tissues responsible for the movement of the isotope across the capillary barrier. The potential error of this approach was noted by Pappenheimer, Renkin, and Borrero [27], who correctly argued that although the arterial concentration might reflect the difference in concentration between blood and tissues at the arterial end of the capillary at an early time, this did not mean that this concentration difference was sustained along the entire capillary. Obviously, if the capillary is very permeable to the injected indicator, the concentration difference between the blood and tissues would diminish rapidly down the length of the vessel. These considerations had been fully realized some forty years before by Bohr [28] and Krogh [29], who characterized the movement of gases across capillaries in terms of concentration gradients that declined with distance along the capillaries. The general principles had not been applied, however, to studies of isotopic solute movement.

Pappenheimer's solution to the problem of measuring an "average" blood-tissue concentration difference along the capillary was particularly ingenious since it apparently required no mathematical modeling of the sort Bohr and Krogh used. Since the Pappenheimer procedure depends on osmotically active quantities of indicator instead of tracer amounts, we shall discuss it later.

The simplicity and physiologically benign nature of the isotope approach appealed to Pappenheimer's coworker Renkin, who introduced an alternative method of estimating the concentration difference between the blood and tissues [30]. Crone and others later modified this procedure [31, 32] and used it for measurements of capillary permeability in a variety of organs including the brain, lung, and skeletal and cardiac muscle.

Each of these tracer techniques is based on one or another model of how indicator concentrations decline along the capillary length. The mathematical complexity of the model is largely related to the number and kinds of assumptions made about the way in which the indicator passes into the tissue. The simplest approach of this sort was devised by Renkin and Crone. Most of the following discussion is concerned with the assumptions and limitations of this procedure.

Using an experimental approach similar to that of Chinard et al. [33, 34], Crone compared the emergence of a diffusible indicator in the outflow from an organ with that of a reference indicator which did not diffuse out of the vascular compartment. He assumed that the relative concentrations of the reference indicator in the collected blood represented what the concentrations of the diffusible indicator would be if this indicator had not diffused into the tissues. The indicators are administered together in a small volume of a solution which is rapidly injected into the blood flowing into the lung. Blood is collected from the pulmonary outflow (generally from the aorta), and the concentrations observed in this blood for the vascular and diffusible indicators are then divided by the injected doses to yield comparable "fractional concentrations" (w, in units of ml^{-1}, see Fig. 1). The observed venous fractional concentrations of the diffusible indicator are initially less than the fractional concentrations of the vascular indicators, and this is attributed to passage of the diffusible indicator into the tissues. The extraction E of indicator is calculated from the equation

$$E = \lim_{t \to a} (1 - w_d/w_v) \tag{1}$$

where the subscripts d and v refer to the diffusible and vascular indicators, and the limit indicates that it is desirable to obtain data as early as possible (a represents the appearance time). Crone actually used the average extraction

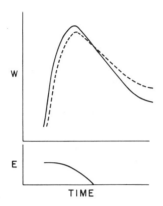

FIGURE 1   Crone experiment. Fractional concentrations w of the vascular indicator (continuous line) and of the diffusible indicator (interrupted line) are plotted against time in the upper panel and the corresponding extraction values E are shown in the lower panel.

observed over the upslope and the use of the limiting values was introduced by Martin and Yudilevich [35]. More recently, Bassingthwaighte has proposed use of maximal extraction whenever this occurs [36].

It was hoped that by using early data it would be possible to avoid any appreciable increase in the tissue concentrations of indicator. However, even the earliest samples may be misleading in this respect, since as Pappenheimer has pointed out, the diffusible indicator may become equilibrated between blood and tissues before the end of the capillary is reached. Renkin [30], and thereafter Yudilevich and Martin [37], recognized this situation but further reasoned that such equilibration could be detected simply by changing the rate of tissue perfusion. If the extraction of indicator remained constant as flow increased, then the rate at which indicator was cleared from the vessels should obviously increase linearly with flow ("clearance" equals the product of flow and extraction). This is illustrated by points A and B in Figure 2. Under such circumstances, the delivery of indicator to the tissues is limited only by the rate of flow. If on the other hand, the extraction of indicator diminished in such a way that the clearance approached a constant value as flow increased (C, D, and F in Fig. 2), it could obviously be concluded that delivery of indicator is limited by some other factor besides blood flow—presumably by the permeability of the capillary bed.

Evidence that indicator clearance did tend to reach maximal values in skeletal muscles was interpreted by Renkin to mean that at rapid flows significant differences in the blood and tissue concentration of indicator could be sustained along the length of the capillaries [30].

At extremely high flows, point F, the decline in the concentration of indicator along the capillaries should become negligible, at which time the clearance of indicator is maximal and determined exclusively by the capillary permeability. This is equivalent to the model intuitively assumed by the

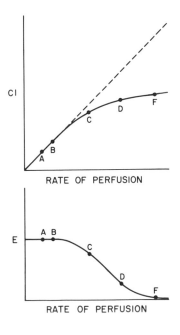

FIGURE 2 Flow and permeability limitation. Clearance Cl and extraction E values are plotted against rate of perfusion. Points A and B are in the flow-limited range: indicator extraction is proportional to flow. In the Crone model, extraction in this region should be complete (equal to 1.0) and indicator clearance and blood flow should be equivalent. Points C, D, and F show that as flow is increased further, indicator clearance approaches a constant value determined by the permeability-surface area product.

earlier investigators who relied on arterial concentrations. Aside from problems of attaining such flows in practice, without altering the organ, it is undesirable to increase flow to this extent since the extraction of indicator tends to diminish to unmeasurably small levels. It is therefore preferable to operate at a flow at which clearance is not exclusively flow-limited or permeability-limited.

Interpreting indicator extraction data requires a model that describes how the concentration gradient declines along the capillary. The simplest model, which both Renkin and Crone used, is based on the following assumptions:

1. The early loss of diffusible indicator from the bloodstream is not accompanied by a significant rise in tissue concentration.

2. Diffusion from the blood phase to the tissue is limited only by the capillary wall. It is assumed that mixing within the capillary is rapid and that there are no concentration gradients between the center and the periphery of the capillary.

3. There is no diffusion of indicator from the arterial to the venous ends of the circulation within either the capillaries or the tissues.

Indicator delivery to the capillaries and washout therefrom are accomplished exclusively by convective flow within the vessels.

4. Indicator extraction is uniform throughout the organ.

If this somewhat unrealistic set of assumptions is granted, it can be shown that the extraction E of indicator will be related to the blood flow F, permeability P, and surface area S of the pulmonary capillaries by the equation

$$E = 1 - \exp(-PS/F). \tag{2}$$

Solving for the product of permeability and surface area gives

$$PS = F \ln[1/(1 - E)]. \tag{3}$$

A confusing variety of units have been used for both permeability P and filtration constant P_f data. For simplicity, most investigators have adopted the cm/sec unit for both parameters. This abstract unit is equivalent to the more obvious but cumbersome term "(moles of solute or water per second) per (moles per cubic centimeter of concentration difference) per (square centimeter of surface area)." One can see the equivalence of these units by abbreviating the latter to $(mol/sec) (mol/cm^3)^{-1} (cm^2)^{-1}$.

It is convenient to discuss the permeability of the pulmonary capillaries to small molecules relative to those substances that remain essentially extracellular during a single circulation through the lungs (e.g. ions and sugars) and those that readily cross the cell walls (e.g. lipid soluble molecules and labeled water). The distinction is somewhat arbitrary, since given enough time, solutes such as urea and potassium will enter the endothelial and epithelial cells of the lung, and other substances (a variety of weak acids and bases) contain both poorly diffusible (ionic) and very diffusible (non-ionized) moieties.

It is generally assumed that "extracellular" indicators exchange with the pulmonary interstitium by way of the interendothelial junctions and that "cellular" indicators readily traverse both endothelial and epithelial cell membranes as well as the interendothelial junctions, to become distributed within the entire water content of the lung. In this model, the junctions and endothelial cells provide parallel pathways for diffusion of water and solutes out of the capillaries. Interest has been primarily directed towards the permeability of the capillary wall to extracellular indicators, since these might be expected to give information about the permeability of the 4-nm junctions between the cells. Recently, however, studies of the cellular indicators have been extended so that the diffusion of solutes through the postulated small pore system can be characterized.

B. Extracellular Solutes

In single-passage studies of pulmonary capillary permeability, Chinard et al. and Crone found that the extraction of small hydrophilic solutes is limited and that the extravascular volume calculated from the mean transit times of these indicators is very small [31,33,34,38,39]. Three explanations could be responsible for these observations: (1) The pulmonary capillaries are relatively impermeable to these solutes. (2) The volume of distribution accessible to $^{22}Na^+$ is limited. (3) The low extractions reflect the high perfusion of pulmonary tissue and the small volumes are due to the failure to properly extrapolate the indicator dilution curves.

Interpreting these "transient" studies is complicated by several factors:

1. The size of the pulmonary capillary bed is uncertain and depends on blood flow [40]. On the basis of an assumed capillary surface area of 500 cm^2 per gram of wet weight tissue, Chinard et al. [39] have calculated that the pulmonary capillary permeability to $^{22}Na^+$ is 2.4×10^{-5} cm/sec. They have compared this with a value of 5.5×10^{-5} cm/sec for skeletal muscle capillaries and attributed the greater extraction in skeletal muscle mainly to the relatively longer transit times of skeletal muscle capillaries. Staub has questioned this explanation, citing evidence that muscle capillary transit times are little more than twice those in the lung and not enough to explain the reported differences in extraction [22,41].

2. To show that extraction measurements provide an index of permeability, it must be shown that extraction diminishes with flow (see Equation (2)). Data bearing on this question are very limited. Perl et al. [39] found that the extraction of ethylene glycol did appear to diminish with flow. However, since the longer-chain diols enter the pulmonary cells during a single passage, it is possible that increased extraction at lower flows is due to passage of ethylene glycol directly into the endothelial cells. If ethylene glycol enters cells, then it would presumably be the permeability of the endothelial cell membrane rather than permeability of the interendothelial junction that is measurable by the single-passage procedure. The presence or absence of cellular equilibration should be determined by perfusing the lungs with ethylene glycol for several minutes and determining tissue concentrations.

Recently we have found that the extraction of $^{22}Na^+$ in an isolated perfused lung preparation is unaltered by very large changes in perfusion [50]. Furthermore, the volume of distribution of $^{22}Na^+$ calculated from the single-pass studies represents only one-third of the volume measured when the organ is perfused with $^{22}Na^+$ for 2 min. These observations suggest that $^{22}Na^+$ rapidly enters a small volume not accessible to protein-bound indicators. It was not possible to increase perfusion rates to levels that would decrease indicator extraction and thereby provide a measure of the rate of entry of $^{22}Na^+$ into this space. One compartment that might permit rapid entry of small solutes but not protein would be the "calveoli," or pinocytotic vesicles that line the luminal surface of the endothelial cells. These vesicles are covered by an attenuated membrane that apparently permits access of polypeptides such as angiotensin I [51] but that may exclude larger molecules such as proteins. It should be noted that the similarity of outflow patterns of $^{22}Na^+$ and $^{36}Cl^-$ suggest that surface charge has little effect on diffusion into this compartment (Fig. 3).

Even at very low perfusion rates (well below those that could be expected in vivo), the extraction of $^{22}Na^+$ and its volume of distribution remained small. This suggests that entry into the remainder of the accessible tissue compartment by $^{22}Na^+$ is simply too slow to measure in a single-passage study. In a series of in vivo perfusion studies, Wangensteen et al. [44] have found that the half-time required for entry of labeled sucrose into the lung is 15 sec, or perhaps 20 times as long as the normal capillary transit time (about 0.75 sec). Although constant infusion studies of this kind are probably more satisfactory for measurements of pulmonary capillary permeability to extracellular solutes, several uncertainties remain. Equilibration of local regions may be delayed if perfusion to these areas is diminished and the arrival of indicator depends on diffusion from more distant vessels. Furthermore, an appropriate model for equilibration must be chosen: the model Wangensteen selected [44,52] assumes that mixing in the extravascular compartment is instantaneous. If this were the case, the extracellular indicator would arrive in the pulmonary outflow in advance of the vascular indicator, an event that has not been observed in the lung.

3. Even if solute extraction can be shown to be determined by capillary permeability, it is not clear whether the calculated value would be representative of the lung as a whole. The extraction of $^{22}Na^+$ diminishes as the peak of the vascular indicator curve is approached, presumably because of back-diffusion from the tissue to the vasculature. To avoid the effects of back-diffusion, extraction at the earliest time should be used. However, selective use of early data involves the risk that only vessels with high flow or small volumes are represented, a situation that might lead to erroneously low extractions. The consequences of heterogeneous vascular beds on permeability measurements have been considered by Levitt [53] and Friedman [54].

4. The validity of the Crone approach depends partly on the assumption that there is no longitudinal diffusion in the direction of the blood flow within the tissues. Although direct diffusion from arterial to venous vessels has been noted in the kidney (note the diffusion-convection model of Perl and Chinard [55]), it is less likely that this is an important factor in the lungs.

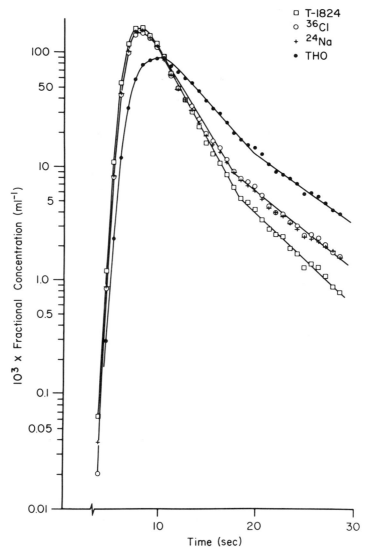

FIGURE 3 Crone study of [^{125}I] albumin, ^{24}Na, ^{36}Cl, and THO in the per-fused rabbit lung. Recirculation was not permitted in these studies. None of the indicators had monoexponential outflow patterns. The close proximity of the ^{24}Na and ^{36}Cl curves was maintained over a pH range between 6.8 and 8.0.

5. Another assumption of the Crone equations is that there are no con-centration gradients between the blood at the periphery and blood in the

central part of a vessel. Taylor showed that such gradients are to be expected in vessels and would tend to alter the relative outflow patterns of large and small moleculess [56]. Evidence for such effects has been obtained in the brain [49].

With these reservations in mind, a summary of reported values for capillary permeability of a variety of organs is presented in Table 1. Several studies have suggested that extraction of extracellular solutes may be increased by circum-

TABLE 1   Capillary Permeability Parameters of Extracellular Solutes and Water

Solute Permeability P (10^{-5}cm/sec)

Solute	D[a,k]	Lung	Skeletal muscles[b]	Brain[c,l]
Sodium	2.00	2.4–4.4[d]	7.4	
Urea	1.95		6.1	0.44
Hexose	0.90		2.7 (glucose)	0.15 (fructose)
Sucrose	0.70	1.1[e]	1.8	Undetectable
Raffinose	0.64		1.1	
Inulin	0.21–0.26		0.27	

Filtration Coefficient P_f (10^{-2}cm/sec)

	Lung	Skeletal muscle (leg)	Brain
Lymph studies	0.2[f]		
Weight studies	2–10[g]	4.4[h]	
Volume studies			0.024[i]

Reflection Coefficients σ_d

	Lung[g]		Skeletal muscle[h]	Brain[i]
Sodium Chloride	0.3		0.16	
Urea	0.3	0.018	0.21	0.44
Glucose	0.48	0.026	0.22	0.89
Sucrose	0.39	0.044	0.29	0.98
Raffinose	0.35		0.30	1.00
Inulin			0.54	

SOURCE: [a]Perl [15]. [b] Trap-Jensen and Lassen [42]. [c]Crone [43]. [d]Perl [39]. [e]Wang-ensteen et al. [37]. [f]Staub [22]. [g]Perl et al. [45]; Taylor and Gaar [46]. [h]Pappenheimer et al. [27]; Perl [15]. [i]Fenstermacher and Johnson [47]; Fenstermacher [48]. [j]Taylor and Gaar [46]; Perl et al. [45]. [k]Free diffusion coefficient in water at 25°C (10^{-5} cm^2/sec). [l]These values may be in error because significant Taylor diffusion is evident in brain studies [49].

stances that produce pulmonary edema [57–60]. There is no way of telling from these data whether these changes in extraction were due to alterations of capillary permeability or an increase in the volume of some extravascular compartment.

It is difficult to use the rate of entry of small solutes into lymphatic fluid from the vasculature to calculate values for pulmonary capillary permeability. Interpreting such data is complicated by the contribution of bronchial vasculature, delay in transport to the collection site by the lymphatics and exchange with vessels in the nodes. Normand et al. found that lymphatic sucrose concentrations reached half equibration values in 4.26 min in fetal lambs [61]. Selinger et al. reported that full equilibration of sucrose was attained in 8.5 minutes [23].

C. Cellular Indicators

Chinard et al. [34, 37, 62] have shown that the permeability of the pulmonary capillaries to solutes is largely governed by lipid solubility. This is best shown with the aliphatic amides and terminal diols. The permeability of the pulmonary capillaries to these solutes generally parallels the length of the aliphatic chain and the corresponding oil-to-water solubility coefficient. The only exception noted to this rule has been for formamide and acetamide. Although the oil-water coefficient of acetamide is greater, formamide appeared to be more diffusible through the capillary wall. Chinard et al. suggest, in effect, that passage of formamide into the tissues is accomplished through small pores in the cellular membrane as well as through the interendothelial junctions. The larger size of acetamide restricts passage through the small-pore pathway. The movement of propionamide and the higher aliphatic amides presumably occurs to an increasing extent by the lipid pathway.

These observations agree with a large body of information that suggests that the cell membranes contain hydrophilic pores of approximately 0.4-nm diameter embedded in a hydrophobic lipid barrier (see above). The formamide and acetamide data seem to be contrary to the earlier suggestion by Chinard that the cellular membrane is homogeneous [63, 64]. It should be noted, however, that in some cells small amides can be transported differently from water [65]. The amides may therefore not be suitable for evaluating aqueous pores.

Increase in the solubility of the indicator in lipid may increase the calculated volume of distribution of the indicator and complicate the interpretation of permeability data. Consider, for example, two very diffusible, flow-limited indicators. If it is assumed that equilibration of each occurs along most of the length of the capillary during a single pass, then the relative concentrations of that indicator which is distributed into a larger volume or pool within the tissue will be less both within the tissue and at the capillary outflow.

It would be of particular interest to measure the permeability of the pulmonary capillaries to labeled water. Diffusion of labeled water through the cell membranes of the heart and skeletal muscles appears to be very rapid and delivery to these tissues is limited by the rate of blood flow rather than permeability barriers [66]. Pappenheimer's estimate of the permeability of hind limb capillaries to water was based on extrapolation of small-solute data rather than direct measurements and predicts the movement of a hypothetical extracellular indicator of the same size as a water molecule [27]. Recently, Eichling et al. [67] reported experiments that suggest that at high flows, the extraction of $H_2^{15}O$ is incomplete and limited by capillary permeability in the brain. This conclusion was prompted by the discovery that as flow increased, the fraction of the $H_2^{15}O$ that traversed the brain with the same half-life as labeled red cells also increased, with restriction of as much as 40% of the water to the vascular compartment. It is possible that the normally rapid perfusion of lung tissue may permit a similar measurement of water permeability. Chinard et al. [39] did find that the extraction of octanediol exceeds extraction of tritiated water, suggesting that the octanediol may diffuse through the cells more rapidly than water. Confirmation that the permeability of the pulmomary capillaries can be measured at attainable blood flows must, however, await more complete correlation of water and octanediol extraction with changes in blood flow.

One of the most persuasive arguments for the existence of separate lipid pathways for the passage of lipid-soluble solutes in capillary beds is the finding that by the simple process of cooling to 15°C, the passage of these solutes through capillaries can be blocked in both skeletal muscle and the lung, whereas the movement of the labeled sodium is relatively unchanged [68, 69]. It appears that under these circumstances, the lipid pathway has become gelled and transit through the cells is effectively blocked.

D. Weak Electrolytes

From a respiratory point of view, carbon dioxide (in the form of carbonic acid and bicarbonate) represents the most important weak acid in plasma. Although dissolved CO_2 readily diffuses through cellular membranes, it represents only 5% of the CO_2 which can be derived from plasma. Nearly 95% is in the form of bicarbonate, and a very small fraction is carbonic acid and other moieties.

It can be expected that the pulmonary parenchymal membranes are considerably less permeable to bicarbonate ion than to carbon dioxide gas. That such is indeed the case was shown by Chinard et al. in a series of studies with labeled carbon dioxide and bicarbonate [70, 71]. They found that following intravenous injections, each of these indicators traversed the lung in essentially the same way. Carbon dioxide in the form of dissolved gas or bicarbonate had a mean transit time from the vein to a peripheral artery exceeding that of tritiated water, suggesting distribution into a volume exceeding that of the water space of the lung. It is likely that some of the label entered the alveolar gas phase (and perhaps, to a lesser extent, some entered the lipid compartment of the lung) only to return to the capillary blood flow at a later time. Loss of CO_2 label to the expired air amounted to about 5% of that injected.

Inhibition of carbonic anhydrase had a dramatic effect on the transit of both dissolved CO_2 and bicarbonate through the lung. The mean transit times of both materials were diminished to values quite comparable with those of the vascular indicator. Furthermore, losses of dissolved CO_2 from the circulation were greater than losses of bicarbonate. Chinard et al. concluded that whereas bicarbonate and dissolved CO_2 were rapidly converted by carbonic anhydrase into one another between the point of injection and the pulmonary capillaries, the interconversion of these forms of CO_2 was not completed in the presence of inhibitor. It is likely, however, that a very significant amount of the dissolved carbon dioxide was converted to bicarbonate, since the mean transit time of carbon-14 injected as dissolved CO_2 was similar to the mean transit time of bicarbonate and considerably shorter than before the inhibitor was introduced. Presumably that portion that had become bicarbonate was confined to the vascular volume and perhaps the interstitial volume.

We have recently completed a series of studies of isolated rabbit lungs in which red cells and carbonic anhydrase were excluded from the perfusion fluid. The tissue volume of distribution of $^{14}CO_2$ was from 5 to 70 times greater than that of $H^{14}CO_3^-$ when carbonic anhydrase was inhibited. These studies suggest the presence of carbonic anhydrase in the pulmonary vasculature and also confirm that the pulmonary tissues are much more permeable to $^{14}CO_2$ than to $H^{14}CO_3^-$.

Because cell membranes are relatively impermeable to the ionic forms of conjugate acid-base pairs, concentration gradients of these indicators can be maintained between the cellular and extracellular compartments. This phenomenon, referred to as nonionic diffusion or hydrogen ion trapping, results in the preferential distribution of cationic acids (i.e., acids of the form $R\text{-}NH_3^+ \leftrightharpoons R\text{-}NH_2 + H^+$) within the relatively acid cellular environment and the reciprocal concentration of anionic acids (i.e., acids of the type $RH \leftrightharpoons R^- + H^+$) in the extracellular fluids [72, 73]. Evidence has been obtained by indicator dilution techniques that in the lung nonionic diffusion helps govern the distribution of weak acids and bases between the blood and tissues as it does in other organs [74, 75]. These studies are based on the principle that the distribution ratio of any indicator between these compartments that would prevail during a constant infusion of indicator can be calculated from mean transit time data obtained with a sudden injection (transient) study.

The methodology underlying these procedures is outlined elsewhere [74]. It was found that the distribution of a variety of cationic indicators (viz., amines) and anionic indicators (viz., barbiturates) were altered by changes in arterial pH. These changes in distribution were consistent with the hypothesis that (1) diffusion is primarily restricted to the nonionized moiety, (2) the extravascular contents of the lung are more acid than the plasma, and (3) changes in cellular pH are less than changes induced in plasma pH.

On the basis of the plasma pH and of the observed distribution of these indicators between the plasma and tissues, values can be calculated for the tissue pH. For a variety of reasons, tritiated nicotine was chosen as the most appropriate pH indicator in the lung and pH values of 6.69 were calculated for the pulmonary extravascular space. It was not possible to distinguish between the interstitial and cellular compartments in these studies because traditional extracellular indicators such as sodium ion and sucrose do not enter the pulmonary interstitium in sufficient amounts before recirculation begins. Respiratory and metabolic changes in arterial pH result in parallel though lesser changes in extravascular pH. Changes in CO_2 tension at constant arterial pH (maintained with infusions of Na_2CO_3 or HCl) did not appear to appreciably alter extravascular pH when these measurements were obtained after 20 to 30 min. These findings were somewhat unexpected since in a variety of other organs, there is evidence that regardless of arterial pH, acute changes in CO_2 tension may produce rapid and pronounced changes in cellular pH. It was postulated that the pH of the lung is largely maintained by the buffers derived from the blood. Although the amount of buffer within the lung tissue at any one moment probably exceeds the amount in the pulmonary capillaries [76], the amount delivered to the lung by the flow of blood is considerably greater. The lung is rapidly perfused by the entire cardiac output and is consequently linked to the acid-base-regulating mechanisms of the body as a whole. Since CO_2 enters the cells more rapidly than bicarbonate, a transient fall in cellular pH is likely. Recovery of tissue pH to normal values within the 20 to 30-min observation interval presumably reflects subsequent entry of buffer into the lung tissue. The rise in plasma bicarbonate produced by the infusion of Na_2CO_3 may promote entry of bicarbonate into the cells (e.g., by an exchange of bicarbonate for chloride, or alternatively, accelerated hydrogen ion secretion from the cells). The rapidity with which the process occurs in the lung, compared with muscle, brain, and heart tissues, may reflect the large surface area and short diffusion distance that characterize much of the pulmonary mass (endothelial and type I alveolar cells) and the rapid perfusion of the lung tissues.

These observations suggest that, as in other cells, CO_2 enters much more rapidly than bicarbonate. However, the exchange of bicarbonate with cells may be relatively rapid in the lung because of the unusual relation of pulmonary parenchyma and blood flow, wherein rapid diffusion and exchange are encouraged. From a teleological point of view, the rapid buffering of tissue pH in the face of a changing CO_2 tension may be of advantage since it could moderate changes in cellular pH due to increase in alveolar P_{CO_2} following regional or general variations in ventilation.

The available studies of the passage of weak acids and bases into the lung tissue are primarily based on analysis of mean transit times and distribution volumes. No studies of the Renkin-Crone approach to initial indicator extraction are available at this time. Of importance is the apparent failure of the pH indicator DMO to enter lung tissues in significant quantities during a single circulation. This seems to contradict the general assumption that the passage of the neutral form of this weak acid across tissues is for all practical purposes instantaneous.

IV. Filtration Coefficient

The rate at which fluid flows across a membrane in response to an increase in hydrostatic pressure is referred to as the filtration coefficient (P_f). The formation of pulmonary edema involves fluid flow across two discrete cellular barriers: the endothelial membrane and the alveolar epithelial membrane. Measurements of the filtration coefficients of these tissue layers are beset by many practical as well as conceptual problems, some of which we shall consider.

The significance of the filtration coefficient in the microcirculation can be best understood in terms of a modified Starling equation:

$$J_v = \frac{v_w P_f S}{RT} (\Delta p - \overset{i}{\Sigma} \sigma_i \Delta \pi_i) \tag{5}$$

J_v refers to the flow of fluid across the capillary surface and S is the capillary surface area. The symbol Δp designates the hydrostatic pressure difference between the capillary lumen and the interstitium. Neither of these pressures can be measured directly, although changes in capillary pressures can be estimated from isogravimetric studies, and pleural pressures have been used as an index of interstitial pressure. The symbol v_w is the molar volume of water.

The symbol $\Delta\pi_i$ designates the osmotic pressure that would be exerted by the ith solute across a membrane that is permeable to water but completely impermeable to this solute. An ideal membrane with these properties is designated semipermeable. In general, $\Delta\pi_i$ can be calculated from the Van't Hoff law:

$$\Delta\pi_i = RT\,\Delta c_i \tag{6}$$

where R is the gas constant, T is the absolute temperature, and Δc_i is the concentration difference across the membrane. (Van't Hoff behavior can be expected only at low concentrations. At physiological concentrations, the term on the right must be multiplied by an osmotic coefficient g to predict osmotic pressures. For simplicity, we assume that g equals 1.) The symbol σ_d designates the solute reflection coefficient, which provides a measure of the effect leakage of solute through the capillary wall has on the osmotic flow induced by the solute. (Discussion of this parameter is deferred until the next section.) For solutes that do not diffuse through the membrane, σ_d equals 1.

Referring to Equation (5), we can see that the filtration coefficient can be measured in either of two ways. The hydrostatic pressure gradient across the capillary can be increased in the presence of constant solute concentrations. Alternatively, the solute concentration gradient between the blood and the tissues can be altered at constant vascular and interstitial hydrostatic pressures. The latter procedure requires the additional knowledge of the reflection coefficient of the solute, information that must ultimately be based on reference to flows induced by hydrostatic pressure gradients (see next section), or some assurance, if it is assumed that the reflection coefficient is 1.0, that the molecule is in solution but remains confined to the vascular compartment.

Measurements of J_v have been made by collecting lymph fluid draining from the lung or from studies of lung weight [77, 78]. The first approach has several distinct advantages: (1) measurements are obtained in vivo, and in some cases have been made in unanesthetized animals; (2) fluid movement is selectively monitored between the vascular and interstitial compartments; (3) information is obtained about the solute concentration as well as about the volume of fluid transferred. It is by no means clear, however, to what extent the flow of lymph reflects total net movement of fluid between the vasculature and the interstitium. Under conditions in which the flow of fluid into the interstitium is rapid, the ability of the lymphatics to remove fluid from the lungs may be overwhelmed. Filtration coefficients determined from increases in organ weight in studies in vitro are generally greater than coefficients determined from lymph flows by a factor of as much as 10 (see Table 1 and Staub's review [22]). The relatively high concentrations described for lymph protein in the lung may reflect some water reabsorption between the capillaries and site of lymphatic fluid collection, though it has been argued that this does not occur [22].

The alternative approach for determining the flow of fluid from the capillaries is accomplished by directly measuring the accumulation or loss of fluid within the lungs. This has been accomplished in the intact animal by increasing left atrial pressures and decreasing plasma protein concentrations and measuring the increase in the wet weight to dry weight ratio of the excised lung. Guyton and Lindsey [79], Levine et al. [80], Mellins et al. [81], and Uter et al. [82] used this procedure to obtain estimates of pulmonary capillary filtration coefficients; they ranged from 0.2×10^{-2} to 10×10^{-2} cm/sec. The principal disadvantage of this approach is the failure to account for lymphatic drainage from the lung, although Levine et al. could find no change in the measured filtration coefficient following occlusion of the thoracic duct. This suggests that lymph flow accounted for a relatively small fraction of the filtration constant. Errors of this kind are more pronounced when fluid accumulation is gradual [22].

Increases in organ weight can be followed continuously if the organ is excised, perfused, and mounted on a balance or a calibrated load cell. These procedures tend to promote edema formation and increased pulmonary vascular resistance. Even under what should be steady state conditions, progressive increases in organ weight may occur [45]. It is difficult to be sure whether increases in organ weight are due to changes in the water content of the vascular, interstitial, cellular, and alveolar compartments [22]. Characteristically, after an abrupt increase in pulmonary outflow pressure, a rapid weight gain is observed, followed by a more prolonged, slow and fairly constant increase in organ weight. It is generally assumed that the initial phase reflects largely vascular distension [83] whereas the latter phase represents interstitial expansion, although this interpretation has been challenged [84].

Increases in pulmonary venous pressure during filtration studies are generally greater than the capillary pressure increases they produce. Since it is the capillary pressure that is responsible for fluid movement, a correction for this difference should be made. Pappenheimer and Soto-Rivera [85], in their early studies, developed a procedure that makes it possible to estimate changes of capillary pressure in the perfused, excised organ. The technique is referred to as isogravimetric, because it provides a measure of the capillary pressure necessary to keep the organ weight from changing at any given plasma and interstitial protein concentration and interstitial hydrostatic pressure. The measurement is accomplished by diminishing arterial pressures and increasing venous pressures in such a way that organ weight remains the same. The value to which these pressures converge (a value at which flow could cease) represents the hydrostatic pressure (p_c) that just balances the forces tending to move fluid out of the capillaries and those tending to return it to the capillaries. Under isogravimetric conditions,

$$p_c = p_v + RF \tag{7}$$

where p_c and p_v are the capillary and venous pressures, R designates the resistance between the capillary and vein, and F is the flow of blood. Provided that resistance remains constant as venous pressure is then changed by Δp_v, the corresponding rise in capillary pressure Δp_c can be calculated at the new blood flow F':

$$(p_c + \Delta p_c) = (p_v + \Delta p_v) + RF'. \tag{8}$$

It is assumed that the vascular volume remains unchanged, an assumption which may be particularly risky in the lung because the pulmonary vasculature is large and distensible.

As fluid movement into the interstitium proceeds, interstitial hydrostatic pressure should rise and interstitial protein concentrations should fall. Both of these events should favor the return of fluid to the vasculature. That this is indeed the case is suggested by the observation that the isogravimetric pressure increases as pulmonary edema proceeds [86]. In other words, as fluid accumulates in the interstitium, there is an increasing tendency for the fluid to return to the capillaries. Evidence has been obtained, however, that distension of the interstitial compartment may facilitate the flow of fluid. Levine et al. [87] found that at higher filtration pressures, the filtration coefficient was increased. (Filtration pressure was used to designate the difference between the plasma hydrostatic and plasma protein osmotic pressures.) This increase did not appear to be the result of vascular distension since no change in filtration occurred at higher vascular hydrostatic pressures provided that the filtration pressure was not changed. Guyton et al. have reported that the accumulation of fluid within the interstitium of subcutaneous tissue results in a marked increase in the rate at which fluid flow through the interstitium proceeds [88]. Levine et al. have suggested that a similar phenomenon may be occurring in the lung. The rate at which fluid enters the lung may be determined partly from the filtration characteristics of the interstitium and not just from the capillary wall alone. Of course rupture of fluid into the alveoli may also occur at high filtration pressures.

Mellins et al. used pleural pressures in estimating interstitial hydrostatic pressure [81]. They concluded that this approximation improved their ability to predict filtration rates with the Starling equation (however, see Ref. 22). They also found that increases in alveolar pressure did not inhibit, but rather encouraged, the accumulation of fluid within the lung. The authors suggest that in lungs inflated to higher pressures, the capillary surface area is increased, with more rapid filtration thereby permitted. They also suggest that the accumulation of fluid in edematous alveoli increases the surface tension of the air-fluid space, an effect that would tend to bring about a decline in interstitial pressure. The rate of filtration was markedly diminished when ventilation with plasma, instead of air, was used, an observation consistent with the concept that the surface tension of the air-fluid interface within lungs acts to increase filtration. More recent information suggests that ventilation at high volumes can deplete surfactant within the lung and thereby promote alveolar flooding [89].

The presence of solutes that do not readily cross the capillary wall tends to diminish filtration rates. This phenomenon is referred to as osmotic buffering. (Its significance is discussed after consideration of capillary reflection coefficients.)

V. Reflection Coefficients

The conceptual need for the reflection coefficient arose with the consideration of membranes that are not ideally "semipermeable" and permit leakage of solute from the more concentrated to the less concentrated solution. From an experimental point of view, there are two different reflection coefficients. This distinction is frequently confused and an effort will be made to characterize each, and to relate them to studies of pulmonary capillary permeability.

A. Solute Reflection Coefficient

The first reflection coefficient was alluded to in the discussion of the filtration constant (Eq. 5) and was designated the solute reflection coefficient (σ_d). Let us consider a vessel of water that is divided into two compartments by a membrane with a filtration coefficient P_f (see Fig. 4). The value of P_f can easily be measured by increasing the hydrostatic pressure in compartment A and watching the flow of water to B (Fig. 4a). In this case, Equation (5) reduces to

$$J_{v,p} = \frac{v_w P_f S}{RT} \Delta p. \qquad (9)$$

Now consider what the effect would be if solute is added to compartment A, and hydrostatic pressure is equal in both compartments (Fig. 4b). Let us further assume that the solute behaves in the ideal Van't Hoff relation (activity coefficients are 1.0) and that it does not traverse the membrane ($\sigma_d = 1.0$). Then

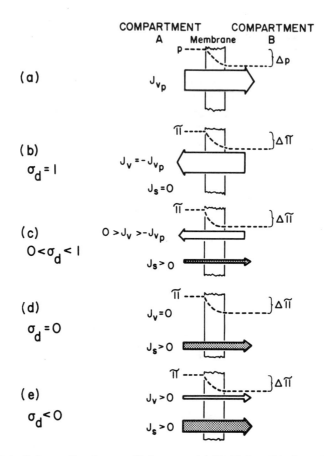

FIGURE 4   Solute reflection coefficient σ_d. (a) Fluid flow (J_{v_p}) produced by a hydrostatic pressure gradient Δp. Below this, the magnitude and direction of flow produced by equivalent osmotic pressure gradients $\Delta \pi$ are shown for solutes with reflection coefficients between 1.0 and an amount less than zero (b, c, d, e).

$$J_v = -\sigma_d \frac{v_w P_f S}{RT} \qquad \Delta \pi = -\sigma_d v_w P_f S \, \Delta c = -v_w P_f S \, \Delta c. \qquad (10)$$

The negative sign is used to indicate that the pressure Δp and $\Delta \pi$ result in opposite flows.

If solute leaks across the membrane, then the flow of water will be diminished (Fig. 4c). If the experiment is repeated with equivalent hydrostatic and osmotic pressures ($\Delta \pi = \Delta p$), σ can be calculated:

$$\sigma = \frac{-J_v}{J_{v,p}} \tag{11}$$

It must be emphasized that solute leakage affects osmotic flow at the very first moment, before there has been any time for the concentration difference between the compartments Δc to diminish. The flow of solution from B to A is diminished by two factors [90, 91]. The movement of solute from A to B interferes with the flow of water from B to A. This is described in terms of a "frictional" interaction of solute and solvent in the membrane. The second factor is generally not so important and simply represents the volume of the solute that is leaking from A to B, thereby diminishing the volumetric flow from B to A.

As indicated above, if the solute does not leak through the membrane, then $\sigma_d = 1.0$ and $J_v = J_{v,p}$. If adding solute to A results in no fluid movement, then $J_v = 0$ and $\sigma_d = 0$ (Fig. 4d). If adding solute to A actually results in the movement of fluid from A to B (because of a very rapid movement of solute in this direction), then σ_d must be negative (Fig. 4e).

Values for σ_d for cardiac muscle capillaries were initially obtained by Vargas and Johnson [92]. The rate of dehydration in a perfused organ was followed after the infusion of a hypertonic solution by watching the decline in organ weight. This rate of fluid flow was compared with the rate at which organ weight decreased following injections of albumin. (They assumed that the reflection coefficient of albumin is 1.0.) Studies were subsequently performed by Taylor and Gaar [46] and Perl et al. [45] on the lungs during which comparisons were made with flows induced by hydrostatic pressure changes, and by Fenstermacher and Johnson on the brain [47], in which sucrose and raffinose were assumed to have reflection coefficients of 1.0.

As noted in Table 1, values for σ_d that Taylor and Gaar obtained were considerably less than the values Perl et al. obtained. Although the reasons for this difference are not clear at this time, there are numerous factors that would tend to lead to erroneously low values of σ_d. It is tacitly assumed that the initial loss of weight following infusion of hypertonic solutions represents loss of fluid from the entire lung. The likelihood that this is indeed the case largely depends on whether the hypertonic solution arrives at all of the capillaries at the same time and whether the fluid extracted from these capillaries arrives at the outflow together. Perl suggested that the fluid extracted from the tissues pushed out blood from the pulmonary vein in a pistonlike fashion. Thus, the loss of weight by the organ seemed to occur at the very time that water was leaving the lung tissue and entering the capillary compartment. More recent studies by these investigators (personal communication) suggest that this is not the case; they suggest that the loss of weight occurs at about the same time that the extracted fluid reaches the outflow, and that mixing of this fluid with blood not containing the tissue fluid would yield diminished rates of weight loss.

Not only should the hypertonic solution reach all the capillaries simultaneously, but it should not become diluted by the perfusion fluid that precedes it. In order to avoid dispersion of the hypertonic solution, the distance between the site of injection and the pulmonary artery should be diminished. The effects of nonuniform and dispersed delivery of solute to the capillaries and nonuniform delivery of extracted fluid to the outflow will tend to be minimized as blood flow is increased. The observation that the rate of loss of weight following infusions of hypertonic solutions increased with flow could partly be due to just such a phenomenon [45].

An alternative method of measuring the rate of the dehydration produced by infusions of hypertonic solutions was provided by studies in vivo by the author [93]. Dilution of the pulmonary blood flow by tissue fluid was measured, instead of following changes of organ weight. The hypertonic solution was injected intravenously as a bolus and the osmolality and the concentrations of hemoglobin and albumin in the arterial blood were monitored. The concomitant flow of blood was also measured. It was possible to calculate from these data the rate of fluid flow out of the lung tissue. On the assumption that the osmotic bolus and extracted water traverse the pulmonary veins in much the same way, the product $\sigma_d P_f S$ was calculated. This procedure has several advantages. The quantity of fluid removed from the lung is matched with a plasma osmolality that corresponds to it. Any dilution of the solute by mixture with blood from capillaries that have not yet received the solute should be approximately equivalent to the dilution experienced by extracted tissue fluid. In addition, tissue fluid flows can be clearly distinguished from flows of blood, since the former contains no hemoglobin and little plasma protein (to be described). There is always some ambiguity in wieght experiments since changes in weight may reflect changes of vascular or extravascular fluid. A third advantage is the obvious benefit of using an intact animal. Unfortunately, the procedure also entails several drawbacks. The dilution of the blood by tissue fluid flows is relatively low and the osmotic bolus must be highly concentrated to elicit a measurable response. Neither ultrafiltration produced by increasing hydrostatic pressure nor tissue dehydration caused by increasing protein osmotic pressures have been detected with this technique.

Values for $\sigma_d P_f S$ calculated from the in situ data appear to match the perfused lung data of Chinard et al. and are not consistent with the data of Taylor and Gaar (see Table 1). This suggests that errors in the Chinard study associated with heterogenous solute delivery and water discharge are small and that changes in organ weight were correctly identified with loss of extravascular fluid. The correspondence also suggests that the differences in changes of osmolality of the two preparations (as little as 5 mosm/kg in the study in situ and as much as 300 mosm/kg in the study in vivo) have relatively little effect on the calculated value of $\sigma_d P_f S$. The response therefore appears quite linear.

Because tissue fluid flows are relatively small compared with blood flow, the osmolality of the perfusion solution does not change by very much as it is in transit between the pulmonary artery and the pulmonary vein. An exponential decline in concentration was assumed by the author. In all these studies, there is much more uncertainty about tissue osmolality. The assumption that changes in tissue osmolality remain negligible at an early time after the hypertonic solution has traversed the capillaries is at best speculative. It may be supposed that at one extreme blood flow is relatively slow and that local equilibration between blood and tissues is complete at these early times. Under these circumstances, the rate of tissue dehydration reflects the rate of blood flow. At the other extreme (generally assumed in these studies), the rate of fluid extraction can be independent of blood flow and limited strictly by the rate of water flow across capillaries. The increase in the rate of pulmonary dehydration that Perl et al. produced at high flows could represent some degree of flow limitation, and calculated values of $\sigma_d P_f S$ and of σ_d could therefore be too low. As noted above, the observed increase in $\sigma_d P_f S$ with flow may also be the result of a more uniform delivery of solute and extraction of fluid. A third explanation for this rise may be the tendency for capillary surface area to increase with increases of blood flow.

No consistent change in the filtration constant–surface area product ($P_f S$) with blood flow was found in the experiments of Perl et al. Nor was a consistent change found in calculated values of σ_d obtained by dividing the osmotic data ($\sigma_d P_f S$) by the filtration data ($P_f S$). Since $\sigma_d P_f S$ does rise significantly with flow, it is likely that the scatter in $P_f S$ data is too great for us to be sure that calculated values of σ_d do not also change with blood flow.

B. Solvent Drag Reflection Coefficient

Leakage of solute through membranes can be monitored by measuring the concentration of solute in fluid filtered through the membranes. If the membrane is relatively impermeable to the solute, the fluid traversing the membrane will contain lower concentrations than the fluid entering the membrane. This process of separating solvent and solute is termed ultrafiltration, and the relative leakiness of the membrane is measured by what is referred to as the sieving, or solvent drag, reflection coefficient (σ_f):

$$J_s = (1 - \sigma_f)c_m J_v \qquad (12)$$

where J_s represents the solute flux in the filtrate, c_m is the average solute concentration of the filtrate in the membrane, and J_v is the flow of fluid through the membrane. It is assumed in this equation that there is no net diffusion of solute across the membranes, a condition that can be met if the concentrations of solute are kept the same. This can be accomplished by continuously renewing the fluid on either side of the membrane with fluid containing the initial solute concentration c_0. If differences in concentrations are permitted (if $\Delta c \neq 0$), then diffusion must be expected, and Equation (12) must be expanded to include diffusional flux of solute:

$$J_s = (1 - \sigma_f)c_m J_v + PS \, \Delta c_i. \tag{13}$$

The properties of σ_f are much the same as the properties of σ_d. If the membrane does not leak solute, then σ_f and σ_d will approach 1.0. On the other hand, if the solute concentration in the filtrate equals that in the filtrate, then $\sigma_f = 0$. If the membrane leaks the solute as readily as this, no osmotic flow of fluid should be expected when a concentration gradient is established across the membrane and σ_d will also be zero. It can be predicted that under the limiting conditions of a sufficiently small concentration gradient and a uniform membrane, the solute and sieving reflection coefficients will be the same:

$$\sigma_d = \sigma_f. \tag{14}$$

This relation is based on statistical mechanical considerations and is referred to as the Onsager reciprocity theorem [91]. Although there has been some question whether these criteria can be met in biological membranes, experimental as well as theoretical justification for using the theorem has been advanced [94–97].

Very little information is available about the σ_f value of the capillary walls. In what is probably the earliest study of this kind, Starling showed that as blood pressure is diminished during hemorrhage, fluid mobilized from the tissues is approximately isotonic (determined from freezing-point depression), suggesting that the solvent reflection coefficients of most of the constituents of the interstitial fluid are close to zero [3]. Starling proposed that there is a constant flow of fluid that leaves the arterial end of the capillary, moves through the interstitium, and then returns to the blood at the venous end of the capillary. He suggested that concentrations of small solutes are nearly equal in this fluid and plasma but that protein is sieved from fluid crossing the capillary wall, i.e., σ_f for protein approaches 1.0. A clear perivascular space around peripheral capillaries has been described [98, 99] but estimates of the flow through this region remain uncertain [100]. The most striking example of such extravascular flow may be found between the glomerular and peritubular capillaries.

Zweifach and Intaglietta have recently modified the Starling hypothesis by suggesting that extravascular flows may proceed from capillaries with high hydrostatic pressures to other, lower-pressure vessels in the mesenteric circulation [7]. The magnitude of extravascular flows will depend on the relative resistance of the vascular and extravascular routes. Consideration must be given to the intrinsic resistance of the interstitial space as well as to the vascular walls. There is some evidence that with the onset of interstitial edema, this resistance may diminish. Information is also needed about the gradient of hydrostatic pressure along the capillary length and within the interstitial space. On the basis of a sheet flow hypothesis, Fung [101] has suggested that pressures along the capillary bed may be relatively uniform.

It is generally felt that diffusion is much more important than convection (filtration with concomitant solvent drag) in the delivery of small solutes to the extravascular compartment [102]. These comparisons are based on estimates of diffusion calculated from measurements of solute permeability and coresponding estimates of filtration and solvent drag. In support of these calculations, Pappenheimer could find no evidence that increasing the hydrostatic pressure between the artery and the vein of the hind limb increased the rate of solute delivery despite the fact that filtration and solute delivery should thereby be increased [26]. Again, the glomerular capillaries represent an important exception to this rule, since solute movement out of these vessels is mostly by solvent drag.

Measurements of sieving reflection coefficients may be frustrated by concomitant diffusional fluxes. With increases in capillary hydrostatic pressure, transudation of fluid containing relatively low concentrations of less permeable molecules (i.e., molecules with high sieving reflection coefficients) occurs through the endothelial cells. Since there is no way of preventing this dilution, some degree of diffusion is inevitable. Pappenheimer et al. found that although the sieving coefficient (originally expressed in terms of sieving factors, where $s = 1 - \sigma_f$) of inulin was 0.7 in the leg, and the concentration of inulin traversing the capillary wall during ultrafiltration should be only 30% of plasma concentrations, inulin concentrations actually amounted to 70% of plasma concentrations. They attributed the movement of extra solute to concomitant diffusion in the direction of filtration. If a local concentration gradient is established, the osmotic difference will tend to slow filtration by osmotic buffering (to be described). As ultrafiltration is increased, dilution of the transudated fluid should become more apparent. A decline in protein concentration from both the lungs and the body as a whole has been noted when lymph flow is increased, but no similar dilution has been reported for small-solute concentrations [22]. This is not surprising, since any concentration difference of, for example, sodium ion that might be expected would not be greater than 1 milliequivalent per liter (with corresponding osmotic pressure equivalent to 40 mmHg if anion and cation concentrations are considered) and would be undectable. The presence of reduced protein concentrations in pulmonary edema secondary to congestive heart failure presumably represents a similar process of sieving [103].

An additional problem associated with increasing capillary pressures deserves comment. When ultrafiltration is induced by raising capillary hydrostatic pressure, there is always some risk that the intercellular junctions will be enlarged, a phenomenon Shirley et al. referred to as the stretched pore phenomenon [104]. This would result in a decline in the selectivity of the membrane to solutes and sieving reflection coefficients would be underestimated. Morphologic evidence for this phenomenon was described earlier.

VI. Osmotic Buffering

As far back as 1937, Ancel Keys [105] suggested that filtration of fluid through the capillary walls is slowed by the presence of small lipophobic solutes in the plasma. Ultrafiltration results in the entry of fluid deficient in these solutes into the interstitium, with a corresponding accumulation within the vascular space. The consequence of such a concentration gradient is that an osmotic force contrary to the hydrostatic-pressure gradient is generated and the observed filtration constant is lower than what would be characteristic in the absence of impermeant solute. This effect was referred to by Keys as osmotic buffering. Chinard later suggested that osmotic buffering may be important in moderating the rate of water filtration across glomerular and capillary membranes [106]. More recently, the phenomenon has been studied in artificial membranes [107] and is referred to as "concentration polarization" in the membrane literature.

Two recent publications suggest that osmotic buffering by small solutes such as sodium chloride, urea, and sugars may be significant in slowing fluid transport across capillary beds in the lung [45] and heart [108]. Perl et al. [45] have calculated that with an increase of capillary pressure by 2 mmHg, the flow of fluid into the pulmonary parenchyma will be slowed by 25% by the normal plasma concentrations of small salts (300 mosm/kg). This figure is arrived at by assuming that the concentration of the fluid crossing the capillary wall c_f will dilute the interstitial fluid until the concentrations in the interstitium c_i and in the entering fluid are the same ($c_i = c_f$). It is further assumed that the concentration difference between the interstitium (c_i) and plasma (c_p) remains relatively small compared to the plasma osmolality, so that the average concentration in the membrane c_m can be approximated by either c_i or c_p. Then Equation (13) becomes

$$\Delta c = \frac{\sigma_f J_v c_p}{PS}. \tag{15}$$

Perl et al., using their data to approximate the flow expected with a 2-mmHg increase in pressure, σ_f (assumed equal to σ_d) and PS, caldulated that the interstitium should be at 299.91 mosm/kg at a time when the plasma osmolality is 300 mosm/kg [45]. Although this fall in osmolality seems minute, it is equivalent to a hydrostatic pressure of 0.51 mmHg, which is fully one-fourth the driving force. This would result in a proportionate fall in the rate of filtration (osmotic buffering).

Perl et al. did not calculate how long it would take for this fall in interstitial osmolality to occur, but suggested that osmotic buffering can help prevent passage of fluid into the lungs during the increase in capillary pressure that accompanies a single cardiac contraction. It can be calculated—from Equations (5) and (13) and from normal tissue volumes—that the buffering effect requires about 10 sec to become fully apparent. If increases in hydrostatic pressure distend capillaries and increase capillary permeability, the osmotic buffering effect will diminish.

A steady state flow through the capillary wall will be established when the concentration of fluid in the interstitium is diluted to the concentration of fluid crossing the capillary wall. The relation between the initial and the steady state flows across the capillary wall that are produced by raising capillary pressure is illustrated in Figure 5. It is assumed that the sieving and solute reflection coefficients are equal. If the reflection coefficient (σ) of the solute in the plasma is 1.0 (Fig. 5a), then the steady-state flow ($J_{v_{ss}}$) will be significantly less than the initial flow (J_{v_o}). This decline in flow is due to the creation of a concentration difference between the plasma and interstitium (Δc) and represents osmotic buffering. If σ is less than 1, the degree of buffering will be diminished (Fig. 5b) and when σ equals zero, osmotic buffering will vanish (Fig. 5c). Osmotic buffering should increase as the concentrations of solutes with reflection coefficients greater than zero are increased. It might therefore be expected that increases in plasma sodium chloride concentrations or infusions of mannitol might be useful in lowering the rate of formation of pulmonary edema in the lung. Increases in solute concentrations might, however, also lower the rate of fluid reabsorption and possibly alter the permeability of the capillary wall; in any case, osmotic buffering across the capillary wall is probably of relatively little clinical importance since it can moderate but not prevent or correct edema formation.

In a model calculation based on cardiac data, Grabowski also concluded that osmotic buffering will diminish calculated values of both the filtration coefficient and the reflection coefficient of electrolytes [108].

Osmotic buffering by small solutes may be more important in slowing the flow of water across the alveolar barrier than the capillary wall since the solute permeability of the epithelium appears to be significantly less than that of the endothelium. Although osmotic buffering by protein molecules is limited by

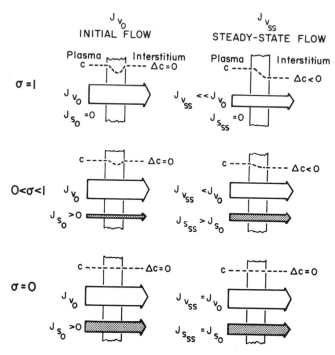

FIGURE 5 Osmotic buffering. The influence of the reflection coefficient on the movement of fluid and solute across the capillary wall is shown (σ_d and σ_f are assumed equal). The flow of fluid is produced by a rise in hydrostatic pressure in the plasma compartment. The symbols J_{v_0} and $J_{v_{ss}}$ represent the flow of solution through the wall at time zero and when a steady state flow has been achieved. Similarly, J_{s_0} and $J_{s_{ss}}$ represent the corresponding initial solute fluxes across the capillary wall. Note that σ does not initially alter fluid flow. The flow of fluid is maximally decreased when a steady state concentration gradient Δc across the membrane has been established, a phenomenon referred to as osmotic buffering. Furthermore, osmotic buffering is greatest when σ is 1.0, and it falls to zero when σ is zero. If $0 < \sigma < 1$, the movement of solute across the membrane will be maximal during the steady state, when the concentration gradient is maximum. Not shown is the expectation that osmotic buffering will increase as plasma solute concentrations increase.

the low osmolalities of these molecules in the plasma, it is conceivable that local concentration differences during filtration are not appreciated.

Perl also hypothesized that osmotic buffering would attenuate the flow of water from the tissues that follows infusion of hypertonic solutions. For example, following an infusion of hypertonic sucrose, water will be extracted from the tissues and concentrations of resident solutes such as sodium and chloride ions will become elevated in the tissues and correspondingly diluted in the plasma. Under these circumstances, the observed rate of tissue dehydration should be lower than the rates that would be found with no resident solute. Once again it is apparent that the magnitude of this effect depends on the duration of filtration. Perl et al. make no distinction between intracellular and extracellular solutes. Very little movement of solute across cell membranes occurs during hypertonic dehydration, and resident solute concentrations rise progressively as dehydration proceeds. This effect is simply equivalent to what must be considered in all permeability studies: To what extent has tissue and blood equilibrated during the study, thereby diminishing the driving force (in this case osmotic) between the vascular and tissue compartments? Under the best of circumstances, data are obtained before significant increases in tissue osmolality has occurred.

Perl et al. found that within 5 sec after the hypertonic solution had begun to cause the lung to lose weight, the weight of the preparation attained a new steady state. The loss of weight appeared to correspond with what would be expected had the fluid been extracted from both the interstitial and the cellular compartments. It is therefore likely that equilibration occurs rapidly throughout the lung. Since the movement of water across cellular membranes is considerably faster than movement of the injected solutes, equilibration presumably involves shifts of water from cell to interstitium and thereafter into plasma.

VII. Isogravimetric and Baseline Dilution Studies

Rather than use tracer studies to measure the solute permeability of the capillaries of the cat leg, Pappenheimer et al. chose an isogravimetric approach, using hypertonic solutions [17]. The loss of weight that followed infusions of hypertonic solutions of low-molecular-weight solutes was blocked by simultaneously increasing capillary hydrostatic pressure.

The average osmotic difference between plasma and tissues was calculated from the imposed hydrostatic pressure that just managed to prevent tissue dehydration. Because the hydrostatic-pressure gradient provided an estimate of the average concentration difference, a description of the decline in concentration gradients from arterial to venous ends of the capillary was unnecessary. In this respect, the procedure appeared superior to the tracer approach, which required some such model.

The concept of solute reflection coefficient was introduced by Staverman [109] about the same time as the publication of the original study of small solutes by Pappenheimer et al. The latter investigators incorrectly assumed that the hypertonic solutions exerted the full van't Hoff hydrostatic pressure. The concentration gradients of solute between plasma and tissue were consequently underestimated by a factor of 3 or more and the solute permeabilities were overestimated by the same factor.

Pappenheimer et al. [27], Vargas and Johnson [92], and Taylor and Gaar [46] tacitly assumed that infusions of hypertonic solutions of small solutes principally resulted in interstitial dehydration. Evidence that this assumption was also erroneous was provided by studies of the author [93]. In these studies, evidence was obtained that the extracted fluid contained very low concentrations of Na^+, K^+, and urea. Since these moieties and associated anions represent the major part of the extravascular osmotic material, it is reasonable to assume that the fluid removed from the lungs by these concentrated solutions is distinctly hypotonic. This observation could be explained by a parallel pathway model, illustrated in Figure 6.

It is assumed that the capillary wall comprises a parallel array of endothelial cells and intercellular junctions. It is further assumed that the cells are highly impermeable to both small and large molecules and that $\sigma_d = \sigma_f = 1$ for all solutes. It is assumed that the junctions are highly impermeable to large molecules for which $\sigma_d = \sigma_f = 1$ but permeable to small molecules for which reflection coefficients approach zero. Water flow may occur through both cells and intercellular junctions.

Consider first what occurs when the capillary hydrostatic pressure increased (Fig. 6a). Water is forced through both the endothelial cells and the junctions. Estimates have been made that junctional flow represents at least half the total flow [110-112, 115]. Because essentially no solute accompanies the flow of water through the cells (reflection coefficients equal zero), it can be expected that dilution of interstitial fluid will be particularly evident just outside the endothelial cell. If mixing with the interstitium is not complete, then it can be expected that osmotic buffering will tend to decrease the proportion of fluid flow that occurs through the cell as the steady state condition is approached.

If protein concentrations within the plasma are increased, then an opposite but otherwise similar movement of water and solute can be expected (Fig. 6b). If the concentrations of small solutes are increased, however, a very different situation can be expected (Fig. 6c). Because the cell is relatively impermeable to the small solute and $\sigma_d = 1$, the flow of water through the cell will be similar to the flow produced by an equivalent increase in protein concentration. Since the cell does not permit the small solutes within the tissue to accompany the flow of water, solute will not be present in the extracted fluid. Because the reflection

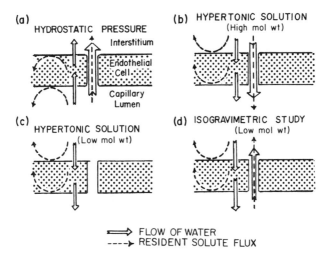

FLOW OF WATER
RESIDENT SOLUTE FLUX

FIGURE 6 Parallel flow hypothesis. (a) When capillary hydrostatic pressure is increased, only water crosses the endothelial cells whereas both solute and water traverse the intercellular junction. Dilution of the fluid outside the endothelial cell should result in osmotic buffering with the fraction of flow through the junction increasing as a steady state is approached. (b) When plasma concentrations of large molecules (σ_d at both cell and junction equals 1.0) are increased, solute and water flows should be produced that are opposite to those produced by equivalent hydrostatic pressure gradients. (c) When plasma concentration of a small lipophobic solute (σ_d at cell equals 1.0 and σ_d at junction is close to zero) is increased, there is initially no flow through the junction but there is flow of water without solute through the cell. (d) Isogravimetric studies are characterized by equal and opposite flows of water through the cells and solution (containing solute) through the junctions. Reproduced from R. M. Effros, *J. Clin. Invest.*, **54**:935-947 (1974), by courtesy of the publishers.

coefficient for the solute at the junction is very low, very little fluid movement through the junction will occur and no solute will be delivered by solvent drag into the plasma. The extracted fluid will therefore be distinctly hypotonic. (This concept of small-solute osmosis is presented in a formal manner elsewhere [93].)

It is proposed that the initial response to these hypertonic solutions is endothelial dehydration. This is followed by interstitial and alveolar cell hydration. Although there is relatively little fluid movement through the junctions under these circumstances, it is somewhat surprising that small solutes already present in the interstitium do not diffuse from the interstitium to the blood as interstitial concentrations increase. The failure to find interstitial solute in the extracted fluid may merely reflect the difficulty with which relatively small fluxes of solute are detected in these experments. Alternatively, it is possible that the injected solute produces an "anomalous" flow of fluid and solute through the junctions into the interstitium and thereby impairs solute diffusion from the interstitium to the blood. Anomalous membrane phenomena of this nature have been described for both artificial and living membranes [113-115]. A third explanation would be that contraction of the interstitium is prevented by the structural matrix of the interstitium, which tends to keep this volume open. Guyton [116] has provided evidence that the interstitial volume is non-compliant under normal circumstances and that interstitial hydrostatic pressure falls rapidly below atmospheric pressures as extracellular dehydration occurs.

In general it is difficult to produce significant movement of any solute out of the tissue with concentrated solutions of substances having similar reflection coefficients. This is shown by the following simple example. Let us assume that the solute reflection coefficient of the injected solute and the sieving reflection coefficient of the resident solute are the same ($\sigma_d = \sigma_f$). If it is assumed that diffusion and interaction between the injected and resident solute flows are negligible, then the movement of resident solute out of the tissue J_s will be described by Equation (12). The value of J_v will in turn be determined by Equation (5). Combining these equations, we obtain the relation

$$J_s = (\sigma - \sigma^2) c_m v_w P_f S \, \Delta c. \tag{16}$$

As noted in Figure 7, the movement of solute out of tissue is maximal if σ is 0.5, and under these circumstances solute flow is only one-quarter of the flux ($J_{s_{max}}$) that would be obtained if the solute reflection coefficient of the injected solute were one and that of the resident solute were zero. It can be predicted that very little movement of resident protein from tissues to blood will be produced by injections of similar proteins into the blood perfusing the organ.

The hypotonic nature of fluid extracted from the lungs with hypertonic solutions of small solutes suggests that these solutions act primarily to dehydrate the cellular compartments of organs. That a considerable portion of the water is derived from cells is also suggested by the osmotic volume studies of Perl et al. (Eq. 4) [45], described previously. These investigators also found that the quantity of fluid removed from the lungs by hypertonic solutions is not materially affected by rapid development of edema. This finding is consistent with the premise that most of the fluid extracted with hypertonic solutions is cellular in origin, since the increase in junctional permeability (specifically a decline in the junctional reflection coefficient) would otherwise result in a detectable decline in the rate of interstitial dehydration.

It is interesting that West found that hypertonic solutions of urea tended to decrease pulmonary vascular resistance in edematous lungs and attributed this to "interstitial dehydration" [117]. This observation was obscured by the observation that hypertonic solutions of other solutes resulted in apparent increases in vascular resistance [118, 119]. It subsequently became clear that these alternative solutions resulted in a loss of red cell deformability and consequent vascular obstruction [119-121]. When cell-free perfusates are used, hypertonicity with all agents appears to reduce vascular resistance, and in recent studies by the author (unpublished), hypotonicity correspondingly increases pulmonary vascular resistance. Cellular rather than interstitial dehydration may have been responsible for the decline in vascular resistance West observed following infusions of hypertonic urea. Furthermore, a decline in resistance with hypertonic urea can be found in both normal and edematous lungs.

Despite the lack of net transfer of fluid between the plasma and tissues during isogravimetric experiments, there may be considerable convectional flows of fluid extracted through the cell membranes into the blood compensated by movement of fluid into the interstitium through the intercellular junctions (see Fig. 6d). Among the effects of such a circulation is the inevitable drag of some solute from the plasma into the tissues [122]. Perl estimated that in the lung, isogravimetric measurements would yield values for the capillary permeability that are 2.4 times as great as those determined by a tracer study in which convectional flows were not carrying additional solute into the interstitium. Grabowski has made similar calculations for myocardial exchange [108].

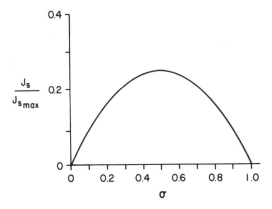

FIGURE 7   Solute movement produced by osmotic gradients of similar solutes. The symbol J_s represents the flux of a "resident" solute from the tissue produced by the rise in plasma concentration of an injected solute. It is assumed that the σ_f, the resident solute, equals the σ_d coefficient of the injected solute (Eq. 16). The symbol $J_{s_{max}}$ represents the solute flux that would be seen if the σ_f of the resident solute were zero and the σ_d of the injected solution were 1.

VIII. Permeability of the Alveolar Epithelium

Three kinds of data show that the permeability of the alveolar epithelial membrane separating blood from gas in the lung is considerably lower than the permeability of the endothelial layer. The first kind is morphologic and is related to the passage of relatively large molecules, which can be detected in electron micrographs. Whereas arterial pressures of 50 mmHg sufficed to permit the passage of hemoglobin (64,500 daltons) through the interendothelial junctions, fully 70 mmHg pressure was required before the hemoglobin began to appear in the airways in perfused dog lungs [12, 13]. Similary, expansion of the vascular space in the mouse resulted in the passage of horseradish peroxidase (40,000 daltons) into the interstitium by way of the interendothelial junctions but the indicator did not enter the alveolar space [11]. Following intranasal instillation, peroxidase was taken up by pinocytotic vesicles and tubules by the flat alveolar cells but none appeared to traverse the epithelium [11].

Freeze-fracture studies show that the epithelial junctions are joined by a much more complex network than the endothelial junctions [123]. The latter are connected by only one or two strands which are discontinuous in some areas and may therefore leak small solutes.

Studies of solute transfer also suggest that the epithelial barrier is considerably less permeable than the endothelial barrier. Early studies of fresh-water and seawater drowning indicated that although water rapidly traversed the alveolar-capillary barrier, the movement of salts and urea was very much slower [124–127]. Chinard found that following intratracheal instillation, hydrophilic solutes such as [^{14}C]urea, ^{22}Na, and ^{36}Cl appeared in the blood much more slowly than labeled water [128]. Chinard also discovered that $^{14}CO_2$ crossed the alveolar capillary barrier more rapidly than $H^{14}CO_3^-$ when carbonic anhydrase was inhibited with acetazolamide [128, 71]. In these same studies, Chinard found that when the indicator was placed in a hypertonic solution (seawater), its transfer into the blood was impaired. Three factors could have been responsible for this observation: (1) The flow of water from blood to the alveolar phase may have directly slowed solute transfer by solvent drag. (2) Entry of water into the alveolar space would tend to dilute the labeled sodium and carry some of it up the bronchioles and away from the principal exchange site, viz. the alveolar membrane. (3) The dilute solutions may have increased the permeability of the alveolar membranes more than the concentrated solutions, endothelial and epithelial swelling and distortion might be expected with the former. All these studies are susceptible to artifacts introduced by filling the alveoli with fluid.

The problems of ensuring that the indicators within the alveoli are well mixed and presented to a known amount of pulmonary membrane surface have not been resolved. The mathematical models used by both Taylor et al. [129] and Wangensteen et al. [44] assume that both compartments are well mixed, and these studies depended on data obtained over the entire time course of solute transfer. Taylor et al. may have avoided the mixing problem to some degree by introducing the indicator into the blood and following its emergence in the alveolar space. Data obtained in this way yielded very much higher values for permeability than subsequent studies in which indicators were instilled intratracheally. Although presentation to the surface of the alveolar-capillary membrane is probably much more uniform when the indicator arrives in the blood phase, the creation of local concentration gradients within the alveolar phase will tend to slow solute transfer unless early data are stressed.

Measurements of alveolar-capillary solute reflection coefficients have provided a third form of evidence that the alveolar epithelial membrane is much less permeable than endothelium. Taylor and Gaar [46] measured the loss of weight produced by increasing the perfusion osmolality of isolated perfused dog lobes that had been degassed and flooded with Tyrode's solution. They found that the flow of water out of these lungs was very much greater than the corresponding flow observed in lungs not containing fluid; and by comparing these data with the rate at which fluid enters the lung with increase of hydrostatic pressure, they were able to calculate solute reflection coefficients. The solute reflection coefficients for urea, glucose, and sucrose were 0.59, 0.72, and 0.81. These values were very much higher than the values obtained for capillary reflection coefficients (described previously).

Several caveats are warranted for interpreting these data. The ability to withdraw more water from the fluid-filled lung may represent, in part, the availability of less water in the air-filled lung. Osmolality may rise more rapidly in the air-filled lung and therefore diminish the rate of dehydration. In addition, it is by no means clear to what extent measurements of filtration coefficients provide information on the endothelial and epithelial membranes, and comparisons with these data may be misleading.

In both the permeability and reflection coefficient studies, the passage of lipid soluble substances and water was much more rapid than the passage of salts and sugars and urea. Furthermore, the alveolar membrane was more permeable to smaller lipophobic solute molecules than to the larger ones. Taylor et al. [129] found that compared with sodium, urea crossed the barrier three times more rapidly despite the similarity of the diffusion coefficients of each in water. They concluded that diffusion of sodium through the barrier was restricted by the small dimensions of the junctions. Wangensteen et al. [44] could not confirm this observation and suggested that the open junctions were very few compared with those of endothelial beds, but of similar size. More recent data suggest the existence of a variety of "pore" populations with a wide range of dimensions [130].

The fetal lung provides a unique opportunity to study alveolar permeability in a preparation normally filled with fluid. A number of studies by Strang and his colleagues have clearly indicated that the epithelial barrier is considerably less permeable than the endothelial barrier [131]. Boyd et al. [132] followed the transfer of labeled polyvinylpyrrolidone fractions of various molecular weights from the blood to lymph and concluded that in addition to pores of 9 nm in the newborn lamb and 15 nm in fetal lambs, it was necessary to postulate the existence of a small population of large leaks over 100 nm in diameter. It is possible that some of this leakage may have occurred through the bronchial vessels. In contrast, the passage of large molecules through the alveolar walls is very slow. On the basis of exchange between lung capillaries, lymph and alveoli, Normand et al. [61] and Olver and Strang [133] have calculated epithelial pore diameters of 0.55 nm to 0.61 nm. Both Gatzy [134] and Olver and Strange [133] have obtained evidence for active Cl^- transfer across the epithelial barriers, though transport across the bronchial epithelium cannot be excluded since similar transport has been documented across the tracheal mucosa [135].

More recently, Egan et al. have provided evidence that alveolar pores transiently enlarge at birth and may thereby promote absorption of alveolar fluid [136, 137]. Egan has also reported that pore size may be increased by distending the alveoli [137].

IX. Conclusions

Many investigators have hoped that measuring permeability of pulmonary capillaries to small hydrophilic solutes could be accomplished in the clinical setting as well as in the laboratory. The transient procedures of Crone and Chinard et al. appeared to provide just such an opportunity. Unfortunately, careful interpretation of both the assumptions on which these procedures are based and the data gathered in this fashion suggest that only qualitative information can be obtained in this way regarding the entry or exclusion of solutes from the extravascular compartments of the lung. Steady state measurements of indicator diffusion into lung tissues (either invasively or by scanning procedures) might be more informative than single-passage studies for important solutes such as Na^+, K^+, Cl^-, and HCO_3^-.

A wide variety of studies suggest that the alveolar epithelial barrier is much less permeable than the endothelial barrier. This property of the lung may be responsible for the common observation that early edema may be confined to the interstitial compartment. It is possible that "osmotic buffering" is more important across the alveolar membrane than across the endothelium. Entry of fluid into the alvcoli may be slowed both by the the lower filtration constant of the epithelium (by no means proven), as well as the low permeability of this barrier to the normal interstitial solutes of the lung (primarily sodium and associated anions). This can be a double-edged sword since solute already within the alveoli may inhibit reabsorption of fluid. In view of the greater permeability of the pulmonary endothelium, it is unlikely that small solutes will significantly slow solute transfer between the capillaries and tissues of the lung.

Alterations in plasma protein concenration should be reflected primarily by changes in the interstitium. In contrast, alterations in plasma concentrations of small solutes should result in cellular volume changes. For example, it can be expected that doubling the plasma protein osmotic pressure from 20 to 40 mmHg will reduce the interstitial volume by one-half if this volume is sufficiently compliant. Because this represents an increase in total serum osmolality of only 1 mosm/kg or about 0.3%, changes in cellular volume will be undetectable. When small solute concentrations are doubled, cellular volume will decrease by approximately one-half (provided that the cell acts as a perfect osmometer and does not permit entry of any of this solute). It has been difficult to show even transient decreases in interstitial volume with increases in small solute concentrations, and it can be predicted that the interstitial volume will tend to return to its normal size within a short time after such changes have occurred. Although small solutes within the plasma or interstitium may moderate the rate of fluid flow across the capillary wall, this effect is probably small.

The usefulness of dehydrating the interstitial and alveolar compartments in pulmonary edema is obvious. The potential advantages of dehydrating the cellular compartment remain uncertain. Cellular swelling is well documented in various forms of pulmonary edema [138, 139]. It is tempting to speculate that impairment of sodium pumping and swelling of both the endothelial and epithelial cells occur with exposure to blood-borne or gaseous toxins. Distortion of these cells may result in widening of the intercellular junctions with increases in permeability to water and solutes and impairment of blood flow. Hypertonic solutions of small solutes have been found useful in promoting blood flow in kidneys in the setting of shock and potential acute tubular necrosis [140], in the edematous brain [141], and in the ischemic heart [142]. These results have been attributed partly to the salutary effect of cellular hydration, and it is conceivable that such solutions might be helpful in the edematous lung if over-expansion of the vascular volume can be avoided. If the integrity of the epithelial membrane can be restored, such infusions might also promote removal of fluid already present within the alveoli. Unfortunately, experimental studies with hypertonic mannitol have failed to demonstrate any benefit from cellular dehydration [143].

Although some information has been obtained about solute and water transport through the endothelial and epithelial barriers of the lung, very little is known about electrolyte exchange between the cells composing these barriers and the extracellular fluid. Leakage of sodium ions and associated anions across the enormous surface areas of the endothelial and epithelial type I cells may be considerable and active extrusion of sodium ion could be partly responsible for the impressive energy requirements of the lung [144]. Aside from volume considerations, even maintenance of the highly organized and attenuated shape of these cells may require expenditure of energy, a phenomenon described for biconcave red cells that contain actin and myosinlike molecules in their membranes [145, 146]. The recent report by Young and Knelson [147] that both spontaneous pulmonary edema and the edema induced by NO_2 are associated with increased glucose metabolism could reflect increased energy requirements of damaged and deformed cells that have become more permeable to electrolytes. It seems safe to predict that the attention of investigators of pulmonary edema will be devoted increasingly to the integrity of the pulmonary cells relative to their metabolic needs and their electrolyte and water balance.

References

1. E. H. Starling, On the absorption of fluids from the connective tissue, *J. Physiol.*, (London), **19**:312-316 (1896).
2. E. H. Starling, The Arris and Gale lectures on the physiological factors involved in the causation of dropsy. Lecture I. The production of lymph, *Lancet,* **1**:1267-1270 (1896).
3. E. H. Starling, The absorption of the inerstitial fluids. In *Fluids of the Body.* Herter Lectures, Keener, 1909, pp. 67-68.
4. P. Ehrlich, *Sauerstoff-Bedürfnis des Organismus. Eine Farbenanalytische Studie,* pp. 69-72. Berlin, 1885. (Cited in L. Bakay, *Blood-Brain Barrier.* Springfield, Ill., Charles C Thomas, 1956).
5. G. M. Bohm, Vascular permeability changes during experimentally produced pulmonary edema in rats, *J. Pathol. Bacteriol.*, **92**:151-161 (1966).
6. T. F. Whayne, Jr., and J. W. Severinghaus, Experimental hypoxic pulmonary edema in the rat, *J. Appl. Physiol.*, **25**:729-732 (1968).
7. B. W. Zweifach and M. Intaglietta, Mechanics of fluid movement across single capillaries in the rabbit, *Microvasc. Res.*, **1**:83-101 (1968).
8. G. G. Pietra, J. P. Szidon, M. M. Leventhal, and A. P. Fishman, Histamine and interstitial pulmonary edema in the dog, *Circ. Res.*, **29**:323-337 (1971).
9. M. J. Karnovsky, Morphology of capillaries with special reference to muscle capillaries. In *Capillary Permeability.* Edited by C. Crone and N. A. Lassen. Copenhagen, Munksgaard; New York, Academic Press, 1970, pp. 341-350.

10. E. E. Schneeberger-Keeley and M. J. Karnovsky, The ultrastructural basis of alveolar capillary membrane permeability to peroxidase used as a tracer, *J. Cell Biol.,* **37**:781-793 (1968).

11. E. E. Schneeberger and M. J. Karnovsky, The influence of intravascular fluid volume on the permeability of newborn and adult mouse lungs to ultrastructural protein tracers, *J. Cell Biol.,* **49**:319-334 (1971).

12. G. G. Pietra, J. P. Szidon, M. N. Leventhal, and A. P. Fishman, Hemoglobin as a tracer in hemodynamic pulmonary edema, *Science,* **166**:1643-1646 (1969).

13. G. G. Pietra, J. P. Szidon, E. J. Callahan, and A. P. Fishman, Permeability of the alveolo-capillary membrane to proteins, *J. Clin. Invest.,* **50**:73 (1971). Abstract.

14. C. C. Michel, Direct observations of sites of permeability to ions and small molecules in mesothelium. In *Capillary Permeability.* Edited by C. Crone and N. A. Lassen. Copenhagen, Munksgaard; New York, Academic Press, 1970, pp. 628-642.

15. W. Perl, Modified filtration-permeability model of transcapillary transport—A solution of the Pappenheimer pore puzzle? *Microvasc. Res.,* **3**: 233-251 (1971).

16. E. Overton, Uber die allgemeinen osmolischer Eigenschaften der Zelle, ihre vermutlichen Ursachen und ihre Bedeutung für die Physiologie, *Vjechr. Naturforsch. Ges.,* Zurich, 1899, pp. 44-88.

17. E. Overton, Beitrage zur allgemeinen Muskel- und Nervenphysiologie, *Pflug. Arch.,* **92**:115-280, 346-386 (1902).

18. R. Collander, The permeability of *Nitella* cells to non-electrolytes, *Physiol. Planlarum,* **7**:420-445 (1954).

19. D. A. Goldstein and A. K. Solomon, Determination of equivalent pore radius for human red cells by osmotic pressure measurement, *J. Gen. Physiol.,* **44**:11-17 (1960).

20. G. Grotte, Passage of dextran molecules across the blood lymph barrier, *Acta Clin. Scand. Suppl.,* **211**:1-84 (1956).

21. A. C. Guyton, *Textbook of Medical Physiology.* 3rd ed. Philadelphia and London, W. B. Saunders, 1966, pp. 419-422.

22. N. C. Staub, Pulmonary edema, *Physiol. Rev.,* **54**:678-811 (1974).

23. S. L. Selinger, R. D. Bland, R. H. Demling, and N. C. Staub, Distribution volumes of [^{131}I]albumin, [^{14}C]sucrose, and ^{36}Cl in sheep lung, *J. Appl. Physiol.,* **39**:773-779 (1975).

24. E. H. Bergofsky, Ions and membrane permeability in the regulation of the pulmonary circulation. In *The Pulmonary Circulation and Interstitial Space.* Edited by A. P. Fishman and H. H. Hecht. Chicago, University of Chicago Press, 1969, pp. 269-286.

25. E. D. Robin, J. D. Smith, A. R. Tanser, J. S. Adamson, J. E. Millen, and B. Packer, Ion and macromolecular transport in the alveolar microphage, *Biochim. Biophys. Acta,* **241**:117-128 (1971).

26. L. B. Flexner, D. B. Cowie, and G. J. Vosburgh, Studies on capillary permeability with tracer substances, Cold Spring Harbor Symposium, *Quant. Biol.,* **13**:88-98 (1948).

27. J. R. Pappenheimer, E. M. Renkin, and L. M. Borrero, Filtration diffusion
     and molecular sieving through peripheral capillary membranes. A contri-
     bution to the pore theory of capillary permeability, *Amer. J. Physiol.*,
     167:13-46 (1951).
28. C. Bohr, Uber die spezifische Tätigkeit der Lungen bei der respiratorischen
     Gasaufnahme und ihr Verhalten zu derdurch die Alveolarwand stall-
     findenen Gasdiffusion, *Skand. Arch. Physiol.*, 22:221-280 (1909).
29. A. Krogh, *The Anatomy and Physiology of Capillaries*. New Haven, Yale
     University Press, 1936.
30. E. M. Renkin, Transport of potassium 42 from blood to tissues in
     isolated mammalian skeletal muscles, *Amer. J. Physiol.*, 197:1205-1210
     (1959).
31. C. Crone, The permeability of capillaries in various organs as determined
     by use of the "indicator diffusion" method, *Acta Physiol. Scand.*, 58:
     292-305 (1963).
32. *Capillary Permeability*. Edited by C. Crone and N. D. Lassen. Copenhagen,
     Munsgaard; New York, Academic Press, 1970.
33. F. P. Chinard, G. J. Vosburgh, and T. Enns, Transcapillary exchange of
     water and of other substances in certain organs of the dog, *Amer. J.
     Physiol.*, 183:221-234 (1955).
34. F. P. Chinard and T. Enns, Transcapillary pulmonary exchange of water in
     the dog, *Amer. J. Physiol.*, 178:197-202 (1954).
35. P. Martin de Julian and D. I. Yudilevich, A theory for the quantification of
     transcapillary exchange by tracer dilution curves, *Amer. J. Physiol.*, 207:
     162-168 (1964).
36. J. B. Bassingthwaighte, T. J. Knopp, and J. B. Hazelrie, A concurrent flow
     model of capillary-tissue exchanges. In *Capillary Permeability*. Edited by
     C. Crone and N. A. Lassen. Copenhagen, Munsgaard; New York,
     Academic Press, 1970, pp. 60-80.
37. D. L. Yudilevich and P. Martin de Julian, Potassium, sodium and iodide
     transcapillary exchange in the dog heart, *Amer. J. Physiol.*, 208:959-967
     (1965).
38. F. P. Chinard, W. Perl, R. M. Effros, F. Silverman, R. Dumpys, and A. C.
     Delea, Lung water: Significance of capillary permeability. In *Central
     Hemodynamics and Gas Exchange*. Edited by C. Giuntini. Turin, Italy,
     Minerva Medica, 1971, pp. 191-206.
39. W. Perl, F. Silverman, A. C. Delea, and F. P. Chinard, Permeability of lung
     endothelium to sodium, diols, and amides, *Amer. J. Physiol.*, 230:1708-
     1721 (1976).
40. L. A. Danzer, J. E. Cohn, and W. F. Zechman, Relationship of D_m and V_c
     to pulmonary diffusing capacity during exercise, *Resp. Physiol.*, 5:250 258
     (1968).
41. E. Ericksson and R. Myrhage, Microvascular dimensions and blood flow in
     skeletal muscle, *Acta Physiol. Scand.*, 86:202 (1972).
42. J. Trap-Jensen and N. A. Lassen, Capillary permeability for smaller hydro-
     philic tracers in exercising skeletal muscle in normal man and in patients
     with long-term diabetes mellitus. In *Capillary Permeability*. Edited by

C. Crone and N. A. Lassen. Copenhagen, Munsgaard; New York, Academic Press, 1970, pp. 135-152.

43. C. Crone, The permeability of brain capillaries to nonelectrolytes, *Acta Physiol. Scand.*, **64**:407-417 (1965).

44. O. D. Wangensteen, L. E. Wittmers, Jr., and J. A. Johnson, Permeability of the mammalian blood-gas barrier and its components, *Amer. J. Physiol.*, **216**:719-727 (1969).

45. W. Perl, P. Chowdhury, and F. P. Chinard, Reflection coefficients of dog lung endothelium to small hydrophilic solutes, *Amer. J. Physiol.*, **228**: 797-809 (1975).

46. A. E. Taylor and K. A. Gaar, Jr., Estimation of equivalent pore radii of pulmonary capillary and alveolar membranes, *Amer. J. Physiol.*, **218**: 1133-1140 (1970).

47. J. D. Fenstermacher and J. A. Johnson, Filtration and reflection coefficients of the rabbit blood-brain barrier, *Amer. J. Physiol.*, **211**:341-346 (1966).

48. J. D. Fenstermacher, The osmotic flow of water across the blood-brain barrier. In *Capillary Permeability*. Edited by C. Crone and N. A. Lassen. Copenhagen, Munsgaard; New York, Academic Press, 1970, pp. 434-446.

49. N. A. Lassen and C. Crone, The extraction fraction of a capillary bed to hydrophilic molecules; theoretical considerations regarding the single injection technique with a discussion of the role of diffusion between laminar streams (Taylor's effect). In *Capillary Permeability*. Edited by C. Crone and N. A. Lassen, Copenhagen, Munsgaard; New York, Academic Press, 1970, pp. 48-59.

50. R. M. Effros, R. S. Y. Chang, and P. Silverman, Comparison of single transit and equilibration studies of $^{22}Na^+$ distribution in the lung, *Chest*, **71S**:296-298 (1977).

51. J. W. Ryan, V. Smith, and R. S. Niemeyer, Angiotension I. Metabolism by plasma membrane of lung, *Science*, **176**:64-66 (1972).

52. J. A. Johnson and T. A. Wilson, A model for capillary exchange, *Amer. J. Physiol.*, **210**:1299-1303 (1966).

53. D. G. Levitt, Quantitation of error of the E_0 method of measurement of capillary permeability for certain capillary and organ models. In *Capillary Permeability*. Edited by C. Crone and N. A. Lassen. Copenhagen, Munsgaard; New York, Academic Press, 1970, pp. 81-103.

54. J. J. Friedman, Muscle blood flow and ^{86}Rb extraction: ^{86}Rb as a capillary flow indicator, *Amer. J. Physiol.*, **214**:488-493 (1968).

55. W. Perl and F. P. Chinard, A convection-diffusion model of indicator transport through an organ, *Circ. Res.*, **22**:273-298 (1968).

56. G. I. Taylor, Dispersion of soluble matter in solvent flowing slowly through a tube, *Proc. Roy. Soc. A*, **219**:186-203 (1953).

57. A. Bauman, M. A. Rothschild, R. S. Yalow, and S. A. Berson, Pulmonary circulation and transcapillary exchange of electrolytes, *J. Appl. Physiol.*, **11**:353-361 (1957).

58. M. L. Pearce, Sodium recovery from normal and edematous lungs studied by indicator dilution curves, *Circ. Res.*, **24**:815-820 (1969).

59. F. E. Gump, Y. Mashima, S. Jorgensen, and J. M. Kinney, Simultaneous
     use of three indicators to evaluate pulmonary damage in man, *Surgery*,
     70:262-270 (1971).
60. W. A. Crosbie, S. Snowden, and S. Parsons, Changes in lung capillary
     permeability in renal failure, *Brit. Med. J.*, 918:388-390 (1972).
61. I. C. S. Normand, R. E. Olver, E. O. R. Reynolds, L. B. Strang and K.
     Welch, Permeability of lung capillaries and alveoli to non-electrolytes in
     the foetal lamb, *J. Physiol. (Lond.)*, 219:303-330 (1971).
62. F. P. Chinard, The permeability characteristics of the pulmonary blood-gas
     barrier. In *Advances in Respiratory Physiology*. Edited by C. G. Caro.
     London, Arnold, 1966, pp. 106-147.
63. F. P. Chinard, Exchanges across the alveolar-capillary barrier. In *The
     Pulmonary Circulation and Interstitial Space*. Edited by A. P. Fishman
     and H. H. Hecht. Chicago, University of Chicago Press, 1969, pp. 79-98.
64. F. P. Chinard, Permeability of the pulmonary blood-gas barrier. In *Capil-
     lary Permeability*. Edited by C. Crone and N. A. Lassen. Copenhagen,
     Munsgaard; New York, Academic Press, 1970, pp. 605-613.
65. R. M. Hays, Independent pathways for water and solute movement across
     the cell membrane, *J. Membr. Biol.*, 10:367-371 (1972).
66. J. A. Johnson, H. M. Caver, and N. Lifson, Kinetics concerned with distri-
     bution of isotopic water in insoluted perfused dog heart and skeletal
     muscle, *Amer. J. Physiol.*, 171:687-693 (1952).
67. J. O. Eichling, M. E. Raichle, R. L. Grubb, Jr., and M. M. ter Pogossian,
     Evidence of the limitations of water as a freely diffusible tracer in the
     brain of the rhesus monkey, *Circ. Res.*, 35:358-364 (1974).
68. E. M. Renkin, Capillary and cellular permeability to some compounds
     related to antipyrine, *Amer. J. Physiol.*, 173:125-130 (1953).
69. F. P. Chinard, W. Perl, and R. M. Effros, Pulmonary endothelial membrane
     characteristics; temperature effects, *Fred. Proc.*, 33:412 (1974). Abstract.
70. F. P. Chinard, T. Enns, and M. F. Nolan, Contributions of bicarbonate ion
     and of dissolved CO_2 to expired CO_2 in dogs, *Amer. J. Physiol.*, 198:78-
     88 (1960).
71. F. P. Chinard, Permeability of the alveolar-capillary barrier to dissolved
     carbon dioxide and to bicarbonate ion. In CO_2: *Chemical and Biochemical,
     and Physiological Aspects*. NASA SP-188.
72. J. Orloff and R. W. Berliner, The mechanism of the excretion of ammonia
     in the dog, *J. Clin. Invest.*, 35:223-235 (1956).
73. W. J. Waddell and R. G. Bates, Intracellular pH, *Physiol. Rev.*, 49:285-329
     (1969).
74. R. M. Effros and F. P. Chinard, The in vivo pH of the extravascular space
     of the lung, *J. Clin. Invest.*, 48.1983-1996 (1969).
75. R. M. Effros, N. Corbeil, and F. P. Chinard, Arterial pH and distribution
     of barbiturates between pulmonary tissue and blood, *J. Appl. Physiol.*,
     33:656-664 (1972).
76. A. B. Dubois, W. O. Fenn, and A. G. Britt, CO_2 dissociation curve of lung
     tissue, *J. Appl. Physiol.*, 5:13-16 (1952).

77. A. J. Erdmann, III, T. R. Vaughan, Jr., W. C. Woolverton, K. L. Brigham, and N. C. Staub, Effect of increased vascular pressure on lung fluid balance in unanesthetized sheep, *Circ. Res.*, **37**:271-284 (1975).

78. N. C. Staub, Steady-state pulmonary transvascular water filtration in unanesthetized sheep, *Circ. Res.*, **28/29** (Suppl. 1):135-139 (1971).

79. A. C. Guyton and A. W. Lindsey, Effect of elevated left atrial pressure and decreased plasma protein concentration of the development of pulmonary edema, *Circ. Res.*, **7**:649-657 (1959).

80. O. R. Levine, R. B. Mellins, R. M. Senior, and A. P. Fishman, The application of Starling's law of capillary exchange to the lungs, *J. Clin. Invest.*, **46**:934-944 (1967).

81. R. B. Mellins, O. R. Levine, R. Skalak, and A. P. Fishman, Interstitial pressure in the lungs, *Circ. Res.*, **24**:197-212 (1969).

82. P. Uter, U. Kotzerke, R. Rufer, and W. Schoedel, Kolloidosmotischer Druck und Filtration von Flüssigkeit durch die Alveolar-Capillar-Schranke in der Hundelunge, *Arch. Ges. Physiol.*, **294**:1-16 (1967).

83. P. K. M. Lunde and B. A. Waaler, Transvascular fluid balance in the lung, *J. Physiol.*, **205**:1-18 (1969).

84. T. Sato, S. M. Yamashiro and F. S. Grodins, Dynamic analysis of gravimetric response of isolated dog hindlimb, *Amer. J. Physiol.*, **228**:1236-1244 (1975).

85. J. R. Pappenheimer and A. Soto-Rivera, Effective osmotic pressure of the plasma proteins and other quantities associated with the capillary circulation in the hindlimbs of cats and dogs, *Amer. J. Physiol.*, **152**:471-491 (1948).

86. K. A. Gaar, Jr., A. E. Taylor, and A. C. Guyton, Effect of lung edema on pulmonary capillary pressure, *Amer. J. Physiol.*, **216**:1370-1373 (1969).

87. O. R. Levine, R. B. Mellins, R. M. Senior, and A. P. Fishman, The application of Starling's law of capillary exchange to the lungs, *J. Clin. Invest.*, **49**:934-944 (1967).

88. A. C. Guyton, K. Scheel, and D. Murphree, Interstitial fluid pressure. III. Its effect on resistance to tissue fluid mobility, *Circ. Res.*, **19**:412-419 (1966).

89. H. H. Webb and D. F. Tierney, Experimental pulmonary edema due to intermittent positive pressure ventilation with high inflation pressure. Protection by positive end-expiratory pressure, *Amer. Rev. Resp. Dis.*, **110**:555-565 (1974).

90. J. Dainty and B. Z. Gingburg, Irreversible thermodynamics and frictional models of membrane processes with particular reference to the cell membrane, *J. Theor. Biol.*, **5**:256-265 (1963).

91. A. Katchalsky and P. F. Curran. *Nonequilibrium Thermodynamics in Biophysics*. Cambridge, Mass., Harvard University Press, 1965.

92. F. Vargas and J. A. Johnson, An estimate of reflection coefficients for rabbit heart capillaries, *J. Gen. Physiol.*, **47**:667-677 (1964).

93. R. M. Effros, Osmotic extraction of hypotonic fluid from the lungs, *J. Clin. Invest.*, **54**:935-947 (1974).

94.   E. H. Bresler and R. P. Wendt, Diffusive and convective flow across membranes: Irreversible thermodynamic approach, *Science,* **163**:944-945 (1969).
95.   J. A. M. Smit and A. J. Staverman, Comments on "Onsager's reciprocal relation. An example of its application to a simple process," *J. Phys. Chem.,* **74**:966-967 (1970).
96.   R. P. Wendt and E. H. Bresler, Reply to communication of Smit and Staverman, *J. Phys. Chem.,* **74**:967-968 (1970).
97.   W. Perl, A friction coefficient, series-parallel channel model for transcapillary flux of nonelectrolytes and water, *Microvasc. Res.,* **6**:169-193 (1973).
98.   H. Heimberger, Kontrakile Function und anatomischer Basa der menschlichen Kapillaren, *Z. Zellforsch.,* **4**:713 (1926).
99.   W. P. Gibson, P. Bosley and R. Griffiths, Photomcirographic studies on the nail bed capillary networks in human control subjects, *J. Nerv. Ment. Dis.,* **123**:219 (1956).
100. J. T. Howe and Y. S. Scheaffer, On the dynamics of capillaries and the existence of plasma flow in the pericapillary lymph space, NASA TN-D, 3497, 1966.
101. V. C. Fung, Fluid in the interstitial space of the pulmonary alveolar sheet, *Microvasc. Res.,* **7**:89-113 (1974).
102. S. Middleman, *Transport Phenomena in the Cardiovascular System,* New York, Wiley-Interscience, 1972, pp. 140-145.
103. S. Nitta and N. C. Staub, Lung fluids in acute ammonium chloride toxicity and edema in cats and guinea pigs, *Amer. J. Physiol.,* **224**: 613-617 (1973).
104. H. H. Shirley, Jr., C. G. Wolfram, K. Wasserman, and H. S. Mayerson, Capillary permeability to macromolecules: Stretched pore phenomenon, *Amer. J. Physiol.,* **190**:189-193 (1957).
105. A. Keys, The apparent permeability of the capillary membrane in man, *Trans. Faraday Soc.,* **33**:930-943 (1937).
106. F. P. Chinard, Derivation of an expression for the rate of formation of glomerular fluid (GFR). Applicability of certain physical and physiochemical techniques, *Amer. J. Physiol.,* **171**:578-586 (1952).
107. S. Sourirajan, *Reverse Osmosis.* New York, Academic Press, 1971.
108. E. F. Grabowski, Osmotic weight transients in myocardium: A convective diffusion model. *Proceedings of the Summer Computer Simulation Conference,* Houston, Texas, July 1974, pp. 678-687.
109. A. J. Staverman, The theory of measurement of osmotic pressure, *Rec. Trav. Chim. Pays-Bas,* **70**:344-352 (1951).
110. D. C. Tosteson, Discussion. In *Capillary Permeability.* Edited by C. Crone and N. A. Lassen. Copenhagen, Munsgaard; New York, Academic Press, 1970, pp. 658-664.
111. N. Lifson, Revised equations of the osmotic transiet method. In *Capillary Permeability.* Edited by C. Crone and N. A. Lassen. Copenhagen, Munsgaard; New York, Academic Press, 1970, pp. 302-305.

112. J. R. Pappenheimer, Osmotic reflection coefficients in capillary membranes. In *Capillary Permeability*. Edited by C. Crone and N. A. Lassen. Copenhagen, Munsgaard; New York, Academic Press, 1970, pp. 278-290.

113. H. H. Ussing, Anomalous transport of electrolytes and sucrose through the isolated frog skin induced by hypertonicity of the outside bathing solution, *Ann. N.Y. Acad. Sci.*, **137**:543-555 (1966).

114. H. H. Ussing and B. Johansen, Anomalous transport of sucrose and urea in toad skin, *Nephron.*, **6**:317-328 (1969).

115. J. T. van Bruggen, J. D. Boyett, A. L. van Bueren, and W. R. Galey, Solute flux in a homopore membrane, *J. Gen. Physiol.*, **63**:639-656 (1974).

116. A. C. Guyton, H. J. Granger, and A. E. Taylor, Interstitial fluid pressure, *Physiol., Rev.*, **51**:527-563 (1971).

117. J. B. West, C. T. Dollery, and B. E. Heard, Increased pulmonary vascular resistance in the dependent zone of the isolated dog lung caused by pulmonary edema, *Circ. Res.*, **17**:191-206 (1965).

118. L. Binet and M. Burstein, Sur l'action vasoconstrictrice du serum sale hypertonique au niveau de la petite circulation, *C. R. Soc. Biol. (Paris)*, **145**:1766-1770 (1951).

119. R. C. Read, J. A. Johnson, J. A. Bick, and M. W. Meyer, Vascular effects of hypertonic solutions on the pulmonary circulation, *Circ. Res.*, **7**: 1011-1017 (1959).

120. P. W. Rand and E. Lacomb, Effects of angiocardiographic injections of blood viscosity, *Radiology*, **84**:1022-1032 (1965).

121. R. M. Effros, Impairment of red cell transit through the canine lungs following injections of hypertonic fluids, *Circ. Res.*, **31**:590-601 (1972).

122. A. Katchalsky and O. Kedem, Thermodynamics of flow processes in biological systems, *Biophys. J.*, **2**:53-78 (1962).

123. E. E. Schneeberger, Ultrastructural basis for alveolar-capillary permeability to protein. In *Lung Liquids*. Amsterdam, North-Holland Publishing Co., Elsevier Excerpts Medica, 1976, pp. 3-28.

124. A. R. Moritz, Chemical methods for the determination of death by drowning, *Physiol. Rev.*, **24**:70-88 (1944).

125. H. G. Swann, Body salt and water changes during fresh and sea water drowning, *Texas Rept. Biol. Med.*, **9**:356-382 (1951).

126. J. A. Klystra, Lavage of the lung, *Acta Physiol. Pharmacol. Neerlandica*, **7**:163 (1958).

127. C. E. Cross, P. A. Rieben, and P. F. Salisbury, Urea permeability of alveolar membrane; hemodynamics effects of liquid in the alveolar spaces, *Amer. J. Physiol.*, **198**:1029-1031 (1960).

128. F. P. Chinard, T. Enns, and M. F. Nolan, The permeability characteristics of the alveolar capillary bed, *Trans. Assoc. Amer. Phys.*, **75**:253-261 (1962).

129. A. E. Taylor, K. Gaar and A. C. Guyton, Na^{24} space, D_2O space, and blood volume in isolated dog lung. *Amer. J. Physiol.*, **211**:66-70 (1966).

130.   S. J. Enna and L. S. Shanker, Absorption of saccharides and urea from the rat lung, *Amer. J. Physiol.*, 222:409-414 (1972).

131.   L. B. Strang, The permeability of lung capillary and alveolar walls as determinants of liquid movements in the lung. In *Lung Liquids*. Edited by C. J. Dickinson. Amsterdam, North-Holland Publishing Co., Elsevier Excerpta Medica, 1976, pp. 49-64.

132.   R. D. H. Boyd, J. R. Hill, R. W. Humphreys, I. C. S. Normand, E. O. R. Reynolds, and L. B. Strang, Permeability of lung capillary to macro-molecules in foetal and newborn lambs and sheep, *J. Physiol. (Lond.)*, 201:567-588 (1969).

133.   R. E. Olver and L. B. Strang, Ion fluxes across the pulmonary epithelium and the secretion of lung liquid in the foetal lamb, *J. Physiol. (Lond.)*, 241:327-357 (1974).

134.   J. T. Gatzy, Bioelectric properties of the isolated amphibian lung, *Amer. J. Physiol.*, 213:425-431 (1967).

135.   R. E. Olver, B. Davis, G. Marin, and J. A. Nadel, Active transport of Na^+ and Cl^- across the canine tracheal epithelium in vitro, *Amer. Rev. Resp. Dis.*, 112:811-815 (1975).

136.   E. A. Egan, R. E. Olver, and L. B. Strang, Changes in the non-electrolyte permeability of alveoli and the absorption of lung liquid at the start of breathing in the foetal lamb, *J. Physiol. (Lond.)*, 219:303-330 (1975).

137.   E. A. Egan, Effect of lung inflation on alveolar permeability to solutes. In *Lung Liquids*. Edited by C. J. Dickinson. Amsterdam, North-Holland Publishing Co., Elsevier Excerpta Medica, 1976, pp. 101-114.

138.   T. G. H. Yuen and R. P. Sherwin, Hyperplasia of type II pneumocytes and nitrogen dioxide (10 ppm) exposure: A quantitation based on electron photomicrographs, *Arch. Environ. Health*, 22:178-188 (1971).

139.   M. Bachofen and E. R. Weibel, Basic pattern of tissue repair in human lungs following unspecified injury. Sixteenth Aspen Lung Conference. *Chest*, 65:14S-19S (1974).

140.   J. Flores, D. R. DiBona, C. H. Beck, and A. Leaf, The role of cell swelling in ischemic renal damage and the protective effect of hypertonic solute, *J. Clin. Invest.*, 51:118-126 (1972).

141.   R. C. Cantu and A. Ames, III, Experimental prevention of cerebral vasculature obstruction produced by ischemia, *J. Neurosurg.*, 30:50-54 (1969).

142.   J. T. Willerson, W. J. Powell, Jr., T.E. Guiney, J. J. Slark, C. A. Sanders, and A. Leaf, Improvement in myocardial function and coronary blood flow in ischemic myocardium after mannitol, *J. Clin. Invest.*, 51:2989-2998 (1972).

143.   M. E. Relf, J. R. McCurdy, J. J. Coalson and L. J. Greenfield, Effects of mannitol and dextran on interstitial pulmonary edema, *J. Surg. Res.*, 12:234-239 (1972).

144.   D. F. Tierney, Lung metabolism and biochemistry. *Ann. Rev. Physiol.*, 36:209-231 (1974). Edited by J. H. Comroe, R. R. Sonenchein, and K. L. Zierler, Palo Alto, Calif.

145.   M. Nakao, T. Nakao, S. Yamazoe, and II. Yoshikawa, ATP and shape of erythrocytes, *J. Biochem. (Tokyo)*, **49**:487-492 (1961).
146.   T. Ohnishi, Extraction of actin and myosin proteins from erythrocyte membrane, *J. Biochem. (Tokyo)*, **52**:307-314 (1962).
147.   S. Young and J. Knelson, Increased glucose uptake by rat and lung with onset of edema, *Physiologist*, **16**:494 (1973). Abstract.

Part Three

PULMONARY EDEMA
Mechanisms and Theories

9

Lung Edema Due to Increased Vascular Permeability

KENNETH L. BRIGHAM

Vanderbilt University School of Medicine
Nashville, Tennessee

I. Introduction

According to Starling's hypothesis describing the transvascular movement of fluid [1], edema in any organ occurs either because the net transmural pressure gradient in exchanging vessels is high enough in the direction of filtration that the fluid cannot be drained away adequately by lymphatics or because the nature of the filtering membrane is altered so that vessels leak excessively. Pulmonary edema can occur by both mechanisms [2,3].

When lung edema develops because of leaky vessels, it is usually called permeability edema, but the term *permeability* used this way is ambiguous. The net amount of fluid filtered from the vascular bed is a function of two interrelated equations, one describing the movement of water and the other

---

Some of the original work reported in this chapter was supported by grants numbered HL-08195, HL-18261, and HL-18210 from the National Heart and Lung Institute, by General Research Support Grant HEW 5S01RR05424-13, and by a grant from the Parker B. Francis Foundation. Dr. Brigham is an Established Investigator of the American Heart Association.

describing the movement of solutes. The first equation as written by Kedem and Katchalsky [4] is

$$J_f = L_p [(P_{mv} - P_{pmv}) + \sigma(\pi_{pmv} - \pi_{mv})] \tag{1}$$

where J_f is net fluid filtration from the vascular bed, P_{mv} and P_{pmv} are hydrostatic pressures inside and outside exchanging vessels, respectively, σ is the reflection coefficient, and π_{pmv} and π_{mv} are osmotic pressures outside and inside exchanging vessels, respectively. This is the general form of the equation Starling described. The second equation is

$$J_s = \omega_s(\pi_{pmv} - \pi_{mv}) + (1-\sigma_s)\bar{C}_s J_f \tag{2}$$

where J_s is the net flux of solute s out of the vascular bed, ω_s is the diffusional permeability for solute s, the value $1 - \sigma_s$ is the sieving coefficient for solute s, and $\bar{C}_s$ is the mean concentration of solute s across the membrane.

From these equations, it is apparent that there are three coefficients that determine the amount of fluid and solutes allowed to cross the walls of exchanging vessels: L_p, hydraulic conductance; σ, reflection coefficient; and ω, diffusional permeability. The three coefficients are interrelated, but used strictly, *permeability* refers only to the diffusive movement of solute. While it is difficult to imagine a passive mechanism by which permeability for solutes could be increased without an increase in hydraulic conductance, it is possible that the reverse could occur, that is, an increase in L_p without an increase in permeability. In this chapter, I use *permeability* in a general sense, and by *permeability edema* I mean edema resulting from a decrease in the resistance of the walls of exchanging vessels to the passage of fluid and solutes.

Figure 1 is an oversimplified conceptual model of the fluid-exchanging

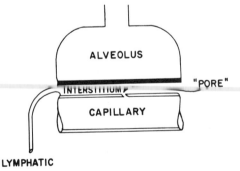

FIGURE 1   Conceptual diagram of the fluid-exchanging unit in the lung. The diagram is greatly oversimplified, as discussed in the text.

unit in the lung. Many investigators have shown alveolar epithelium to be highly impermeable even to small solutes under normal conditions [5,6], so that in terms of fluid exchange, it is usually considered an impenetrable barrier. Fluid and solutes move across the semipermeable exchanging vessel walls into the interstitial space according to the forces already described. Although the vessel in Figure 1 is called a capillary, there is some evidence that other microvessels may participate in fluid and solute exchange [7]. It has also been suggested that the capillary bed is more accurately represented as a thin sheet of blood than as a network of tubes [8]. Transvascular fluid exchange usually has been described as occurring through equivalent pores [9,10], and the concept is useful although perhaps not strictly accurate in an anatomical sense. The interstitial space is not limited to the alveolar wall interstitium, as shown in the diagram, but includes the loose connective tissue potential spaces around larger vessels and airways. In fact, when fluid accumulates in the lung as a result of either increased vascular pressures or increased vascular permeability, it appears in perivascular and peribronchial spaces very early [11]. Like other organs, the lung is drained by lymphatics [12–14]. Evidence is accumulating that the capacity of lung lymphatics for draining away excess filtered fluid, thereby preventing edema, is large [15]. Conceptually, the disorders here discussed are those in which either the pores, as shown in Figure 1, are enlarged or more pores are formed, or both.

II.   Consequences of Increased Lung Vascular Permeability

When lung microvessels are normal, vascular pressure can be elevated substantially without pulmonary edema resulting. Guyton and Lindsey found no lung fluid accumulation in anesthetized dogs until left atrial pressure exceeded about 25 torr [16]. In unanesthetized sheep, we have demonstrated two reasons for this tolerance to increased pressure. First, when pressure is increased, lung lymph flow increases, draining away the filtered fluid at a higher rate. Second, when pressure is increased, interstitial protein concentration falls; the result is an increase in the transmural osmotic gradient in favor of reabsorption, partially offsetting the effect of increased vascular hydrostatic pressure [17]. Figure 2 shows the linear relation between steady state lung lymph flow and protein concentrations (interstitial protein concentrations) over a wide range of lung vascular pressures in normal unanesthetized sheep.

When lung vascular permeability is increased, each unit increase in vascular hydrostatic pressure should cause a larger-than-normal increase in fluid filtration, and because proteins leak from microvessels more easily, the protec-

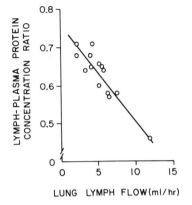

FIGURE 2 Relation between steady state lung lymph flow and lymph–plasma protein concentration ratio in unanesthetized sheep. Different lymph flows were achieved by inflating a balloon in the left atrium. Reproduced from K. Brigham and P. Owen, unpublished.

tion offered by a decrease in interstitial protein osmotic pressure is reduced or eliminated. Thus, the slope of the line relating filtration to vascular pressure should be steeper than normal, and edema should occur at a lower vascular pressure [11,18]. Figure 3 is a set of hypothetical curves showing the rela-

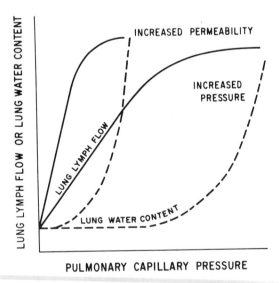

FIGURE 3 Hypothetical relations among lung lymph flow, lung water content and pulmonary capillary pressure under normal conditions and when vascular permeability is increased. Although lymph flow is shown approaching a maximum value, such a maximum has not been demonstrated. Changes in other variables may have important effects on those relations.

tions of lymph flow (net transvascular filtration) and of lung water content to hydrostatic pressure in exchanging vessels. Increased permeability steepens the lymph flow curve, shifts it to the left, and causes the rise of the lung water content curve to occur at a lower pressure. The magnitude of the shift in the curves from normal depends on the degree to which permeability is changed. The illustration shows water beginning to accumulate as lymph flow approaches a maximum, but in reality, a maximum value for lung lymph flow has not been demonstrated [3]. By available data, these relations seem rational, but they remain speculative, since changes in alveolar epithelial permeability, interstitial compliance, direct effects on the lymphatic pumping action and perhaps other changes could have important effects.

The amount by which increased vascular permeability affects the gas-exchanging function of the lung depends on the capacity of lymphatics to drain away the fluid and on the capacity of the lung interstitium to hold fluid. Both these factors act to keep fluid from flooding alveoli, the most important event affecting gas exchange [19]. Although maximum lung lymph flow has not been achieved, we obtained flows greater than 10 times baseline when permeability was high in sheep following *Pseudomonas* bacteremia [15,20], at a time when little excess lung water had accumulated. Thus, relatively large increases in fluid filtration resulting from increased vascular permeability can be handled adequately, and the occurrence of pulmonary edema in such situations is an end-stage manifestation of the pathologic process.

III. Methods for Studying Vascular Permeability in the Lung

A. General

To conclude that lung vascular permeability is increased, it is necessary to show not only that transvascular fluid and solute movement are increased, but also that the changes cannot be accounted for by increased driving pressures. Pressure in exchanging vessels cannot be measured directly but must be inferred from upstream and downstream pressures, and changes in the distribution of vascular resistance between pre- and postcapillary vessels often complicate the distinction between permeability and pressure effects [21-23].

Measuring lung vascular permeability quantitatively is extremely difficult. With the current state of the art, it is impossible to design an experiment in which all the important variables can be measured. Microvascular and perimicrovascular protein osmotic pressures can probably be estimated accurately from plasma and lymph protein concentrations [24-26], but hydrostatic pressure inside and outside exchanging vessels cannot be accurately measured [21-23,27]. In addition, all these variables must be integrated over the exchanging vessel membrane surface area for the hydrostatic field occupied by the lung. So far, all efforts to arrive at quantitative data about the lung's vascular exchanging membrane involve numerous assumptions, many of which are untested [15,24,28].

B. Fluid Accumulation

One experimental approach to detecting increased permeability is to compare the rate of lung fluid accumulation resulting from increased vascular hydrostatic pressure with the rate resulting from some manipulation that is thought to increase vascular permeability [29,30]. Methods for estimating lung water content include indicator dilution techniques [31,32], postmortem desiccation [33], and continuous weighing of isolated perfused lungs [27, 29]. Studies based solely on indicator dilution estimates of lung water content are difficult to interpret because of the baseline variability of the method and because the fraction of total lung water measured by this method is different under different circumstances [33]. The advantages of a method applicable to living animals (including humans) are considerable, however, and this area needs to be developed.

All studies based on increased lung water content as a criterion for increased microvascular filtration are necessarily insensitive. In response to increased vascular pressure, filtration (as reflected in lung lymph flow) increases with moderate pressure increases (Fig. 4), but fluid does not accumulate until pressures are substantially elevated [16]. Under some circumstances, when vascular permeability is increased, microvascular filtration may increase ten-

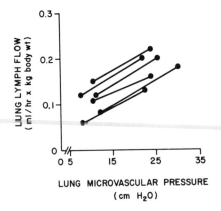

FIGURE 4   Effects of moderate increases in lung microvascular pressure on lung lymph flow in six unanesthetized sheep. Microvascular pressure was calculated assuming 0.4 of the resistance downstream to exchanging vessels. Lines connect steady state baseline and steady state increased pressure values. Lymph flow always increased when pressure was increased. Reproduced from K. Brigham and P. Owen, unpublished.

fold without an increase in lung water content [15]. Pulmonary edema (i.e., fluid accumulation) is only the tip of the iceberg.

Although microvascular pressure can be estimated more accurately for isolated perfused lungs than for intact animals [27,34,35], even such estimates are indirect and mean pressure integrated over the exchanging-vessel surface area at each hydrostatic level is still unknown. Unfortunately, many substances thought to increase permeability also increase pulmonary vascular resistance [21–23], a change that may alter the relations among pulmonary arterial, pulmonary arterial wedge, left atrial, and microvascular pressures [36,37]. The magnitude of the alteration is usually unknown, and this can lead to large errors in estimating pressure in exchanging vessels. The problem is especially difficult with intact animal preparations.

C. Lymph Flow

If the conceptual model shown in Figure 1 is essentially correct, then under steady state conditions, lung lymph flow represents the net volume of fluid leaving exchanging vessels and lymph protein concentration represents perimicrovascular protein concentration. Several investigators have exploited this concept experimentally in the lung [13,15,17,28,38] and other organs [24–26,39,40]. Such experimental preparations provide much more information about transvascular exchange than measurements of vascular pressure and lung fluid content alone.

Following Drinker's pioneering work [41], a modicum of information about the response of right lymphatic duct lymph in anesthetized dogs to pulmonary vascular manipulations has accumulated [38,42]. The more recent studies of Strang and coworkers in anesthetized lambs and sheep represent a considerable advance in technique because they took care to eliminate systemic lymph from their collections [28,43].

In the past few years, we have used a chronic unanesthetized sheep preparation developed by Staub [44], in which pulmonary and systemic vascular pressures can be recorded and manipulated independently and essentially pure lung lymph can be collected [15,17,20]. In sheep, about two-thirds of the lung lymph drains through the pulmonary ligaments to a single long node in the caudal part of the posterior mediastinum (caudal mediastinal node), and a single efferent duct from this node usually traverses the posterior mediastinum for several centimeters before entering the thoracic duct [45]. Although some abdominal lymph enters the caudal end of the node, it can be largely eliminated by resecting the tail of the node below the inferior pulmonary ligaments [15,44,46]. We prepare sheep by a series of three thoracotomies, during which we resect the tail of the caudal mediastinal node, put catheters

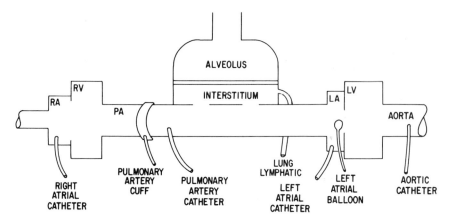

FIGURE 5   Block diagram of a sheep lung lymph preparation showing location of catheters, balloon, and cuff.

into the left atrium, main pulmonary artery, superior vena cava, and thoracic aorta, put a Foley balloon catheter in the left atrium, put an inflatable latex cuff around the main pulmonary artery, and cannulate the caudal mediastinal node efferent duct. Figure 5 is a block diagram of the preparation. We do most experiments without anesthesia, since at least some anesthetics, especially barbiturates, are known to depress lymphatic function [47]. With this preparation, we can test for the presence of systemic lymph by inflating the pulmonary artery cuff and increasing systemic venous pressure. Lymph flow does not increase in properly prepared sheep, indicating that systemic lymph has been effectively eliminated [46]. To assess the effects of agents on vascular permeability, we compare the effects of such agents on lung vascular pressures, lymph flow, and lymph and plasma protein concentrations during a steady state experiment with the effects on the same variables in the same sheep of a prolonged steady state increase in lung vascular pressure made by inflating the left atrial balloon [15,20,48].

   The problems with any lung lymph preparation are (1) estimation of hydrostatic pressure in exchanging vessels, as discussed earlier; (2) unknown perimicrovascular hydrostatic pressure, and possible variation of the pressure with experimental manipulation [49]; and (3) possibility that some exchange occurs across lymphatics or in transit through nodes so that lymph protein concentration does not reflect perimicrovascular protein concentration. Although there is considerable evidence that exchange of protein does not occur across peripheral lymphatics [25] and lymph nodes [26], the information needed is a direct comparative measurement of proteins in interstitial lung fluid and in lung lymph collected at the same time. So far, technical difficulty has precluded collecting lung interstitial fluid directly, but it should be done.

D. Multiple Indicator Dilution Curves

Indicator dilution methods have been used to measure capillary transport in living animals. They are used for measuring extravascular lung water in humans and animals. Also, capillary permeability-surface area (P-S) products (the techniques do not permit separating these two parameters) have been calculated from indicator dilution curves of an intravascular indicator and indicators that escape across microvascular walls only with difficulty in a single pass across the circulation ("barrier-limited" substances) [50–53]. The idea is that the differences between the indicator that does not escape at all from the vascular compartment and the indicator that does escape but is "barrier-limited" (that is, limited in where it can go primarily by hindrance at the capillary wall) is a measure of the rate of escape of the permeable substances from the microcirculation. Several different analytical methods have been used for calculating P-S products from such studies [51], and there is no general agreement about which method is best. We found P-S products for [^{14}C] urea calculated by Crone's method [51] quite variable even under baseline conditions in the lungs of anesthetized dogs [54]. In the lung circulation, most hydrophillic molecules, even sodium ions and urea, are essentially confined to the vascular space in a single transit. This means that they differ very little from the intravascular indicator and this may lead to large errors in P-S product estimates [55]. A systematic comparison of the precision of the several techniques for calculating P-S products might be helpful.

We compared transpulmonary indicator dilution curves for [^{51}Cr] erythrocytes, [^{125}I] albumin, [^{14}C] urea, and [^{3}H] water in the lungs of anesthetized dogs under baseline conditions and during pulmonary edema induced by alloxan (increased vascular permeability), volume overload (high pressure, high flow), or inflation of a left atrial balloon (high pressure, low flow) [54]. Because of the variability of the P-S products calculated from our baseline data, we calculated mean transit time volumes for each of the indicators by the method of Chinard and coworkers [31] and compared the difference between the mean transit time volumes of [^{14}C] urea and [^{51}Cr] erythrocytes with the difference between the mean transit time volumes of [^{51}Cr] erythrocytes and [^{125}I] albumin. We found that under baseline conditions and with high-pressure edema induced either by volume overload or by a left atrial balloon that the urea volume did not exceed the albumin volume. However, with alloxan edema, where permeability was increased, urea volume exceeded albumin volume. The urea volume calculation is likely an underestimate since urea recovery was incomplete, but we believe that this approach offers promise as a qualitative test for vascular integrity in intact animals.

The dog studies showed that indicator methods could distinguish between gross edema resulting from increased permeability and gross edema resulting from high pressure, but they did not show that the methods were sensitive enough to detect increased permeability before gross edema occurred. We now have preliminary evidence suggesting that they may be. I shall subsequently show data from sheep lymph studies indicating that 4-hour intravenous histamine infusions in unanesthetized sheep cause lung vascular permeability to increase and cause moderate pulmonary edema. Figure 6 shows the change from baseline [^{14}C] urea permeability–surface area products caused by a 4-hour increase in left atrial pressure to 15 to 20 cm H$_2$O produced by in-

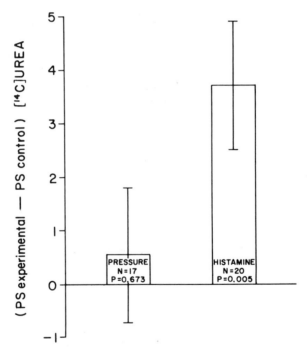

FIGURE 6   Change in lung permeability-surface (PS) product for [^{14}C] urea caused by elevated pressure and by histamine infusion in unanesthetized sheep. Bars show mean ±SEM. Permeability-surface products were calculated from multiple single-pass indicator dilution curves by a technique suggested by Goresky et al. [32]. Intravenous histamine infusion caused PS product to increase while increased pressure did not. Based on data from Harris and Brigham, unpublished.

flating a left atrial balloon and the change caused by a 4-h histamine infusion
(4 μg kg^{-1} min^{-1} histamine phosphate). The P-S products in this case were
calculated from a model suggested by Goresky [56], in which capillary transit
times are constant and large-vessel transit times vary, since we have found such
calculations more precise than several others [57]. The P-S product went up
with histamine although the permeability change was not severe enough to
cause gross pulmonary edema. This suggestion of sensitivity to small permeability changes should encourage further theoretical and experimental work.

Probably the most important question to ask about indicator methods is
whether they can give useful information about the integrity of the lung's
microvascular bed in humans. We have approached this question initially by
studying patients undergoing cardiac surgery [58]. Figure 7 compares the
ratio of the differences between [^{14}C] urea and [^{51}Cr] erythrocyte mean transit
time volumes (excess urea volume) to the differences between [^{125}I] albumin

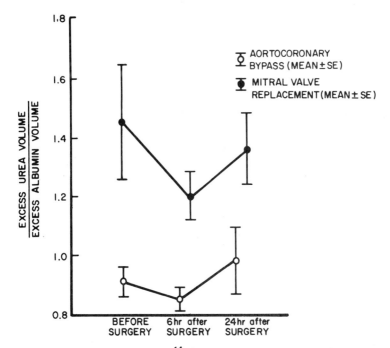

FIGURE 7   Ratio of excess lung [^{14}C] urea distribution volume to excess
[^{125}I] albumin volume, calculated from single-pass multiple indicator dilution
curves for patients having aortocoronary bypass and patients having mitral valve
replacement. In the latter group, urea volume exceeded albumin volume at all
three study times. Reprinted from K. Brigham et al., *Circulation*, **53**:369–376
(1976), by courtesy of the publisher.

and [51Cr] erythrocyte mean transit time volumes (excess albumin volume) before and 6 and 24 hr after surgery in 7 patients undergoing aortocoronary bypass for arteriosclerotic disease with the values for 8 patients undergoing prosthetic mitral valve replacement for mitral stenosis or insufficiency or both. We initially planned the studies expecting to see an effect of cardiopulmonary bypass on lung vascular permeability (bypass time was similar in the two groups). What we found, however, was that urea volume was slightly less than albumin volume in the aortocoronary bypass patients before and after surgery, and that in the mitral valve replacement group, urea volume consistently exceeded albumin volume both before and after surgery. The results in the mitral group are like those we saw with alloxan edema in dogs [54]; but more work is needed to determine whether these results in humans are specific for increased permeability. Specifically, two kinds of indicator dilution studies are needed. First, a variety of "barrier-limited" indicators should be tested in several clinical settings, and second, more theoretical work is needed to define the most precise and accurate analytical techniques to apply to the data [57].

E. Protein Turnover

Aviado [59] and more recently Gorin and coworkers [60] have tried to assess lung vascular permeability by comparing counts of labeled red cells and of labeled macromolecules accumulating in the lung over time. The Gorin group showed that the time course of extravascular [113]Indium-labeled transferrin accumulation (estimated by difference between red-cell and transferrin counts) compared favorably with the time course of equilibration in lung lymph. This technique should be applicable to humans, and it has the advantage of being noninvasive.

The concentrations of macromolecules in pulmonary edema fluid have been compared with concentrations in peripheral blood plasma. Robin and coworkers followed the time course of the appearance of labeled macromolecules in edema fluid after intravenous injection [61]. More studies of this kind are needed, although they give only qualitative information about vascular integrity. Because alveolar epithelium is normally completely impermeable to proteins [5,6], the appearance of protein in edema fluid means either that the fluid gets into alveoli by some other route or that the epithelial barrier is damaged. It is not known whether proteins are partially sieved by the epithelial barrier as fluid goes from interstitium to alveoli, or whether fluid is absorbed or added in transit up the tracheobronchial tree. These problems, and the fact that gross edema is a severe, unsteady perturbation, make it difficult to equate edema-fluid protein concentrations with protein concentrations in the microvascular filtrate. The ideal would be to sample peripheral blood, interstitial fluid, lung lymph, and edema fluid simultaneously.

F. Other

There are some quantitative techniques for studying microvascular exchange that have been used effectively in other organs but not in the lung. In the kidney, micropuncture studies have provided direct measurements of single-nephron glomerular filtration rates [62,63] and have demonstrated the response of the renal microvasculature to many experimental manipulations [64]. The same kind of data for the pulmonary microcirculation would be a tremendous advance towards understanding lung fluid homeostasis and the factors that change it. Lung anatomy may be less convenient for micropuncture studies than the kidney, but it should be possible to do such studies in the lung with existing technology. This approach should also yield direct measurements of interstitial fluid composition.

Studies in vitro of biologic membranes have also yielded much information about the processes involved in membrane transport [65]. In particular, studies of the transport characteristics of the isolated toad bladder have given valuable clues about the function of the renal microcirculation [66,67]. If it were possible to obtain a sheet of endothelium from lung exchanging vessels without altering its transport characteristics, then it could be precisely characterized in vitro over a range of transmembrane pressures, and responses to changes in the chemical environment could be measured. In fact it is impossible to get sheets of microvascular endothelium. One alternative would be to study large-vessel endothelium, for example from the pulmonary artery. At least in sheep, and probably in other large animals, it is technically possible to dissect out fairly large pieces of pulmonary artery intima with little connective tissue. It would be useful to characterize the transport functions of such membranes in vitro and to test the effects of agents that may alter these functions even though it is not possible to know a priori that microvascular endothelium should behave similarly. Recent advances in the engineering of such measurements make it possible to eliminate the influence of boundary layer transport and therefore to define membrane parameters quite exactly [68].

Another approach to measuring microvascular transport directly would be to study isolated capillaries. Wagner and associates [69] have isolated what appear morphologically to be intact capillaries from adipose tissue (Figure 8). If such preparations could be made from the lung, it should be possible by micropuncture techniques to measure their filtration characteristics.

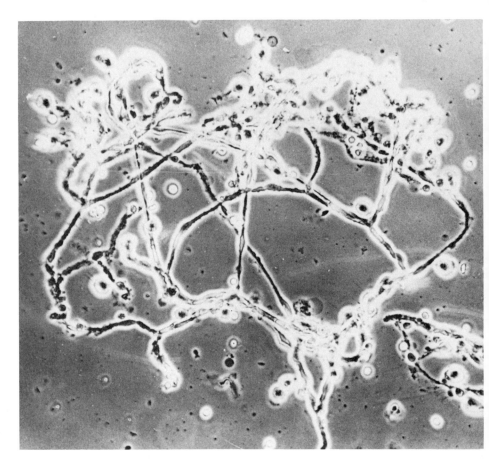

FIGURE 8   Phase-contrast photomicrograph of capillaries isolated from adipose tissue ×272. Reprinted from R. Wagner et al., *Proc. Nat. Acad. Sci.*, **69**: 3175–3179 (1972), by courtesy of the publisher.

The problem whether the vessels are altered during isolation would require comparisons with studies in vivo.

An ideal method for assessing lung vascular permeability has not been developed, and the lack of a reliable method that can be used in living animals and humans seriously impedes study of the abnormality in the clinical setting. Criteria for an ideal method would include (1) applicability to living humans and other animals; (2) enough sensitivity to detect increased permeability before pulmonary edema develops; (3) noninvasive character; (4) ability to distinguish between the effects of increased vascular hydrostatic pressure and increased vascular permeability; (5) quantitative results; and (6) speed and reproducibility.

IV. Causes of Increased Lung Vascular Permeability

It is clear that some toxic chemicals disrupt the endothelium of lung exchanging vessels enough to produce fatal pulmonary edema in the presence of normal or near normal vascular pressures. The two most widely studied such chemicals are alloxan and α-naphthylthiourea (ANTU). Staub and coworkers showed that alloxan produced severe edema in the presence of normal lung vascular pressures, without increasing capillary blood volume, as measured by gas inhalation techniques in anesthetized dogs [11]. Other investigators have used alloxan edema in anesthetized dogs as an experimental model of increased permeability edema. The main difficulty with alloxan is that it produces severe, usually fatal edema and it is not known whether the edema is mechanistically related to the clinical syndromes in which increased lung vascular permeability occurs. We have some evidence that the alloxan effect on the lung may vary among species, since we have not been able to produce the lesion in sheep. Also, when alloxan has been given to humans with pancreatic islet cell tumors, pulmonary edema has not been an observed complication [70].

Since pulmonary edema and respiratory failure sometimes accompany gram-negative bacterial septicemia in humans, many investigators have looked at the effects of *E. coli* bacterial endotoxin on the lung in experimental animals. In sublethal doses, this agent causes pulmonary edema in barbiturate-anesthetized dogs [30], but it also causes pulmonary vascular pressures to increase [71]. While it has been generally stated that vascular permeability is increased in endotoxin edema [61], there has been little experimental basis for the statement.

We have recently compared the effects of mechanically increased lung vascular pressures with the effects of *Pseudomonas aeruginosa* bacteremia on lung fluid dynamics in the unanesthetized sheep preparation described earlier [15,20]. The effects of intravenous *Pseudomonas* infusion on vascular pressures, lymph-to-plasma protein concentration ratios and lung lymph flow are shown for one experiment in Figure 9. We saw two phases to the reaction: an initial period with fever, chills, pulmonary arterial hypertension, and increased lung-lymph flow with decreased lymph-to-plasma protein concentration ratios, and a late phase beginning four hours after *Pseudomonas* was given when lung lymph flow increased, but vascular pressures and lymph-to-plasma protein concentration ratios were similar to those in the baseline period. This

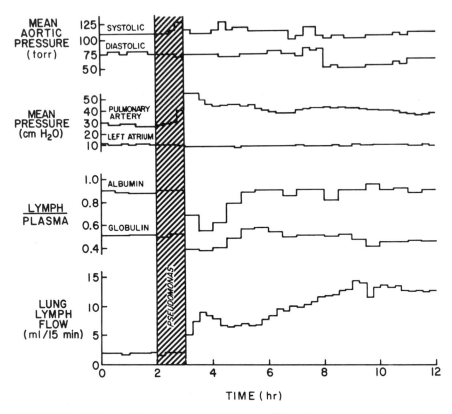

FIGURE 9   Effects of an intravenous infusion of *Pseudomonas aeruginosa* on vascular pressures, lymph-plasma protein concentration (L/P) ratio and lung lymph flow in an unanesthetized sheep. Initially, pulmonary arterial pressure rose, L/P ratios fell, and lymph flow increased. About 4 hr after the infusion, there was a marked and prolonged increase in lymph flow while L/P ratios remained high and vascular pressures were near baseline. This late phase is interpreted as increased vascular permeability. Reprinted from K. Brigham et al., *J. Clin. Invest.*, **54**:792–804 (1974), by courtesy of the publishers.

delayed phase of increased lymph flow lasted for many hours, gradually returning to baseline over 24 to 72 hr. Although an occasional sheep died of fulminant pulmonary edema during the late phase of the reaction, most animals appeared completely well during that period; and except for the animals with severe edema, postmortem studies showed minimal accumulation of fluid in the lung. Figure 10 is a histologic section from the lung of a sheep killed 6 hr after a *Pseudomonas* infusion, while lymph flow was ten times baseline (87 ml/hr) but the sheep appeared well. Although there is marked dilation of lymphatics, only minimal interstitial edema is present and there is no evidence

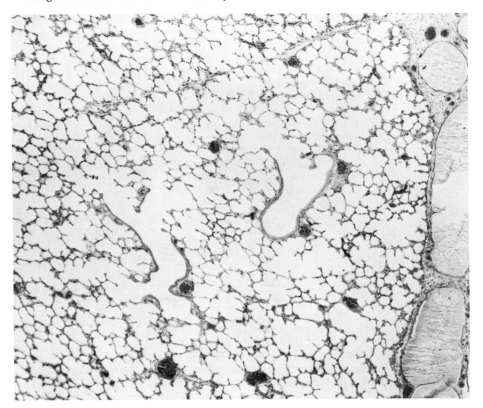

FIGURE 10 Photomicrograph (X25) of a section of lung from a sheep killed 6 hr after a *Pseudomonas* infusion while lung lymph flow was 10 times baseline. There are markedly dilated lymphatics along the right-hand margin of the figure, but only minimal perivascular edema and no alveolar flooding. Reprinted from K. Brigham et al., *J. Clin. Invest.*, **54**:792-804 (1974), by courtesy of the publishers.

of alveolar flooding. Figures 11 and 12 show the relations between lung lymph flow and lung lymph protein flow (lymph flow times lymph protein concentration) and estimated microvascular pressure for studies in sheep where a steady state increase in pressure was produced by inflating a balloon in the left atrium and for the steady state late phase reaction to *Pseudomonas* bacteremia. Both lung lymph flow and lung lymph protein flow were consistently higher in the *Pseudomonas* studies. These findings show that vascular permeability to fluid and protein are increased by *Pseudomonas*. Besides showing that *Pseudomonas* causes lung vascular permeability to increase in sheep, these studies also show that lung lymphatics have a large capacity to

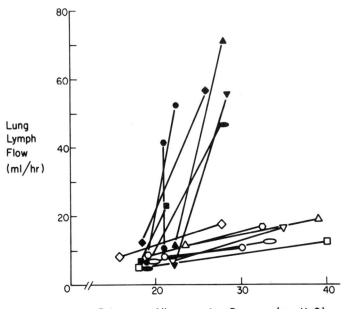

FIGURE 11   Relation between steady state lung lymph flow and estimated microvascular pressure (assuming 0.4 of the resistance downstream to exchanging vessels) in seven sheep during mechanically increased pressure and after *Pseudomonas* infusion. Lines connect steady state baseline and experimental observations in a single experiment. Open symbols are increased pressure studies; closed symbols are *Pseudomonas* studies and a different-shaped symbol is used for each animal. Lymph flow increased much more after *Pseudomonas* was introduced than with increased pressure. Reprinted from K. Brigham et al., *J. Clin. Invest.*, **54**:792–804 (1974), by courtesy of the publisher.

remove excess filtered fluid and thus prevent pulmonary edema when vascular permeability is increased. In most of these experiments, the only evidence that permeability was increased was the increase in lymph flow and lymph protein flow; blood gases were normal, and postmortem measurements of extravascular lung water were usually normal. We think this preparation is a good one for studying lung fluid dynamics because it may be relevant to human diseases and the long period of steady state increased vascular permeability provides an ideal opportunity to test the effects of potentially useful therapies.

Several other chemicals including 3-methyl indole [72] and 4-ipomeanol and its derivatives [73,74] have been shown to cause pulmonary edema in animals and are thought to act by damaging vascular endothelium; their mech-

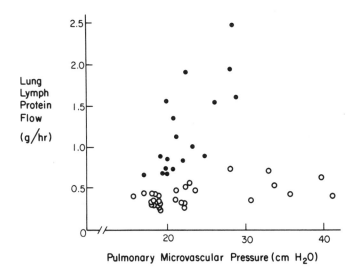

FIGURE 12   Steady state lung lymph protein flow (lymph flow X lymph protein concentration) as a function of microvascular pressure (see legend to Figures 4 and 11, this chapter) during baseline and increased pressure (open circles) and after *Pseudomonas* infusion (closed circles). Protein flow was much higher during the *Pseudomonas* reaction, indicating that vascular permeability was increased. Reprinted from K. Brigham et al., *J. Clin. Invest.*, **54**:792–804 (1974), by courtesy of the publisher.

anisms of action need further clarification, however, and the relevance of these observations to clinical syndromes in animals or man remains to be demonstrated. The direction of research in this area in the immediate future should be towards developing experimental models of clinical syndromes that permit sensitive measurement of transvascular fluid and protein movement in which comparisons with mechanical pressure manipulations can be made. The sheep model we are using is one approach, but others need to be developed.

The effects of inhaled high concentrations of oxygen and noxious gases on lung fluid homeostasis have clear relevance to clinical disease. It has been shown that the initial morphologic lesion in oxygen toxicity in the lung is in the capillary endothelium, and the clinical findings are compatible with increased vascular permeability as a primary abnormality [75,76]. Nitrogen dioxide [77] and sulfur dioxide [78] cause pulmonary edema, and ozone causes pulmonary edema with morphologic lesions in endothelium compatible with increased vascular permeability [79]. All these substances and also other air pollutants that may damage microvessels in the lung should be studied in a preparation in which filtration can be measured more sensitively than by measuring only accumulated lung water. For example, it would be of great benefit to know the dose-response relations between inhaled oxygen and lung vascular damage and also the natural history of the lesion in physiological terms. Pharmacologic approaches to prevention and reversal of the lesions also need to be studied in a physiologic preparation.

In their recent review, Robin et al. list thirteen clinical settings in which the primary pulmonary lesion is thought to be an increase in microvascular permeability [2]. In fact, there is very little hard evidence that any of the disorders they list result primarily from lung microvascular damage. The reason is that there is no specific test for detecting increased lung vascular permeability in humans. The development of such a test would open a vast area of clinical research aimed at clarifying the altered microvascular function in each of the disorders for which increased permeability is suspected. Until such information is available, therapy in these disorders will necessarily be empirical or nonspecific.

Spencer, in a classic book on lung pathology, presents the theory that some subacute and chronic interstitial lung diseases may result from increased microvascular permeability to protein with chronic interstitial edema which organizes to produce fibrosis [80]. Because of the lack of a test for detecting increased permeability in living humans, physiologic evidence for or against this hypothesis is nonexistent. It is an exciting idea, because it would link the pathogenesis of several acute lung diseases with the subacute and chronic states to which they sometimes progress, and might provide important clues to mechanism and therapy. It is quite possible that there is a whole spectrum of clinical syndromes that have as their basis a primary or a secondary pulmonary "microvasculopathy."

The biggest impediment to elucidating the role of increased lung vascular permeability in human diseases is the lack of a way of measuring the abnormality. The indicator dilution and external scanning methods are promising, but they have disadvantages and limitations. Much more work is needed.

V.   Mechanisms Involved in Altering Lung Vascular Permeability

A.   General

Fluid and solute filtration across microvessels is probably passive and it should be possible to describe the process in physical terms. It should be possible to describe, in terms of physical changes in the filtering membrane, the changes in microvessels that cause them to leak excessively. Ideally, it should also be possible to demonstrate morphologic changes in microvessels that are consistent with the quantitative description of the physical processes involved. In fact this has not been the case.

The usual approach to a mathematical description of fluid and solute filtration in microvessels is to describe fluxes in terms of the equations Kedem and Katchalsky have presented [4], and to characterize membrane transport as occurring through "equivalent pores." These "pores" are thought to be through endothelial intercellular junctions, and the process of arriving at an equivalent pore structure for the microvascular membrane compatible with experimental data is called modeling. The details of such approaches are discussed by Blake in Chapter 5. An advantage of the equivalent-pore approach is that the equations describing fluid and solute movement through such pores are well known. The geometry of the passageway between vascular lumen and interstitium is actually unknown, and it is quite possible that the pore concept is not physically accurate. But if such a model can consistently predict experimental data, it is a useful way to describe the membrane structure conceptually.

The question to ask about a model that is relevant to understanding increased permeability is, What is the physical change in the filtering membrane structure necessary for predicting the degree of increased permeability observed? Only a few investigators have tried to answer this question [15,81]. Using data from the sheep lymph preparation described above, we found that baseline and increased pressure data in the lung could not be described by a single-pore model, but that a model consisting of numerous small pores that completely exclude proteins per one intermediate pore of 125-Å radius described the data well [15,82]. During increased permeability after *Pseudomonas* bacteremia, it was only necessary to approximately double the area of the small pores and to increase the radius of the intermediate pores to 150 Å in order to predict the large increases in lymph flow and lymph protein flow that were observed experimentally [15]. Although the increases in filtration after *Pseudomonas* were large, the changes in the filtering membrane structure necessary to predict such changes were small. Figure 13 shows the effect of increasing intermediate-pore radius on predicted lung lymph flow (net fluid filtration) and on lymph-plasma albumin and globulin ratios in our equivalent-pore model. The important conclusion is that large increases in filtration are predicted for slight changes in membrane pore structure. This is consistent with the observation in sheep *Pseudomonas* studies that the lesion was usually reversible and only occasionally caused significant interference with gas exchange [15]. We think this is a very important observation because it points out that it is not necessary to postulate wholesale destruction of endothelial cells to explain tremendous increases in transvascular fluid and protein movement. The implication is that in clinical diseases in which lung vascular per-

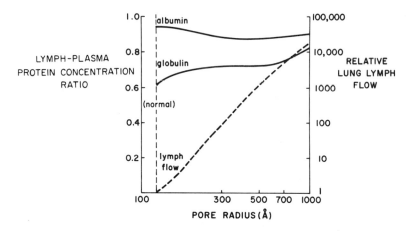

FIGURE 13   Effects of increasing equivalent-pore radius on lung lymph flow and lymph-to-plasma protein concentration ratios in a theoretical model of sheep lung microvessels. The broken vertical line is the pore radius most consistent with normal lung. Small increases in pore radius cause large increases in lymph flow. Reprinted from K. Brigham et al., *J. Clin. Invest.*, **54**:792–804 (1974), by courtesy of the publisher.

meability is increased, perhaps even in the presence of fulminant edema, damage to lung vascular endothelium may be minimal and reversible, and that even temporary support of the lung's gas-exchanging function may permit recovery. These results also emphasize that the search for morphologic changes produced by agents that increase permeability may be difficult and may require very refined techniques since the changes may be small.

Several investigators, in an effort to demonstrate the physical lesion, have made electron micrographs of lung tissue when vascular permeability was apparently increased. Cottrell and coworkers compared the ultramicroscopic changes produced by alloxan with those caused by increased pressure edema in dogs, showing apparent complete destruction of endothelial cells in alloxan edema (increased permeability), but intact endothelium in high-pressure edema [83]. Cunningham and Hurley saw endothelial blebs and gaps in ANTU edema [84], but Hovig et al. saw no endothelial abnormalities when permeability was increased in isolated perfused lungs by depleting the perfusate of divalent cations [85]. Our own ultrastructural studies of alloxan edema in dogs [86] show changes more like those shown by Cunningham and Hurley in ANTU edema than the alloxan changes described by Cottrell and associates. Figure 14 compares our findings in alloxan edema with those of Cunningham and Hurley in ANTU edema. The approach of Hyde [79] may offer considerably greater sensitivity in detecting small changes, and more re-

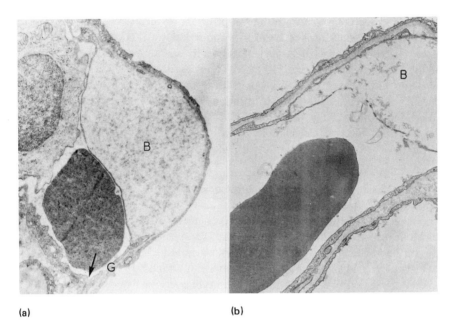

(a)   (b)

FIGURE 14   Electron photomicrographs of lung capillaries from (a) a rat with
α-naphthylthiourea edema and (b) a dog with alloxan edema. The letter B marks
an endothelial bleb in each picture. In (a), an arrow points to an endothelial
intercellular junction, and G marks an endothelial gap. Magnification of (a) illustration is X20,400 and (b) X30,000. Picture (a) reprinted from A. Cunningham and J. Hurley, *J. Pathol.*, **106**:25–35 (1972), by courtesy of the publisher;
picture (b) from Blake and Brigham, to be published.

fined techniques will likely make it possible to reconcile eventually the exchanging membrane structure predicted from theoretical models with what is
seen morphologically. More anatomic studies need to be made, in which careful physiologic data are collected at the time the tissue samples are taken.

    Some studies suggest that the geometry of passageways between micro-
vascular lumens and interstitium may not be fixed. Shirley and associates
proposed several years ago that capillary pores stretch in response to increased
vascular hydrostatic pressure [87]. It is almost certainly possible to raise
vascular pressure high enough to disrupt vessels, and since exchanging microvessels have less connective tissue and muscular support in their walls than
large vessels, they might be the first to break, but it is not at all clear that the
dimensions of interendothelial junctions increase in response to increases in
pressure of the magnitude that might be expected to occur in living animals.
In the unanesthetized sheep lung lymph preparation, we have found that

lymph-plasma protein concentration ratios invariably decrease when vascular pressure is mechanically increased to moderate levels. This change is predictable over a broad range of vascular pressures by a static equivalent pore model of the exchanging membrane [15,82]. Teleologically, it seems disadvantageous for pores to increase in size when pressure is high, since this would greatly magnify the effect of pressure on filtration rate (Fig. 3) and make pulmonary edema much more likely [88]. More data are needed that allow quantitative assessment of the possible relations between vascular pressure and permeability in the lung before this question can be answered definitely.

B.   Endogenous Vasoactive Substances

The lung is a rich source of vasoactive substances [89,90] that may be released in response to a variety of stimuli [91,92], and reactions producing increased microvascular permeability in other organs are generally thought to be mediated by endogenous release of vasoactive substances [93]. The question whether increased lung microvascular permeability is mediated this way is unanswered.

Histamine

Histamine increases permeability in peripheral vascular beds [39,94] and causes endothelial gaps to appear in systemic venules [95,96]; it has thus been considered a probable mediator of increased systemic vascular permeability in several reactions. Studies in isolated perfused lungs and isolated fluid-filled lung lobes have failed to show, however, any effect from histamine on transvascular filtration [97,98]. Pietra and associates showed that histamine could cause large carbon particles to leak from bronchial venules, but they saw no such effect in pulmonary vessels [99]. We have recently investigated the effect of prolonged steady state histamine infusions on lung fluid dynamics in the sheep lung lymph preparation described earlier [46,100]. Figure 15 shows the effects of histamine on pulmonary vascular pressures and lung lymph flow. When we infused histamine intravenously at the rate of $4\mu g$ kg^{-1} min^{-1} for 4 hr, left atrial pressure fell, pulmonary artery pressure did not change substantially, and lymph flow increased and remained high for the duration of the infusion. Figure 16 shows steady state lymph-plasma protein concentration ratios during baseline and experimental periods for increased pressure studies and for histamine studies in the same unanesthetized sheep. When pressure was increased mechanically, lymph flow increased but lymph-plasma protein concentration ratios invariably fell. During the histamine infusions, although lymph flow was high, lymph-plasma protein concentration ratios did

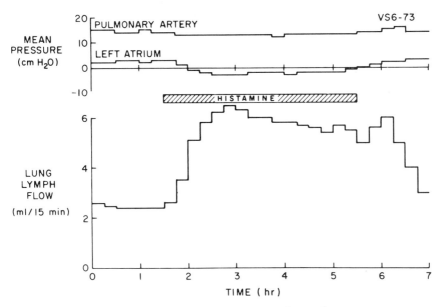

FIGURE 15   Effects of a 4-hr intravenous 4 μg kg^{-1} min^{-1} histamine phosphate infusion on lung vascular pressures and lymph flow in an unanesthetized sheep. Reprinted from K. Brigham and P. Owen, *Circ. Res.*, **37**:647–657 (1975), by courtesy of the publisher.

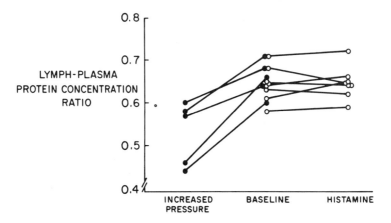

FIGURE 16   Effects of increased pressure and histamine infusion on steady state lymph-to-plasma protein (L/P) ratio in unanesthetized sheep. L/P ratios always fell with increased pressure, but did not fall during histamine infusion. Reproduced from K. Brigham and P. Owen, previously unpublished illustration.

not change from baseline. The histamine effect on lymph flow was dose-related and intravenous infusions always caused a bigger lymph flow increase than infusions in the left atrium in the same animals. We conclude from these studies that in awake sheep, histamine causes a dose-related increase in lung vascular permeability to protein. We have found the classic antihistamine, diphenhydramine, capable of preventing and reversing the histamine effect on permeability. The difference between these studies and those that others reported may be the result of a difference in experimental preparation and design, and perhaps of a difference among animal species in their response to histamine. Lung lymph is a much more sensitive measure of increased transvascular fluid movement than measurements of accumulated lung water, and the magnitude of the structural changes necessary to cause the increase in lymph flow with histamine are probably small, so that carbon particles might not leak from lung microvessels as a result [99]. Histamine should be considered a possible mediator of increased lung vascular permeability and because of the therapeutic implications, this possibility needs further study.

Serotonin

Serotonin (5-hydroxytryptamine) is another vasoactive substance contained in the lung. It has been suggested as a possible mediator of increased microvascular permeability in the lung [22] and other organs [95,96]. The effects of serotonin infusion on sheep lung vascular pressures and lymph flow are illustrated in Figure 17. Lymph flow increases with intravenous serotonin infusion, but lung vascular pressures also increase. Figure 18 shows lymph-to-plasma protein concentration ratios as a function of lung lymph flow in the sheep preparation for studies where vascular pressure was mechanically increased and during steady state histamine and serotonin infusions. Lymph-to-plasma protein ratios during high lymph flow produced by serotonin are indistinguishable from the protein ratios for a similar lymph flow produced by increasing pressure. These data indicate that histamine increases lung vascular permeability to protein, whereas the main effect of serotonin on fluid and protein filtration is a result of an increase in the transmural hydrostatic pressure gradient in exchanging vessels [17,82]. It is possible that in some reactions, both histamine and serotonin are released, and this would have a much greater effect on filtration than either agent alone because the effect of an increase in microvascular pressure would be magnified by a concomitant increase in vascular permeability. Serotonin may contribute to pulmonary edema when permeability is high, but at least in sheep, it does not appear to affect permeability directly.

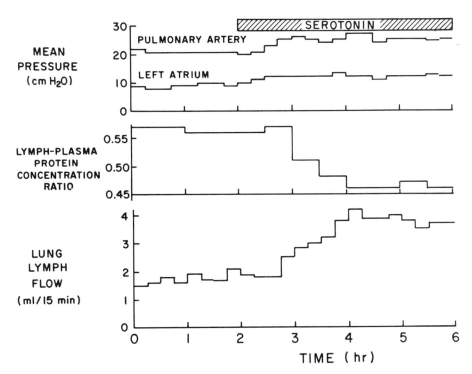

FIGURE 17   Effects of 4 μg kg^{-1} min^{-1} serotonin creatinine sulfate infusion
on lung vascular pressures, lymph/plasma protein (L/P) ratios and lung lymph
flow. Serotonin caused pulmonary arterial and left atrial pressure to increase,
L/P ratios to fall, and lymph flow to increase. Reprinted from K. Brigham and
P. Owen [117], *Circ. Res.*, **36**:761–770 (1975), by courtesy of the publisher.

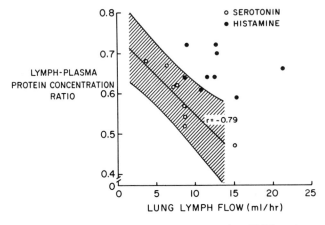

FIGURE 18   Lymph-to-plasma protein concentration (L/P) ratios as a function
of steady state lung lymph flow in unanesthetized sheep. The regression line
and 95% confidence limits (shaded area) are for increased pressure. L/P ratios
were higher for a given lymph flow during histamine infusion but not during
serotin infusion. From K. Brigham and P. Owen, previously unpublished
illustration.

Prostaglandins

A recent, burgeoning interest in prostaglandins has led to the postulate that
they may be involved in mediating increased capillary permeability in the systemic circulation [101]. Since the lung is rich in prostaglandins and the enzymes necessary for their synthesis and degradation [101–104], and since
prostaglandins and their precursors are released from the lung under some
experimental conditions [91,92,104], it is tempting to think that they may be
related in some way to microvascular permeability in the lung. There is very
little evidence relevant to such a hypothesis, and the effects of these agents on
lung fluid dynamics should be studied. We have found some interesting responses to salicylate (a potent inhibitor of prostaglandin synthetase, the enzyme group involved in synthesizing prostaglandins from arachidonic acid) in
the sheep lung lymph preparation. Figure 19 shows the responses of lung
lymph and vascular pressures in a sheep to an intravenous infusion of 600 mg
acetylsalicylate dissolved in phosphate-bicarbonate buffer. Salicylate caused

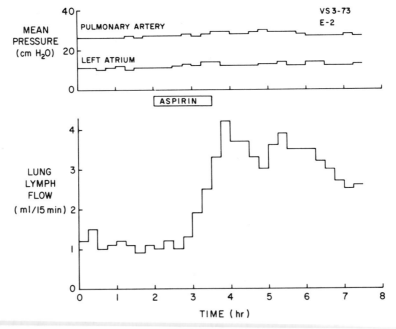

FIGURE 19   Changes in lung vascular pressures and lymph flow caused by
aspirin in an unanesthetized sheep. Intravenous infusion of 600 mg acetylsalicylate dissolved in phosphate-bicarbonate buffer caused a marked increase in
lymph flow but affected pressure very little. From K. Brigham, previously unpublished illustration.

lung lymph flow to increase dramatically and the high lymph flow persisted for a long period with very little change in pulmonary vascular pressures. This experiment suggests that salicylate caused an increase in lung vascular permeability. It is quite possible that the effect is unrelated to the inhibition of prostaglandin synthetase, and studies of other inhibitors of this enzyme need to be done, but it is also possible that in the lung prostaglandins are in some way related to the maintenance of normal vascular integrity. Thus the release of prostaglandins from the lung in reactions in which permeability is increased could be interpreted as an attempt to restore the microvessels to normal. In this regard, it is interesting that pulmonary edema has been reported as a complication of salicylate toxicity [105]. Our preliminary studies with indomethacin (another prostaglandin synthetase inhibitor) suggest that qualitatively it has an effect on lung lymph flow resembling the effect of salicylates. These data are preliminary and are insufficient for drawing any firm conclusions, but the hypotheses suggested should be carefully investigated.

Other Substances

Increases in lung microvascular permeability could be mediated by a slow-reacting substance of anaphylaxis [106] or any of numerous other vasoactive substances that have been isolated, or by some still unidentified substance. If there are endogenous mediators of increased lung vascular permeability, the goal should be to identify them, isolate them, characterize them biochemically and develop antagonists that could be used in humans.

Allergic reactions in the lung appear to involve cyclic nucleotides as second messengers in the release of vasoactive substances from mast cells [89, 106]. Increases in water movement across isolated toad bladders also involve cyclic nucleotides [107], and several effects of histamine appear to be mediated through cyclic nucleotides [108]. Although it has not been demonstrated that the effect of histamine on microvascular permeability is mediated in this way, if the permeability effect is a result of endothelial cell contraction, as has been suggested [95], it could be analogous to histamine-induced contraction of smooth muscle, which is mediated through cyclic nucleotides. Although I know of no evidence to support such a hypothesis, it is possible that reactions in which lung vascular permeability is increased involve cyclic nucleotides in the biochemical sequence of events, either as second messengers in the release of vasoactive substances or as second messengers in mediating the effect of vasoactive substances on vascular endothelium, or both. Aminophylline, an inhibitor of cyclic nucleotide phosphodiesterase, has long been used in the therapy of pulmonary edema of any cause, and isoproterenol, a stimulator of adenylate cyclase has been thought beneficial in the therapy of shock, where pulmonary complications are common. We have done some anecdotal experiments that suggest that cyclic nucleotides could be involved in the reaction of the sheep lung lymph preparation to *Pseudomonas* bacteremia. Figures 20 and 21 show the effects of a *Pseudomonas* infusion on lung vascular pressures and lymph flow without (Fig. 20) and during an infusion of isoproterenol (Fig. 21). Without isoproterenol the reaction was similar to that described earlier, that is, both lymph flow and lung vascular pressures increased during the early phase, then vascular pressures fell, and lymph flow rose, remaining higher than baseline for many hours. If the *Pseudomonas* infusion was given during an isoproterenol infusion that was maintained throughout the experiment, both the pulmonary vascular pressure response and the effect on lymph flow were diminished. As shown in Figure 22, aminophylline had an effect similar to isoproterenol in the same sheep. Thus both aminophylline and isoproterenol appear to diminish the effect of *Pseudomonas* on lung vasculature in sheep. We do not have sufficient data to determine whether the isoproterenol and aminophylline effects were solely due to the lower vascular pressures or whether they also diminish the permeability response, and these studies do not prove that cyclic nucleotides are involved in the reaction. That possibility is suggested, however, and this area should be thoroughly investigated because of the possible therapeutic implica-

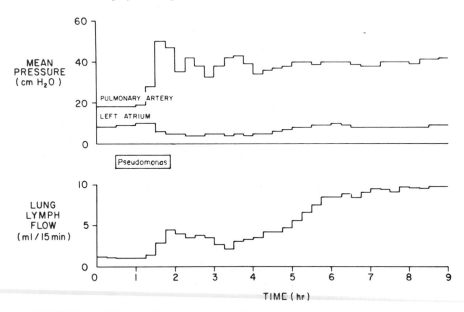

FIGURE 20 Effects of *Pseudomonas* infusion on lung vascular pressures and lymph flow in a sheep. This is the same animal as in Figures 24 and 25. This figure is to be compared with those figures. From K. Brigham and P. Owen, previously unpublished illustration.

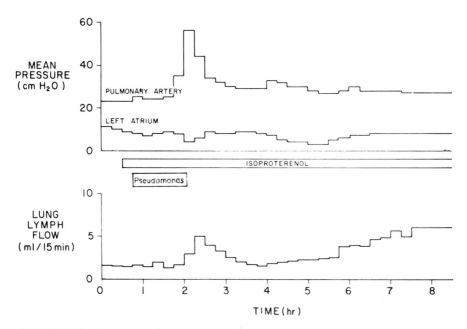

FIGURE 21 Lung vascular pressure and lymph flow responses to a *Pseudomonas* infusion given during a prolonged isoproterenol ($2 \mu g \ kg^{-1} \ min^{-1}$) infusion. The late-phase pulmonary artery pressure and lymph flow were less when isoproterenol was given than with *Pseudomonas* alone in the same animal (Figure 23). From K. Brigham and P. Owen, previously unpublished illustration.

tions. It has recently been suggested that the lung is an important source of circulating cyclic nucleotides [109], and we have preliminary evidence that both histamine and isoproterenol infusions may increase the release of cyclic AMP into the systemic circulation by the lung [110]. Whether this has anything to do with microvascular changes remains to be seen.

Some reactions in which lung vascular permeability may be increased (for example, gram-negative sepsis) may be accompanied by intravascular coagulation with release of fibrin degradation products into the circulation, and it is possible that these substances affect permeability either directly or indirectly. Also, we have demonstrated that the transient leukopenia and arterial hypoxemia that may occur in patients undergoing hemodialysis is probably a result of leukostasis in pulmonary microvessels resulting from complement activation [111]. Since these phenomena are also seen in gram-negative sepsis [15], it is possible that release of lysozymes or other leukocyte toxins in the pulmonary microcirculation may cause increased permeability. It has also been suggested that lung vascular permeability may be increased in adult respiratory distress syndromes via neural rather than humoral mechanisms [112].

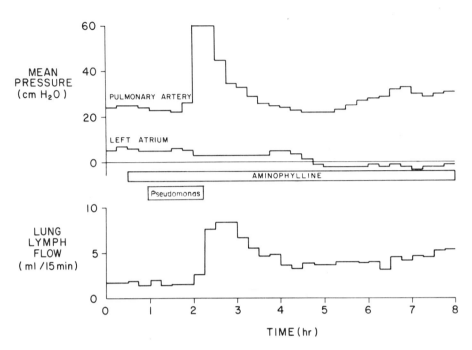

FIGURE 22   Lung vascular pressures and lymph flow responses to a *Pseudomonas* infusion given during a prolonged aminophylline (500 mg/hr) infusion. As with isoproterenol (Figure 24), the late-phase pulmonary artery pressure and lymph flow were less than that resulting from *Pseudomonas* infusion alone in the same sheep (Figure 23). From K. Brigham and P. Owen, previously unpublished illustration.

One suggestion that may have some use in designing experimental studies of the biochemical mechanisms involved in increased lung vascular permeability is that there may be "permeability receptors" on the lung vascular endothelium [113]. Such receptors might involve sulfhydryl bonds [114], and the effects of alloxan on the lung circulation in dogs may involve sulfhydryl groups [115]. The increased permeability of frog islet cells caused by alloxan apparently involves a similar mechanism [116]. In fact, it has even been suggested that cellular permeability under some circumstances may involve a sort of "trap door" with sulfhydryl groups as the handle [114]. Experiments could be designed to test the effects of agents with strong affinity for sulfhydryl groups on lung vascular permeability, and the interaction of these agents with others that are sulfhydryl donors. The involvement of sulfhydryl bonds in increased permeability reactions would not be incompatible with other first or second messengers discussed earlier, and it could provide another site of pharmacologic attack on the lesion.

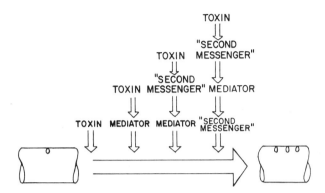

FIGURE 23   Some possible biochemical sequences involved in altering vascular permeability. The more complicated sequences may be harder to clarify experimentally but offer more sites of therapeutic attack.

Figure 23 illustrates several hypothetical levels of complexity that could characterize the biochemical sequence of events leading to increased lung vascular permeability. It is largely unknown which, if any, of these suggested sequences occurs. Although the more complicated sequences are more difficult to delineate experimentally, they would offer a greater opportunity for attacking the problem therapeutically, since there are more sites at which the reaction might be interrupted.

The goal for research into the mechanisms involved in increased lung vascular permeability should be to define both the physical and biochemical changes that are involved and to synthesize both kinds of data into a coherent integrated hypothesis that can be tested further experimentally.

VI. Prevention and Reversal of Increased Lung Vascular Permeability

The most pragmatic question to ask about increased lung vascular permeability is, How can it be prevented and reversed in humans? The answer is unknown because there is not enough information about the lesion. I believe there are several other questions that must be answered before effective therapy can be rationally developed. These questions can be answered experimentally with existing technology.

Question 1   Is there a "final common pathway" for reactions where lung vascular permeability is increased?

Answer   This question needs to be answered both for the physical changes in the microvascular filtering membrane that result in increased permeability and for the biochemical sequence of events involved in these reactions. It is not known whether all these reactions affect the theoretical equivalent pore structure of exchanging vessel walls similarly or whether some basically similar change underlies the divergent morphology that has been shown by electron microscopy. Nor is it known whether there is some single mediator that all the reactions have in common. This is an extremely important question, since if there is some common denominator it should be possible to develop a single therapy that would be of benefit in disorders with a wide variety of etiologies.

Question 2   Does increased lung vascular permeability result from an effect on endothelial cells or from a direct effect on intercellular junctions, or both?

Answer   There is experimental evidence to suggest that the effect of histamine on permeability in the systemic circulation is a result of the contraction of endothelial cells and pulling apart of intercellular junctions [95,96]. If this effect is so produced, and if other agents of increased permeability act in the same way, it is very important to delineate the mechanisms of this contraction and develop ways to prevent or interrupt it. On the other hand, if some agents cause permeability to increase as a result of a direct effect on the "intercellular cement," then the biochemical characteristics of this substance must be understood so that we may learn to reverse the permeability change. These are two basically different approaches to the problem, and this question should be answered in order to provide a rationale for further research. It is also possible that some reactions affect the permeability of endothelial cells themselves, which would suggest still another basic approach to the problem.

Question 3   Are there mediators of increased vascular permeability, and if so, what are they and where do they come from?

Answer   I presented some experimental evidence to suggest that there are at least some candidate mediators of increased permeability in the lung, but it has not been established whether there are any clinical syndromes in which the reaction is mediated by endogenous release of vasoactive substances. This question is critical to development of possible therapy as well as understanding the pathogenesis of the lesion. There may be several mediators, with different ones participating in different syndromes, or several substances may be released at once with synergistic effects on filtration. If mediators and their sources were identified, it would provide a more solid basis for developing effective therapy.

Question 4   If there are mediators, what is their release mechanism?

Answer   There is much evidence indicating that the release of vasoactive substances from the lung in allergic reactions is mediated through a cyclic nucleotide system. Identifying this or some other release mechanism involved in increased lung vascular permeability reactions would provide another site for a pharmacologic approach to therapy.

Question 5 Is it feasible to take a physical approach to therapy of increased vascular permeability?

Answer There are two possible specific ways in which increased vascular permeability could be reversed. First, if the biochemical sequence of events were sufficiently clarified, agents could be used or developed that would interrupt the sequence. Second, it might be possible to alter the physical structure of the membrane in such a way as to make it less permeable. Robin et al. thought that high-molecular-weight dextran decreased the rate of filtration in a human with severe pulmonary edema apparently resulting from gram-negative sepsis [61]. They suggested that the mechanism may have been a physical "plugging" of the pores in the microvascular walls. As far as I know, such an approach has not been investigated further, but it might be possible to develop substances that would not have severe systemic effects and that would stick in the microvascular pores and impede filtration of fluid and protein. This would likely be a temporary effect, but if as we suggested [15], many of the reactions are temporary, even a transient decrease in filtration would be beneficial.

References

1. E. Starling, On the absorption of fluids from the connective tissue spaces, *J. Physiol.*, **19**:312–326 (1895–1896).
2. E. Robin, C. Cross, and R. Zelis, Pulmonary edema, *N. Engl. J. Med.*, **288**: 239–304 (1973).
3. N. Staub, Pulmonary edema, *Physiol. Rev.*, **54**:678–811 (1974).
4. L. Kedem and A. Katchalsky, Thermodynamic analysis of the permeability of biological membranes to nonelectrolytes, *Biochem. Biophys. Acta*, **27**: 229–246 (1958).
5. A. Taylor and K. Gaar, Estimation of equivalent pore radii of pulmonary capillary and alveolar membranes, *Am. J. Physiol.*, **218**:1133–1140 (1970).
6. D. Wagensteen, L. Wittmers, and J. Johnson, Permeability of the mammalian blood-gas barrier and its components, *Am. J. Physiol.*, **216**:719–727 (1969).
7. L. Iliff, Extra-alveolar vessels and edema development in excised dog lungs, *Circ. Res.*, **28**:524–532 (1971).
8. Y. Fung and S. Sobin, Theory of sheet flow in the lung alveoli, *J. Appl. Physiol.*, **26**:472–488 (1969).

9. J. Pappenheimer, E. Renkin, and L. Borrero, Filtration, diffusion and molecular sieving through peripheral capillary membranes. A contribution to the pore theory of capillary permeability, *Am. J. Physiol.*, **167**:13–46 (1951).

10. E. Landis and J. Pappenheimer, Exchange of substances through capillary walls, In *Handbook of Physiology, Circulation*. Vol. 2. Edited by W. Hamilton and P. Dow. Washington, D. C., American Physiological Society, 1962, pp. 961–1034.

11. N. Staub, H. Nagano, and L. Pearce, Pulmonary edema in dogs, especially the sequence of fluid accumulation in lungs, *J. Appl. Physiol.*, **22**:227–240 (1967).

12. W. Miller, Das Lungenlappchen, seine Blut and Lymphgefasse, *Arch. Anat. Physiol.*, **179**:197–228 (1900).

13. C. Drinker, *Pulmonary Edema and Inflammation*. Cambridge, Mass., Harvard University Press, 1945.

14. J. Lauweryns and Boressauce, The ultrastructure of pulmonary lymphatic capillaries of newborn rabbits and of human infants, *Lymphology*, **2**:108–129 (1974).

15. K. Brigham, W. Woolverton, L. Blake, and N. Staub, Increased sheep lung vascular permeability caused by *Pseudomonas* bacteremia, *J. Clin. Invest.*, **54**:792–804 (1974).

16. A. Guyton and A. Lindsey, Effect of elevated left atrial pressure and decreased plasma protein concentration on the development of pulmonary edema, *Circ. Res.*, **7**:649–657 (1959).

17. J. Erdmann, T. Vaughan, W. Woolverton, K. Brigham, and N. Staub, Regulation of lung transvascular water flow by perimicrovascular protein osmotic pressure in sheep, *Fed. Proc.*, **31**:305 (1972). Abstract.

18. C. Drinker and E. Hardenbergh, Acute effects upon the lungs of dogs of large intravenous doses of alpha-naphthyl thiourea (ANTU), *Am. J. Physiol.*, **156**:35–43 (1949).

19. M. Visscher, F. Haddy, and G. Stephens, The physiology and pharmacology of lung edema, *Pharmacol. Rev.*, **8**:389–434 (1956).

20. K. Brigham, W. Woolverton, and N. Staub, Reversible increase in pulmonary vascular permeability after *Pseudomonas aeruginosa* bacteremia in unanesthetized sheep, *Chest*, **65**:51S–52S (1974).

21. R. Gilbert, L. Hinshaw, H. Kuida, and M. Visscher, Effects of histamine, 5-hydroxytryptamine and epinephrine on pulmonary hemodynamics with particular reference to arterial and venous segment resistances, *Am. J. Physiol.*, **194**:165–170 (1958).

22. S. Kabins, C. Molina, and L. Katz, Pulmonary vascular effects of serotonin (5-OH-tryptamine) in dogs: Its role in causing pulmonary edema, *Am. J. Physiol.*, **197**:955–958 (1959).

23. J. Glazier and J. Murray, Sites of pulmonary vasomotor reactivity in the dog during alveolar hypoxia and serotonin and histamine infusions, *J. Clin. Invest.*, **50**:2550–2558 (1971).

24. E. Renkin, Transport of large molecules across capillary walls, *Physiologist*, 7:13–28 (1964).

25. D. Garlick and E. Renkin, Transport of large molecules from plasma to interstitial fluid and lymph in dogs, *Am. J. Physiol.*, 219:1595–1605 (1970).

26. H. Mayerson, R. Patterson, A. McKee, S. LeBrie, and P. Mayerson, Permeability of lymphatic vessels, *Am. J. Physiol.*, 203:98–106 (1962).

27. K. Gaar, A. Taylor, L. Owens, and A. Guyton, Pulmonary capillary pressure and filtration coefficient in the isolated, perfused lung, *Am. J. Physiol.*, 213:910–914 (1967).

28. R. Boyd, J. Hill, P. Humphreys, I. Normand, E. Reynolds, and L. Strang, Permeability of lung capillaries to macromolecules in foetal and newborn lambs and sheep, *J. Physiol.*, 210:568–588 (1969).

29. G. Grega, R. Daugherty, J. Scott, D. Radawski, and F. Haddy, Effects of pressure, flow and vasoactive agents on vascular resistance and capillary filtration in canine fetal, newborn and adult lung, *Microvasc. Res.*, 3:297–307 (1971).

30. J. Snell and L. Ramsey, Pulmonary edema as a result of endotoxemia, *Am. J. Physiol.*, 217:170–175 (1969).

31. F. Chinard, T. Enns, and M. Nolan, Pulmonary extravascular water volumes from transit time and slope data, *J. Appl. Physiol.*, 17:179–183 (1962).

32. C. Goresky, R. Cronin, and B. Wangel, Indicator dilution measurements of extravascular water in the lungs, *J. Clin. Invest.*, 48:487–501 (1969).

33. L. Pearce, B. Yamashita, and B. Beazell, Measurement of pulmonary edema, *Circ. Res.*, 16:482–488 (1965).

34. K. Gaar, A. Taylor, and A. Guyton, Effect of lung edema on pulmonary capillary pressure, *Am. J. Physiol.*, 216:1370–1373 (1969).

35. E. Agostoni and J. Piiper, Capillary pressure and distribution of vascular resistance in isolated lung, *Am. J. Physiol.*, 212:1033–1036 (1962).

36. H. Hellems, F. Haynes, L. Dexter, and T. Kinney, Pulmonary capillary pressure in animals estimated by venous and arterial catherization, *Am. J. Physiol.*, 155:98–105 (1948).

37. S. Rao and N. Sissman, The relationship of pulmonary venous wedge to pulmonary arterial pressures, *Circulation*, 44:565–574 (1971).

38. H. Uhley, S. Leeds, J. Sampson, and M. Friedman, Right duct lymph flow in experimental heart failure following acute elevation of left atrial pressure, *Circ. Res.*, 20:306–310 (1967).

39. F. Haddy, J. Scott, and G. Grega, Effects of histamine on lymph protein concentration and flow in the dog forelimb, *Am. J. Physiol.*, 223:1172–1177 (1972).

40. R. Carter, W. Joyner, and E. Renkin, Effects of histamine and some other substances on molecular selectivity of the capillary wall to plasma proteins and dextran, *Microvasc. Res.*, 7:31–48 (1974).

41. C. Drinker, Lane Medical Lectures. The lymphatic system, its part in

regulating composition and volume of tissue fluid, *Med. Sci.*, 4:135–235 (1942).

42. H. Uhley, S. Leeds, J. Sampson, and M. Friedman, Some observations on the role of lymphatics in experimental acute pulmonary edema, *Circ. Res.*, 9:668–693 (1961).

43. P. Humphreys, I. Normand, E. Reynolds, and L. Strang, Pulmonary lymph flow and the uptake of liquid from the lungs of the lamb at the start of breathing, *J. Physiol.*, 3:1–29 (1967).

44. N. Staub, Steady state pulmonary transvascular water filtration in unanesthetized sheep, *Circ. Res.*, 28/29 (Suppl. 1):I-135–139 (1971).

45. A. Lascelles and B. Morris, Surgical techniques for the collection of lymph from unanesthetized sheep, *Q. J. Exp. Physiol.*, 46:199–205 (1961).

46. N. Staub, R. Bland, K. Brigham, R. Demling, A. Erdmann, III, and W. Woolverton, Preparation of chronic lung lymph fistulas in sheep, *J. Surg. Res.*, 19:315–320 (1975).

47. J. Yoffey and F. Courtice. *Lymphatics, Lymph and the Lymphomyeloid Complex.* London, Academic Press, 1970.

48. K. Brigham, Effects of histamine on lung transvascular fluid and protein movement in awake sheep, *Chest*, 67:50S–51S (1975).

49. A. Pandeli, W. Neely, and J. Hardy, Interstitial fluid pressure changes in endotoxin shock, *Surgery*, 63:938–941 (1969).

50. R. Sheehan and E. Renkin, Capillary interstitial and cell membrane barriers to blood-tissue transport of potassium and rubidium in mammalian skeletal muscle, *Circ. Res.*, 30:588–607 (1972).

51. *Capillary Permeability.* Alfred Benzon Symposium 2. Edited by D. Crone and N. Lassen. New York, Academic Press, 1970.

52. T. Harris and E. V. Newman, A comparative analysis of the proposed mathematical models of circulatory indicator dilution curves, *J. Appl. Physiol.*, 28:840–850 (1970).

53. W. Perl and F. Chinard, A convection-diffusion model of indicator transport through an organ, *Circ. Res.*, 22:273–298 (1968).

54. K. Brigham and J. Snell, *In vivo* assessment of pulmonary vascular integrity in experimental pulmonary edema, *J. Clin. Invest.*, 52:2041–2052 (1973).

55. F. Chinard, Exchanges across the alveolo-capillary barrier. In *The Pulmonary Circulation and Interstitial Space.* Edited by A. Fishman and H. Hecht. Chicago, University of Chicago Press, 1969, pp. 79–98.

56. C. Goresky, W. Ziegler, and G. Bach, Capillary exchange modelling: Barrier limited and flow limited distribution, *Circ. Res.*, 27:739–764 (0000).

57. T. Harris, D. Rowlett, and K. Brigham, The assessment of pulmonary capillary permeability by multiple-indicator experiments: The effects of capillary pressure, alloxan and mathematical technique, *Fed. Proc.*, 34: 437 (1975). Abstract.

58. K. Brigham, S. Faulkner, D. Fisher, and H. Bender, Lung water and vascular permeability: Comparisons after mitral valve replacement and aorto-coronary bypass operations, *Circulation*, 50:164 (1974). Abstract.

59. D. Aviado, Pathogenesis of alloxan pulmonary edema investigated by phosphorus 32 and iodine 131, *Fed. Proc.*, **12**:299 (1953). Abstract.

60. A. Gorin, R. Demling, J. Weidner, and N. Staub, Noninvasive measurement of pulmonary transvascular protein flux in sheep, *Clin. Res.*, **23**:138A (1975). Abstract.

61. E. Robin, L. Carey, A. Grenvik, F. Glauser, and K. Gaudio, Capillary leak syndrome with pulmonary edema, *Arch. Intern. Med.*, **130**:66–71 (1972).

62. B. Brenner, J. Troy, and T. Daugherty, The dynamics of glomerular ultra-filtration in the rat, *J. Clin. Invest.*, **50**:1776–1780 (1971).

63. W. Dun, C. Robertson, and B. Brenner, A model of glomerular ultrafiltration in the rat, *Am. J. Physiol.*, **223**:1178–1182 (1972).

64. V. Andreucci, J. Herrera-Acosta, F. Rector, and D. Seldin, Effective glomerular filtration pressure and single nephron filtration rate during hydropenia, elevated arterial pressure and acute volume expansion with isotonic saline, *J. Clin. Invest.*, **50**:2230–2234.

65. H. Ussing and K. Zerahm, Active transport of sodium as the source of electric current in the short-circuited isolated frog skin, *Acta Physiol. Scand.*, **23**:110–127 (1951).

66. J. Orloff and T. Handler, The similarity of effects of vasopressin, adeno-sine-3′,5′-phosphate (cyclic AMP) and theophylline on the toad bladder, *J. Clin. Invest.*, **41**:702–709 (1962).

67. A. Ozer and G. Sharp, Effect of prostaglandins and their inhibitors on osmotic water flow in the toad bladder, *Am. J. Physiol.*, **222**:674–680 (1972).

68. A. Kozinski and A. Lightfoot, Protein ultrafiltration: A general example of boundary layer filtration, *A. I. Ch. E. J.*, **18**:1030–1040 (1972).

69. R. Wagner, P. Kreiner, R. Barnett, and M. Bitensky, Biochemical charac-terization and cytochemical localization of catecholamine-sensitive adenylate cyclase in isolated capillary endothelium, *Proc. Natl. Acad. Sci.*, **69**:3175–3179 (1972).

70. A. Brunschwig, J. Allen, F. Owens, and T. Thornton, Alloxan in treatment of insulin producing islet cell carcinoma of pancreas, *JAMA*, **124**:212–216 (1944).

71. L. Thomas, The physiological disturbances produced by endotoxins, *Ann. Rev. Physiol.*, **16**:467–490 (1954).

72. J. Curlson, M. Yokoyama, and E. Dickinson, Induction of pulmonary edema and emphysema in cattle and goats with 3-methylindole, *Science*, **176**:298–299 (1972).

73. B. Wilson, M. Boyd, T. Harris, and D. Yang, A lung edema factor from mouldy sweet potatoes (*Ipomeu Batatas*), *Nature*, **231**:52–53 (1971).

74. B. Wilson, D. Yang, and M. Boyd, Toxicity of mould-damaged sweet potatoes (*Ipomeu Batatas*), *Nature*, **227**:521–522 (1970).

75. K. Remod, Nature of pulmonary damage produced by high oxygen pres-sures, *J. Appl. Physiol.*, **9**:1–4 (1956).

76. J. Balentine, Pathologic effects of exposure to high oxygen tension: A re-view, *N. E. J. Med.*, **275**:1038–1040 (1966).

77. A. Durvell, K. Kilburn, and P. Pruitt, Short-term exposure to nitrogen dioxide. Effects on pulmonary ultrastructure, compliance and the surfactant system, *Arch. Intern. Med.*, **128**:74–80 (1971).

78. G. Heuter and M. Fitzhand, Oxidants and lung biochemistry, *Arch. Intern. Med.*, **128**:48–53 (1971).

79. D. Hyde, A freeze-fracture study of ozone-induced morphological change in primate lung. In *31st Annual Proceedings of the Electron Microscopy Society of America*. Edited by C. Arceneaux. Baton Rouge, Louisiana State University Press, 1973.

80. H. Spencer. *Pathology of the Lung.* 2nd ed. London, Pergamon Press, Ltd., 1968, p. 243.

81. J. Diana, S. Long, and H. Yao, Effect of histamine on equivalent pore radius in capillaries of isolated dog hindlimb, *Microvasc. Res.*, **4**:413–437 (1972).

82. L. Blake and N. Staub, Modeling of steady state pulmonary transvascular fluid and protein exchange in unanesthetized sheep, *Physiologist*, **15**:88 (1972). Abstract.

83. T. Cottrell, R. Levine, R. Senior, J. Wiener, D. Spiro, and A. Fishman, Electron microscopic alteration at the alveolar level in pulmonary edema, *Circ. Res.*, **21**:783–797 (1967).

84. A. Cunningham and J. Hurley, Alpha-naphthyl thiourea-induced pulmonary edema in the rat: A topographical and electron-microscope study, *J. Pathol.*, **106**:25–35 (1972).

85. T. Hovig, A. Nicolaysen, and G. Nicolaysen, Ultrastructural studies of the alveolar-capillary barrier in isolated plasma-perfused rabbit lungs. Effects of EDTA and of increased capillary pressures, *Acta Physiol. Scand.*, **82**: 417–432 (1971).

86. M. Blake and K. Brigham, unpublished observations, 1976.

87. H. Shirley, C. Wolfram, K. Wasserman, and H. Mayerson, Capillary permeability to macromolecules: Stretched pore phenomenon, *Amer. J. Physiol.*, **190**:189–197 (1957).

88. G. Pietra, P. Szidon, M. Leventhal, and A. Fishman, Hemoglobin as a tracer in hemodynamic pulmonary edema, *Science*, **166**:1643–1646 (1969).

89. M. Kaliner and K. Austen, A sequence of biochemical events in the antigen-induced release of chemical mediators from sensitized human lung tissue, *J. Exp. Med.*, **138**:1077–1094 (1973).

90. S. Karim, M. Sandler, and E. Williams, Distribution of prostaglandins in human tissues, *Brit. J. Pharmacol. Chemother.*, **31**:340–344 (1967).

91. P. Piiper and J. R. Vane, The release of prostaglandins from lung and other tissues, *Ann. N. Y. Acad. Sci.*, **180**:363–385 (1971).

92. S. Said, T. Yoshida, S. Katamura, and C. Vicini, Pulmonary alveolar hypoxia: Release of prostaglandins and other humoral mediators, *Science*, **185**:1181–1183 (1974).

93. W. Spector and D. Willoughby, The inflammatory response, *Bacterial Rev.*, **27**:117–154 (1963).

94. R. Carter, W. Joyner, and E. Renkin, Effects of histamine and some other substances on molecular selectivity of the capillary wall to plasma proteins and dextran, *Microvasc. Res.*, 7:31–48 (1974).

95. G. Majno, V. Gilmore, and M. Leventhal, On the mechanism of vascular leakage caused by histamine-type mediators, *Circ. Res.*, 21:833–847 (1967).

96. G. Majno and G. Palade, Studies on inflammation: I. Effect of histamine and serotonin on vascular permeability: An electron microscopic study, *J. Biophys. Biochem. Cytol.*, 11:571–605 (1961).

97. G. Grega, R. Daugherty, J. Scott, D. Radawski, and F. Haddy, Effects of pressure, flow and vasoactive agents on vascular resistance and capillary filtration in canine fetal, newborn and adult lung, *Microvasc. Res.*, 3: 297–307 (1971).

98. B. Goetzman and M. Visscher, The effects of alloxan and histamine on the permeability of the pulmonary alveolo-capillary barrier to albumin, *J. Physiol.*, 204:51–61 (1969).

99. G. Pietra, P. Szidon, M. Leventhal, and A. Fishman, Histamine and interstitial pulmonary edema in the dog, *Circ. Res.*, 29:323–337 (1971).

100. K. Brigham, Increased lung vessel permeability in awake sheep caused by histamine, *Clin. Res.*, 22:500A (1974). Abstract.

101. D. Willoughby, Effects of prostaglandins F_2 and E on vascular permeability, *J. Path. Bact.*, 96:381–387 (1968).

102. B. Fanberg, Prostaglandins and the lung, *Amer. Rev. Resp. Dis.*, 108: 482–489 (1973).

103. E. Anggard and B. Sammuelson, Prostaglandins and related factors 28. Metabolism of prostaglandin E in guinea pig lungs: The structure of two metabolites, *J. Biol. Chem.*, 239:4091–4096 (1964).

104. S. Ferriera and J. R. Vane, Prostaglandins: Their disappearance from and release into the circulation, *Nature*, 216:868–879 (1967).

105. C. Toshima and M. Rose, Pulmonary edema and salicylates, *Ann. Intern. Med.*, 81:274 (1974).

106. R. Orange, M. Kaliner, P. La Raiu, and K. F. Austen, The immunological release of slow reacting substance of anaphylaxis from human lung. II. Influence of cellular levels of cyclic AMP, *Fed. Proc.*, 30:1725–1729 (1971).

107. A. Ozer and G. Sharp, Effect of prostaglandins and their inhibitors on osmotic water flow in the toad bladder, *Am. J. Physiol.*, 222:674–680 (1972).

108. T. Dousa and C. Code, Effect of histamine and its methyl derivatives on cyclic AMP metabolism in gastric mucosa and its blockage by an H_2 receptor antagonist, *J. Clin. Invest.*, 53:334–337 (1974).

109. R. Wehmann, L. Blonde, and A. Steiner, Sources of cyclic nucleotides in plasma, *J. Clin. Invest.*, 53:173–179 (1974).

110. P. Hammitt and K. Brigham, unpublished observations, 1976.

111. P. Craddock, J. Fehr, K. Brigham, and H. Jacob, Pulmonary capillary

leukostasis: A complement-mediated complication of hemodialysis, *Clin. Res.*, **23**:402A (1975). Abstract.

112.   G. Moss, C. Staunton, and A. Stein, The centrineurogenic etiology of the acute respiratory distress syndrome, *Am. J. Surg.*, **126**:37–41 (1973).

113.   A. Gregory, Inhalation toxicology and lung edema receptor sites, *Amer. Industr. Hyg. Assoc. J.*, **31**:454–459 (1970).

114.   S. Sahaphong and B. Trump, Studies of cellular injury in isolated kidney tubules of the flounder, *Am. J. Path.*, **63**:277–290 (1971).

115.   C. Gruzhit, B. Peralta, and G. Moe, The pulmonary arterial pressor effect of certain sulfhydryl inhibitors, *J. Pharm. Exp. Ther.*, **101**:107–118 (1951).

116.   D. Watkins, S. Cooperstein, and A. Lazarow, Effect of sulfhydryl reagents on permeability of toadfish islet tissue, *Am. J. Physiol.*, **219**:503–509 (1970).

117.   K. Brigham and P. Owen, Mechanisms of the serotonin effect on lung transvascular fluid and protein movement in unanesthetized sheep, *Circ. Res.*, **36**:761–770 (1975).

10

Acute and Chronic Clearance
of Lung Fluids, Proteins, and Cells

EDWARD C. MEYER

Mercy Catholic Medical Center
Darby, Pennsylvania

I. Introduction

In the lung, as in any tissue, the composition of exudative edema fluid depends not only on the degree of microvascular injury, but also on the time elapsing after the injury. The most significant component of early exudative edema is plasma protein, and the concentration of protein in the fluid is a rough indicator of the severity of the injury. Older exudative edema, however, contains a variety of white blood cells and histiocytes, which enter the field of injury in phases. Finally, there is the additional presence of degraded tissue components, including fibrillar and nonfibrillar ground substance, and these components may have significant, though undiscovered, roles in the ultimate outcome of the repair process.

What distinguishes the lung from all other organs is the presence of two extravascular spaces for the accumulation of exudate: the airspace and the interstitium. The clinical significance of the airspace is obvious to anyone who has observed acute pulmonary edema. The interstitium stands between

This work was supported in part by Grant HL 13596 from the National Institutes of Health.

the vascular space and the airspace, and has clinical significance for two reasons. First, regional airspace filling occurs only after regional interstitial fluid clearance is exceeded [1], and second, the chronic accumulation of exudate in the interstitium leads to tissue changes, which include pulmonary fibrosis [2].

Before clearance rates and routes from both extravascular spaces are described, some comment on the need for exudative edema removal is warranted.

II. Need for Exudate Removal

A. Minimal Capillary Membrane Alterations

Very few studies have been directed at the effects of chronic fluid and protein accumulations in the lung. Most of the work has involved fluid and solute flux changes, and ultrastructural capillary membrane changes, in acute lesions. It appears, however, that even minor chronic accumulations of fluid and proteins in the interstitium invoke a tissue response. As seen in chronic mitral stenosis, there is a proliferation of collagen, reticular, and elastic fibers with thickening of basement membranes [3]. This change was described as *gefässlose Organisation* by Eppinger [4] to separate it from other interstitial lesions associated with capillary ingrowth. Whether it is caused by the fluid or the protein is not known; but if it is related to interstitial protein concentration, there is little safety factor. Pulmonary lymph-to-plasma steady state protein concentrations are quite high. The ratio for albumin is 0.8 to 0.9 [5], for globulin 0.6 [6], and for fibrinogen, approximately 0.2 (unpublished observations). There is considerable controversy whether pulmonary lymph adequately reflects corresponding interstitial fluid. For dogs, we calculated mean interstitial fluid albumin concentration as 74% that in corresponding lung lymph [5]. The problem is whether the albumin is evenly distributed in the interstitial fluid. Even if it is, the concentration is high compared with concentration in the body as a whole [7]. Currently, we are studying comparable steady state interstitial "globulin" and fibrinogen concentrations.

Increases in pulmonary venous pressure may offset the narrow protein concentration gradient. As Renkin predicted [8], for constant permeability of the capillary membrane to protein, there is an inverse relation between net transcapillary water flux (reflected in lymph flow) and protein concentration [9]. Further chronic (steady state) studies of pulmonary venous hypertension in terms of quantitative tissue change are needed. These should be directed also at all plasma proteins, particularly fibrous proteins such as fibrinogen, which appear to be so important in tissue change.

B. Important Capillary Membrane Alterations

Coupling of Coagulation and Exudate Formation

Following serious vascular membrane injury, all plasma proteins may leak into the extravascular space at their corresponding plasma concentrations. There is little doubt that this occurs by convection only. Aschheim and Zweifach have demonstrated that in systemic tissue the bulk flow of plasma precedes capillary dilatation and stasis [10].

The resulting exudate can coagulate, and this is initiated not only by activation of the plasma thromboplastic system (intrinsic system) but also by release of tissue thromboplastins from injured cells (extrinsic system). The latter is particularly interesting in that the thromboplastic activity appears to be bound to particulate matter at the site of injury, thus limiting entrance into the general circulation or extension to other normal extravascular sites [11]. When the fibrinous coagulum retracts, serum may be expelled and absorbed by lymph. This serum contains coagulation-enhancing factors, which may enter the circulation and produce intravascular clotting elsewhere [12]. Finally, the modification of extravascular tissue proteins by the injury may trigger the inflammatory reaction [13] and modify glycosaminoglycans sufficiently to alter the sol-gel phases of ground substance and interfere with convective clearance of proteins. This aspect has not been studied but together with fibrin deposition may interfere with clearance mechanisms.

Control of Fibrin Deposition

Although the production of a fibrinous "hemostatic plug" represents the first tissue defense to injury, all fibrin must be removed if tissue restoration to normal is to occur. Various factors including components of the intrinsic system and inhibitors of these components [11] may interfere with the formation of fibrin. Persistent fibrin on the other hand serves as a matrix for proliferating fibroblasts, capillaries, and epithelial cells [14]. Thus, the removal of fibrin prevents connective tissue overgrowth, and this is accomplished by activation of the plasminogen-plasmin fibrinolytic system. Although humoral activators participate in this process [15], tissue activators are probably more important in the lung. The lung is particularly rich in tissue plasminogen activator [16],

and this significantly affects the amount of exudative edema following microvascular injury. In an unpublished experiment, we induced exudative pulmonary edema with α-naphthylthiourea (ANTU) (20 mg/kg body weight) in two
groups of 20 rats. One group had ε-aminocaproic acid (EACA) added to their
drinking water to inhibit fibrinolysis. This group had a 75% mortality rate
within 24 h, and the mean lung-to-body weight ratio was 0.74 ± 0.04 (SE).
By comparison, the group not receiving EACA had a 100% mortality rate
within 24 h, and the mean lung-to-body weight ratio was 0.92 ± 0.04 (SE).
The edema fluid contained more fibrin in the EACA-treated rats, and the
fibrin not only surrounded capillaries in the interalveolar septa, but was more
prominent in alveolar fluid. Apparently, therefore, some tissue activator
passes into alveoli with the fluid. It must be rapidly depleted because fibrin
in alveolar spaces appears to persist long enough for invasion by macrophages
(Section III.B).

With lysis, fibrin-fibrinogen degradation products increase capillary permeability and attract leukocytes [17]. Leukocytes, however, may have little
part in the resolution of fibrin. Opie [18] noted the disappearance of leukocytes in fibrinous pleurisy before the fibrin was removed. More recently,
Kwaan and Astrup noted the same in homologous plasma clots implanted
subcutaneously in rats [19]. In the absence of fibrinolysis, ultimate tissue
repair was characterized by fibroblastic proliferation and capillary ingrowth.
This has been demonstrated also in burns [20], corneal inflammatory disease
[21], and experimental glomerulonephritis [22]. The renal cortex has low
fibrinolytic activity [23], and fibrin deposits in the glomerular urine space not
only persist, but are associated with fibroepithelial cellular proliferations.
These proliferations appear as crescents within glomeruli, and usually indicate
a predictably rapid deterioration of renal function. In humans, this lesion is
called rapidly progressive glomerulonephritis [24]. It has been simulated experimentally in rabbits by injecting heterologous nephrotoxic antiserum [25].
It is interesting that anticoagulating the animals before injecting the antiserum
prevented crescent formation even though deposition of the antibody in basement membranes still occurred [25]. These experiments therefore link cellular proliferations to persistent fibrin deposits.

Capillary ingrowth into fibrinous deposits does represent one important
cellular mechanism of lysis. As seen by the fibrin plate histological technique,
endothelial cells of veins and venules have high fibrinolytic activity [26].
Similar activity has been seen in young proliferating capillaries, and this
activity decreases when these vessels involute to scar formation [27]. The
ultimate products of fibrinolysis are fibrinogen and fibrin split products.

Cellular digestion of these products may be significant in their removal.
MacFarlane [28] has demonstrated that radioiodinated fibrinogen injected

subcutaneously in rabbits is retained principally at the site of injection, only small amounts returning to the circulation. This contrasts sharply with the action of albumin and globulins, and raises the question whether fibrinogen is bound in extravascular tissues following the trauma of injection. In this regard, the half-life of tagged albumin injected subcutaneously is 20 to 40 h [29,30]. Mutschler [31] noted that subcutaneously injected tagged fibrinogen disappeared locally with a half-life of 3 days in rats. When the rats were given EACA in their drinking water, the half-time approached 2 weeks [31]. This is consistent with removal mechanisms hinging on local fibrin-fibrinogen lysis.

Several other studies emphasize this fact. Mutschler [32] showed that radioiodinated fibrinogen injected intravenously in rats is cleared with a half-life of 1.2 days. This clearance rate, and whole body clearance rate, were not affected by EACA. When turpentine abscesses were induced, however, the abscess uptake of the tagged fibrinogen was higher when EACA was given, and its clearance from the abscess markedly impaired. Kwaan and Astrup [33] noted a marked fibroblastic proliferation into homologous plasma clots implanted subcutaneously when inhibitors of fibrinolysis were incorporated into the clot. Polyvinyl sponges implanted into the peritoneal cavity have delayed connective tissue ingrowth when intraperitoneal infusion of heparin or anti-thrombin was given [34].

How can these studies be extrapolated to the lung? Unfortunately most descriptive pathology deals with lungs at an end stage of chronic disease. There is some convincing evidence, however, that failure to clear extravascular fibrin results in tissue change. Spencer [35] theorizes that persistent alveolar and interstitial fibrin masses undergo organization resulting in "chronic interstitial pneumonia." There is difficulty distinguishing between alveolar and interstitial sites at end stages. Persistent intra-alveolar fibrin masses may be covered by proliferating epithelial cells, and appear as "interstitial" tissue masses later. On the other hand, they may be organized by intra-airway proliferation of a vascular fibroblastic tissue. This results in bronchiolar-alveolar fibrous plugs—the *bourgeons conjonctifs* of Masson et al. [36].

There is some other evidence of lung fibrosis associated with fibrinolysis failure. Uremic lung contains fibrinous edema fluid [37]. Heard suggested that it might be caused by inactivation of fibrinolysis [38], and MacLeod et al. proved this in a single patient [39]. Posttraumatic pulmonary insufficiency, or "shock lung," consists of diffuse exudative edema including intra-alveolar hyaline masses composed principally of fibrin. The cause is uncertain, although proposed theories suggest diffuse pulmonary capillary microemboli [40], changes in pulmonary capillary permeability to protein [41], and lysosomal tissue damage from degenerating neutrophiles. Rammer and Saldeen [42] note strong inhibition of the fibrinolytic system in patients dying with this syndrome. Demling et al. [43] present evidence from sheep that hemorrhagic shock itself does not cause an immediate increase in pulmonary capillary permeability to albumin. At any rate, treatment consists of supportive measures to improve gas exchange. These may include the use of extracorporeal oxygenation [44]. With extracorporeal oxygenation, only a cleanup operation is left to the lungs. Astrup et al. [16] have shown that mammalian lung is rich in tissue plasminogen activator, so that in the absence of inhibitors, the degradation of coagulation products may be quite efficient. Interestingly, however, a potent inhibitor of tissue activator has been identified in bovine lung, and Astrup et al. suggest that this may be the cause of bovine brisket disease [45]. Guinea-pig lung is low in fibrinolytic activity, but is low in tissue thromboplastin also [16]. Thus the balance between coagulation and fibrinolysis appears critical not only in the developing phases of flooding exudative edema, but also in the clearance of clot products and ultimate tissue repair.

III.   Clearance Mechanisms in the Lung

A.   Interstitial Space

Interstitial fluid contains all plasma proteins that have passed through the microvascular membrane in the direction of their concentration gradients. Net removal from the interstitial space must occur by lymph drainage [46], endocytosis, or metabolic degradation. The fact that radioiodinated proteins injected intravenously appear rapidly in lymph suggests that lymph drainage is the main route of interstitial protein clearance. The intra- and extrapulmonary lymphatic pathways have been reviewed in detail by Staub [47].

Pulmonary Lymph Flow

Normal

The anatomy of pulmonary lymphatics renders total collection of lung lymph impossible. The technique of Uhley et al. [48] ignores any contribution of lung lymph to the thoracic duct (TD). Humphreys et al. [49] proved that lung lymphatics enter the *intrathoracic* TD in fetal lambs. However, in an attempt to exclude all *infradiaphragmatic* lymph from TD collections in their experiments, they ligated the TD at the diaphragm. Lung lymphatics do pass below the diaphragm into the cisterna chyli in humans [50], so the data of Humphreys et al. on total flow of lung lymph in lambs neglects potential collateral trunks passing from the lungs below the diaphragm into the TD. Incidentally, it is common to find anthracotic (pigmented) lymph nodes below the diaphragm in surgical specimens.

The best extrathoracic source of pulmonary lymph is the right lymphatic duct (RLD). Drinker's group first identified it [51,52], and its extrapulmonary contributions have been described in detail [53].

Various lung lymph fractions to the RLD have been reported. Said et al. [54] estimated that 50% RLD flow came from the lungs. We estimated that 80% of RLD lymph originated in the lungs [55]. Both studies used RLD lymph oxygen tensions to indicate lymph origin. One would expect small molecules such as respiratory gases to equilibrate with lymph node blood since molecules as large as albumin cross the lymph node-blood interface [56].

Recently we demonstrated that [^{131}I] albumin washin into RLD lymph of dogs is the same as [^{131}I] albumin washin into pulmonary interstitial fluid [5]. This rate constant, for all practical purposes, is the same as the rate constant for cardiac interstitial fluid [57]. Thus, in terms of steady state lymph-to-plasma albumin ratios, the RLD is a good source for representative lung lymph. Using a simple convective model of plasma-to-lymph albumin transport, we estimated that RLD lymph accounted, on an average, for 28% of pulmonary interstitial fluid.

The main question is, What is lung lymph flow normally? Since it is reasonable to assume that the albumin, which has passed from plasma to interstitial fluid, is not consumed by cells or other extravascular structures but passes into lymph by bulk flow, we can use the rate constant of pulmonary interstitial albumin equilibration to estimate lymph flow. Unfortunately, the transport process by which albumin passes from plasma to interstitial fluid must be defined. There are two models for this: diffusion and convection.

A diffusion model assumes that the capillary membrane is ideally semipermeable for albumin, that is, that the osmotic reflection coefficient [58] for albumin is unity. This model therefore predicts small equivalent pores in the capillary membrane. By first-order kinetic compartmental analysis, the rate constant for albumin K_A in pulmonary interstitial fluid is [59]

$$K_A = \frac{PS + L}{V_i} \tag{1}$$

where PS is the permeability–surface area product, in ml/min, of the capillary membrane for albumin, and V_i is the interstitial fluid volume in ml. It can be shown also that

$$PS = \frac{K_A A_i V_p}{A_p} \tag{2}$$

where A_i is the albumin mass in interstitial fluid and A_p is the albumin mass in plasma, and V_p is the plasma volume. Substituting Equation (1) into Equation (2), and defining $A_p/V_p = C_p$ (plasma albumin concentration), and $A_i/V_i = C_i$ (interstitial albumin concentration), we get

$$\frac{PS}{L} = \frac{C_i/C_p}{1 - C_i/C_p} \tag{3}$$

This is identical to the Renkin equation [8] if $C_i/C_p = R$ (steady state lymph-to-plasma albumin concentration). There is no definite information whether pericapillary fluid is identical to lymph in albumin concentration, or whether it has an albumin concentration equal to A_i/V_i, where V_i is the extravascular (sucrose) volume. Measured A_i and V_i depend on accurate measurement of plasma volume in lung homogenates. Our measurements used the method of Pearce et al. [60], which probably overestimated plasma significantly. Marshall [61] has shown that the only accurate method uses radioiodinated albumin as a plasma tag. By applying appropriate corrections to our data [5], we estimate $A_i = 4.5 \times 10^{-2}$ g/kg body weight, and $V_i = 3.4$ ml/kg body weight. From Equation 2, therefore, $PS = 6 \times 10^{-2}$ ml/min for a 14-kg dog. Assuming that dog pulmonary capillary area is 33 m^2 [62], we estimate the "permeability" coefficient to be 0.03×10^{-7} cm/sec, which is quite small [47]. Incidentally, this is a maximal value since it is based only on diffusional microvascular albumin transport. Assuming that extravascular albumin is not evenly distributed in extravascular water but distributed in a volume relative to lymph, one can solve Equation (3) for $L = 1.5 \times 10^{-2}$ ml/min for a 14-kg dog. This is the lowest estimate for lymph flow.

A convection model assumes that albumin passes from plasma by hydrodynamic flow through pores that impose frictional resistance to albumin, resulting in molecular sieving [7]. The pores are large enough to account for all unidirectional albumin flux, diffusional flux approaching zero. With this model, $K_A = L/V_i$, resulting in $L = 8.4 \times 10^{-2}$ ml/min for a 14-kg dog. This is a maximal value.

Which is the best estimate? The equations of Kedem and Katchalsky [63] based on irreversible thermodynamics predict that albumin passes from plasma by both diffusion and convection depending on its osmotic reflection coefficient, on the true permeability coefficient of the membrane, and on the hydraulic conductivity of the membrane. Staub [47] notes that since lymph flow and albumin concentration vary inversely (as predicted by the Renkin equation), diffusion must be a significant component. If convection predominated (as suggested by the high R), the capillary pores would have to decrease in size as the intracapillary pressure increased, to account for a reduction in lymph albumin concentration.

Viewing the capillary membrane as an inert structure may be shortsighted. Transport may involve enzymatic activity, and this has been shown to account partially for the blood-brain barrier. At any rate, it is likely that diffusion and convection both contribute to transcapillary solute flux. Staub's model of pulmonary capillary albumin flow predicts a very low permeability coefficient, and a fairly high albumin osmotic reflection coefficient (0.8) [47].

We have estimated that approximately one-third lung lymph flows into the RLD in dogs [55]. If oxygen tension data are correct, approximately 80% of RLD flow comes from the lungs. Mean RLD flow in a 14-kg dog is 2.1×10^{-2} ml/min [5], and this implies that approximately 1.7×10^{-2} ml/min comes into the RLD from the lungs. Total lung lymph flow may be estimated, therefore, as $(1.7 \times 10^{-2}) \times 3 = 5.1 \times 10^{-2}$ ml/min in a 14-kg dog. This estimate lies between those prediced for diffusion and convection models. This estimate, within a range, appears reasonable. It is the best estimate short of collecting all lung lymph.

Edema

Acute Many investigators have measured RLD lymph flow in acute pulmonary edema [47]. In most instances, RLD flow increases from five to ten times basal rates, and this is true following acute increases in pulmonary capillary hydrostatic pressure or following capillary damage. It is difficult to use the relations between normal lung lymph flow and RLD flow that were stated in the previous section for estimating maximal lung lymph flow rates. This is because edema fluid is oriented in gravity-dependent lung zones, and may not be reflected in RLD increases. With this limitation in mind, however, we estimate that a 10-fold increase in RLD flow represents a 13-fold increase in lung lymph flow (80% of RLD lymph originating in the lung, and all RLD increases coming from the lung). We know that this is the upper limit of lymph pumping rate because significant interstitial fluid accumulations occur. In actual flow, this is approximately 0.6 ml/min in a 14-kg dog. This maximal flow rate is very low compared with edema formation rate.

We have measured interstitial exudative edema volumes by morphometric techniques in dogs 90 min after alloxan [64]. Although the number of dogs is small, there is a correlation between total edema volume and interstitial edema volume, both measured morphometrically. These data are presented in Figure 1, and there appears to be a maximal interstitial volume capacity of approximately 7 ml/kg body weight. For a 14-kg dog, this represents 100 ml fluid,

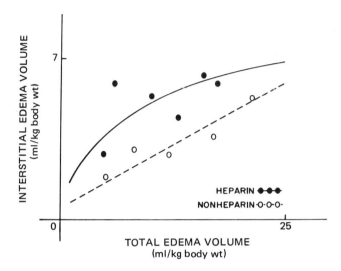

FIGURE 1   Relation between interstitial and total pulmonary edema volumes measured morphometrically in dogs 90 min after alloxan. For any given total edema volume, more interstitial fluid is present in heparinized dogs. The interstitial compartment consists of interalveolar, peribronchial, and perivascular spaces.

and approaches pulmonary blood volume. With estimated maximal lymph flow rates, this could be cleared in 2.5 hr.

The obstacle facing the lymph pump is the rate at which edema fluid forms. If the interstitial edema fluid after alloxan leaked at a constant rate, this might be well within maximal lymph flows. However, all studies of alloxan edema indicate that the appearance is very rapid after a delay period exceeding one hour [65,1]. This is clear since alveolar flooding occurs. Staub et al. [1] have shown conclusively that alveolar filling occurs only after the capacity of the interstitial space is exceeded. This does not mean that the entire lung interstitium must be filled before alveolar flooding occurs in some regions.

Our estimates of interstitial volume capacity are greater than those Hughes et al. have presented [66]. They noted a weight increase in excised perfused lung averaging 30% due to interstitial edema. In the absence of alveolar flooding, however, interstitial collections may not be maximal. Our data suggest that interstitial fluid can increase wet lung weight by 70%.

Chronic   The ability of lung lymphatics to hypertrophy in response to a chronic load has not been tested adequately. Sampson et al. [67] believe that their experiments prove pulmonary lymphatic expansion even to the point of preventing edema (see the references in Ref. 67). Their dog model was one of chronic cardiac failure in which thoracic duct lymph flow increased also, and they never accounted for the opening of collateral TD-to-RLD lymphatic trunks. A better experiment would involve isolated chronic pulmonary venous hypertension.

This is difficult to achieve. In 1960, Rabin and I [68] attempted to snare the mitral annulus, and slowly constrict it over a period of weeks. Unfortunately most snares ruptured the annulus, resulting in bacterial endocarditis. More recently Vasko et al. [69] described an ingenious method. They inserted a plug of Ameroid into the left atrial appendage, and invaginated the appendage into the mitral annulus. Unfortunately, the appendage and plug must be held in this position, and this requires a holding suture emerging through the left ventricle. Theoretically this may become infected. Their hemodynamic data demonstrate an ideal animal model of chronic mitral stenosis as the Ameroid swells.

Other methods have been described [70]. The current ease with which heart-lung bypass is used should encourage even more imaginative techniques of inducing slow mitral leaflet symphysis.

Experiments of this sort are needed badly to help explain the steady state compensation for increased lung interstitial fluid in chronic mitral stenosis. In addition to potential hypertrophy of lung lymphatics, the changes in perivascular ground substance might impose significant alterations in transcapillary water and solute flux. It is important to remember that capillary "membranes" consist not only of endothelial cells but also of basement membranes.

Interstitial Lymph Transport

Composition of Interstitial Ground Substance

Extravascular ground substance consists of glycosaminoglycans, long-chained molecules of random configuration and varying charge. The most studied molecule is hyaluronic acid. The osmotic pressure that this molecule exerts is very non-ideal increasing far more rapidly than albumin as a function of concentration [71]. Through water binding, the intercellular matrix consists of gel and fluid phases. The permeation of this matrix by plasma proteins depends on the volume occupied by glycosaminoglycans (exclusion effect) and the effective pores that exist between the molecular coils (sieving effect). Studies in vitro suggest that during convective flow of proteins through the matrix, smaller proteins may diffuse into the matrix, the larger ones passing more rapidly via the effluent [71]. This shorter transit time of larger molecules as opposed to smaller ones forms the basis of separation by gel chromatography.

This effect might increase convective transport of fibrous proteins in vivo, and limit their possible local deleterious effects (Section II). Garlick and Renkin [9] found no different transit times of various dextran molecules transported from interstitial fluid to lymph in dog legs but the steady state lymph concentrations of the dextrans were uncertain. At any rate, there is every reason to believe that transit times may be different. Productive investigations should be done to map the transit of various molecular species through pulmonary interstitial ground substance both in normal states and in abnormal states.

Protein Pumping in the Interstitial Space

Pappenheimer and Soto-Rivera [72] stated that because the free-diffusion coefficients of plasma proteins are low, considerable concentration gradients exist in the interstitial space in the absence of bulk flow. They concluded that 20 min would be required to obtain 90% equilibration across a distance of 50 μm in the absence of a convective force.

Garlick and Renkin challenged this [9]. They noted that the distribution volumes of popliteal lymph, which the kinetics of plasma-to-lymph transport of dextrans of different molecular weight determined, varied directly with molecular weight. They concluded that the smaller molecules were transported by diffusive as well as convective components. It is difficult to evaluate these conclusions since a small error in steady state concentration drastically affects distribution volume [5].

In general, it is difficult to interpret lymph experiments. As Grotte pointed out [73], the actual tissue volume a lymph trunk drains is uncertain. Furthermore, since lymph trunks contain lymph from innumerable terminal lymphatics arranged in parallel, there is no certainty that solute washin rate constants in all terminal lymphatics will be equal. Albumin washin in dog RLD is monoexponential up to at least 1/e experimental time, and data points fit quite well with a simple, first-order kinetic model (Fig. 2). However, careful analysis of "experimental noise" in Figure 2 suggests that the model may be too simple. The data points cycle too regularly. Similar cycles appear in the data Demling et al. present for sheep [43]. This is an interesting phenomenon, and appears to represent an albumin pulse in lymph. Figure 3 summarizes a typical experiment, in which [^{125}I]albumin was injected intravenously into a dog and allowed to equilibrate with intra- and extravascular albumin over several days. Subsequently, with the experimental animal under pentobarbital anesthesia, the RLD was cannulated, and [^{131}I]albumin injected intra-

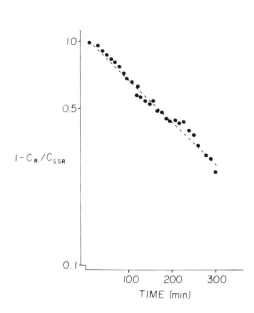

FIGURE 2   Semilogarithmic plot of right lymphatic duct lymph washin for [^{131}I] albumin from plasma. C_R = instantaneous [^{131}I] albumin concentration in right duct lymph. C_{ssR} = steady state concentration. The value C_{ssR} was determined by injecting [^{125}I] albumin several days earlier to allow total equilibration. Since plasma [^{131}I] albumin concentration was maintained constant, C_{ssR} = lymph [^{131}I] albumin concentration X lymph [^{125}I] albumin concentration/plasma [^{125}I] albumin concentration. Reprinted from E. C. Meyer and R. Ottaviano, *Circ. Res.*, 35:197–203 (1974), by courtesy of the American Heart Association, Inc.

venously. Over several hours' observation, the concentration of [^{125}I] albumin cycled regularly every 45 min, and these cycles were in phase with [^{131}I] albumin cycles. There was no concomitant cycling in RLD flow. Possibly this signal represents binding of albumin to glycosaminoglycans to a "saturation point" and then rapid expulsion into the interstitial effluent. This is highly speculative—but the pulse is very persistent. Incidentally, noncovalent protein-hyaluronic acid complexes may exist [74], but whether the binding is reversible is not known.

The concept of a pulmonary interstitial albumin pulse gains further support from experiments in which radioiodinated albumin, instilled into alveoli, appears in plasma and lymph (Fig. 4). The pulses in lymph and plasma need not be in phase, since the transit time necessary for lymph to pass into RLD cannulas is a factor. It is apparent, therefore, that the albumin first enters the pulmonary interstitial space from alveoli, and then passes into plasma and lymph. Experiments directed at interstitial transport of macromolecules are important and needed. Most interstitial spaces are quite inaccessible for the primary injection of tracer molecules. The pulmonary interstitial space may be an exception, since alveolar instillation of small amounts of macromolecular solutions produces no morphologic injury.

Other experimental evidence supports the diffusion of labeled macromolecules from the interstitium to plasma. Normand et al. [75] instilled

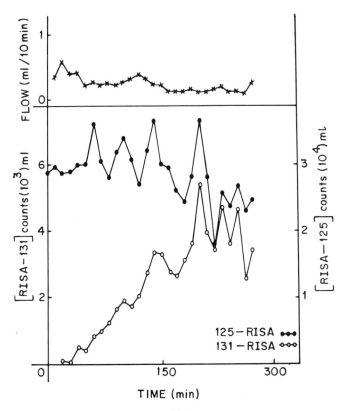

FIGURE 3 An experiment in which [^{125}I] albumin was injected intravenously in a dog and allowed to equilibrate over several days. Subsequently, with the subject under general anesthesia with the right lymphatic duct (RLD) cannulated, [^{131}I] albumin was injected intravenously at zero time. The upper graph shows RLD flow. The lower graph shows RLD lymph concentrations of [^{125}I] albumin ([125-RISA] right ordinate) and [^{131}I] albumin ([131-RISA] left ordinate). Both signals pulsed regularly at 45-min intervals. The fractional change of [125-RISA] with each pulse exceeded the changes of [131-RISA], so that the pulses were not related to errors in sample volumes. A graph of [^{131}I] albumin specific activity ([131-RISA]/[125-RISA]) therefore will also demonstrate pulses.

polyvinylpyrrolidones (PVP) of various molecular weights into lung fluid of fetal lambs. There was no appearance in blood or lung lymph before positive pressure ventilation was begun. After ventilation, however, PVP entered plasma and lymph. Polyvinylpyrrolidones of the same molecular radius as albumin entered both lymph and plasma from the extra-alveolar interstitial

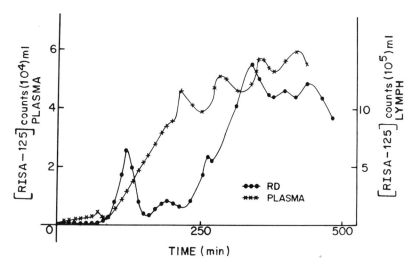

FIGURE 4   An experiment in which isoosmolar [^{125}I]albumin (125-RISA) was instilled into alveoli of a dog with the right lymphatic duct (RD) cannulated. The concentrations of 125-RISA in plasma (left ordinate) and RD lymph (right ordinate) pulsed at 70 to 90-min intervals. Note that RD lymph concentration is 10 times the concentration of plasma.

space. Bensch and Dominguez [76] noted the passage of alveolar-instilled horseradish peroxidase (HRP) into the interstitial space, and then into plasma directly by endothelial pinocytosis. Gonzalez-Crussi and Boston [77] had similar results when HRP was instilled into lung liquid of fetal lambs. These studies do not indicate a reversal of *net* albumin transport from plasma to the interstitial space, but simply that there is bidirectional albumin flow between both spaces, the net flux being from plasma.

Pinocytotic vesicles normally exist in endothelial and epithelial cells. Their large size (500 to 700 Å diameter) suggests that transport of large macromolecules might be through them as opposed to a few large equivalent pores [9]. Their actual part in transport is uncertain, since they appear to move within cytoplasm by Brownian motion [78] and are evenly distributed at the luminal, abluminal, and intermediate portions of cytoplasm [79]. Karnovsky [80] has pointed out the problems involved in interpreting transport of macromolecular tracers by pinocytotic vesicles.

Following pulmonary edema induced by α-thionaphthylurea (ANTU) in rats, membranous pneumocytes develop large vesicles (3000-Å diameter) apparently containing coagulation products (Fig. 5). The function of these vesicles in transport is not known.

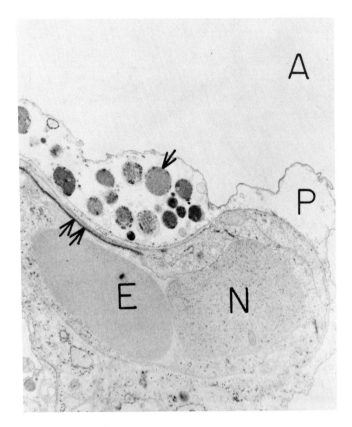

FIGURE 5   Rat lung three days after receiving ANTU (20 mg/kg body weight) in conjunction with continuous EACA. Alveolar septum is lined by swollen cytoplasmic extensions of membranous pneumonocytes (P). The capillary contains an erythrocyte (E) and a neutrophil (N). The epithelium contains numerous large vesicles (arrow) measuring up to 3000 Å in diameter. They appear to be filled with coagulation products. The epithelial cytoplasm containing these vesicles lies over a thin layer of fibrin (arrows) beneath the capillary endothelium. No fibrin is seen in the alveolar airspace (A). Electron photomicrograph (X8200).

Exudate Coagulation and Lymph Flow

Menkin, in his classic description of the localization of inflammation, claimed that coagulation of exudate both in the interstitial space and in the lymphat ics constituted the chief defense against septic processes [81]. Glenn et al. [82] made the same observation for sterile inflammation (burns). Miles and Miles [83] noted that india ink passed from injured sites into terminal lym- phatics, suggesting that "fixation" of the injured site is caused by physiochemical changes of the tissue itself. There is clinical evidence favoring Menkin's theory. Streptococcal lymphangitis is related to streptokinase produced by the bacteria, and *Clostridium welchii,* which produces hyaluronidase, causes a devastating interstitial septic process.

Pores exist between fibrin strands, and fibrin strands contract expelling serum. The interaction between fibrin masses and ground substance has not been investigated satisfactorily, and experiments should be directed at this.

These effects are particularly important in the lung. The fact that airway is one component of extravascular fluid clearance stresses the importance of the lymph pump. We have studied the distribution of pulmonary exudate in relation to fibrin [64]. The results indicate three facts. First, in a flooding pulmonary exudative edema produced by alloxan, fluid inevitably enters alveoli. When the alveolar exudate clots, the flow of edema fluid up the airways is minimized. When the exudate does not clot, it rapidly passes into bronchi and blocks ventilation. Second, when alveolar exudate clots, interstitial fluid accumulations and lymph flow rates are greater for any given total edema volume. This suggests that there is little resistance to airway extravascular exit of fluid compared with the resistance lymphatics impose [84]. Third, the absence of fibrin in interstitial exudate as opposed to alveolar exudate suggests that pulmonary tissue activator lyses interstitial fibrin rapidly and efficiently.

We have some unpublished data confirming this third fact by analyzing RLD lymph for fibrin split products. The fibrinolytic reaction has been described in detail [85]. The earliest fibrin degradation product (fdp) is a large fragment (fragment X^0) that is capable of spontaneous polymerization. Usually this does not occur because it forms soluble complexes with later degradation products of fibrinogen [86] or with fibrinogen itself [87]. Protamine sulfate apparently causes a dissociation of these complexes, permitting fragment X^0 to polymerize to strand formation. This "paracoagulation reaction" of protamine sulfate forms the basis of detecting fdp [88]. Continued plasmin digestion results in the formation of fibrinogen degradation products (FDP). The largest of these (fragment X) can be polymerized by the action of thrombin, but not spontaneously, like fragment X^0. Further plasmin digestion produces other FDP that have smaller molecular weights than fibrinogen and are not polymerized by thrombin. These products (fragments D and E) possess anticoagulative properties, and leukotactic properties [17], but are antigenically similar to fibrinogen. This antigenic similarity forms the basis for detection by an antigen-antibody reaction [89]. Fragment X^0 is larger than fibrinogen and fragments X, D and E are progressively smaller. Fragment E has a molecular weight slightly greater than the molecular weight of albumin. The action of lung tissue plasminogen activator thus may become extremely important in the digestion of large fibrinogen like molecules to smaller ones for better clearance by lymphatics.

Tests for these split products are done usually on plasma samples in the search for syndromes of diffuse intravascular coagulation and primary fibrinolysis. However, the concentration of these products in lymph should be much greater when they result from extravascular plasmin digestion. We have observed the appearance of fragment X^0 in right lymphatic duct lymph approximately 60 min after alloxan pulmonary edema development. Table 1 shows the semiquantitative amounts of fragment X^0 in plasma, and lymph from the TD and RLD in three dogs with similar alloxan edema volume (16 ml/kg). One dog was nonheparinized (N), another heparinized (H), after surgery, and a third given EACA (E) before surgery. Following the surgery necessary to cannulate both lymph ducts, significant quantities of fdp appeared in plasma in the N and H dogs, but little to none in the E dog. Since electrocoagulation was used for hemostasis, numerous intravascular thrombi apparently were induced, and these underwent lysis, appearing as fdp in plasma throughout the prealloxan and postalloxan periods. Following introduction of alloxan, significant fdp appeared in RLD lymph and TD lymph in the N dog. The H dog had no fdp in RLD or TD lymph, indicating satisfactory anticoagulation. No significant fdp were found in the plasma, TD, or RLD in the E dog. We believe that these data indicate rapid extravascular fibrinolysis in the lung. They also seem to indicate that protein molecules even larger than fibrinogen can pass into lymph following tissue edema although the actual quantitative clearance is unknown.

Fibrin split products are not the only large molecules in the interstitial space following microvascular injury. Tissue proteins, particularly collagen, are damaged by proteases, and with subsequent contact with serum proteins can activate the complement system [13]. Willoughby and DiRosa [13] recently reviewed the sequential mediators involved in inflammation; they suggest that contact between altered tissue proteins and plasma proteins may be the trigger mechanism.

Interstitial Cell Accumulations

Whenever vascular endothelium is damaged, it becomes "sticky" for various formed blood elements. The subsequent emigration of white cells is a sign of the inflammatory process [90]. The earliest emigrating cells are neutrophils, but except in bacterial infections, they disappear soon from the extravascular space. The common notion that death of the cells with release of lysosomal proteases provides the stimulus for mononuclear cell emigration has been challenged by Willoughby and Spector [91]. They showed that agranulocytic animals can generate an inflammatory reaction, and their experiments indicate

TABLE 1 Concentrations (mg/100 ml) of Fibrin Split Products (Fragment X^0) Following Alloxan Pulmonary Edema in Dogs

	Plasma			TD Lymph			RLD Lymph		
	N	H	E	N	H	E	N	H	E
Presurgery[a]	10	10	20			100			0
		Post heparin	Post EACA		Post heparin	Post EACA		Post heparin	Post EACA
Post surgery									
30 min	50–100	50–100	20	0	20	0	0	0	0
60 min	50–100	50–100		50–100	50		0	0	0
90 min	50–100	50–100		10	10		0	0	0
Post alloxan									
30 min	50–100	50–100	0	0	0	50–100	10–20	0	0
60 min	50–100	50–100	0	50–100	0	0	50–100	0	0
90 min	50–100	50–100	0	50–100	0	0	>200	0	0

Note: N = non-heparinized dog; H = heparinized dog; E = aminocaproic acid (EACA), treated dog; alloxan = 80 mg/kg body weight injected intravenously.

[a]Surgery = cannulations of thoracic duct (TD) and right lymphatic duct (RLD).

that some other mediator incites mononuclear cellular infiltration of the injured site.

Neutrophils are end cells. We do not know the absolute size of their tissue pool. Kinetic studies indicate that this pool has a turnover rate of a few days only, so that, as Hirsch [92] notes, approximately 10^{11} neutrophils must disappear daily. No "graveyard" has been identified, and he suggests that passage through intestinal mucosa may be one clearance route. In bacterial pneumonia, a constant stimulus for neutrophil emigration apparently exists, so that alveolar collections are seen for many days. These probably are cleared through the airway. Following sterile injury to pulmonary capillaries by ANTU, there is an impressive accumulation of neutrophils sticking to capillary endothelium, a few entering alveolar spaces. Within three days, most neutrophils have disappeared. Some undergo dissolution while still adherent to endothelium, and others are cleared through the airway. Increased numbers of macrophages then appear in the field of injury. Macrophage emigration characterizes the inflammatory process. There is good evidence that pulmonary macrophages are derived from circulating monocytes [93], but an intermediate residence in pulmonary tissue is required before final conversion [94]. A great many resident cells must be present, because the immediate recruitment of macrophages is not affected by marrow irradiation [95].

Little is known about the clearance of these cells. We have not seen them in lymphatics. Brundelet [96] made a detailed study of macrophage engulfment of dyes instilled into alveoli of rats. The macrophages not only moved directly towards the mucociliary escalator, but penetrated alveolar epithelium into interstitial connective tissue at six different points of the alveolar surface. These were (a) the last bifurcation of the terminal bronchiole, (b) alveolar ducts, (c) interalveolar walls, (d) alveolar walls to perivascular connective tissue, (e) alveolar walls into peribronchiolar connective tissue, and (f) alveolar walls into the periphery of peribronchial lymphoid tissue foci. In the last instance, the macrophages penetrated the lymphoid tissue directly into bronchi. Von Hayek [97] noted that these lymphoid foci resembled "diverticula of the mucous membrane of the small bronchi and bronchioles." These lymphoid cells penetrate the bronchial mucosa by infiltrating muscle, and come to lie beneath the epithelium. At certain points, the epithelium becomes discontinuous, the bronchiolar lumen communicating directly with the lymphoid tonsil. Von Hayek referred to these structures as lymphoepithelial organs, since lymphocytes appear to be released into the bronchiolar lumen. Brundelet [96] observed that many cells entering the lumen from these foci are macrophages, and recently Green [98] concluded that these foci represent a shortcut for alveolar macrophages to enter the bronchociliary escalator. Green links macrophage movement to bulk fluid flow, and suggests that the centripetal and centrifugal movements of alveolar macrophages are compatible with lymph drainage pathways and alveolar fluid flow that Staub described as "liquid veins" of the lung [99]. Centrifugal fluid flow may bring macrophages into subpleural tissues, which may represent long-term storage depots. Likewise, peribronchiolar and perivascular connective tissue spaces receiving fluid flow may represent long-term storage depots. Strict clearance analysis of various macrophage deposits is impossible. Morrow et al. [100] in their study of radioactive particle clearance from human lungs observed at least three exponentials, the longest with a half-life of approximately 65 days.

This is an important subject, because wherever macrophages accumulate (granulomas), fibroblasts appear. Spector [101] believes that macrophages stimulate fibroblasts by cell death. He notes that fibroblastic proliferation is greater in "high-turnover granulomas" (rapid macrophage cell division and death) than in "low-turnover granulomas." Khouri et al. [102] believe that macrophages transform into fibroblasts, but Ross et al. [103] have more convincing evidence that fibroblasts originate from connective tissue cells. In the lung, these cells exist principally in perivascular connective tissue.

To what extent do macrophages contribute to protein clearance in the lung? It is known that macrophages engulf altered collagen following tissue injury [104], but the clearance rates from the various lung interstices are not known. In the case of inhaled particles, macrophages take various routes away

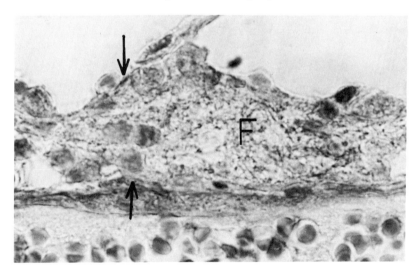

FIGURE 6 Same experiment as Fig. 5. The perivenular connective tissue space (arrows) is filled with a network of fibrin (F), which persisted for 3 days. There was no cellular invasion of the fibrin. Light photomicrograph (X550).

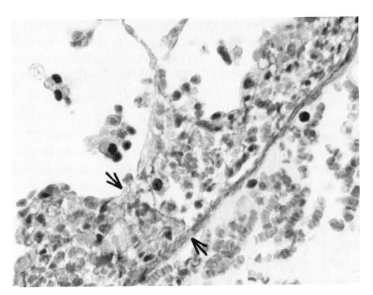

FIGURE 7   Rat lung 7 days after ANTU in association with EACA as described in Fig. 5. The perivenular connective tissue space (arrows) is filled with macrophages. Although no fibrin fibrils can be identified, cytoplasmic inclusions of the macrophages stain positively for fibrin. Light photomicrograph (×400).

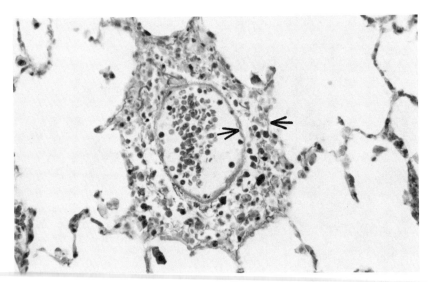

FIGURE 8   Rat lung 6 months after receiving ANTU in association with aminocaproic acid. The ANTU was given in weekly doses of 3 mg/kg for 2 months, and the rat killed 4 months later. The perivenular connective tissue space (arrows) is filled with mononuclear cells, most of which are macrophages. Light photomicrograph (×140).

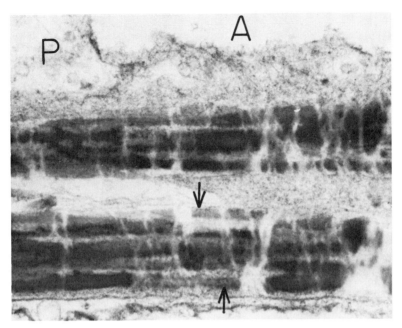

FIGURE 9 Rat lung 3 days after ANTU in association with EACA, as described in Fig. 5. A thin portion of the alveolar septum is covered by epithelial cytoplasmic extensions of injured membranous pneumonocytes (P) showing indistinct cell membranes facing the alveolar airspace (A). The basement membrane is disrupted by sheets of material staining deeply with phosphotungstic acid and uranyl acetate. Although this material is largely amorphous, separate portions show a distinct periodicity of 250 Å (arrows). This material appears to be fibrin. There are pinocytotic vesicles measuring to 750 Å diameter in the epithelial cytoplasm, but no large vesicles as seen in Fig. 5. Electron photomicrograph (×52,000).

from alveoli, some of which carry them into the interstices. But will macrophages preferentially enter these spaces to engulf proteins? Preliminary evidence suggests they will. When exudative edema is induced in rats with ANTU at the same time that fibrinolysis is inhibited by EACA, perivascular fibrin deposits persist for at least several days (Fig. 6). Within one week these deposits are invaded by macrophages (Fig. 7). The ultimate fate of these macrophages is uncertain; cellular collections persist for at least six months (Fig. 8).

Within the alveolar septa, persistent fibrin deposits appear as packed layers of material resembling elastic tissue through the electron microscope. The material is not amorphous but has the distinct periodicity of 250 Å characteristic of fibrin (Fig. 9). Some of this fibrin may pass through alveolar

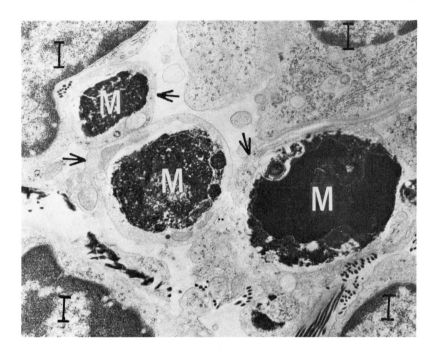

FIGURE 10   Rat lung 7 days after ANTU in association with EACA, as described in Fig. 5. A portion of an alveolar septum is thickened by numerous interstitial cells (I). They surround amorphous material (M), presumably old fibrin, staining deeply with phosphotungstic acid and uranyl acetate. The interstitial cells have cytoplasmic extensions (arrows), which surround the coagulation products and appear to be removing them by phagocytosis. Electron photomicrograph (×11,200).

epithelium (Fig. 5) for subsequent alveolar clearance. The remaining material loses the morphologic characteristics of fibrin, and by one week is surrounded by cytoplasmic extensions of interstitial cells apparently removing the material by endocytosis (Fig. 10). The clearance rate of these cells is not known. Perhaps they pass into alveoli as mature alveolar macrophages.

When fibrinolysis is not inhibited, these cellular collections do not occur after single injuries. After repetitive injury, induced by ANTU given in small weekly doses, perivascular cellular collections do occur. This suggests that tissue activator may be depleted. Definite identification of fibrin deposits in tissue sections is not easy. A worthwhile experiment to identify old fibrin would involve electron microautoradiography. An animal could be given radio-labeled fibrinogen just before the production of exudative edema. At the time of maximal edema, the circulating tracer fibrinogen could be removed by blood or plasma exchange. All fibrin deposits would contain labeled fibrinogen, and subsequent autoradiographs would indicate which fibril was fibrin. Unfortunately, in the case of ^{125}I labeling, the bonding is not tight.

Further studies of the pulmonary tissue response to extravascular proteins are needed. Important questions about the possible depletion of tissue activator and its relation to cryptogenic pulmonary fibrosis need answers. The knowledge that involuting scar tissue is almost devoid of activator suggests that repetitive exudate formation in the lung, by depleting tissue activator, might set the stage for fibroblastic proliferation, subsequent further reduction in the amount of activator, and a vicious cycle resulting in pulmonary fibrosis.

B. Alveolar Space

It is an oversimplification to assume that all intra-alveolar-fluid protein is cleared by expectoration. One never sees sputum volume equal exudate volume in pneumonitis, particularly considering that a human pulmonary lobe can hold more than 500 ml of exudate. Drinker first studied alveolar protein removal over 30 years ago. He enumerated three mechanisms: (1) airway clearance, (2) direct lymphatic removal, and (3) intra-alveolar protein digestion by macrophages with the production of smaller moieties able to penetrate alveolar epithelium and enter blood or lymph or both. Drinker believed that of the three, airway clearance was most efficient, since his numerous experiments indicated the inadequacy of pulmonary lymph flow at keeping pace with fluid formation [105], and the apparent impermeability of alveolar epithelium to protein [106]. His conclusions regarding alveolar epithelial permeability were based on experiments in which protein mixtures containing albumin tagged with T-1824 dye were instilled into the tracheas of anesthetized, ventilated, supine dogs [106]. The dogs were tilted from the horizontal to assist the passage of solutions into the terminal bronchial tree. Small quantities of bovine and egg albumin appeared in the RLD soon after instillation; none appeared in lymph from the TD or in blood plasma. Dyed, heparinized dog plasma appeared nonabsorbable; that is, none appeared in plasma or lymph from either the TD or RLD during 5 hr after instillation. However, when the chest was opened, and heparinized dyed plasma injected by needle directly into pulmonary tissue, dye promptly appeared in RLD lymph. Drinker and Hardenbergh thus concluded that alveolar epithelium was nearly impermeable

to proteins, which had to be split to smaller moieties to penetrate the epithelium and enter the interstitial space.

Courtice and Simmonds proved otherwise [107]. They also tagged albumin in protein mixtures with T-1824 dye and instilled the solutions into
the tracheas of rabbits. With the use of precipitin reactions, they demonstrated that intact protein did pass the alveolar epithelium, eventually appearing in plasma. They believed that the proteins entered the plasma from the
lymphatic system, and that rate of appearance of the dye-protein in the
plasma depended on the ventilatory status of the animals. Appearance was
rapid when the animals were awake. When the animals were supine and under
general anesthesia, plasma concentration of dye-protein increased slowly, but
linearly. They criticized Drinker and Hardenbergh's use of anesthesia, believing
that depressed ventilation impaired the flow of lymph, and thus, absorption of
instilled protein from the lung.

Schultz et al. [108] suggested that protein solutions instilled into the
trachea may not pass to the surface of maximal absorption in the lung. In
their experiments on anesthetized, supine dogs, radioiodinated albumin was instilled into the lung through a long 2-mm-diameter cannula passed through the
trachea into a wedged position in the distal bronchial tree. Peripheral plasma
radioactivity increased linearly for nearly 24 hr. By estimating plasma volume,
they concluded that 15% of the instilled albumin was present in plasma by 24
hr, half of it unchanged. In a later study on isolated perfused lungs [109] in
which all lymphatics were divided, they reported that over 6% of instilled
radioiodinated albumin appeared in the blood perfusate by 5 hr. This study
demonstrated not only that albumin was absorbed from alveoli directly into
blood, but also that the appearance rate in blood was the same as that in the
experiments of Courtice and Simmonds, in which they assumed that lymphatics were intermediaries.

All these studies, however, suffered from the uncertainty of determining
absorption rate only by the carriage of tagged protein in plasma. Dominguez
Liebow, and Bensch [110] determined the amount of radioactivity remaining
in lungs in order to define absorption rate. They instilled radioiodinated albumin in guinea pigs and dogs by the method of Schultz et al. [108]. The
animals were allowed to recover from anesthesia, and were sacrificed at varying intervals. The lungs were homogenized, and the remaining radioactivity
measured. Approximately 50% of the albumin was removed from the lungs of
the dogs by 24 hr; this rate of removal was independent of the concentration
of albumin instilled. Possible airway clearance was not considered in their
experiments.

Airway clearance also was not avoided in the experiments of Gillespie
and Lee [111]. They instilled radioiodinated albumin into dogs through a

catheter in the wedged position. Lymph cannulations were successful in only three experiments. They also noted predominant plasma carriage of the isotope, and this was even greater in induced cardiac failure. In a single animal with balloon obstruction of the ipsilateral pulmonary artery, they noted an appearance rate of radioactivity in blood comparable to that in control dogs. They presented blood absorption by calculating total plasma radioactivity. By 5 hr, 6.6% of instilled albumin was present in plasma. Meyer et al. [112] instilled radioiodinated albumin into the right diaphragmatic lobe of anesthetized, supine dogs maintained with positive pressure ventilation. The TD and RLD were cannulated, and by diverting all lymph from the animals, the investigators were able to compare the radioactivity in the blood compartment with the radioactivity in the lymphatic compartment. The data indicated that pulmonary blood absorbs 11 times as much albumin from alveoli as pulmonary lymph does. In 5-hr experiments, the amount of instilled albumin present in plasma was the same as that reported by others, but by homogenate analysis, roughly 30% of instilled albumin had disappeared from the lungs.

Tagged albumin delivered by aerosol appears to have different clearance kinetics in different lung regions. Sanchis et al. [113] demonstrated that in normal human subjects [^{131}I] albumin-saline droplets of 3 μm median diameter were cleared most rapidly from the perihilar region, presumably by mucociliary action. In the peripheral (bronchiolar-alveolar) region, there was an initial increase ($t_{1/2} = 1$ hr), followed by a decrease ($t_{1/2} = 23$ hr). Although they felt that these data were at variance with the data of Dominguez et al. [110], the Dominguez data did show a similar 50% 24-hr clearance of instilled albumin from alveoli of awake dogs. Our experiments [112] showed a $t_{1/2}$ of approximately 8 hr (in experiments lasting only 5 hr) when general anesthesia and positive pressure ventilation were used. Comparisons between aerosol and instillate clearances must consider not only the optimum particle size necessary for reaching and striking alveolar walls, but also the alveolar surface area available to instillates of several milliliters.

Water instilled into alveoli is rapidly absorbed. Humphreys et al. [49] quote Colin's experiments [114] in which 25 liters of water were instilled into the trachea of a horse over a 6-hr period with no ill effects. More recently Acevedo and Robin [115] noted proportional increases in right lymphatic duct lymph flow following instillations of 5 ml/kg and 10 ml/kg distilled water into the lungs of anesthetized, ventilated dogs. Humphreys et al. [49] correlated increased pulmonary lymph flow in fetal lambs with absorption of lung fluid following artificial ventilation. In mature fetuses, approximately 40% of the lung fluid was accounted for in lymph flow. Although alveolar water appears to pass into the pulmonary interstitial space, it is not certain whether this occurs by diffusion or hydrodynamic flow. Apparently alveolar surface tension has some effect, since in immature fetal lambs having lung fluid surface tensions 10 times larger than those of mature fetuses, absorption of lung water after ventilation was slower.

Evidence for molecular sieving through alveolar epithelium was obtained by Normand et al. [75] for fetal lambs. They instilled PVP of various molecular radii into alveolar liquid. Before positive pressure ventilation with 50 to 100% oxygen was instituted, no PVP appeared in lung lymph or plasma. Following ventilation, PVP passed through alveolar epithelium and appeared in lymph and plasma. There was evidence of molecular sieving, but this varied among animals. They suggested that positive pressure opened gaps in alveolar epithelium that imposed restricted diffusion for the macromolecules. The gaps were smaller in mature fetuses. In a later study [116], the same investigators studied passage rates of smaller water-soluble molecules (equivalent spherical radii ranging from 1 to 13 Å). From kinetic analyses, they concluded that fetal lambs have effective pulmonary capillary pores of 150 Å and alveolar epithelial pores of 5.5 Å. They suggested that the small alveolar pores protect against plasma proteins entering the alveolar space. In computing effective alveolar pore dimensions, however, the investigators used data from both studies that were not comparable. The experiments with PVP included positive pressure ventilation; those with smaller molecules used no ventilation. Thus the "gaps" that appeared after ventilation were not present for the smaller molecules in the fluid-filled lungs.

This distinction between air-filled and fluid-filled lungs must also be applied to the studies of Taylor and Gaar [117]. They estimated pulmonary capillary and alveolar effective pore radii in excised fluid-filled dog lung lobes by computing the osmotic reflection coefficient of each membrane for urea, glucose, and sucrose. With isogravimetric lung lobe preparations, they concluded that pulmonary capillaries have equivalent pore radii of 40 to 58 Å, and the alveolar membrane, 6 to 10 Å. These data agree closely with the data of Normand et al. [116], but like all fluid-filled lung experiments, do not take into account surface-tension effects on alveolar epithelium. Alveolar pore radii of this dimension would exclude albumin, but numerous previously cited studies indicate that albumin-sized molecules do pass the alveolar membrane. The experiments with horseradish peroxidase [76,77] suggest that transport occurs by pinocytosis, but the kinetics of PVP transport [75] seem to rule out pinocytosis as the principal process, and favor diffusion through epithelial gaps. Therefore, these gaps must be larger than 6 to 10 Å in air filled lungs.

The inconsistencies among studies are complicated even more by the studies of Goetzman and Visscher [118] and Goodale, Goetzman, and Visscher [119]. These investigators studied the alveolar-capillary permeability to radio-iodinated albumin in fluid-filled, perfused, isolated dog-lung lobes. Assuming passage by diffusion, they reported $t_{1/2}$ removal rates of approximately 79 hr by one technique [118], and 140 hr by another [119]. The difference was related to the models of diffusion. The earlier study assumed vascular uptake from a constant alveolar source [118]. The later study assumed two-compartment kinetic transfer [119]. Although the second model is superior, the data were analyzed without accounting for a possible partition coefficient of albumin between alveolar fluid and capillary plasma, i.e., molecular sieving. They used the equations of Taylor et al. [120] for small molecules with partition coefficients close to unity. Thus the $t_{1/2}$ of 140 hr was an overestimate, and this resulted in an underestimated permeability coefficient. I have calculated their permeability surface area product as 6.2×10^{-3} ml/min, which is only 10% of the product calculated for pulmonary capillary endothelium alone, assuming pure diffusional transport (Section III.A). Since the alveolar and capillary membranes represent series diffusion barriers, it is unlikely that their values correlate with living lungs. Furthermore, the possibility that the albumin leaked from perivascular tissues and lymphatics into the fluid bath in which the lobe was suspended was not evaluated. These investigators did show that alloxan [118] or iodoacetic acid [119] added to the alveolar fluid drastically increased estimated alveolar-capillary permeability. Since alveolar-capillary damage is the initial lesion leading to collections of alveolar exudate, more studies of permeability characteristics following pathologic lesions are sorely needed.

All studies of alveolar permeability, therefore, have suffered from uncertainties relating to experimental models. In living animals, alveolar clearance of macromolecules probably occurs by all three mechanisms enumerated by Drinker. We have begun studying this in intact dogs by the methodology demonstrated in Figure 11. In anesthetized dogs with cuffed endotracheal tubes (to inhibit airway clearance), [^{125}I] protein (125-P) is instilled into alveoli (Alv.). Simultaneously, [^{131}I] protein (131-P) is injected intravenously. An external detector (Detector) is placed over the site of 125-P. We use a 2-in. detector with a multihole collimator. At the focus (8 cm) the system has a fractional response (modulation transfer function [121]) of 0.48 at a spatial frequency of 0.5 cycle/cm for ^{125}I. If the detector axis is placed perpendicular to the bronchial axis, airway displacement of the instilled protein results in a rapid decay of the detector signal. Data are collected from four sites: specific activities of 131-P and 125-P are determined in plasma, TD, and RLD lymph as functions of time; the clearance of 125-P from alveoli is monitored with the use of the external detector. The clearance of 125-P represents both passage of 125-P through alveolar epithelium, and convective airway transport proximally away from alveoli. At the end of the experiment the lungs are homogenized and residual 125-P Alv. determined (anatomic lung). Convective

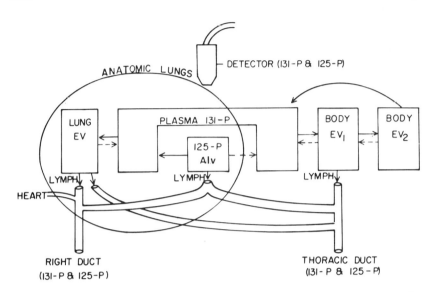

FIGURE 11   Schema of experiment to identify clearance rate and routes of
[^{125}I]protein (125-P) instilled into alveoli (ALV). Lymph clearance is identified
by collecting all drainage from the right and thoracic ducts since lymph flow
from 125-P Alv may enter both. A portion of 125-P in lymph represents direct
absorption, and the remainder appears as a transfer from plasma. The transferred
quantity is estimated by simultaneously injecting [^{131}I] protein (131-P) into
plasma and analyzing the plasma-to-lymph transport kinetics (Fig. 12a and b).
Blood clearance of 125-P consists of three quantities: the quantity transported
from plasma to lymph, the quantity residing in the body extravascular space or
spaces (body EV_1 and body EV_2) and the lung extravascular space (Lung EV),
and the quantity present in circulating plasma. An external detector (Detector),
monitoring the disappearance of 125-P Alv, measures both proximal airway dis-
location and absorption through microairway epithelium with subsequent clearance from the interstitium.

airway clearance is estimated by the total detector 125-P Alv. decay minus the
quantity absorbed. The quantity absorbed is calculated in the following way.
Assuming that the plasma-to-lymph transports of 131-P and 125-P are the
same, the total quantity of plasma-absorbed 125-P in body extravascular
lymph and lung extravascular lymph compartments are analyzed in terms of
sums of exponentials appropriate to the kinetics of compartment models
Direct lymph removal of 125-P is analyzed by comparing the difference between the expected plasma-lymph transport signal and measured amounts.
This is done by a simple graphic application of the convolution principle

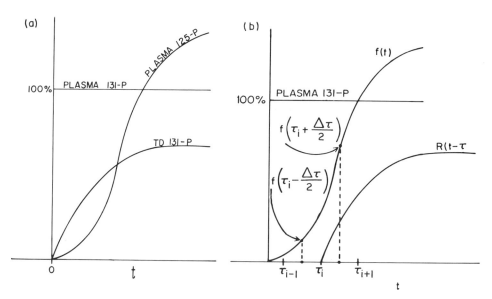

FIGURE 12 (a) Graphic application of the convolution principle in estimating the quantity of 125-P in lymph as a transfer from plasma. Plasma 131-P concentration is plotted as a step function of time t, and lymph 131-P concentration (TD 131-P) at each t is plotted as a percentage of the step function. (b) If superposition linearity is assumed, the concentration of 125-P in plasma (plasma 125-P) is converted into a series of incremental step functions at each τ_i; τ therefore becomes a time variable, moving from 0 to time = t. Each incremental step increase of plasma 125-P will produce a corresponding increase in lymph 125-P at time t, according to the relation between plasma 131-P and TD 131-P. The TD 131-P curve is shifted so that it originates at each τ_i at which the corresponding step increase in 125-P occurs. All incremental increases in lymph 125-P concentration are summed at time t to give a value representing transfer from plasma.

(superposition linearity) as shown in Figures 12a and 12b. Figure 12a presents plasma 131-P concentration as a step function, and thoracic duct lymph 131-P and plasma 125-P (directly absorbed) as percentages of the step function. In Figure 12b, τ is established as a moving variable in which plasma 125-P has a value at each τ, and the thoracic duct lymph 131-P concentration becomes a function of $(t - \tau)$. The predicted thoracic duct lymph 125-P concentration $(g(t))$ corresponding to each t is represented by multiplying the slope of $f(t)$ at each τ by $R(t - \tau)$ and integrating to the specific t (convolution integral, Eq. 4).

$$g(t) = \int R(t - \tau) \left[\frac{df(\tau)}{d\tau}\right] d\tau \qquad (4)$$

$$\cong \sum_i R(t - \tau_i) \left[f\left(\tau_i + \frac{\Delta\tau}{2}\right) - f\left(\tau_i - \frac{\Delta\tau}{2}\right)\right] \qquad (5)$$

This integral has an approximate solution by a series summation (Eq. 5), where $\Delta\tau$ is equal to a short collection period. In Figure 12b, $\Delta\tau$ is greatly exaggerated. Application of this solution in a typical dog, in which P was radioiodinated albumin, is shown in Figure 13. This demonstrates that direct blood absorption of albumin is significant, representing approximately half the absorbed albumin present in TD lymph. By comparison, the albumin is highly concentrated in RLD lymph, only a small portion appearing as a transfer from plasma.

Compartmentation of total albumin absorbed poses several problems. First, although total plasma quantity is simply plasma concentration multiplied by plasma volume, the quantity transferred from plasma to interstitial fluid is not known. Staub (personal communication) simplifies this by noting that the quantity lies between zero (no transfer) and twice the plasma quantity (total equilibration), since in the case of albumin, the total body mass of al-

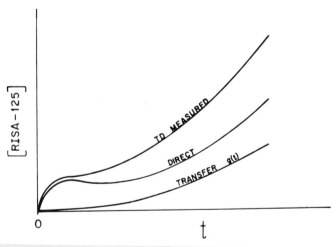

FIGURE 13   The concentration of $[^{125}I]$ albumin (125-RISA) in thoracic duct lymph following instillation into alveoli of a dog. The upper curve represents total TD lymph concentrations in collection samples. The middle curve represents the concentration component related to direct lymph absorption. The lower curve represents the concentration component related to transfer from plasma (Eqs. 4 and 5 in text). The symbol t = time.

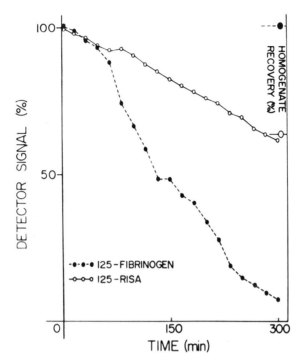

FIGURE 14 Comparison between external detector decay and actual lung recovery of [^{125}I] albumin (125-RISA) and [^{125}I] fibrinogen (125-Fibrinogen) instilled into dogs' alveoli. The proteins were 1% isoosmolar solutions, and were instilled into separate dogs. The rapid decay in detector signal for 125-Fibrinogen suggests rapid proximal airway transport.

bumin is twice the intravascular mass [122]. This quantity therefore diminishes as plasma concentration decreases. Computing this quantity by compartmental analysis is complicated by the wide distribution of interstitial fluid to lymph albumin washin rate constants as reflected in thoracic duct lymph. This suggests that total-body extravascular, extracellular space is described in its simplest form (Fig. 11) by two compartments in series, body EV_1 and body EV_2, with potential reversibility (dashed arrows), and a closed-loop forced-flow sequence of albumin around the compartments (solid arrow). Both body EV_1 and body EV_2 may be represented by a series of parallel arrangements of other compartments. The lung extravascular compartment (Lung EV, Fig. 11) appears to be a single space with a single albumin washin rate constant (Fig. 2).

The second problem in compartmentation of total albumin absorbed is the quantity in lymph ducts that has not passed into collection tubes. This could be estimated only after lymph concentrations have reached a steady state. Reference to Figure 13 suggests that experiments must be prolonged greatly to achieve steady state values. Finally, it is important to correct homogenate residuals of instilled proteins by the quantity in lung plasma. With dual isotopic labeling of proteins, one must find another plasma label to measure homogenate lung plasma volume. We have used T-1824 dye for this purpose. The results of these analyses are presented in Table 2. The percentage of absorbed albumin is separated into detector signal (A_D) and homogenate analysis (A_H). In most instances, these values are fairly close, as suggested in Figure 14. On the other hand there are marked exceptions (dogs 1,4, and 5 in Table 2). Homogenate analyses in these animals indicated near total absorption, and the lymph concentrations of tagged albumin were also greatest. It is likely that the detectors were focusing on the cisterna chyli or other lymph pool, but this is speculative and merely indicates some measurement difficulties with external detectors. The percentage of recovery is based on absorption as defined by homogenate analysis A_H, and is divided into plasma and lymph compartments. The quantity in the lymph compartment includes direct lymph absorption plus that transferred from plasma g(t) in Equations (4) and (5). The absorbed albumin present in plasma is divided into body and lung compartments. On the average, we could account for less than 50% of the absorbed albumin by summing the plasma and lymph quantities. These data neglect absorbed albumin in body extravascular com-

TABLE 2   Absorption of Tracer Albumin from Alveoli

| Dog | Time | % Absorbed | | % Recovery of Absorbed (A_H) | | | | |
| | | | | Plasma | | Lymph | | |
		A_H	A_D	Body	Lung	TD	RLD	Total
1	3.0	98.7	80.7	0.94	0.04	7.95		8.94
2	3.5	17.2	14.7	11.80	0.42	0.22		12.44
3	4.4	36.7	34.5	50.40	3.49	0.50	0.60	55.00
4	5.0	99.4	28.4	1.31	0.10	5.80	21.70	28.90
5	5.0	98.0	46.0	15.00	1.10	17.20	9.30	42.60
6	5.0	26.5	25.0	57.40	2.60	0.80		60.80
7	5.0	36.0	46.0	22.6	1.10	0.31	0.30	24.31
8	5.0	13.0	10.6	15.62	1.10	0.40	6.50	23.62
9	5.0	18.5	35.5	20.44	1.00	4.50	7.00	32.94
10	6.0	43.8	31.3	9.5	0.30	1.90	3.04	16.90
11	8.0	39.5	39.0	43.70	3.10	2.40	3.20	52.40

Note: Time = hours following instillation of isoosmolar [^{125}I] albumin. A_H = absorption determined from lung homogenates. A_D = absorption determined from external detector signal. TD = thoracic duct. RLD = right lymphatic duct.

partments or in undrained lymph trunks. The latter may be a significant amount.

It is extremely important to instill isoosmolar protein solutions into the distal bronchial tree. Previous studies have not specified the osmolarity of the solutions. This is not important in isolated fluid-filled lung experiments, but is critical in our experiments. Hyperosmolar albumin solutions are washed rapidly out of the detector focus, and are not absorbed. Presumably this indicates proximal convective airway clearance. Since all radioiodinated protein solutions should be dialyzed to remove free iodide, the choice of buffered dialysate is important. Furthermore, osmolarity measurements of the instillate should be performed and compared to plasma osmolarity before instillation. This is important because early pulmonary exudate is nearly isoosmolar with respect to plasma.

Airway clearance is more dramatic with instillations of isoosmolar radio-iodinated fibrinogen. Even though analyses of residual homogenate fibrinogen indicate that virtually none is absorbed, detector signals indicate a rapid movement out of the detector focus. Figure 14 indicates this dramatically, and suggests that fibrinogen is displaced proximally. A possible mechanism for this might involve inactivation of surfactant by fibrinogen [123], and subsequent alveolar closure resulting in bulk ejection of the fibrinogen solution proximally towards terminal bronchioles and the mucociliary escalator. The same implication resides in the experiments of Normand et al. [75] in which PVP were instilled into fetal lambs before ventilation. In ventilated immature lambs with high lung fluid surface tensions, much less PVP was absorbed. These macromolecules might have been displaced into bronchioles where absorption is minimal. Proof of this theory will require several external detectors stationed on a line from alveoli towards the major bronchi or the use of a gamma camera. These experiments suggest, therefore, that convective airway transport of fibrinogen constitutes an efficient removal mechanism. Albumin, on the other hand, appears to be removed largely by transport through alveolar epithelium. Significant studies of other proteins, particularly partially degraded ground substance fibrils, are needed to define these processes.

Polymerized fibrinogen (fibrin) in alveoli poses several theoretical threats to the lung. First, it is apparent that alveolar fibrin masses are fixed to alveolar walls [2] for a period at least exceeding several days. Since the fibrin is derived from injured capillaries, the strands extend through alveolar epithelium into the capillaries themselves. One may speculate that lung tissue plasminogen activator lyses those portions of strands passing through alveolar walls, leaving a fibrin matrix in alveoli alone. However, these tangled knots probably do not pass proximally on fluid films as protein solutions do. Second, the persistence of fibrin in distal air spaces may cause fibroblastic proliferation and epithelial proliferation. Spencer [3] notes that alveolar plugs of fibrin may be reepithelialized, after which they become components of the inter-alveolar septa. There are difficulties in assessing the volume of alveolar fibrin in lungs fixed with the transbronchial infusion of fixatives. The fibrin appears to be washed out in the process. Better fixation methods involve the formalin steam method [124], which we have used to measure pulmonary exudative edema volume [64]. By this method, it is apparent that fibrinous edema fluid is cleared, leaving fibrin skeletons in alveoli. The mechanism by which this occurs is unknown, but apparently the proteins either are absorbed through larger alveolar epithelial pores, or are transported proximally by a fluid tide. This emphasizes the need for alveolar epithelial permeability studies in lungs following capillary injury.

The principal clearance process for alveolar fibrin occurs by macrophage engulfment. It has been suggested that alveolar fibrin is lysed by tryptic en-zymes released from degenerating neutrophils [3], but as already noted, this probably does not occur. Alveolar macrophages readily ingest fibrin (Fig. 15), and by light microscopy, the intracytoplasmic fibrin residues stain a brilliant red with Lendrum's Yellowsolve II method [125]. The macrophages then pass toward the bronchiolar mucociliary blanket. Kilburn [126] believes that an alveolar fluid tide carries the macrophages and that they do not reach bronchioles through random movement. The clearance rate is rapid—approximately 2×10^6 cells/hr in rat lungs [127]. Obviously, patent alveolar blood vessels are necessary to bring monocyte-macrophages into alveolar fibrin collections. This aspect of fibrin clearance has not been studied, but one can speculate that once pulmonary capillaries are obliterated, macrophage recruitment may not be possible. Thus, the intra-alveolar and interalveolar septal masses of granulation tissue described as chronic "mural alveolitis" in human lungs may represent macrophage delivery failure.

Plasma proteins and fibrin are not the only proteins in alveoli following injury. Elastic and collagen fibers may fragment, and extrude into the alveolar space. Great caution must be exercised in interpreting residues seen micro-scopically. Lendrum [125] observed that fibrin, sheltered from lysins, under-goes a metamorphosis, ultimately appearing and staining like collagen. He called old fibrin "pseudocollagen," and suggested that fibrin actually becomes collagen in time. Biochemically this probably is not possible. One might speculate that the collagen that Lendrum saw was collagen residue resulting from the initial injury. If this is true, one can speculate further that intra alveolar clearance of collagen may be extremely inefficient. Almost nothing is known about the clearance of fibrillar and nonfibrillar ground substance, but Lynn (personal communication) has identified hydroxyproline residues in lung

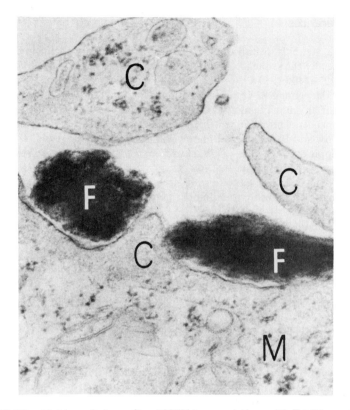

FIGURE 15 Rat lung 3 days after ANTU in association with EACA, as described in Fig. 5. An alveolar macrophage (M) appears to be removing fibrin masses (F) by phagocytosis. Cytoplasmic extensions (C) are surrounding the fibrin. Electron photomicrograph (X52,000).

washings from patients with alveolar proteinosis. The complex protein residues found suggest that altered fibrillar ground substance is present in considerable quantity. Obviously further biochemical analyses of lung washings in experimental animals following microvascular membrane injury are needed. Most interesting would be analyses at varying intervals following the injury to identify the clearance rates of various exudate constituents. Perhaps macrophages are needed to clear these tissue fragments. If so, further electron-microscopic and biochemical analyses of macrophage inclusions are needed. Since macrophages are obtained readily by lung lavage, experiments dedicated to this problem should be very fruitful.

References

1. N. C. Staub, H. Nagano, and M. L. Pearce, Pulmonary edema in dogs, especially the sequence of fluid accumulation in lungs, *J. Appl. Physiol.,* 22:227–240 (1967).
2. E. C. Meyer and R. Ottaviano, Pulmonary fibrosis in relation to interstitial fibrin: an animal model, *Amer. Rev. Resp. Dis.,* 109:738 (1974). Abstract.
3. H. Spencer, Chronic interstitial pneumonia. In *The Lung.* Edited by A. Liebow and D. Smith. Baltimore, Williams and Wilkins, 1968.
4. H. Eppinger. *Die Permeabilitatspathologie als die Lehre von Kranksheits-beginn.* Vienna, Springer, 1949.
5. E. C. Meyer and R. Ottaviano, Right lymphatic duct distribution volume in dogs: Relationship to Pulmonary interstitial volume, *Circ. Res.,* 35: 197–203 (1974).
6. N. C. Staub, Steady state pulmonary transvascular water filtration in un-anesthetized sheep, *Circ. Res.,* 28/29 (Suppl. 1):135–139 (1971).
7. E. M. Landis and J. R. Pappenheimer, Exchange of substances through the capillary walls. In *Handbook of Physiology.* Circulation. Vol. 2. Washington, D.C., American Physiological Society, 1963, p. 984.
8. E. M. Renkin, Transport of large molecules across capillary walls, *Physiologist,* 7:13–28 (1964).
9. D. G. Garlick and E. M. Renkin, Transport of large molecules from plasma to interstitial fluid and lymph in dogs, *Amer. J. Physiol.,* 219:1595–1605 (1970).
10. E. Aschheim and B. W. Zweifach, Quantitative studies of protein and water shifts during inflammation, *Amer. J. Physiol.,* 202:554–558 (1962).
11. T. Astrup, Blood coagulation and fibrinolysis. In *Thrombosis: Mechanisms and Control.* Edited by K. M. Brinkhous. Stuttgart, F. K. Schattauer Verlag, 1973, p. 87.
12. S. L. Wessler, D. G. Reiner, S. M. Freiman, and M. Lertzman, Serum-induced thrombosis, *Circulation,* 20:864-874 (1959).
13. D. A. Willoughby and M. DiRosa, A unifying concept for inflammation: A new appraisal of some old mediators. In *Immunopathology of Inflammation.* Edited by B. K. Forscher and J. C. Houck. Amsterdam, Excerpta Medica, 1971.
14. G. Odland and R. Ross, Human wound repair. I. Epidermal regeneration, *J. Cell. Biol.,* 39:135–151 (1968).
15. G. R. Fearnley. *Fibrinolysis.* London, Edward Arnold Ltd., 1965.
16. T. Astrup, P. Glass, and P. Kok, Thromboplastic and fibrinolytic activity in lungs of some mammals, *Lab. Invest.,* 22:381–386 (1970).
17. M. I. Barnhart, L. Sulisz, and G. B. Bluhm, Role for fibrinogen and its derivatives in acute inflammation. In *Immunopathology of Inflammation.* Edited by B. K. Forscher and J. C. Houck. Amsterdam, Excerpta Medica, 1971.
18. E. L. Opie, Experimental pleurisy—resolution of a fibrinous exudate, *J. Exp. Med.,* 9:391–413 (1907).

19. H. C. Kwan and T. Astrup, Fibrinolytic activity of reparative connective tissue, *J. Path. Bact.*, **87**:409–414 (1964).
20. R. S. McCleery, W. R. Schaffarzick, and R. A. Light, The experimental study of the effect of heparin on the local pathology of burns, *Surgery*, **26**:548–564 (1949).
21. S. B. Aronson, J. H. Elliott, T. E. Moore, Jr., and D. M. O'Day, Pathogenetic approach to therapy of peripheral corneal inflammatory disease, *Amer. J. Ophthalmol.*, **70**:65–90 (1970).
22. J. Kleinerman, Effects of heparin on experimental nephritis in rabbits, *Lab. Invest.*, **3**:495–508 (1954).
23. O. Myrhe-Jensen, Localization of fibrinolytic activity in the kidney and urinary tract of rats and rabbits, *Lab. Invest.*, **25**:403–411 (1971).
24. R. H. Heptinstall, Rapidly progressive glomerulonephritis. In *Pathology of the Kidney*. Boston, Little Brown, 1974.
25. P. Vassalli and R. T. McCluskey, The pathogenic role of the coagulation process in rabbit masugi nephritis, *Amer. J. Path.*, **45**:653–657 (1964).
26. A. S. Todd, The histological localization of fibrinolysis activator, *J. Path. Bact.*, **78**:281–283 (1959).
27. H. I. Peterson, A. Peterson, and B. Zederfeldt, Fibrinolytic activity in healing wound, *Acta Chir. Scand.*, **135**:649–652 (1969).
28. A. S. McFarlane, In vivo behavior of [I^{131}] fibrinogen, *J. Clin. Invest.*, **42**:346–361 (1963).
29. H. Langgard, The subcutaneous absorption of albumin in edematous states, *Acta Med. Scand.*, **174**:645–650 (1963).
30. J. Kroll, Lysis of ^{131}I-labelled plasma clots in human subcutaneous tissue in vivo, *Scand. J. Clin. Lab. Invest.*, **19**:1–3 (1967).
31. L. E. Mutschler, Anti-fibrinolytic effect of E-aminocaproic acid as measured by in vivo clot lysis, *Proc. Soc. Exp. Biol. Med.*, **115**:1019–1024 (1964).
32. L. E. Mutschler, Effect of E-aminocaproic acid on deposition of radioiodinated fibrinogen and antibodies to fibrinogen in turpentine-induced abscesses of the rat, *Proc. Soc. Exp. Biol. Med.*, **115**:1024–1028 (1964).
33. H. C. Kwan and T. Astrup, Tissue repair in presence of locally applied inhibitors of fibrinolysis, *Exp. Mol. Path.*, **11**:82–88 (1969).
34. D. C. Triantaphyllopoulos and E. Triantaphyllopoulos, Fibrin deposition and growth of connective tissue, *Thromb. Diathes. Haemorrh.*, **21**:144–150 (1969).
35. H. Spencer, Chronic interstitial pneumonia. In *The Lung*. Edited by A. A. Liebow and D. E. Smith. Baltimore, Williams and Wilkins, 1968.
36. P. Masson, J. L. Riopelle, and P. Martin, Poumon rheumatismal, *Ann. Anat. Path.*, **14**:359–382 (1937).
37. H. Spencer, *Pathology of the Lung*. 2nd ed. New York, Pergamon Press, 1968, p. 679.
38. B. E. Heard, Fibrous healing of old iatrogenic pulmonary edema ("hexamethonium lung"), *J. Path. Bact.*, **83**:159–164 (1962).

39. M. MacLeod, A. L. Stalker, and D. Ogston, Fibrinolytic activity of lung tissue in renal failure, *Lancet,* 1:191–192 (1962).

40. T. Saldeen, On the pathogenesis of the microembolism syndrome. In *New Aspects of Trasylol Therapy–The Lung in Shock.* Edited by G. L. Haberland and D. H. Lewis. Stuttgart, F. K. Schattauer Verlag, 1973.

41. C. M. Derks and R. M. Peters, The role of shock and fat embolus in leakage from pulmonary capillaries, *Surg. Gynecol. Obstet.,* 137:945–948 (1973).

42. L. Rammer and T. Saldeen, Inhibition of fibrinolysis in post-traumatic death, *Thromb. Diathes. Haemorrh.,* 24:68–75 (1970).

43. R. H. Demling, S. L. Selinger, R. D. Bland, and N. C. Staub, Effect of acute hemorrhagic shock on pulmonary microvascular fluid filtration and protein permeability in sheep, *Surgery,* 77:512–519 (1975).

44. J. D. Hill, J. L. Ratliff, R. J. Fallat, H. J. Tucker, M. Lamy, H. P. Dietrich, and F. Gerbode, Prognostic factors in the treatment of acute respiratory insufficiency with long-term extracorporeal oxygenation, *J. Thorac. Cardiovasc. Surg.,* 68:905–917 (1974).

45. T. Astrup, P. Glas, and P. Kok, Lung fibrinolytic activity and bovine high mountain disease, *Proc. Soc. Exp. Biol. Med.,* 127:373–377 (1968).

46. C. K. Drinker and M. E. Field, The protein content of mammalian lymph and the relation of lymph to tissue fluid, *Amer. J. Physiol.,* 97:32–39 (1931).

47. N. C. Staub, Pulmonary edema, *Physiol. Rev.,* 54:678–811 (1974).

48. H. N. Uhley, S. E. Leeds, J. J. Sampson, and M. Friedman, Right lymph duct flow in dogs measured by a new method, *Dis. Chest,* 37:532–534 (1960).

49. P. W. Humphreys, I. C. S. Normand, E. O. R. Reynolds, and L. B. Strang, Pulmonary lymph flow and the uptake of liquid from the lungs of the lamb at the start of breathing, *J. Physiol.,* London, 193:1–29 (1967).

50. K. K. Meyer, Direct lymphatic connections from the lower lobes of the lung to the abdomen, *J. Thor. Surg.,* 35:726–733 (1958).

51. M. F. Warren and C. K. Drinker, The flow of lymph from the lungs of the dog, *Amer. J. Physiol.,* 136:207–221 (1942).

52. M. F. Warren, D. K. Peterson, and C. K. Drinker, The effects of heightened negative pressure in the chest, together with further experiments upon anoxia in increasing the flow of lung lymph, *Amer. J. Physiol.,* 137:641–648 (1942).

53. J. M. Yoffey and F. C. Courtice. *Lymphatics, Lymph, and the Lymphomyeloid Complex.* London, Academic, 1970.

54. S. I. Said, R. K. Davis, and C. M. Banergee, Pulmonary lymph: Demonstration of its high oxygen tension relative to systemic lymph, *Proc. Soc. Exp. Biol. Med.,* 119:12–14 (1965).

55. E. C. Meyer and R. Ottaviano, Pulmonary collateral lymph flow: Detection using lymph oxygen tensions, *J. Appl. Physiol.,* 32:806–811 (1972).

56. H. S. Mayerson, R. M. Patterson, A. McKee, S. L. LeBrie, and P. Mayerson, Permeability of lymphatic vessels, *Amer. J. Physiol.,* 203:98–106 (1962).

57.   N. H. Areskog, G. Arturson, and G. Grotte, Studies on heart lymph, *Acta Physiol. Scand.,* **62**:209–217 (1964).
58.   A. J. Staverman, The theory of measurement of osmotic pressure, *Rec. Trav. Chim.,* **70**:344–352 (1951).
59.   J. A. Johnson, Capillary permeability, extracellular space estimation, and lymph flow, *Amer. J. Physiol.,* **211**:1261–1263 (1966).
60.   M. L. Pearce, J. Yamashita, J. Beazell, Measurement of pulmonary edema, *Circ. Res.,* **16**:482–488 (1965).
61.   B. E. Marshall, Determination of the blood content of lungs in vitro, *J. Appl. Physiol.,* **31**:643–645 (1971).
62.   E. R. Weibel, Morphological basis of alveolar-capillary gas exchange, *Physiol. Rev.,* **53**:419–495 (1973).
63.   O. Kedem and A. Katchalsky, A physical interpretation of the phenomenological coefficients of membrane permeability, *J. Gen. Physiol.,* **45**:143–179 (1961).
64.   E. C. Meyer and R. Ottaviano, The effect of fibrin on the morphometric distribution of pulmonary exudative edema, *Lab. Invest.,* **29**:320–328 (1973).
65.   D. M. Aviado and C. F. Schmidt, Pathogenesis of pulmonary edema by alloxan, *Circ. Res.,* **5**:180–186 (1957).
66.   J. M. Hughes, J. B. Glazier, J. E. Maloney, and J. B. West, Effect of extra-alveolar vessels on distribution of blood flow in the dog lung, *J. Appl. Physiol.,* **25**:701–712 (1968).
67.   J. J. Sampson, S. E. Leeds, H. N. Uhley, and M. Friedman, The lymphatic system and pulmonary disease. In *Lymph and the Lymphatic System.* Edited by H. S. Mayerson. Springfield, Ill., Charles C Thomas, 1968.
68.   E. R. Rabin and E. C. Meyer, Cardiopulmonary effects of pulmonary venous hypertension with special reference to pulmonary lymphatic flow, *Circ. Res.,* **8**:324–335 (1960).
69.   J. S. Vasko, R. C. Elkins, T. J. Fogarty, and A. G. Morrow, The experimental production of chronic mitral valvular obstruction, *J. Thor. Cardiovasc. Surg.,* **53**:875–880 (1967).
70.   A. Hawe, A. G. Tsakiris, D. C. McGoon, and G. C. Rastelli, Experimental production of graded mitral valve stenosis, *J. Thor. Cardiovasc. Surg.,* **60**:559–564 (1970).
71.   T. C. Laurent, The structure and function of the intercellular polysaccharides in connective tissue. In *Capillary Permeability.* Edited by C. Crone and N. A. Lassen. New York, Academic Press, 1970.
72.   J. R. Pappenheimer and A. Soto-Rivera, Effective osmotic pressure of the plasma proteins and other quantities associated with the capillary circulation in the hind limbs of cats and dogs, *Amer. J. Physiol.,* **152**:471–491 (1948).
73.   G. Grotte, Passage of dextran molecules across the blood-lymph barrier, *Acta Chir. Scand.* (Suppl.), **211**:1–84 (1956).
74.   T. C. Laurent, Structure of hyaluronic acid. In *Chemistry and Molecular*

Biology of the Intercellular Matrix. Vol. 2. Edited by E. A. Balasz. New York, Academic Press, 1970.

75. I. C. S. Normand, E. O. R. Reynolds, and L. B. Strang, Passage of macro-molecules between alveolar and interstitial spaces in foetal and newly ventilated lungs of the lamb, *J. Physiol.* (London), **210**:151–164 (1970).

76. K. G. Bensch and E. A. Dominguez, Studies on the pulmonary air-tissue barrier. Part IV: Cytochemical tracing of macromolecules during absorp-tion, *Yale J. Biol. Med.*, **43**:236–241 (1971).

77. F. Gonzalez-Crussi and R. W. Boston, The absorptive function of the neo-natal lung—ultrastructure study of horseradish peroxidase uptake at the onset of ventilation, *Lab. Invest.*, **26**:114–121 (1972).

78. S. M. Shea and M. J. Karnovsky, Brownian motion: A theoretical explana-tion for the movement of vesicles across the endothelium, *Nature* (London), **212**:353–355 (1966).

79. R. R. Bruns and G. E. Palade, Studies on blood capillaries. II. Transport of ferritin molecules across the wall of muscle capillaries, *J. Cell. Biol.*, **37**:244–276 (1968).

80. M. J. Karnovsky, Morphology of capillaries with special reference to muscle capillaries. In *Capillary Permeability*. Edited by C. Crone and N. Lassen. New York, Academic Press, 1970.

81. V. Menkin, Biology of inflammation: Chemical mediators and cellular in-jury, *Science*, **123**:527–534 (1956).

82. W. W. L. Glenn, D. K. Paterson, and C. K. Drinker, The flow of lymph from burned tissue, with particular reference to the effects of fibrin forma-tion upon lymph drainage and composition, *Surgery*, **12**:685–693 (1942).

83. A. A. Miles and E. M. Miles, The state of lymphatic capillaries in acute in-flammation lesions, *J. Path. Bact.*, **76**:21–35 (1958).

84. M. Papp, G. B. Makara, and B. Hajtman, The resistance of in situ perfused lymph trunks and lymph nodes to flow, *Experientia*, **27**:391–392 (1971).

85. N. U. Bang, Physiology and biochemistry of fibrinolysis. In *Thrombosis and Bleeding Disorders: Theory and Methods.* New York, Academic Press, 1971.

86. B. Lipinsky, Z. Wegrzynowicz, A. Z. Budzynski, M. Kopec, Z. S. Latallo, and E. Kowalski, Soluble unclottable complexes formed in the presence of fibrinogen degradation products (FDP) during the fibrinogen-fibrin con-version and their potential significance in pathology, *Thromb. Diathes. Haemorrh.*, **17**:65–77 (1967).

87. J. R. Shainoff and I. H. Page, Significance of cryoprofibrin in fibrinogen-fibrin conversion, *J. Exp. Med.*, **116**:687–707 (1962).

88. S. Niewiarowski and V. Gurewich, Laboratory identification of intravascu-lar coagulation, *J. Lab. Clin. Med.*, **77**:665–676 (1971).

89. E. J. Melliger, Detection of fibrinogen degradation products by use of anti-body coated latex particles, *Thromb. Diathes. Haemorrh.*, **23**:211–227 (1970).

90. L. Grant, The sticking and emigration of white blood cells in inflamma-

tion. In *The Inflammatory Process.* Vol. 2. Edited by B. Zweifach, L. Grant, and R. T. McCluskey. 2nd ed. New York, Academic Press, 1973.

91. D. A. Willoughby and W. G. Spector, Inflammation in agranulocytotic rats, *Nature* (London), **219**:1285 (1969).

92. J. G. Hirsch, Neutrophil leukocytes. In *The Inflammatory Process.* Vol. 1. Edited by B. Zweifach, L. Grant, and R. T. McCluskey. 2nd ed. New York, Academic Press, 1973.

93. D. H. Bowden, The alveolar macrophage, *Curr. Top. Path.,* **55**:1–36 (1971).

94. D. H. Bowden and I. Y. R. Adamson, The pulmonary interstitial cell as immediate precursor of the alveolar macrophage, *Amer. J. Path.,* **68**:521–528 (1972).

95. D. A. Bowden, I. Y. R. Adamson, W. G. Gratham, and J. P. Wyatt, Origin of the lung macrophage: Evidence derived from radiation injury, *Arch. Path.,* **88**:540–546 (1969).

96. P. J. Brundelet, Experimental study of the dust-clearance mechanism of the lung, *Acta Pathol. Microbiol. Scand.,* **175** (Suppl.):1–141 (1965).

97. H. Von Hayek. *The Human Lung.* New York, Hafner, 1960.

98. G. M. Green, Alveolobronchiolar transport mechanisms, *Arch. Intern. Med.,* **131**:109–114 (1973).

99. N. C. Staub, The "liquid veins" of the lung, *Physiologist,* **9**:294 (1966). Abstract.

100. P. E. Morrow, F. R. Fibb, and K. M. Gazioglu, A study of particulate clearance from the human lungs, *Amer. Rev. Resp. Dis.,* **96**:1209–1221 (1967).

101. W. G. Spector, The granulomatous inflammatory exudate, *Int. Rev. Exp. Pathol.,* **8**:1–55 (1969).

102. J. Khouri and O. Ancheta, Transformation of macrophages into fibroblasts, *Exp. Cell. Res.,* **71**:168–176 (1972).

103. R. Ross, N. B. Everett, and R. Tyler, Wound healing and collagen formation. IV. The origin of the wound fibroblast studied in parabiosis, *J. Cell. Biol.,* **44**:645–654 (1970).

104. P. F. Parakkal, Involvement of macrophages in collagen resorption, *J. Cell. Biol.,* **41**:345–354 (1969).

105. C. K. Drinker. *Pulmonary Edema and Inflammation.* Cambridge, Mass., Harvard University Press, 1950.

106. C. K. Drinker and E. Hardenbergh, Absorption from the pulmonary alveoli, *J. Exp. Med.,* **86**:7–18 (1947).

107. F. C. Courtice, W. J. Simmonds, Absorption from the lungs, *J. Physiol.,* **109**:103–116 (1949).

108. A. L. Schultz, J. T. Grismer, and F. Grande, Absorption of radioactive albumin from the lungs of normal dogs, *J. Lab. Clin. Med.,* **61**:494–500 (1963).

109. A. L. Schultz, J. T. Grismer, S. Wada, and F. Grande, Absorption of al-

bumin from alveoli of perfused dog lung, *Amer. J. Physiol.*, **207**:1300–1304 (1964).

110. E. A. M. Dominguez, A. A. Liebow, and K. G. Bensch, Studies on the Pulmonary air-tissue barrier. I. Absorption of albumin by the alveolar wall, *Lab. Invest.*, **16**:905–911 (1967).

111. W. J. Gillespie and G. deJ. Lee, Vascular and lymphatic absorption of radioactive albumin from the lungs, *Cardiovasc. Res.*, **1**:42–51 (1967).

112. E. C. Meyer, E. A. M. Dominguez, and K. G. Bensch, Pulmonary lymphatic and blood absorption of albumin from alveoli, *Lab. Invest.*, **20**:1–8 (1969).

113. J. Sanchis, M. Dolovich, R. Chalmers, and M. Newhouse, Quantitation of regional aerosol clearance in the normal lung, *J. Appl. Physiol.*, **33**:757–762 (1972).

114. G. Colin, *Traite de physiologie comparée des animaux.* 2nd ed. Vol. 2. Paris, Balliere et Fils, 1873.

115. J. C. Acevedo and E. D. Robin, Effect of intrapulmonary water instillation on pulmonary lymph flow and composition, *Amer. J. Physiol.*, **223**:1433–1437 (1972).

116. I. C. S. Normand, R. E. Olver, E. O. R. Reynolds, L. B. Strang, and K. Welch, Permeability of lung capillaries and alveoli to non-electrolytes in the foetal lamb, *J. Physiol.* (London), **219**:303–330 (1971).

117. A. E. Taylor and K. A. Gaar, Jr., Estimation of equivalent pore radii of pulmonary capillary and alveolar membranes, *Amer. J. Physiol.*, **218**:1133–1140 (1970).

118. B. W. Goetzman and M. B. Visscher, The effects of alloxan and histamine on the permeability of the pulmonary alveolocapillary barrier to albumin, *J. Physiol.* (London), **204**:51–61 (1969).

119. R. L. Goodale, B. Goetzman, and M. B. Visscher, Hypoxia and iodoacetic acid and alveolocapillary barrier permeability to albumin, *Amer. J. Physiol.*, **219**:1226–1230 (1970).

120. A. E. Taylor, A. C. Guyton, and V. S. Bishop, Permeability of the alveolar membrane to solutes, *Circ. Res.*, **16**:353–362 (1965).

121. W. J. MacIntyre, S. O. Fedoruk, C. C. Harris, D. E. Kuhl, and J. R. Mallard, Sensitivity and resolution in radioisotope scanning. In *Medical Radioisotope Scintigraphy.* Vol. 1. Vienna, International Atomic Energy Agency, 1969.

122. K. Wasserman, J. D. Joseph, and H. S. Mayerson, Kinetics of vascular and extravascular protein exchange in unbled and bled dogs, *Amer. J. Physiol.*, **184**:175–182 (1956).

123. F. B. Taylor and M. E. Abrams, Effect of surface active liprotein on clotting and fibrinolysis, and of fibrinogen on surface tension of surface active lipoprotein with a hypothesis on the pathogenesis of pulmonary atelectasis and hyaline membrane in respiratory distress syndrome of the newborn, *Amer. J. Med.*, **40**:346–350 (1966).

124. E. R. Weibel and R. A. Vidone, Fixation of the lung by formalin steam in

a controlled state of air inflation, *Amer. Rev. Resp. Dis.*, **84**:856–861 (1961).

125.   A. C. Lendrum, D. S. Fraser, W. Slidders, and R. Henderson, Studies on the character and staining of fibrin, *J. Clin. Path.*, **15**:401–413 (1962).

126.   K. H. Kilburn, A hypothesis for pulmonary clearance and its implications, *Amer. Rev. Resp. Dis.*, **98**:449–463 (1968).

127.   A. A. Spritzer, J. A. Watson, J. A. Auld, and M. A. Guetthoff, Pulmonary macrophage clearance—the hourly rates of transfer of pulmonary macrophages to the oropharynx of the rat, *Arch. Environ. Health*, **17**:726–730 (1968).

11

Detection and Measurement
of Pulmonary Edema

RICHARD CASABURI, KARLMAN WASSERMAN,
and RICHARD M. EFFROS

Harbor General Hospital
School of Medicine
University of California, Los Angeles
Torrance, California

I.   Introduction

All too often, the onset of pulmonary edema is a dramatic event with severe subjective distress and obvious physical findings. The physician may note tracheal fluid or foam, moist rales, changes in lung mechanics, evidence of arterial hypoxemia and increases in radiographic density in the affected areas. Unfortunately, these manifestations are signs of the late stages of alveolar flooding and are therefore relatively poor guides to patient management. It has been hoped that by developing sufficiently sensitive techniques, the early stages of pulmonary edema can be detected before respiration is grossly impaired and at a time when treatment would presumably be most effective.

Current research has emphasized both direct and indirect assessments of fluid volume of the lung. Historically, physiologists have directed more attention to measuring blood flow than to measuring organ volumes. It is primarily among pulmonary investigators that systematic attempts at measuring compartmental volumes have been made. It is our objective to describe the current status of methods of measuring pulmonary water volume that are at least potentially applicable to the clinical situation. To this end, destructive measures of lung water will first be briefly reviewed in the context that these are the measures against which any clinical technique must ultimately be compared. These destructive techniques have recently received extensive review by Staub [1]. In somewhat more detail, we shall document the limitations of detection techniques currently available to the physician: physical signs, conventional radiology, lung mechanics, and pulmonary gas exchange. Finally, we shall focus on methods that are the object of active research and represent the most promising procedures from a clinical point of view.

II. Destructive Measures

A.   Gravimetry

Conceptually, the most direct technique for measuring lung water content is to excise the lungs and measure the amount of water they contain. Lung weight increases rapidly after death [2], so that the rapidity and technique of excision are of concern. But even if the excised lung is considered unchanged from the state in vivo, certain considerations are involved before a valid index of pulmonary water content can be extracted.

The simple measure of lung weight has proved of value primarily in studies where serial determinations in isolated perfused lung are made [3,4,5]. Calculating the ratio of excised lung weight to body weight provides a rough way of compensating for variation of lung size among members of a given animal species [6,7,8]. A more precise way to accomplish this involves desiccating the excised lung to obtain the weight of the pulmonary tissues (dry weight). Guyton and Lindsey [8] presented the first extensive series of measurements, though Lambert and Gremels [9] had reported the technique over 30 years earlier. The comparison of wet and dry weights has been reported as a ratio when used to facilitate comparison among individuals [8,9,10]. The difference between the two measures (total lung water) has been used as a yardstick to determine the accuracy of less direct methods [11,12,13].

The distinction between vascular engorgement and pulmonary edema can be made by determining the contained blood volume. Hemingway [14] developed a spectrophotometric technique by which the hemoglobin content of homogenized lung samples could be measured and used to yield the weight of blood in the lungs. It has been pointed out [15], however, that presumably due to streaming effects, lung hematocrit is less than the hematocrit measured in large systemic vessels; a correction may be introduced to avoid underestimating pulmonary blood volume. Thus, extravascular lung water can be calculated as the excised lung weight minus the sum of the dry weight and the blood weight [15, 16, 17].

B. Sterologic Microscopy

Microscopy, particularly electron microscopy, has been shown to be useful not only in detecting the presence of edematous changes, but also in defining the nature of the structural alterations that precede and accompany edema of various etiologies. It has been possible to describe the alterations underlying edematous changes in oxygen toxicity [18], pulmonary vascular hypertension [19,20], and several kinds of chemical insults to the pulmonary vasculature [19,21,22]. It is possible, at least in theory, to obtain quantitative assessments of edematous changes by microscopy. Weibel [23] has described a detailed mathematical construct by which counting procedures can be used to estimate volumetric fractions from electron-photomicrographs (two-dimensional). Kapanci et al. [18] have detected the increase in interstitial fluid consequent to oxygen toxicity by these counting procedures.

Despite the elegance and high level of description of the microscopic technique, several drawbacks are apparent. Not the least is that specimen preparation, fixation, and analysis are difficult, time-consuming, and costly, even in the most expert hands. Obtaining representative samples in anisotropic tissue presents special problems [23]. Also, the fixation of lung tissue is particularly difficult, and may alter normal morphology. The fixative must be infused into either the airways or the vasculature; vascular infusion distorts the features of the airspaces and vice versa [24].

C. Interstitial Hydrostatic Pressure

It is clear that as lung tissue water increases in pulmonary edema, the interstitial hydrostatic pressure will rise in a manner determined by the compliance of this space. Measurement of interstitial pressure would seem to be a valuable index of developing edema; increases in this pressure would be expected to be a necessary precursor of alveolar transudation.

Yet it has proved difficult to measure this pressure. It is surprising that since Starling identified extracapillary hydrostatic pressure as one of the four factors determining transcapillary fluid exchange [25,26], the better part of a century has elapsed without agreement about the magnitude of this component. Two schools of thought exist, each ultimately based on different techniques of measurement.

Investigators have measured hydrostatic pressures in tissues (non lung) by inserting small hypodermic needles subcutaneously, intracutaneously, and intramuscularly. Injecting small volumes of saline has allowed manometric measurement of tissue pressures, and they have been found to range from 1 to 5 mmHg above atmospheric pressure [27,28,29]. However, such methods have received cogent criticism. Guyton [30] pointed out that the diameter of the smallest hypodermic needle is roughly 500 times the width of the interstitial spaces into which the needle is asserted to protrude. Further, sufficient time for absorption of the injected fluid has generally not been allowed [31]. Wiederhielm has attempted to answer these criticisms by developing a micropipette technique [32], which has been used to measure positive interstitial hydrostatic pressures in the free fluid spaces of the wing of the bat [33]. Further, Wiederhielm advanced detailed mathematical simulations of transcapillary fluid exchange that argue in favor of finding positive interstitial pressures [34].

On the other hand, Guyton et al. found that the pressures within implanted capsules are normally subatmospheric. Hollow, perforated spheres about 2 cm in diameter have been implanted in various body tissues [30,31, 35–38], including the lung [38]. During the first week following implantation, the air within the capsule is absorbed and is replaced by fluid. Fibrous tissue grows within the capsule and soon covers the entire wall of the cavity. Guyton has argued that the fluid within the capsule is in hydrostatic equilibrium with the interstitium, and that the pressure measured by inserting small hypodermic needles through the skin and then through one of the capsule perforations represents true interstitial fluid pressure. He has further presented a series of studies that suggest that the negative pressures measured within these capsules are not artifactual [35,38]. However, criticism has been directed against the assumption that fluid exchange across capsule walls is free [34]. The observations of Scholander et al. [39] seem to support Guyton's thesis. Small Teflon catheters in which the tip has been occluded with a cotton wick have allowed measurement of subcutaneous and subperitoneal pressures in the range -1 to -13 mmHg in a variety of species.

Regardless of whether the negative values obtained with tissue capsules represent true interstitial pressures, the capsule measurements may provide a useful index of tissue hydration. In nonedematous tissues, interstitial compliance appears to be low and extreme subatmospheric pressures are needed to withdraw fluid from the interstitium. Only after interstitial pressure exceeds atmospheric pressure does the tissue space become easily distensible and edema readily form [35,36]. Meyer et al. [38], measuring pressures in capsules implanted in lung tissue, found that elevation of left atrial pressure produced an immediate increase in pulmonary interstitial pressures, which preceded the gross manifestations of the resultant pulmonary edema. On the contrary, tissue fluid pressures measured with needles show the compliance of the tissue spaces to be high and fairly constant throughout the progress of edema accumulation [30,35].

D. Lymph Flow

The rate at which lymph flows from the lungs is partly a function of the pulmonary interstitial hydrostatic pressure, and thereby a function of interstitial water content. Although measured lymph flow rate may lag behind interstitial changes [40], relatively modest changes in pulmonary vascular pressures have been found to induce substantial increases in lymph flow [41,42].

The primary difficulty in using pulmonary lymph flow to measure changes in the dynamics of lung water formation is methodologic. Although cannulation procedures have been well described [43–45], it is acknowledged that it is virtually impossible to isolate the entire lymphatic drainage of the lung and to separate lung from nonlung sources [1]. Anesthesia, opening of the chest, and partial catheter blockage are held to markedly reduce lymph flow [43,46]. Extrathoracic approaches to both the right lymphatic duct and the thoracic duct have been developed [44,45,47,48] but the relative fraction of pulmonary drainage ascribable to each route is disputed [40,49].

Staub has recently reported success in measuring the time course of lymph flow and protein content in unanesthetized chronically instrumented sheep [41,42]. Yet the most that can be expected, even from these advanced methods, is that changes in flow and composition of lymph obtained by cannulation reflect proportional changes in pulmonary lymph.

III. Nondestructive Measures

A. Physical Manifestations

Early vascular congestion and interstitial swelling may be manifested only by wheezing, which may be confused with bronchial asthma and inappropriately treated as such. The appearance of bubbly rales at the lung bases remains the most reliable physical sign of pulmonary edema. These sounds are produced by fluid in the small conducting airways of the lung, and if edema progresses unabated, these become coarser in quality and generalized throughout the lung fields, eventually becoming audible without the aid of a stethoscope ("death rattle") and visible as froth composed of fluid containing variable quantities of protein, surfactant, and red cells derived from the alveoli. As the alveoli fill with fluid, the patient may become increasingly cyanotic as pulmonary gas exchange is impaired.

It has been suggested that the severe dyspnea and tachypnea experienced by the patient may be the direct result of stimulation of mechanoreceptors in the pulmonary interstitium (J-receptors) [50].

B. Radiology

As edema fluid is denser than air, pulmonary edema engenders characteristic changes in the x ray of the thorax. Loss of the sharpness of the central vessels on the chest x ray is an early sign of pulmonary edema. The vascular shadows become enlarged and hazy, presumably due to lymphatic engorgement and perivascular edema [51]. A second manifestation is the appearance of septal lines. The secondary lobules are separated by fine fibrous tissue septa containing the small pulmonary veins and the lymphatics draining the lobule. Edema markedly thickens these septa, making them visible radiographically [52,53]. These septal lines appear as dense, well-defined lines, several centimeters long, perpendicular to the pleural surfaces, and usually seen in the basilar portions of the lung [53]. They are called Kerley's B lines [51].

In the more advanced stages of pulmonary edema, irregular alveolar flooding develops. The branching vessels can no longer be identified since the gas spaces that normally highlight them are replaced with fluid. It is hypothesized that the hilar areas flood before the peripheral areas, possibly because of better lymphatic drainage at the periphery [51,54], although the lateral roentgenogram shows that the opacities are rarely of a purely central origin [55]. In any case, bilateral central confluent densities develop a "butterfly," or "batwing," roentgenographic appearance [53,54]. The opacities may shift from lobe to lobe.

Though the inability to quantitate radiographic findings reduce the usefulness of the chest x ray somewhat, it is, in the proper hands, probably the most sensitive aid in the diagnosis of pulmonary edema generally available. Techniques of image focusing and shadow enhancement may serve to make radiologic evidences of early edema more apparent.

C. Lung Mechanics

Intuitively, progressive engorgement of the lung by edema fluid would seem likely to alter lung mechanics, increasing the force necessary for inflation, decreasing contained gas volume, and increasing resistance to airflow. Unfortunately, measurements of lung mechanics have thus far failed to provide a reliable method for detecting early pulmonary edema or for measuring the amount of excess fluid in the lung.

Insight into the reasons why mechanical changes are not manifest until severe edema is present was obtained by Cook et al. [56]. From their studies of excised dog lungs, before and after edema was induced, it is apparent that compliance changes in edema stem predominantly from surface phenomena and not from changes in elastic recoil of lung tissue. Thus, interstitial edema should cause no great change in lung mechanics. It is only when alveolar flooding ensues that changes in the pressure-volume relation become apparent.

Several investigators have compared compliance changes with lung water content changes in studies in which edema was induced in experimental animals. Hughes et al. [57] found that a doubling of lung weight that pulmonary hypertension produced in excised rabbit lungs caused only a 30% decrease in compliance. Pulmonary edema resulting from vagotomy in the guinea pig produced no significant changes in compliance, though a marked shift in the pressure-volume relation shortly before death was noted [58]. Pearce et al. [59] found in dogs subjected to acute large saline infusions that, after an initial decrease, lung compliance returned to control levels despite continued elevation in pulmonary extravascular water measurements. Levine et al. [7] noted that decreases in lung compliance of comparable magnitude could be produced by pulmonary hypertension through pulmonary vascular engorgement whether or not increases in lung water content were actually present. Furthermore, airway resistance was found to be little affected until the edema was manifest by foam in the airways. Guyton et al. [8] found that even in severe pulmonary edema in dogs, no valid assessment of the degree of edema could be obtained by measuring compliance.

Ventilatory mechanics in eight patients with frank pulmonary edema were described by Sharp et al. [60]. Dynamic lung compliance and airway resistance (studied using intraesophageal pressure measurements [61]) averaged, respectively, one-fourth and four times normal. However, these dramatic changes were present in patients with roentgenographic and ausculatory manifestations of late pulmonary edema.

D. Pulmonary Gas Exchange

It is to be expected that pulmonary edema leads to decreased efficiency of gas transport. It seems likely that the sequence of fluid accumulation in the edematous lungs is such that the first encroachment of the airspaces comes when the fluid-filled interstitium overflows into the respiratory bronchioles [42,62]. The earliest deficit in gas exchange would then be a shuntlike effect as respiratory units are blocked by flow of fluid into the alveoli, rather than a true diffusion deficit resulting from a thicker alveolar-capillary barrier.

Studies in animals seem to bear this out. Progressive edematous changes engender widened alveolar-arterial oxygen gradients [63-65] which may lead to severe hypoxemia. Although hyperventilation commonly produces hypocapnia, as edema progresses alveolar ventilation may be compromised and hypercapnia may ensue.

Said et al. [65] measured shunt flow and DL_{CO} in dogs subjected to fluid overload. Postmortem lung weights were obtained, and they showed that edema resulting in doubled lung weight caused roughly a 25% increase in pulmonary venous admixture and a 35% decrease in DL_{CO}. Clearly, pulmonary gas exchange disturbances occur with pulmonary edema. However, these disturbances are hardly specific and may be of limited use in detecting pulmonary edema in its early stages.

E.   Indicator Dilution, Nongaseous

These indicator dilution procedures are distinguished from the soluble gas techniques (to be described in the following section) by their use of nongaseous indicators. In principle, these indicators will not exchange with the alveolar air. The indicators are injected intravascularly and indicator concentrations are measured either in the pulmonary "outflow" (usually approximated by arterial blood) or, in the case of gamma-emitting isotopes, by external probes. The former approach has been much more popular than the latter. Although the "outflow" procedure was originally described by Freinkel et al. [66] and although an appropriate mathematical analysis was not derived until somewhat later [67–69], it is generally agreed that Chinard and Enns [70] deserve principal credit for developing this method of measuring the water content of the lung.

Since the introduction of the outflow procedure, its simplicity from both a mathematical and an experimental point of view has continued to appeal to many investigators. However, despite a good deal of ingenuity and refinement of technique over the past two decades, indicator dilution measurements of lung water have proved frustrating, and the procedure remains an investigative tool rather than a clinical one. To understand the advantages and limitations of the outflow technique and alternative scanning approaches, one must give some consideration to the basic indicator dilution equations. The present derivation is similar to the one of Meier and Zierler [71] though it is generalized for extravascular volumes. Attention will be given primarily to methodology. Comprehensive reviews of data obtained by the outflow procedures in animals and man under normal and pathological circumstances may be found elsewhere [1,72,73].

Outflow Procedures and Total Lung Water

Theory

As devised by Chinard et al. [70], a small volume of fluid containing a "vascular" indicator that remains confined to the vascular volume (e.g., T-1824 or [^{125}I] albumin) and a "water" indicator that readily diffuses into the extravascular compartment of the lung (e.g., tritiated water) is rapidly injected into a peripheral vein and blood is collected in serial samples at approximately 1-sec intervals from a peripheral artery. From the way in which the indicators emerge in the arterial blood, it is possible to calculate both the blood flow through the lung and the extravascular water content of the lung.

The abrupt injection of indicator is intended to imitate a delta function $\delta(t)$. By definition, this function has an infinitesimal duration, an infinite amplitude at time zero, and an area that is unity. Its value is zero at all other times. Of course, such an input can be approached only as a limit. The input $i(t)$ from such an injection is

$$i(t) = m_0\delta(t) \tag{1}$$

where m_0 is the quantity of indicator injected. Injecting the indicator in this way makes it possible to define the fraction $h(t)$ of the injected indicator that appears in the exit at each time after the moment of injection

$$e(t) = \dot{Q}c(t) = m_0 h(t) \tag{2}$$

where $e(t)$ is the rate of indicator emergence in the outflow, $\dot{Q}$ is the blood flow, $c(t)$ is the outflow concentration of indicator, and $h(t)$ is expressed in sec^{-1}.

Once an impulse experiment has been done and $h(t)$ has been thereby determined, the outflow of indicator from the organ can be predicted *regardless* of the form of the injection, provided that this form is known. This is accomplished using the convolution integral:

$$e(t) = \int_0^t h(t-u)\,i(u)\,du = h * i. \tag{3}$$

This formidable-appearing equation simply relates the rate of indicator efflux from the organ $e(t)$ to the rate of indicator influx $i(u)$, and the delay imposed by transit through the organ, indicated by the function h. The term $h(t-u)$ represents the fraction of injected indicator traversing the organ per second during the interval between entry into the organ at time u and at time t. The significance of the equation is illustrated in Figure 1. If one wants to know how much indicator will arrive in the outflow at 5 sec, one must know the quantity of indicator entering the organ at 1 sec, $i(1)$, and multiply this by the fraction that traverses the organ during the remaining 4 sec, $h(5-1) = h(4)$. This figure is added to the product of $i(2)$ and $h(3)$ and successive products are added as noted in Figure 1. This summation is described by the integral expression of Equation (3) and is frequently abbreviated as shown with an asterisk at the right of Equation (3). Indicator efflux for each time t can be calculated in the same manner.

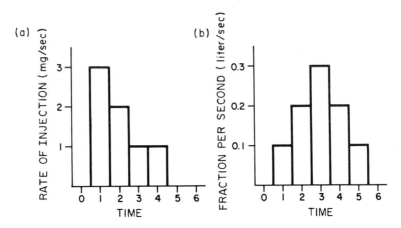

FIGURE 1   Illustration of the convulution integral (finite difference analogy). The form of injection and the distribution of transit times following a bolus injection are shown schematically. The expected outflow of indicator at 5 sec can be calculated as the sum

$$e(5) = i(1)h(5 - 1) + i(2)h(5 - 2) + i(3)h(5 - 3) + i(4)h(5 - 4)$$
$$= (3)(0.2) + (2)(0.3) + (1)(0.2) + (1)(0.1)$$
$$= 1.5 \text{ mg/sec}.$$

Useful information can be obtained from indicator dilution studies only if h, the distribution of transit times, is unchanged by alterations in the amount of indicator injected (linearity) and in the time at which the indicator is injected (stationarity). These basic conditions are assumed in this derivation.

The value of knowing $h(t)$ can be appreciated by considering the consequences of a constant infusion of indicator. If the indicator is infused into the organ at a constant rate i_0, then equation (3) becomes

$$e(t) = \int_0^t h(t - u) i_0 \, du$$

(4)

$$= i_0 \int_0^t h(t) \, dt = \dot{Q}c_0 \int_0^t h(t) \, dt = \dot{Q}c_0 \, H(t) \, dt$$

where c_0 is the concentration of indicator in the blood entering the organ, and $H(t)$ represents the integral $\int_0^t h(t) \, dt$. The total quantity of indicator that has entered the organ by time t should be $M_i(t)$, where

$$M_i(t) = \dot{Q}c_0 t.$$

(5)

The total quantity of indicator $M_e(t)$ that has left the organ by the same time can be calculated by integrating Equation (4):

$$M_e(t) = \int_0^t e(t)\, dt = \dot{Q}c_0 \int_0^t H(t)\, dt. \tag{6}$$

It is assumed that indicator is neither produced nor destroyed within the organ and that there are no other inflows or outflows of indicator from the organ. These assumptions are often referred to as indicator conservation in a single input–single output system. In such a system, the amount of indicator actually present within the organ at time t should be $M(t)$, where

$$M(t) = M_i(t) - M_e(t) = \dot{Q}c_0 \int_0^\infty [1 - H(t)]\, dt. \tag{7}$$

After a sufficiently long infusion of indicator at a rate $\dot{Q}c_0$, the quantity of indicator within the organ should become constant at a value M:

$$M = \dot{Q}c_0 \int_0^\infty [1 - H(t)]\, dt. \tag{8}$$

The integral expression can be integrated by parts by setting $v = 1 - H(t)$ and $du = dt$:

$$uv = \int v\, du + \int u\, dv$$

$$\int v\, du = uv - \int u\, dv$$

$$\int_0^\infty [1 - H(t)]\, dt = \left\{ [1 - H(t)]\, t \right\}_0^\infty + \int_0^\infty th(t)\, dt.$$

The first term on the right is zero. Therefore

$$M = \dot{Q}c_0 \int_0^\infty th(t)\, dt = \dot{Q}c_0 \bar{t} \tag{9}$$

where $\bar{t}$ is referred to as the mean transit time and is defined by the integral expression

$$\bar{t} = \int_0^\infty th(t)\, dt. \tag{10}$$

As noted in Equation (2), $h(t)$ can be obtained from a sudden injection experiment and the value of $\bar{t}$ can be calculated from these data.

On the basis of this analysis, it is clear that (a) we can readily obtain the distribution function h(t) simply by injecting the indicator as a bolus injection and following the concentrations in the outflow, and that (b) by calculating the mean transit time from h(t), we can then *predict* the amount of indicator that would eventually be present within the organ if it were infused at a given constant rate. This prediction depends on the assumptions that the distribution of transit times remains the same (linearity and stationarity), and indicator is neither added nor lost by tissue metabolism or destruction or through entrances or exits other than the artery and vein. The chief advantage of using the bolus injection approach is that it avoids the trouble of ensuring a prolonged and constant rate of infusion and then finding some method of determining just how much indicator remains within the organ.

Now let us assume that we know by some independent means that during constant infusion the indicator becomes uniformly distributed within a certain volume within the organ. For example, let us make the assumption that the activity of tritiated water becomes constant in all the aqueous compartments of the lung during a prolonged constant infusion. Then we may presume that the tritiated water activity [THO] in each milliliter of the aqueous phase of blood and tissues is the same:

$$M_{THO} = [THO] \, V_{EV,W} + [THO] \, V_{B,W} = [THO] \, f_B \dot{Q} \bar{t}_{THO}$$

or

$$V_{T,W} = V_{EV,W} + V_{B,W} = f_B \dot{Q} \bar{t}_{THO} \tag{11}$$

where $V_{EV,W}$ and $V_{B,W}$ represent the aqueous volumes in the extravascular and vascular compartments and f_B represents the volumetric fraction of the blood flow which is actually water. The value f_B can be calculated if the hematocrit (Hct) and the volumetric fractions of water in red cells (f_R) and plasma (f_P) are also known:

$$f_B = Hct \, f_R + (1 - Hct) \, f_P. \tag{12}$$

Values of f_R and f_P have been estimated for isotonic human and dog blood [1,73,74]. Calculations of the blood volume are somewhat more complicated since both the red cell and plasma phases must be considered and the hemocrit in the small vessels of the lung is less than the large vessels [1,73–76]. The problem can be resolved if both red cell and plasma indicators are injected, as indicated in the Appendix of this chapter:

$$V_{EV,W} = \dot{Q} \left\{ [f_R Hct + f_P (1 - Hct)] \bar{t}_{THO} - f_R Hct \, \bar{t}_R - f_P (1 - Hct) \bar{t}_P \right\}. \quad (13)$$

Approximate corrections for studies performed with only the plasma and water indicator can be found elsewhere [1,73-75]. It is assumed that labeled-water exchange between red cells and plasma occurs within a very short interval compared with the time required for traversal of the pulmonary capillary and that the plasma and red cell labels remain within their respective compartments. This assumption is not justified for some indicators and two publications have appeared recently that consider the situation in which exchange of indicator between red cells and plasma takes about the same time as exchange between plasma and tissue [77,78].

Pulmonary blood flow as well as indicator mean transit times must be determined for calculation of indicator dilution volumes. Fortunately, the pulmonary blood flow can be readily calculated from the indicator dilution curves themselves. Provided that none of the indicator is lost in transit between the points of injection and detection, blood flow can be calculated from the area (B) (see Figure 2) under the pulmonary outflow concentration curve:

$$\dot{Q} = \frac{m_0}{\int_0^\infty c(t)\, dt} = \frac{m_0}{B}. \quad (14)$$

It is customary to plot the indicator dilution data in terms of "w," the fraction of the injected dose found in each milliliter of outflow blood. In this way, relative concentrations of different indicators can be compared. The fraction w is sometimes referred to as the fractional concentration; it has units of ml^{-1} and is related to the concentration $c(t)$, the injected mass (m_0), $h(t)$, and $\dot{Q}$ in the following way:

$$w(t) = \frac{c(t)}{m_0} = \frac{h(t)}{\dot{Q}} \quad (15)$$

There has been some confusion in the literature about "alternative" methods of calculating lung water from the same indicator dilution curves. These procedures are based on the assumption that some sort of indicator equilibration occurs within the organ during the transient experiment. In the early studies of Lillienfeld et al. [79] and Anthonisen and Crone [80], it was suggested that at the time when outflow concentrations of the vascular and water indicators become equal (i.e., when the indicator dilution curves intersect], concentrations of the water indicator in the extravascular space are uniform and equal to the outflow concentrations. It is a simple matter to calculate the quantity of water indicator in the extravascular space of the lung at this time with the equation

$$Mt_{eq} = \int_0^{t_{eq}} \dot{Q}(c_B - c_W)\, dt \qquad (16)$$

where t_{eq} is the time at which concentrations become equal at the collection site, M is the quantity of the water indicator in the extravascular space at that time, c_W is the outflow concentration of the indicator at the outflow, and c_B is the concentration of the water indicator that would be observed in the outflow had none of the water indicator entered the extravascular compartment. It was in effect assumed that c_B could be calculated from the observed blood concentrations of the vascular indicator c_V:

$$c_B = c_V \frac{m_B}{m_W} \qquad (17)$$

where m_W and m_B are the quantities of water and vascular indicators in the injection fluid. Provided that c_{eq}, the outflow concentration of the water indicator at time t_{eq}, is indeed the same as the extravascular concentration, then

$$V_{EV} = \frac{M(t_{eq})}{c_{eq}} \qquad (18)$$

where V_{EV} is the extravascular volume.

The suggestion that "water" indicators such as tritiated water and ethyl alcohol do become uniformly distributed throughout the lung at some time after a bolus has been injected is based on the premise that these indicators readily traverse the vascular and cellular barriers of the lung. However, even if outward diffusion of indicator from any point along the pulmonary capillary to the adjacent lung tissue is instantaneous, this does *not* ensure that the concentration of water label is uniform throughout the exchange site at any time after a bolus injection. Goresky has provided both model and experimental evidence (in lung and liver) that following such injections, indicator passage through the organ occurs as a discrete "wave" in which indicator concentrations are never uniform throughout the exchange site [74,81]. Uniform concentrations could only occur if instantaneous equilibration both perpendicular and parallel to the direction blood flow occurred. Under these circumstances, the delivery of the water indicator to the venous outflow from the capillary should precede delivery of the vascular indicator since extravascular diffusion along the length of the capillary would be instantaneous. There is no evidence that standard water labels do precede vascular indicators in the pulmonary outflow. Furthermore, concentrations of the vascular and water indicators in the outflow are equal only momentarily and water concentrations exceed concentrations of the vascular indicator at later times. It should be added that even if uniform concentrations were attained at the exchange site on a local basis, the notorious heterogeneity of tissue perfusion throughout the lung and the delay in indicator delivery and washout from different regions of the lung would make it improbable that uniform concentrations in the organ would ever be established. Since such considerations are unnecessary in the mean transit time formulation, there appears to be little merit in retaining the Lillienfield-Anthonissen-Crone approach.

Although the Lillienfield-Anthonisen-Crone equations resemble equations that Kety originally used for measuring cerebral perfusion [82], the two procedures should not be confused. In the Kety procedure, values for flow per unit of tissue weight or volume (equivalent to the reciprocal of the mean transit time) are obtained after the experimental subject has inhaled a gaseous indicator and measurements are made of cerebral arterial and venous concentrations. Because the inhalation of gas is sustained, equilibration of gas concentrations in the tissue and outflow blood can be expected. Nor should the Kety cerebral perfusion approach be confused with the procedure Kety used for measuring local muscle blood flow [83]. The latter technique assumes initial rapid equilibration of indicator and exponential washout. (It will be discussed with scanning procedures.)

Calculations of mean transit times should be accomplished by some form of equation [10]. A convenient method for joining discrete point data with exponential extrapolation is provided elsewhere [84]. Simpler calculations based on downslope information are difficult to justify on theoretical grounds and do not appear to yield accurate data [67,69].

Although it must be assumed that the concentration of each indicator within its own volume of distribution becomes uniform during constant infusion, it is *not* assumed that equilibration occurs either locally or throughout the organ during the transient study. As stressed previously, this represents the chief advantage of the mean transit time approach.

Some indicators, e.g., pH indicators, become nonuniformly distributed between various compartments of the lung during steady state infusions. Under these circumstances, Equation (9) can be used to derive other information besides indicator dilution volumes. For example, multiple indicator studies with pH indicators have been used to determine extravascular and cellular pH in the intact canine lung and heart [84,85].

Injection Site and Form

Using a vascular indicator as well as a water indicator not only permits calculation of the extravascular water content of the lung but also diminishes the importance of the sites of injection and collection. If only the water indicator were injected in an outflow study, it would be necessary to place the injector catheter in the pulmonary artery and the collection catheter in the pulmonary vein to obtain information on the water content of the pulmonary tissues and blood. By including an indicator that measures the blood volume between the two catheters, the volume of the systemic venous and arterial circulations can be eliminated simply by subtracting this entire vascular volume from the total water volume.

The actual form of the transient study injection is immaterial (although it must involve a change in concentration at some particular time). Impulse injections are the most common because they are relatively easy to do, they provide a direct measure of the function h(t), and they are associated with the largest fractional changes in outflow concentrations. Alternative forms of injection are possible (though without obvious benefit in pulmonary water measurements), e.g., step functions (the commencement of a constant infusion) and ramp functions (constantly increasing inflow concentrations). Each of these alternative forms of injection require additional calculation for the derivation of h(t).

Although the form of the injection is arbitrary, so long as it is defined, the physical manner in which the injected indicator enters the bloodstream is critical. The delivery of both the vascular and the water indicators to all parts of the lung should be in proportion to the blood flow to each of these regions. Such flow-proportional delivery can best be ensured by injecting the indicators into the venous return to the heart and permitting convection in the right ventricle to provide adequate mixing of blood and indicators. Preferential delivery of a *bolus* of indicator to the flow entering the right lung will be analogous to the excessive *infusion* of indicators to the right lung and the concomitant flow of indicator-poor blood to the left lung. Under these circumstances, indicator concentration will *never* become uniform in each lung regardless of the duration of the infusion.

Indicator Collection and Detection

Consideration must also be given to the manner of indicator detection at the outflow. Collection of blood is unavoidable for the analysis of some indicators, e.g., tritiated water. Obviously, if samples are collected primarily from one lung, then the mean transit time data will largely reflect flow through that lung. If the entire output cannot be collected, then a representative sample must be obtained. Adequate mixing from both lungs is more likely if blood is collected downstream from the left ventricle, e.g., from the aorta.

An inevitable problem associated with blood collection is the delay imposed by the collection catheter. In principle, this should provide no special problem. The volume of the collection catheter is measured and divided by the collection flow to yield the mean catheter delay. The mean catheter delay is then subtracted from the total mean transit times to yield the mean transit times from the point of injection to the point of collection. It is best to keep flow through the collection catheter constant and this is commonly achieved by pumping blood through the collection system with a tubing pump of some sort. Unless the delay through the collection catheter is kept as small as possible, the outflow pattern may be severely distorted and extrapolation may thereby be complicated (to be described later). The catheter distortion can in principle be eliminated by characterizing the distribution of transit times through the catheter and deconvoluting the observed curve with this function. Such procedures present serious mathematical and experimental problems, however [86,87].

Problems associated with collection can be avoided if detection is accomplished at the pulmonary outflow itself. This can be done with probes sensitive to heat [88,89], hydrogen concentrations [90], conductivity [88], or even the color of the blood [91,92]. An additional advantage of these probes is that they entail no loss of blood from the patient. Aside from the need for knowing the response time of the probe, which is generally small, and also the need for situating the probe in a representative part of the outflow, such devices can introduce another problem. These probes detect changes of physical variables within a more or less discrete volume in their vicinity. Values obtained for this volume may not appropriately represent indicator outflow from the organ [93,94]. For example, if the monitored volume includes a relatively stagnant pool of blood formed near the catheter, the value may be biased by measured indicator concentrations in this blood.

Pulmonary Perfusion and Correction for Recirculation

If portions of the lung are poorly perfused, it may be technically difficult to obtain accurate mean transit times. Only a small portion of the indicator will enter such regions and emergence of the indicator will be delayed and concentrations will be diminished in the outflow. Even when indicator recovery is nearly complete (and flow measurements correspondingly accurate), mean transit times may be grossly underestimated. It should be understood, however, that if *no* indicator reaches a stagnant area following a sudden injection, then it is assumed that none would reach it during a constant infusion. Otherwise the conditions of stationarity and linearity would not be satisfied.

The emergence of indicator from regions of the lung with slow perfusion tends to be obscured by recirculation. Recirculation represents a particularly serious problem in indicator dilution studies of the lung since essentially all the cardiac output traverses the lung and there is no opportunity for indicator leaving the lung to be diluted by parallel flows from other organs. Traditionally, it is assumed that outflow patterns of each of the indicators are exponential, though there is evidence that such is not the case. One consequence of this practice is that the relative recoveries of labeled water, sodium, and other diffusible indicators are typically incomplete by about 5% compared to the recovery of the vascular indicator [1,95]. It is patently impossible for this 5% deficit to represent an actual loss of fluid from the lung since a persistent net loss of this amount of isotonic fluid would amount to 250 ml/min (if the cardiac output were 5 liters/min) or more than 100 times the loss expected in lymph per minute. The incomplete recovery presumably reflects amputation of the later portions of the diffusible indicator dilution curves by the correction for recirculation.

Standard indicator dilution curves characteristically measure only a fraction (between 40% and 90%) of the fluid present in the lung tissue [1]. It is very likely that these poor results are also partly due to the improper extrapolation of the indicator dilution curves. Those portions of the lungs that are more slowly perfused (e.g., the apices in erect man) [96] presumably empty during the period of recirculation and are not properly evaluated. Indicator dilution volume measurements yield better (higher) estimates of lung water when blood flows are high in awake and exercising animals and man [97,98]. Higher values are also obtained when pulmonary arterial pressures are increased [99]. It is likely that under these circumstances, perfusion of the lung is more uniform and outflow patterns of water and the vascular indicator more closely approximate a monoexponential form.

In theory, problems of recirculation may be better solved by monitoring indicator returning to the pulmonary artery and correcting outflow concentrations by a deconvolution procedure [100,84]. Alternatively, the return of recirculating indicators to the collection site can be determined by injecting a bolus of indicator into the aorta just downstream from the collection site and observing indicator concentrations in the collected blood [101]. Unfortunately, the problems associated with recovering the first-pass information from the observed data in the face of high levels of recirculating "noise" are considerable [102] and it seems unlikely that a practical and reliable deconvolution procedure can be developed for the lung.

A third, intricate procedure that Guintini has suggested depends on deriving a function from early vascular and water data that permits calculating the later portions of the water curve [103]. This procedure assumes that such a function describing the outflow of labeled water from the lung can be derived, an assumption that is particularly vulnerable if tissue perfusion is irregular.

Water Indicators

Although a small fraction of deuterium and tritium labels may exchange with hydrogen ions associated with tissue constituents and although labeled water has slightly different physical properties from those of unlabeled water, water molecules containing hydrogen or oxygen isotopes are probably the best labels available for water measurements. Local diffusion into tissues and alveolar fluid is very rapid and it has been difficult to document measurable barriers to diffusion at the capillary or alveolar surfaces. Even if the label freely diffuses through the pulmonary water, however, diffusion should account for a movement of no more than 0.2 mm during a typical capillary transit time of 1.0 sec [104,73]. It can be concluded that although full equilibration occurs in tissue volumes comparable to the alveolar dimensions during a single circulation, there is inadequate time for equilibration with more distant tissues (e.g., between bronchopulmonary segments) before recirculation occurs.

Some attention has been given to lipid-soluble indicators, such as alcohol and iodoantipyrine, and heat [105], which might be expected to reach some areas of the lung, by way of cellular membranes, more rapidly than labeled water. Indicator dilution volumes obtained with these substances do tend to be larger than such volumes obtained with labeled water, but this observation probably represents, partly at least, distribution in lipid compartments. It is unrealistic to expect that such substances will rapidly reach large volumes of poorly perfused lung tissue before recirculation occurs, and interpretation of such data is complicated by considerations of lipid-solubility and distribution in alveolar gas.

Scanning Procedures and Regional Water Content

The inherent problems associated with outflow procedures of measuring lung water should be evident from the above considerations. One available option is using external scanning in place of outflow analysis. What are the advantages of scanning procedures? Obviously the elimination of arterial catheterization for blood collection would be a distinct asset. Furthermore, scanning procedures may permit a more accurate evaluation of areas of the lung that empty more slowly, and it may be easier to detect the retention of indicators within an area of the lungs with slow washout than to detect the slow emergence of indicator in the outflow. Lastly, scanning procedures should permit measurements of regional water content and might therefore detect regional abnormalities.

Steady State Procedures*

From a technical point of view, it is best to use a gamma-emitting indicator that is retained within the body and equilibrates with the tissue volume. In early studies of Weidner et al. [106], ^{22}Na was used for measuring pulmonary extracellular fluid. Because ^{22}Na loss from the body can be minimized, equilibration with tissue fluids can be expected. If the volume of distribution is assumed equal to the extracellular fluid volume, then when interstitial and plasma activities become equal,

$$V_{EC} = \frac{a_{r,22Na}}{Ec_{22Na}} \tag{19}$$

where $a_{r,22Na}$ represents the activity at any time after equilibration over a discrete volume of the lung, c_{22Na} is the activity per milliliter of plasma (obtained from venous blood), and E is the ratio of efficiency of the external counter to efficiency of the counter used to measure plasma activity. This indicator never became popular for this purpose, presumably because of the considerable radioactive exposure required and uncertainty regarding the actual fraction of the tracer equilibrated with cellular fluids. A water indicator such as [^{131}I]iodoantipyrine [105] or $H_2^{15}O$ [107] might be an adequate *steady state* marker of regional lung water but such studies have not been reported.

Kety Procedure for Measuring Tissue Perfusion

Most of the traditional extracellular indicators except ^{22}Na are lost from the body at a rate largely determined by glomerular filtration. It is therefore not possible to get an equilibrium concentration with these substances (unless a sustaining infusion is used) and some sort of transient analysis is necessary.

Measurements of regional transit times by scanning techniques were introduced by Kety in measuring local muscle perfusion [83]. A dose of ^{22}Na was injected into the tissue and the disappearance monitored with a scintillation probe; Kety assumed that ^{22}Na concentrations became, and remained, uniform after a negligible delay and that loss of indicator from the tissue was accomplished exclusively by local blood flow. Thus, the rate of

---

*Although the indicator can be administered as a bolus injection, activities and concentrations are measured when a "steady state," or equilibrium has been attained.

isotope decline under the probe $(-\frac{dm}{dt})$ must equal the product of indicator concentration $(c(t))$ and blood flow:

$$- \frac{dm}{dt} = \dot{Q} \, c(t) \tag{20}$$

Since the concentration of ^{22}Na is uniform throughout its volume of distribution (V_d) and equal to outflow concentration:

$$c(t) = \frac{m(t)}{V_d} \, .$$

The distribution volume V_d is related to the tissue volume V_i by the factor λ:

$$V_d = \lambda V_i.$$

The symbol λ represents the ratio of tissue to blood concentrations of the indicator during prolonged constant infusion. Thus

$$\frac{dm(t)}{dt} = \frac{\dot{Q}}{\lambda V_i} \, m(t).$$

Integrating yields

$$m(t) = m_0 \, \exp \frac{-\dot{Q}}{\lambda V_i} \tag{21}$$

where m_0 is the initial dose of indicator.

Equation (21) predicts that indicator activity will decline in a monoexponential fashion. Generally the decline of activity is not monoexponential, indicating that the assumption of uniform indicator concentrations is probably unwarranted. Concentration gradients of extracellular indicators such as ^{22}Na can be maintained within tissues by capillary barriers [108]. Moreover, even diffusible gaseous indicators are generally washed out in a multiexponential fashion [109]. This observation has prompted the development of a variety of models in which two or more tissue compartments empty in parallel at different rates. It is difficult to be sure of the appropriate number of compartments and there is no guarantee that each of these actually empties in a monoexponential fashion. Furthermore, if the indicator injection is given at a point distant from the region of the lung seen by the detector, arrival of indicator into the observed tissue may occur throughout a portion of the observation interval, thereby invalidating Equation (21). This problem is discussed further with the Zierler technique.

Zierler Procedure for Measuring Tissue Perfusion

Zierler showed that assuming instantaneous mixing within tissue compartments was unnecessary for measuring perfusion by scanning procedures [110].* Zierler considered the situation in which the probe measures the activity of the entire organ including the site of injection. If the efficiency of the external count is the same throughout the organ and is known, determining the quantity of indicator within the organ at any one time should be possible. Furthermore, the quantity measured by scanning (residue detection) should be the same as the quantity calculated from the outflow concentrations by Equation (9). The equivalence of outflow and residue detection is based on indicator conservation. After an impulse injection, the quantity of indicator remaining in the organ should be

$$M(t) = \underbrace{\frac{a(t)}{E}}_{\substack{\uparrow \\ Residue \\ detection}} = \underbrace{m_0 - M_e(t) = m_0 - \int_0^t e(t)\, dt}_{\substack{\uparrow \\ Outflow \\ detection}} = m_0 \left[1 - H(t) \right]\, dt \qquad (22)$$

where m_0 is the injected dose of indicator, $a(t)$ is the activity measured over the organ and E represents the ratio of the efficiency of residue detection with the external probe to the efficiency of the instrument that measures outflow activity. If Equation (22) is integrated, we obtain

$$\int_0^\infty \frac{a(t)\, dt}{E} = m_0 \int_0^\infty \left[1 - H(t) \right]\, dt = m_0 \bar{t}. \qquad (23)$$

Zierler made the additional suggestion that evaluation of the efficiency of the probe could be avoided if it was assumed that the peak value of the activity a_{max} represented the total injected dose of indicator, and that $a_{max} = Em_0$. Thus, mean transit times were calculated by dividing the area under the curve $(A = \int_0^\infty a(t)\, dt)$ by the peak value of the curve:

$$\bar{t} = \frac{A}{a_{max}} = \frac{V_i}{Q}. \qquad (24)$$

*Reference should be made to the correction noted by Worsham [111].

The ratio $\dot{Q}/V_i$ represents overall "perfusion," or flow per unit volume of tissue. The total blood flow through the organ can be calculated from the organ outflow as described in Equation (14). However, both Lewis et al. [112] and Zierler [110] suggested alternative methods of calculating flow from the scanning and blood data that permit more limited blood sampling and may avoid recirculation corrections.

Regional Volumes

Zierler did not explicitly show that Equation (24) applies to measurements of *regional* perfusion. If only a portion of the organ is monitored or the sites of injection or outflow are not within view of the monitor, Equation (24) will not generally hold unless the peak value over that region represents the total quantity of indicator entering that region. Furthermore, neither the Kety nor the Zierler formulation indicate the way in which regional volumes can be calculated from the indicator dilution curves without the additional information of *local* blood flow. If the indicator injection is given properly (see previous discussion), the delivery of indicator to any one region should be in proportion to the regional blood flow ($\dot{Q}_r$) to this tissue, so that

$$\frac{m_{0,r}}{m_0} = \frac{\dot{Q}_r}{\dot{Q}} \tag{25}$$

where $m_{0,r}$ is the amount of indicator reaching this region, and

$$\int_0^\infty \frac{a_r(t)\, dt}{E} = m_{0,r}\bar{t}_r = \frac{\dot{Q}_r}{\dot{Q}} m_0 \bar{t}_r. \tag{26}$$

The symbols $a_{r,t}$ and $\bar{t}_r$ refer to regional values of activity and mean transit time. Now the regional volume under the probe should equal the product of the local blood flow and the local mean transit time *:

$$V_r = \dot{Q}_r\bar{t}_r = \dot{Q} \int_0^\infty \frac{a_r(t)\, dt}{Em_0}. \tag{27}$$

Thus it is possible to obtain a value for the *regional* volume from the area under the *regional* activity curve and the *total* blood flow. Since the information is regional, the site of injection may be remote from the lung (e.g., a peripheral vein). If the outflow is collected at the same time that activity

*It is assumed that transport of indicator to and from any macroscopic region of the lung is accomplished by blood flow rather than by diffusion from neighboring regions.

over the lung is measured, then blood flow can be calculated from the area
under the outflow curve (B) as described in Equation (14), and

$$V_r = \frac{A_r}{EB}.$$

(28)

Equation (28) may also be justified by direct use of the basic integral indicator equation and the reader is referred to the earlier articles of Bergner and
others [113–116].

It is useful to compare Zierler's perfusion equation (Eq. 24) with the
volume equation (Eq. 28). The perfusion equation does not require information about blood concentrations whereas regional volume measurements do
require blood collection and analysis. Nor is it necessary to obtain information about the efficiency of the external probe in the perfusion measurements,
a procedure that must be accomplished in the volume measurement. On the
other hand, the perfusion equation is based on the assumption that the peak
value of the external activity curve represents the portion of the injected indicator that arrives in the monitored region:

$$a_{max,r} = Em_{0,r}.$$

(29)

Unfortunately, there is little reason to believe that this condition prevails in
the lung. If the injection site is distant from the monitored site (e.g., in a
peripheral vein) or if regional blood flow is slow, the injection bolus will tend
to become dispersed and a_{max} will be diminished. It is not necessary to make
an assumption of this sort in the regional volume measurement. Indeed, it
can be shown that Equation (28) holds regardless of the configuration of the
injection.

Although in principle Equation (28) should permit calculating regional
water content if suitable indicators are used, this approach does not solve the
overriding problem of recirculation. Furthermore, arterial samples must be
obtained, as in the Chinard method. Recently, the procedure has been modified by one of the authors (R.M.E.) in such a way that regional measurements
of pulmonary extracellular water can be obtained that are not influenced by
recirculation and do not require arterial sampling. The study is accomplished
by observing the concomitant decline of lung and plasma activity over a period
as it is lost from the body.

A bolus of the extracellular indicator ^{99m}Tc DTPA (^{99m}Tc diethylenetri-
amine pentaacetate) is injected into a peripheral vein and the activity is measured
at intervals for several hours over the lung and in plasma obtained from another
peripheral vein. These activities are corrected for radioactive decay. During the
observation interval, the corrected activities of both the lung and plasma decline

as indicator distributes into extrapulmonary compartments and is lost from the body. Initially both pulmonary and plasma activities fluctuate rapidly during the first few circulations but these rapid changes diminish and indicator activities then decline more slowly (see Fig. 2). The actual loss of indicator from the body is determined essentially by the glomerular filtration rate. No correction is made for recirculation in any of the measured parameters. The regional activity (corrected for the efficiency of the probe) is designated $M_r(t)$ and is related to the rate of injection $i(u)$ by the equation:

$$M_r(t) = \int_0^t \frac{a_r(t-u)}{m_0 E} \, i(u)du$$

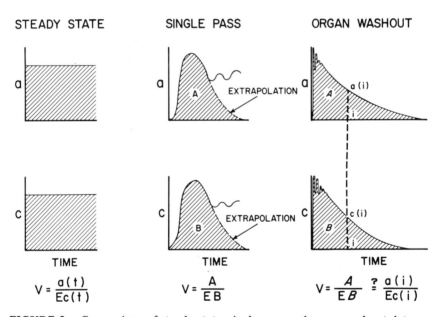

FIGURE 2   Comparison of steady state, single-pass, and organ washout data. The equivalence of the area ratios is shown (see text for the meaning of the symbols). Pulmonary blood flow can be calculated from the area under the single transit curve (B), whereas the clearance of indicator from the body can be calculated from the plasma washout curve (*B*). The usefulness of instantaneous values of activity and concentration obtained during a washout study (dotted line) for volume calculation depends on the rate of tissue equilibration with the blood and the rate of indicator elimination from the monitored region.

where m_0 is the total activity injected and $a_r(t)$ is the timecourse of the regional activity (uncorrected for probe efficiency) after a bolus injection. Italics are used to indicate that there is no recirculation correction.

Consider the effect of a constant infusion, i, of ^{99m}Tc-DTPA into the same venous site. Regional activity should reach a steady-state value of M_r, where:

$$M_r = i \int_0^\infty \frac{a_r(t)dt}{m_0 E} = i\theta \tag{29a}$$

where θ is defined as the integral of the expression and is referred to as the "residence," "sojourn" or "occupancy" time of the recirculating indicator [113-116]. Under these steady state, recirculating conditions, i must equal the rate at which indicator is lost from the system, which in turn equals loss in the urine:

$$i = c\,(C_{99m\,Tc})$$

where $C_{99m\,Tc}$ designates clearance of ^{99m}Tc-DTPA in the urine (this approximates the glomerular filtration rate) and c is the plasma concentration of ^{99m}Tc-DTPA Substituting in Equation (29a) and dividing by the uniform concentration c which would be obtained during a prolonged infusion, we obtain

$$V_{EC,r} = (C_{99m\,Tc})\,\theta. \tag{29b}$$

The magnitude of θ is considerably longer than $\bar{t}$ since θ includes recirculatory indicator data.

Values for $C_{99m\,Tc}$ are easily determined by measuring the plasma activity per milliliter of plasma during the observation interval, correcting for radioactive decay, plotting against time, and determining the area under this curve:

$$C_{99m\,Tc} = \frac{m_0}{\int_0^\infty c\,dt} \tag{29c}$$

Venous samples suffice for this purpose. Substituting Equations (29a) and (29c) into (29b), we obtain an equation that is analogous to (24). (See Fig. 2.)

$$V_{EC, r} = \frac{\int_0^{\infty} a_r(t)\, dt}{E \int_0^{\infty} c(t)\, dt} = \frac{A_{EC, r}}{BE} \tag{29d}$$

where $A_{EC, r}$ represents the area under the regional activity curve divided by m_0 and B represents the area under the curve of the plasma activity per milliliter of plasma. As indicated in Figure 2, the ratios described by Equations (19), (28), and (29d) should be the same for any one indicator.

Preliminary studies from our laboratory suggest that the equilibration of Tc–DTPA with the interstitium of the lung is nearly complete within a minute. Because approximately an hour is needed for indicator concentrations in the plasma and regional activity to decline by one-half, the ratio of activities in tissue to plasma at any one time should closely approximate the ratio between the areas under these curves. Thus, the measurements obtained from the entire washout experiment may indicate that data obtained from individual observations provide a valid measure of regional extracellular lung water content (after the first few minutes) (see Fig. 2).

Only an extracellular indicator is currently being used in these studies and it is therefore not possible to distinguish between the plasma, and the interstitial and alveolar water volumes. Furthermore, measurements of efficiency are required to obtain absolute values for water content. The gamma probe is fitted with a focusing collimator to reduce the contribution of indicator within the extracellular fluid of the thoracic wall. Uncertainty regarding the contribution of thoracic wall activity and the variable efficiency of the probe for detecting regional activities represent the principal problems associated with this and other scanning procedures.

Scanning Studies with Protein Indicators

Because serum protein concentrations are not the same in the plasma, interstitial, and alveolar compartments, they cannot be used for fluid volume measurements. However, pulmonary edema is generally associated with accumulation of serum protein in the extravascular, extracellular compartment of the lung. Two non-invasive approaches, using radioactive labeling of serum protein and external chest counting, are currently being evaluated for detecting the rate of accumulation of protein in the extravascular compartment [117] and the distribution of albumin between the vascular and extravascular compartments [118].

Rate of serum protein leakage   Gorin and his colleagues [117] use two radioactive isotopes, technetium-99m for labeling erythrocytes and indium-113 for labeling the serum protein transferrin. The method requires that both labels be simultaneously injected and that the respective counts of the two radioactive isotopes be monitored over the chest with a collimator-focused scintillation counter. By selective gating of the energy spectra of the two isotopes, the ratio of technetium-99m to indium-113 in the zone of the lung being monitored can be determined. Since the technetium label remains intravascular, the relative counts per minute of the two radioactive isotopes become the measure of the rate of transferrin movement from the circulation into the interstitium. Ordinarily, the transfer rate is established over a 3-hr period by obtaining counts at 15-min intervals.

These investigators studied the transfer rate of indium-113-labeled transferrin in sheep from the vascular into the extravascular compartment by the external counting technique (caudal, posterior chest region) and compared this with the simultaneous appearance of the radioactive label in lung lymph. The two measurements showed good agreement.

This technique implicitly assumes that lung hematocrit remains constant during the period in which the rate of protein transfer into the interstitium is being investigated. The chief technical disadvantages are the need to label the subject's own red cells before performing the test and the requirement that two relatively high energy isotopes be counted. Correction for the relative counting efficiencies of each isotope in different regions of the lungs may be particularly difficult. On the other hand, the flat shape of the human chest represents an advantage over the boat shape of animals and should facilitate regional counting. The rate of protein transfer could be increased by greater capillary permeability to the protein or by solvent drag as bulk fluid flows into the lung.

Distribution of serum albumin between the vascular and extravascular spaces   During the development of pulmonary edema, increases in interstitial and alveolar fluid become proportionately very much greater than any corresponding increase in intravascular fluid. Because edema fluid contains significant amounts of serum protein, the total quantity of albumin within the lungs assumes an increasingly extravascular protein distribution as edema worsens. This is particularly likely to occur if capillary permeability to protein is increased and extravascular protein concentration is thereby elevated, a circumstance that may occur, for example, in certain respiratory distress syndromes [119].

We have used a noninvasive, radioisotope technique in man, which is designed to estimate the fraction of serum albumin in the extravascular space of the lung. Extravascular serum is labeled 24 hr before the measurement by injecting [^{131}I]-labeled human serum albumin. This time is adequate for equilibration of specific activities of serum albumin in the vascular and extravascular space of the lungs in dogs [120] and sheep [1] and apparently in man. Further evidence to this point is that longer periods of equilibration do not result in larger fractions of serum albumin in the extravascular space in normal man. On the other hand, equilibration periods as short as 6–8 hr result in a lower calculated percentage of serum albumin in the extravascular space than is found with the 24-hr equilibration.

An external focusing collimator permits a scintillation crystal to detect the disintegrations from the radioactive albumin in the lung parenchyma, with minimal contribution from the chest wall. The disintegrations represent the albumin in both the vascular and extravascular compartments.

The procedure requires that 24 hr following the initial injection, a venous blood sample (B_0) be drawn to compare the blood radioactivity with the scanned lung radioactivity ($A_{l,0}$). A second injection of the same radioactive-labeled albumin is given, but now only 10 min is allowed for this tag to mix. Thus, its volume of distribution is restricted almost wholly to the vascular compartment. The count over the lungs is again obtained ($A_{l,10}$) and another venous blood sample is counted (B_{10}). The increment in counts over the lung represents an increase in contribution from the vascular compartment ($A_{t,0}$). The venous blood sample (B_{10}) enables determination of the proportion of increase in radioactivity in the vascular compartment of the lung. This test allows estimation of the fraction of the total serum albumin in the lung which

resides in the extravascular compartment of the lung ($\frac{A_{t,0}}{A_{l,0}}$). The measurements may be repeated in 24 hr, after allowing reequilibration of the labeled protein with the extravascular albumin pool.

The mathematical derivation for the computation is presented below. The following nomenclature is used:

A = activity measured over the chest by external counting

B = venous blood activity

Subscripts:

l = total lung activity seen by probe

b = lung blood activity seen by probe

t = lung tissue activity seen by probe

0 = 24 hr after first [131 I] albumin dose

10 = 10 min later

The count determined by scanning at a given time is the sum of blood and lung tissue contributions:

$$A_{l,0} = A_{b,0} + A_{t,0} \tag{30}$$

$$A_{l,10} = A_{b,10} + A_{t,10}. \tag{31}$$

Since 10 min is a short time in relation to equilibrium kinetics for serum albumin between intravascular and extravascular compartments, $A_{t,0} = A_{t,10}$. Thus,

$$A_{l,10} = A_{b,10} + A_{t,0}. \tag{32}$$

The blood contribution to scanned lung activity must be proportional to the simultaneously determined venous blood activity:

$$\frac{A_{b,0}}{A_{b,10}} = \frac{B_0}{B_{10}}. \tag{33}$$

Equations (30), (32), and (33) constitute three equations with three unknowns. They can be solved for $A_{t,0}$ in terms of the measured variables, to yield

$$A_{t,0} = \frac{B_0 A_{l,10} - B_{10} A_{l,0}}{B_0 - B_{10}}. \tag{34}$$

In our laboratory, 19 measurements on 10 normal subjects have yielded a mean value for $A_{t,0}/A_{l,0} = 0.26$ and a standard deviation 0.14. This measurement has potential application in evaluating disorders associated with increased capillary permeability to macromolecules. It is noninvasive (except for peripheral vein injection and blood sampling) and can be repeated, and therefore promises to be a valuable clinical technique.

F. Soluble Gas Absorption

An inhaled gas will leave the lung gas to dissolve in the pulmonary tissues. Those inert gases that are relatively soluble in the pulmonary tissue will become diluted in a larger volume than inert gases that are only slightly soluble. From this difference in dilution, values can be calculated for pulmonary tissue volume. As roughly 80% of pulmonary tissue is water, this measured volume is influenced by changes in pulmonary water content. A complicating factor arises in that all gases that are soluble in pulmonary tissue are also soluble in the blood perfusing the lung. Calculation of tissue volumes therefore requires extrapolation to "zero time" before any of the indicator gas has been carried away from the lung by the pulmonary circulation.

Although Krogh and Lindhard in 1912 [121] and Kety in 1951 [122] pointed out that the disappearance of inert gases from the lung was influenced by the solubility of these gases in lung tissue, it was not until 1959 that Cander and Forster [123] considered quantitative aspects of the lung tissue uptake. The speed of equilibration of an inert gas with the pulmonary parenchyma (including the tissue and the contained blood) is so rapid that it may be considered instantaneous. Thus, the fraction of inert indicator gas in the alveolar air (FA) is immediately reduced to

$$FA_{0+} = FA_0 \frac{VA}{VA + \lambda_p V_p (P_B - 47)/760} \tag{35}$$

where VA is the alveolar volume; V_p is the parenchymal tissue volume, and λ_p is the solubility of the inert gas in the parenchyma; FA_0 is the predicted alveolar concentration resulting from lung gas volume dilution and FA_{0+} is the concentration after further dilution by the parenchymal tissue volume. Thereafter, the inert gas in both the alveoli and the parenchyma is diluted by absorption into blood flowing through the pulmonary capillaries. The flow rate of gas leaving the alveoli equals the flow rate of gas entering the blood:

$$- \frac{d\,FA}{dt} \left(VA + \lambda_p V_p \frac{P_B - 47}{760} \right) = FA\lambda_b \dot{Q}c \left(\frac{P_B - 47}{760} \right) \tag{36}$$

where λ_b is the solubility of the inert gas in blood, and $\dot{Q}_c$ is the capillary blood flow rate. Equation (36) can be solved with the initial condition of Equation (35), to yield

$$FA = FA_0 \frac{VA}{VA + \lambda_p V_p (P_B - 47)/760} \exp \left[\frac{-\lambda_B \dot{Q}_c t}{VA (760/(P_B - 47)) + \lambda_p V_p} \right] \tag{37}$$

Thus, if the indicated solubilities, the alveolar volume, and the time course of alveolar inert gas concentration following a single inhalation of a gas containing an inert gas are known, both the parenchymal tissue volume and the pulmonary capillary blood flow can be determined.

The addition of a relatively insoluble inert gas (such as helium or argon) allows calculation of the initial alveolar concentration of the soluble gas as well as the alveolar volume. Since the insoluble test gas does not leave the lung gas, the ratio between expired and inspired concentrations reflects dilution in alveolar gases. Thus

$$FA_{s_0} = FI_s \frac{FE_i}{FI_i} \qquad (38)$$

where the subscripts i and s indicate the insoluble and soluble inert gases, respectively, and the small capitals I and E refer to inspired and end-expired gas concentrations. The alveolar volume can be determined:

$$VA = (VI - VD) \frac{FI_i}{FE_i} \qquad (39)$$

where VI is the volume of the inspirate (BTPS), VD is the volume of the anatomical dead space, and PB is the barometric pressure.

Cander and Forster [123] suggested that in order to follow the time course of alveolar inert gas concentration, the experimental procedure should consist of a series of sudden inspirations of a given volume of test gas mixture with the breath being held for varying times. The end-expiratory soluble test gas concentration as a function of the length of breath-hold should follow the same time course as the alveolar concentration of a single inhalation.

Cander and Forster discussed further considerations in the measurement. The choice of soluble inert gas is critical. The alveolar concentration of a gas with too low a solubility (for example, helium or SF_6) would not decline measurably during a breath-hold. A gas with too high a solubility (for example, acetone or diethyl ether) would dissolve in significant quantities into the tissues lining the respiratory dead space. Since the concentration of soluble gas in the dead space does not decline with time, the exhaled alveolar sample would be contaminated with this dissolved deadspace gas. Gases of intermediate solubilities avoid both problems; either nitrous oxide or acetylene have been found satisfactory. Equation (36) is valid so long as the blood entering the capillaries does not contain a significant concentration of the inert gas. Clearly, if the breath-hold is of longer duration than the recirculation time, the venous blood will contain the inert species and the decline of alveolar inert gas concentration will no longer be exponential. Although under some circumstances, recirculation may occur in as little as 8 sec [122], significant deviation from an exponential decay is not generally observed until 20 sec have elapsed [124].

Calculating the pulmonary parenchymal volume is typically facilitated by plotting the logarithm of the expired soluble gas fraction versus the length of the breath-hold (as illustrated in Figure 3). A line is fitted to these data; the slope of the line defines the capillary blood flow and the difference between the actual zero-time intercept, and the theoretical zero-time intercept as determined by Equation (38) defines the parenchymal tissue volume. This intercept is an estimate of the fractional alveolar concentration of the soluble gas after absorption of the gas by the parenchymal tissue but before gas is diluted by capillary blood flow (i.e. FA_{0+} in Equation (35)). Substituting Equations (38) and (39) into Equation (35) and solving for V_p yields

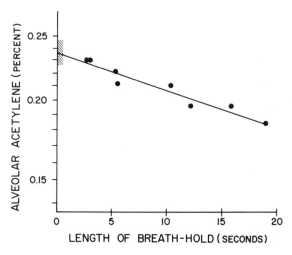

FIGURE 3   Determination of pulmonary parenchymal volume in a normal subject from measurements of alveolar acetylene concentration following breath-holds of varying lengths of a gas mixture containing 0.92% acetylene and 8.6% helium. Equations (41 to 45) permitted determination of the 95% confidence limit of the extrapolated "zero-time" intercept (shaded area). Based on an inspired gas volume of 1000 ml, an anatomic dead space of 150 ml, and the observed helium dilution, Equation (40) allowed calculation of the pulmonary parenchymal volume (see text).

$$V_p = \frac{(VI - VD)}{\lambda_p} \left[\frac{FI_s}{FA_{s_{0+}}} - \frac{FI_i}{FA_i} \right] \left(\frac{760}{P_B - 47} \right). \tag{40}$$

We have found that some confusion exists concerning the appropriate numerical value for the solubility coefficient of the soluble inert gas in the pulmonary parenchyma. There seems to be some uncertainty regarding use of the Ostwald solubility coefficient and the Bunsen solubility coefficient (denoted α and λ). The most widely accepted measurement is that of Cander [125], in which pure soluble gases were equilibrated with blood-free lung homogenate at 37°C. The number of milliliters of gas, reduced to STPD, dissolved in 1 milliliter of lung tissue in equilibrium with pure gas under 760 mmHg tension at 37°C is defined as the Bunsen solubility coefficient and is designated $\alpha_t^{37°}$. The Ostwald solubility coefficient, designated $\lambda_t^{37°}$, differs only in that the gas volume dissolved in a volume of lung homogenate is corrected to BTPS. Clearly, the choice is determined by whether the lung volumes (VI and VD) in Equation (40), typically measured ATPS, are corrected to BTPS or to STPD. The two solubility coefficients are related as $\lambda^{37°} = 1.136\alpha^{37°}$ [122]. Failure to match the volume correction used with the appropriate solubility coefficient would lead to an error of up to 14% in the measured pulmonary parenchymal volume. A second issue relates to the fact that the calculated parenchymal volume includes not only lung tissue, but also the volume of blood contained in the lung at the instant at which the soluble gas is inhaled. Sackner et al. [126] acknowledged this fact by using a solubility coefficient that weighted bloodless lung and blood solubility coefficients in a ratio 4:1, corresponding to the ratio of the volume of pulmonary tissue to capillary blood in the normal lung.* (Capillary blood volume can be measured independently by noninvasive techniques [127, 128]). It appears from the tabulation Butler made [129] that the best available estimate of the Ostwald solubility coefficient appropriate for substitution into Equation (40) is $\lambda_p^{37°} = 0.465$ for nitrous oxide and $\lambda_p^{37°} = 0.086$ for acetylene.

One of the main pitfalls of this soluble gas technique for determining pulmonary tissue volume involves the back extrapolation of the disappearance curve. Intuitively, a calculation involving a back extrapolation might be suspected to be quite sensitive to a variety of measurement errors. In reference to Figure 3, the intercept of the plot can be empirically calculated by minimizing the summed-square errors between the measurements and the best-

---

*Illustrating the confusion about the choice of proper solubility coefficient just referred to, Sackner weighted the *Ostwald* solubility coefficient for blood with the *Bunsen* coefficient for lung tissue!

fitted line on the logarithmic plot. The following relation facilitates this calculation:

$$\ln FA_{int} = \frac{\sum\limits_{j=1}^{N} \ln FA_j}{N} - \frac{\sum\limits_{j=1}^{N} t_j}{N} \frac{N \sum\limits_{j=1}^{N} (t_j \ln FA_j) - \left(\sum\limits_{j=1}^{N} t_j\right)\left(\sum\limits_{j=1}^{N} \ln FA_j\right)}{N \sum\limits_{j=1}^{N} (t_j^2) - \left(\sum\limits_{j=1}^{N} t_j\right)^2} \quad (41)$$

where the number of breath-holds is N and breath-hold j is of length t_j and yields an expired fraction of soluble test gas FA_j.* A measure of the reliability of this estimate is revealed by calculation of the confidence interval of the intercept FA_{int}. If the best estimate of the slope of the logarithmic curve is calculated as

$$m = \frac{\sum\limits_{j=1}^{N} \ln FA_j - N \ln FA_{int}}{\sum\limits_{j=1}^{N} t_j} \quad (42)$$

then the standard error of the estimate of the intercept (in the logarithmic domain) is [131]

$$s = \sqrt{\frac{1}{(N-2)N} \sum\limits_{j=1}^{N} \ln FA_j - \ln FA_{int} - mt_j)^2 \left[1 + \frac{\left(\sum\limits_{j=1}^{N} t_j\right)^2}{N \sum\limits_{j=1}^{N} (t_j - \bar{t})^2}\right]} \quad (43)$$

where $\bar{t} = \sum\limits_{j=1}^{N} t_j/N$. The upper 95% confidence limit for FA_{int} is then

$$FA_{int} \exp s \, t_{0.975} \quad (44)$$

and the lower limit is

$$FA_{int} \exp -s \, t_{0.975} \quad (45)$$

---

*It should be noted that fitting a line to a logarithmic plot inappropriately emphasizes the influence of longer breath-holds to a small extent. To be rigorous, techniques of nonlinear regression might be applied; iterative computer routines are available that are well suited to the task [130].

where t signifies the Student-t statistic with $N - 2$ degrees of freedom. From the measurements depicted in Figure 3, data from the eight breath-holds can be analyzed to yield a tissue volume of 730 ml with an upper confidence limit of 920 ml and a lower confidence limit of 560 ml. We calculate that for a particularly bad case in the recent literature, the estimate of parenchymal volume of 635 ml on the basis of three breath-holds has an upper confidence limit of 30 *liters* and a lower confidence limit of −6 *liters*! We urge that all calculations of pulmonary parenchymal volume derived by the soluble gas technique be accompanied by the confidence limit estimate as just derived.

Demonstration that the calculation of pulmonary parenchymal volume is critically sensitive to error leads to consideration of factors that might occasion systematic error. Certain assumptions underlying the technique must be examined. As a first consideration, cardiac output is implicitly assumed to remain constant over the course of the breath-holds. Estimating the sensitivity of the measurement to this assumption, we calculate that for typical lung and blood flow parameters, if pulmonary parenchymal volume is computed on the basis of two breath-holds of 10 and 15-sec duration, and the cardiac output happens to be 20% higher during the second breath-hold compared with the first, the calculated tissue volume will be in error by 6%. Thus, the technique does not appear to be critically sensitive to cardiac output changes. Yet, it is clearly indicated that maneuvers that would lead to predictable changes in pulmonary blood flow should be avoided. For example, closure of the glottis during the breath-hold (Valsalva maneuver) will lead to errors, since the increased alveolar pressures will reduce filling pressures of the heart [132,133] and transiently decrease cardiac output dramatically [134]. Similar considerations dictate that the volumes of the gas inspired in each breath-hold should be roughly equal so that intrapleural pressure changes will not induce cardiac output changes. Clearly, postural changes during the measurements would have untoward effects [135].

A further assumption underlying the soluble gas technique is that no ventilation-to-perfusion inequalities exist within the lung. In upright man, ventilation per unit alveolar volume decreases with distance up the lung, just as blood flow does, but ventilation has a rate of change only about a third that of blood flow [136]. The observed disappearance curve can be seen to be the sum of curves for regions of differing $\dot{V}A/\dot{Q}$. Unfortunately, the sum of exponential disappearance curves is not an exponential, and distortion of the true parenchymal tissue volume is inevitable. Very rough calculations based on liberal assumptions and on the data of West [136] show that the $\dot{V}A/\dot{Q}$ inequalities present in normal upright man could generate an overestimate of approximately 2%. We conclude that normal $\dot{V}A/\dot{Q}$ distribution in upright man engenders no great error in tissue volume measurement but that the technique can not be applied in a cavalier fashion in the presence of severe maldistribution of either ventilation or perfusion, such as frequently occurs in patients with lung disease.

Several other methods of measurement of pulmonary tissue volume based on ramifications of soluble gas absorption have been described. Feisal et al. [137] and later Sackner et al. [138] reasoned that a pulmonary artery injection of an ether-alcohol solution would cause ether to be eluted into the alveolar air as the bolus reached the pulmonary capillaries. The sudden increase in lung gas volume can be detected by sensitive plethysmographic [137] or pneumotachographic [124, 138] measurements. The main determinants of this volume are the volume of ether injected and the volume of ether taken up due to the solubility of ether in the pulmonary parenchyma. Sackner et al. [126] also has reported a technique for plethysmographic determination of parenchymal volume from comparison of pressure changes accompanying single inhalations of air and a nitrous oxide mixture. The immediate downward shift of the plethysmographic curves for N_2O compared with air is due to pulmonary parenchymal absorption of nitrous oxide and can be interpreted to arrive at an estimate of tissue volume. Both plethysmographic techniques require exquisitely sensitive gas volume measurements; neither has found wide application.

A recently developed application of soluble gas absorption techniques that does seem to show promise of wide application is a rebreathing method reported by Sackner et al. [139]; by this method tissue volume can be assessed by computerized analysis of mass spectrometer tracings. Instead of multiple breath-holds, the subject respires from a bag filled with an acetylene-helium-air mixture. If the time spent at end expiration is negligible relative to the time spent in full inspiration, end-tidal concentrations approximate the time course of alveolar samples [140]. Sackner's subjects respired from a 3.5-liter bag for 15 to 25 sec at a rate of 25 breaths/min while trying to empty the bag on each inspiration. Measurements appear to compare well with breath-holding determinations of tissue volume.

The effect of exercise and of acute pulmonary hypertension on pulmonary parenchymal volume as measured by soluble gas techniques has been reported. Both Cross et al. [141] and Sackner et al. [139] detected significant increases in tissue volume in moderate exercise, but Johnson et al. [142] did not. Glauser et al. [143] found that aortic balloon inflation caused a doubling of tissue volume in anesthetized dogs.

A comprehensive comparison of measured pulmonary parenchymal volume with more direct techniques is not available. It appears that there may be no large systematic difference between soluble gas absorption determinations and lung tissue volumes determined gravimetrically (after the lungs have been stripped of extrapulmonary airways and large blood vessels). Cander and

Forster [123] determined weights and densities of blood-free homogenates of five human lungs; the calculated tissue volumes were of the same order as measured by soluble gas absorption in normal subjects. Glauser et al. [143] obtained paired comparison in seven dogs of acetylene absorption tissue volume obtained just before lung excision and the subsequent measurement of lung weight. Pulmonary venous hypertension edema had been induced before these measurements. The lung tissue volumes determined by the two techniques were not significantly different.

In summary, these soluble gas techniques for determining lung tissue volume appear promising but require further development. A large-scale study to determine the sensitivity and accuracy of the technique, compared with more direct methods, seems in order. We reiterate our suggestion that the determination should be based on more breath-holds than the number that seems to be in vogue (say, a minimum of six or eight) and that the confidence limits of the calculated tissue volumes be reported routinely. The tedious calculations experienced for data reduction should prove amenable to computerization; recent attempts in this direction by Sackner et al. [139] appear very productive.

G.   Transthoracic Impedance

All body tissues are conductors of electric current to a greater or lesser extent. If an alternating voltage is applied across the chest, the current flow will be a function of the conductivity of skin, muscle, fat, intrathoracic blood, and lung. The lung is a unique organ in this regard; air is a very poor conductor, and thus, lung conductivity varies strikingly with inflation and with relative water content. Changes in transthoracic impedance at a given level of inflation therefore should provide an index of pulmonary water content.

In the construction of a practical device for transthoracic impedance measurements, the frequency and intensity of the applied voltage must be considered. The applied voltage particularly must not stimulate excitable tissue within the chest. So that stimulation will be avoided, sinusoidal wavelengths shorter than the chronaxie for the most excitable tissues must be used. At frequencies above 500 Hz, the signal amplitude necessary for stimulation rises sharply [144]. In practice, peak-to-peak currents in the range 20 μA to 20 mA have been used [145], well below the threshold for stimulation. Further, at these frequencies, polarization of the electrodes (in which the electrode and the underlying skin act as plates of a capacitor, thus impeding current flow) is minimized [145]. The impedance of the chest tissues is primarily due to movement of ions in extracellular water [146]. This impedance is composed of a resistance and a capacitive reactance, the resistive component predominating [147–149]. Most studies of transthoracic impedance have used frequencies of 50 kHz or 100 kHz.

The primary difficulty in obtaining an index of lung conductivity from measurements made from electrodes attached to the chest is in distinguishing between lung and nonlung conductivity. Current applied to the chest wall will be shunted around the lung to an extent dictated by the relative resistivities of the thoracic contents. The resistivities of the various body tissues have been measured from excised samples. The lung, due to the insulating properties of the air it contains, has a low conductivity. Lung tissue resistivity averages 1000 Ω-cm in the dog [148,150,151] compared with 150 Ω-cm for blood [151]. Current applied to the chest must first pass through a highly resistive layer of skin and underlying fat. The postural muscles, encountered next, are anisotropic in their conductivity, generally tending to shunt current along the muscle fibers (parallel to the chest wall) rather than into the thorax [152]. The remaining radial current must flow between the nonconducting ribs and through the poorly conducting (but thin) parietal pleura. Consequently, the predominant pathway for current applied to the chest is around the chest wall [152,153]; about 5% actually flows through the lung [154].

Several configurations of electrode placement have been studied to try to make thoracic impedance measurements maximally sensitive to changes in pulmonary impedance. The geometry of the tissue underlying the electrodes dictates their placement [144,155]. Configurations of two electrodes have been found to be highly sensitive to the properties of the tissues nearest the electrodes [152]. This effect is reduced by adding a second pair of electrodes in close proximity to the active electrodes (those across which the voltage is applied). In these four-electrode configurations, transthoracic impedance is measured as the quotient of the potential induced across these "floating" electrodes, and the current is applied through the active electrode. A four-electrode configuration currently finding some favor [156–158] is the vertical electrode array of Kubicek et al. [159]. Conductive strips encircling the upper abdomen and the neck effectively measure the impedance of the chest as a cylinder.

A recent refinement makes transthoracic measurements considerably more sensitive to lung impedance changes. A "guard ring" circumscribing the sensing electrode is driven at such a potential as to cancel voltage gradients between it and the sensing electrode. Lateral current (along the chest wall) is thus induced to flow to the guard ring, rather than to the sensing electrode. The flow path for current arriving at the sensing electrode is primarily through the central core of tissue. The current is said to have been "focused" to reduce the influence of chest wall shunting on transthoracic impedance measurement. The technique, which Graham first described in 1965 [160], was applied to impedance pneumography by Cooley and Longini [153] and to measurement of pulmonary edema by Severinghaus et al. [146]. These authors report that this configuration engenders a tenfold increase in measured transthoracic impedance with respect to the unfocused, two-electrode configuration. Sensitivity to lung inflation has been reported to increase sevenfold [153] and tenfold [160].

The influence of inflation and relative water content on the electrical impedance of the lung has been measured in animal studies in which electrodes were positioned directly on the pleural surface. Witsoe and Kinnen [148] determined that a linear relation described the dependence of lung resistivity on lung inflation and that resistivity was doubled by inflating a collapsed lung to high lung volumes. Rush et al. [150] found that a dog lung, ventilated at a large tidal volume, exhibited a resistivity varying cyclically between 1950 Ω-cm and 2390 Ω-cm. Lambert and Gremels [9] found that a large saline infusion engendering gross pulmonary edema in cats was accompanied by a halving of measured lung resistance. Alloxan-induced edema produced a fourfold reduction in measured impedance of a dog heart-lung preparation [161].

Several reports have appeared describing clinical trials of transthoracic impedance measurement as a means of assessing pulmonary water. In a series of five papers, Swedish investigators studied changes in transthoracic impedance in the newborn [149,155,162–164]. They interpreted a decline in impedance averaging under 3% over the first half-hour of life as reflecting an increased pulmonary interstitial fluid and blood volume somewhat offset by a coincident increase in FRC [163]. Pomerantz et al. [156,161] followed the course of transthoracic impedance in 52 patients. Fluid removal from the chest by thoracentesis or dialysis produced marked increases in transthoracic impedance. In one patient drainage of a 1300 ml pleural effusion was accompanied by a 20% rise in impedance [156]. These studies demonstrated that in trauma, cardiac insufficiency, and respiratory insufficiency, impedance changes paralleled (but did not seem to predict) changes in arterial blood gases, central venous pressure, and radiologic indications.

Studies seeking to correlate transthoracic impedance changes with more quantitative indices of pulmonary water are surprisingly scarce. Lambert and Gremels [9] found that transpulmonary impedance in open-chested cats was well correlated with percentage of water content of small portions of the lung excised while inducing gross pulmonary edema. Leupker et al. [158] reported that an average 8% decrease in transthoracic impedance accompanied a 100% increase in indicator dilution lung water. Severinghaus et al. [146] achieved a 1% fall in transthoracic impedance for each 5% increase in indicator dilution lung water with the guard ring electrode configuration.

It is our opinion that current instrumentation technology is insufficient to allow transthoracic impedance measurements to achieve usefulness as a quantitative index of lung water content. The following problems are evident:

1. It has been generally conceded that it will be impossible to establish a normal range of transthoracic impedance values for a given electrode configuration. Interpersonal variation in chest geometry, and more critically, variation in subcutaneous fat and water content, doom comparison among individuals. The technique is therefore limited to examining trends in measured impedance, with each subject as his own control.

2. Electrode positioning and body surface contact are strong influences on transthoracic impedance. In all reported studies of impedance trends, the electrodes have been left in place through a series of measurements. Though some success has been claimed in obtaining reproducible measurements when the electrodes were precisely repositioned [153,157], it seems likely that repositioning artifacts limit the practicality of impedance measurements for detecting long-term trends in pulmonary water content.

3. It seems essential that in comparing serial measurements of transthoracic impedance, chest geometry should be rigorously controlled. Postural changes strongly influence measured impedance [146]. More important, the variation of transthoracic impedance with tidal breathing is of the same order as the changes induced by the most severe pulmonary edema. Making impedance measurements at end-tidal volume ignores the possibility of shifts in FRC during edema formation. It seems likely that a transthoracic impedance measurement without simultaneous determination of the volume of air contained in the lung is of little value in assessing pulmonary edema development.

4. Finally, there has been no claim that transthoracic measurements are sensitive enough to detect anything but gross pulmonary edema. Although the guard ring concept for decreasing the effect of current shunted around the thoracic wall seems promising, impedance measured at the body surface remains a quite insensitive indicator of moderate changes in pulmonary conductivity.

IV. Conclusions

And since the ideal of quantitative measurement has been to a great degree reached in both chemistry and physics, that ideal is held as the essential aim in biological investigations.

Walter B. Cannon [165]

Recognition that pulmonary edema in man probably occurs quite frequently, even in the absence of congestive heart failure, has lent a new sense of urgency to the development of reliable and simple methods of measuring lung water in vivo. Our critique is motivated in large part by the problems that have been experienced with each of the currently available techniques.

It is difficult to predict whether any of the procedures described will prove useful from a clinical point of view. It is with some reluctance that we must conclude that the detection of rales and changes in the chest x ray remain the most reliable signs of edema formation. Indeed it can be argued that more effort should be made to standardize the routine chest film; the precision with which regional fluid accumulation can be detected by the roentgenogram is unattainable with any of the more recently proposed techniques.

It is our feeling that, rather than simply trying to quantitate the amount of fluid within the lungs, methods should be developed for detecting alterations in the lung which may promote pulmonary edema, such as changes in pulmonary capillary or alveolar permeability. With such techniques it might be possible to alert the physician to the likelihood of a crisis before, rather than after, it has occurred.

Appendix

Derivation of $V_{EV,W}$ from Red Cell, Plasma, and Water Data

Consider the mass of red cell indicator M_R and plasma indicator M_P present within the lung following a prolonged infusion of these indicators at influx rates of I_R and I_P respectively:

$$M_R = I_R \bar{t}_R \tag{46}$$

$$M_P = I_P \bar{t}_P. \tag{47}$$

If a prolonged infusion of the red cell label results in a uniform distribution of label throughout the fraction of the vascular volume occupied by red cells V_R, then

$$M_R = [R] V_R$$

where [R] designates the steady state red cell activity. Since $I_R = [R](Hct)\dot{Q}$, Equation (47) can be divided by [R] to obtain

$$V_R = (Hct)\dot{Q}\bar{t}_R. \tag{48}$$

Similarly,

$$V_P = (1 - Hct)\dot{Q}\bar{t}_P.$$

Now

$$V_{R,W} = f_R V_R$$

$$V_{P,W} = f_P V_P$$

therefore

$$V_{B,W} = f_R Hct \dot{Q}\bar{t}_R + f_P (1 - Hct)\dot{Q}\bar{t}_P. \tag{49}$$

Knowledge of both $V_{T,W}$ and $V_{B,W}$ permits calculating $V_{EV,W}$:

$$V_{EV,W} = \dot{Q}\left\{[f_R Hct + f_P (1 - Hct)]\bar{t}_{THO} - f_R Hct \bar{t}_R - f_P (1 - Hct)\bar{t}_P\right\}. \tag{50}$$

Acknowledgment

The authors are grateful to Linda Gardner for her patient and expert secretarial support in the preparation of this manuscript.

References

1. N. C. Staub, Pulmonary Edema, *Physiol. Rev.,* **54**:678–811 (1974).
2. S. H. Burlacher, W. G. Banfield, and A. D. Bergner, Post-mortem pulmonary edema, *Yale J. Biol. and Med.,* **22**:565–575 (1950).
3. A. Hauge and G. Nicolaysen, Studies on transvascular fluid balance and capillary permeability in isolated lungs, *Bull. Physiopath. Resp.,* **7**:1197–1216 (1971).
4. P. K. M. Lunde and B. A. Waaler, Transvascular fluid balance in the lung, *J. Physiol.,* **205**:1–18 (1969).
5. R. Hughes, A. J. May, and J. G. Widdicombe, Mechanical factors in the formation of edema in perfused rabbits' lungs, *J. Physiol.,* **142**:292–305 (1958).

6. M. B. Visscher, F. J. Haddy, and G. Stephens, The physiology and pharmacology of lung edema, *Pharmacol. Rev.,* 8:389–434 (1956).

7. O. R. Levine, R. B. Mellins, and A. P. Fishman, Quantitative assessment of pulmonary edema, *Circ. Res.,* 17:414–426 (1965).

8. A. C. Guyton and A. W. Lindsey, Effect of elevated left atrial pressure and decreased plasma protein concentrations on the development of pulmonary edema, *Circ. Res.,* 7:649–657 (1959).

9. R. K. Lambert and H. Gremels, On the factors concerned in the production of pulmonary edema, *J. Physiol.,* 61:98–112 (1926).

10. G. S. M. Cowan, L. H. Edmunds, and A. J. Erdman, Analysis of weight gain in reimplanted dog lungs, *Surgical Forum,* 24:269–271 (1973).

11. R. B. Mellins, O. R. Levine, R. Skalak, and A. P. Fishman, Interstitial pressure of the lung, *Circ. Res.,* 24:197–212 (1969).

12. W. A. Murphy, D. M. Nicoloff, and E. W. Humphrey, Factors influencing the measurement of pulmonary extravascular water, *J. Surg. Res.,* 14:331–337 (1973).

13. N. E. O'Connor, J. M. Sheh, R. H. Bartlett, and H. Bass, The relation of extravascular water to gas exchange and pressures in pulmonary edema. In *Central Hemodynamics and Gas Exchange.* Edited by C. Guintini. Turin, Minerva Medica, 1971, pp. 207–222.

14. A. Hemingway, A method of chemical analysis of guinea pig lung for the factors involved in pulmonary edema, *J. Lab. and Clin. Med.,* 35:817–822 (1950).

15. M. L. Pearce, J. Yamashita, and J. Beazell, Measurement of pulmonary edema, *Circ. Res.,* 16:482–488 (1965).

16. W. H. Noble, J. Obdrzalek, and J. C. Kay, A new technique for measuring pulmonary edema, *J. Appl. Physiol.,* 34:508–512 (1973).

17. G. M. Turino, M. B. Pine, S. J. Shubrooks, and J. P. Carey, The volume of extravascular water of the lung in normal man and in disease, *Bull. Physiopath. Resp.,* 7:1161–1179 (1971).

18. Y. Kapanci, E. R. Weibel, H. P. Kaplan, and F. R. Robinson, Pathogenesis and reversibility of the pulmonary lesions of oxygen toxicity in monkeys. II. Ultrastructural and morphometric studies, *Lab. Invest.,* 20:101–118 (1969).

19. T. S. Cottrell, O. R. Levine, R. M. Senior, J. Wiener, D. Spiro, and A. P. Fishman, Electron microscopic alterations at the alveolar level in pulmonary edema, *Circ. Res.,* 21:783–797 (1967).

20. G. G. Pietra, J. P. Szidon, M. M. Leventhal, and A. P. Fishman, Hemoglobin as a tracer in hemodynamic pulmonary edema, *Science,* 166:1643–1646 (1969).

21. A. L. Cunningham and J. V. Hurley, Alpha-naphthyl thiourea induced pulmonary edema in the rat. A topographical and electron microscopic study, *J. Path.,* 106:25–35 (1972).

22. B. Kisch, Electron microscopy of the lungs in pulmonary edema and pneumonia. *Proceedings of the European Regional Conference on Electron Microscopy.* Vol. 2. Delft, 1960, pp. 900–902.

23. E. R. Weibel, Stereological principles for morphometry in electron microscopic cytology, *Int. Rev. Cytology,* **26**:235–302 (1969).
24. J. Gil, Methods for demonstration of interstitial and alveolar edema by electron microscopy. In *Central Hemodynamics and Gas Exchange.* Edited by C. Guintini. Turin, Minerva Medica, 1971, pp. 19–32.
25. E. H. Starling, On the absorption of fluids from the connective tissue spaces, *J. Physiol.,* **19**:312–326 (1895–6).
26. E. H. Starling, On the physiological factors involved in the casuation of dropsy, *Lancet,* **1**:1267–1270, 1331–1334 (1896).
27. G. E. Burch and W. A. Sodeman, The estimation of the subcutaneous tissue pressure by a direct method, *J. Clin. Invest.,* **16**:845–850 (1937).
28. H. S. Wells, J. B. Youmans, and D. G. Miller, Tissue pressure (intracutaneous, subcutaneous and intra-muscular) as related to venous pressure, capillary filtration and other factors, *J. Clin. Invest.,* **17**:489–499 (1938).
29. P. D. McMaster, The pressure and interstitial resistance prevailing in normal and edematous skin of animals and man, *J. Exp. Med.,* **84**:473–494 (1946).
30. A. C. Guyton, Pressure-volume relationships in the interstitial spaces, *Invest. Ophthamology,* **4**:1075–1084 (1965).
31. A. C. Guyton, Interstitial fluid pressure-volume relationships and their regulation. In *Circulatory and Respiratory Mass Transport.* A Ciba Foundation Symposium. Boston, Little, Brown, 1969, pp. 4–24.
32. C. A. Wiederhielm, J. W. Woodbury, S. Kirk, and R. F. Rushmer, Pulsatile pressures in the microcirculation of frog's mesentery, *Amer. J. Physiol.,* **207**:173–176 (1964).
33. C. A. Wiederhielm, The interstitial space and lymphatic pressure in the bat wing. In *The Pulmonary Circulation and Interstitial Space.* Edited by A. P. Fishman and H. H. Hecht. 1970, pp. 29–41.
34. C. A. Wiederhielm, Dynamics of transcapillary fluid exchange, *J. Gen. Physiol.,* **52**:29S–63S (1968).
35. A. C. Guyton, A concept of negative interstitial pressure based on pressures in implanted perforated capsules, *Circ. Res.,* **12**:399–414 (1963).
36. A. C. Guyton, Interstitial fluid pressure. II. Pressure-volume curves of interstitial space, *Circ. Res.,* **16**:452–460 (1965).
37. A. C. Guyton, K. Scheel, and D. Murphress, Interstitial fluid pressure. III. Its effect on resistance to tissue fluid mobility, *Circ. Res.,* **19**:412–419 (1966).
38. B. M. Meyer, A. Meyer, and A. C. Guyton, Interstitial fluid pressure. V. Negative pressure in the lung, *Circ. Res.,* **22**:263–271 (1968).
39. P. F. Scholander, A. R. Hargens, and S. L. Miller, Negative pressure in the interstitial fluid of animals, *Science,* **161**:321–328 (1968).
40. M. F. Warren and C. K. Drinker, The flow of lymph from the lungs of the dog, *Amer. J. Physiol.,* **136**:207–221 (1942).
41. N. C. Staub, The pathophysiology of pulmonary edema, *Human Path.,* **1**:419–432 (1970).

42. N. C. Staub, Pathogenesis of pulmonary edema. State of the Art, *Amer. Rev. Resp. Dis.*, **109**:358–372 (1974).
43. C. K. Drinker. *Pulmonary Edema and Inflammation.* Cambridge, Mass., Harvard University Press, 1945.
44. S. E. Leeds, H. N. Uhley, J. J. Sampson, and M. Friedman, A new method for measurement of lymph flow from the right duct in the dog, *Amer. J. Surgery*, **98**:211–216 (1959).
45. E. C. Meyer, Collection of pulmonary lymph in dogs, *J. Surg. Res.*, **8**:544–550 (1968).
46. F. C. Courtice, Lymph flow in the lungs, *Brit. Med. Bull.*, **19**:76–79 (1963).
47. E. C. Meyer, E. A. M. Dominguez, and K. G. Bensch, Pulmonary lymphatic and blood absorption of albumin from alveoli, *Lab. Invest.*, **20**:1–8 (1969).
48. R. N. Pilon and D. A. Bittar, The effect of positive end-expiratory pressure on thoracic-duct lymph flow during controlled ventilation in anesthetized dogs, *Anesthesia*, **39**:607–612 (1973).
49. E. C. Meyer and R. Ottaviano, Pulmonary collateral lymph flow: Detection using lymph oxygen tensions, *J. Appl. Physiol.*, **32**:806–811 (1972).
50. A. P. Fishman, Pulmonary edema: The water exchanging function of the lung, *Circulation*, **46**:390–408 (1972).
51. L. G. Rigler and E. L. Surprenant, Pulmonary edema, *Seminars in Roentgenology*, **2**:33–48 (1967).
52. R. G. Grainger, Interstitial pulmonary edema and its radiological diagnosis, *Brit. J. Radiology*, **31**:201–217 (1958).
53. R. B. Logue, J. V. Rogers, and B. B. Gay, Subtle roentgenographic signs of left heart failure, *Amer. Heart J.*, **65**:464–473 (1963).
54. F. G. Fleischner, The butterfly pattern of acute pulmonary edema, *Amer. J. Cardiology*, **20**:39–46 (1967).
55. D. C. Gleason and R. E. Steiner, The lateral roentgenogram in pulmonary edema, *Amer. J. Roentgenology*, **98**:279–290 (1966).
56. C. D. Cook, J. Mead, G. L. Schreiner, N. R. Frank, and J. M. Craig, Pulmonary mechanics during induced pulmonary edema in anesthetized dogs, *J. Appl. Physiol.*, **14**:177–186 (1969).
57. R. Hughes, A. J. May, and J. G. Widdicombe, The effect of pulmonary congestion and edema on lung compliance, *J. Physiol.*, **142**:306–313 (1958).
58. R. H. Rech and H. L. Borison, Vagotomy-induced pulmonary edema in the guinea pig, *Amer. J. Physiol.*, **202**:499–504 (1962).
59. M. L. Pearce and M. J. Wong, Interstitial pressure and compliance changes in experimental pulmonary edema in the dog. In *Central Hemodynamics and Gas Exchange.* Edited by C. Guintini. Turin, Minerva Medica, 1971, pp. 181–190.
60. J. T. Sharp, G. T. Griffith, I. L. Bunnell, and D. G. Greene, Ventilatory mechanics in pulmonary edema in man, *J. Clin. Invest.*, **37**:111–117 (1958).
61. J. Mead, Mechanical properties of lungs, *Physiol. Rev.*, **41**:281–330 (1961).

62. N. C. Staub, H. Nagano, and M. L. Pearce, Pulmonary edema in dogs, especially the sequence of fluid accumulation in lungs, *J. Appl. Physiol.*, 22: 227–240 (1967).

63. H. P. Kaplan, F. R. Robinson, Y. Kapanci, and E. R. Weibel, Pathogenesis and reversibility of the pulmonary lesions of oxygen toxicity in monkeys, *Lab. Invest.*, 20:94–100 (1969).

64. M. H. Williams, Effect of ANTU-induced pulmonary edema on the alveolar-arterial oxygen pressure gradient in dogs, *Amer. J. Physiol.*, 174:84–86 (1953).

65. S. I. Said, J. W. Longacher, R. K. Davis, C. M. Banerjee, W. M. Davis, and W. J. Wooddell, Pulmonary gas exchange during induction of pulmonary edema in anesthetized dogs, *J. Appl. Physiol.*, 19:403–407 (1964).

66. N. Freinkel, G. E. Schreiner, and J. W. Athens, A new method for measuring transcapillary exchanges: The transfer of salt and water in the lesser circulation of man, *J. Clin. Invest.*, 31:629 (1952).

67. L. Ramsey, W. Puckett, A. Jose, and W. Lacy, Comparison of slope and mean transit time volumes by use of diffusible and non-diffusible indicators, *Trans. Assoc. Amer. Physicians*, 74:280–289 (1961).

68. F. P. Chinard, T. Enns, and M. F. Nolan, Indicator-dilution studies with "diffusible" indicator, *Circ. Res.*, 10:473–490 (1962).

69. F. P. Chinard, T. Enns, and M. F. Nolan, Pulmonary extravascular volumes from transit time and slope data, *J. Appl. Physiol.*, 17:179–183 (1962).

70. F. P. Chinard and T. Enns, Transcapillary pulmonary exchange of water in the dog, *Amer. J. Physiol.*, 178:197–202 (1954).

71. P. Meier and K. L. Zierler, On the theory of the indicator-dilution method for measurement of blood flow and volume, *J. Appl. Physiol.*, 6:731–744 (1954).

72. P. N. Yu, Lung water in congestive heart failure, *Mod. Cardiovasc. Dis.*, 40: 27–32 (1971).

73. R. M. McCredie, The measurement of lung water. *Progress in Cardiology*. Vol. 3. Edited by P. N. Yu and J. F. Goodwin. Philadelphia, Lea and Febiger, 1974, pp. 331–349.

74. C. A. Goresky, R. F. P. Cronin, and B. E. Wangel, Indicator dilution measurements of extravascular water in the lungs, *J. Clin. Invest.*, 48:487–501 (1969).

75. F. P. Chinard, W. Perl, R. M. Effros, R. Dumphys, and A. C. DeLea, Lung water: Physiological and clinical significance, *Trans. Amer. Clin. Climat. Assoc.*, 81:85–97 (1969).

76. L. E. Bayliss, The rheology of blood. *Handbook of Physiology*. Section 2, Vol. 1. Edited by W. F. Hamilton and P. Dow. Washington, D.C., American Physiological Society, 1960, p. 137.

77. C. A. Goresky, G. G. Bach, and B. E. Nadeau, Red cell carriage of label, *Circ. Res.*, 36:328–351 (1975).

78. W. Perl, Red cell permeability effect on the mean transit time of an indicator transported through an organ by red cells and plasma, *Circ. Res.*, 36: 352–357 (1975).

79. L. S. Lillienfield, E. D. Freis, E. A. Partenope, and A. J. Morowitz, Trans-
     capillary migration of heavy water and ion in the pulmonary circulation of
     normal subjects and patients with congestive heart failure, *J. Clin. Invest.*,
     34:1–8 (1955).

80. P. Anthonisen and C. Crone, Transcapillary migration of ethyl alcohol in
     the pulmonary circulation: Method for determining the water content of
     the lungs in vivo, *Acta Physiol. Scand.*, **37**:370–379 (1956).

81. C. A. Goresky, A linear method for determining liver sinusoidal and extra-
     vascular volumes, *Amer. J. Physiol.*, **204**:626–640 (1963).

82. S. S. Kety and C. F. Schmidt, The determination of cerebral blood flow in
     man by use of nitrous oxide in low concentrations, *Amer. J. Physiol.*, **143**:
     53–66 (1945).

83. S. S. Kety, Measurement of regional circulation by the local clearance of
     radioactive sodium, *Amer. Heart J.*, **38**:321–328 (1949).

84. R. M. Effros, B. Haider, P. O. Ettinger, S. S. Ahmed, H. A. Oldewurtel, K.
     Marold, and T. J. Regan, In vivo myocardial cell pH in the dog. Response
     to ischemia and infusion of alkali, *J. Clin. Invest.*, **55**:1100–1110 (1975).

85. R. M. Effros and F. P. Chinard, The in vivo pH of the extravascular space
     of the lung, *J. Clin. Invest.*, **48**:1983–1996 (1969).

86. C. V. Sheppard, Catheter artifacts in indicator dilution experiments, *Fed.
     Proc.*, **16**:118 (1957).

87. J. M. Gonzalez-Fernandez, R. J. Chessman, and E. H. Wood, Mathematical
     analysis for the recovery of a dye-dilution curve distorted by the sampling-
     recording system, *Physiologist*, **2**:146 (1959).

88. W. H. Noble and J. W. Severinghaus, Thermal and conductivity dilution
     curves for rapid quantitation of pulmonary edema, *J. Appl. Physiol.*, **32**:
     770–775 (1972).

89. W. Ganz and H. J. C. Swan, Measurement of blood flow by the thermo-
     dilution technique. In *Dye Curves: The Theory and Practice of Indicator
     Dilution.* Edited by D. A. Bloomfield. Baltimore, University Park Press,
     1974, pp. 245–266.

90. L. C. Clark, Jr., and L. M. Bargeron, Jr., Left-to-right shunt detection by
     an intravascular electrode with hydrogen as an indicator, *Science*, **130**:
     709–710 (1959).

91. M. L. Polanyi, Fiberoptics in cardiac catheterization. I. Theoretical Con-
     siderations. In *Dye Curves: The Theory and Practice of Indicator Dilu-
     tion.* Edited by D. A. Bloomfield. Baltimore, University Park Press, 1974,
     pp. 267–283.

92. P. F. Hugenholtz, P. D. Verdoaco, and G. T. Meister, Fiberoptics in cardiac
     catheterization. II. Practical Applications. In *Dye Curves: The Theory
     and Practice of Indicator Dilution.* Edited by D. A. Bloomfield. Balti-
     more, University Park Press, 1974, pp. 285–311.

93. C. V. Sheppard, M. P. Jones, and B. L. Couch, Effects of catheter sampling
     on the slope of indicator-dilution curves, mean concentration versus mean
     flux of outflowing dye, *Circ. Res.*, **7**:895–906 (1959).

94. G. W. Roberts, K. B. Larson, and E. E. Spaeth, The interpretation of mean transit time measurements for multiphase tissue systems, *J. Theor. Biol.*, **39**:447–475 (1973).

95. F. P. Chinard, W. Perl, and F. Silverman, Permeability of dog lung endothelium to sodium, diols and amides, *Amer. J. Physiol.*, in press.

96. J. B. West, Topographical distribution of blood flow in the lung. In *Handbook of Physiology, Respiration.* Section 3, Vol. 2. Washington, D.C., American Physiological Society, 1965, pp. 1437–1451.

97. O. R. Levine, R. B. Mellins, and R. M. Senior, Extravascular lung water and distribution of pulmonary blood flow in the dog, *J. Appl. Physiol.*, **28**:166–171 (1970).

98. R. B. Luepker, B. Liander, M. Korsgren, and E. Varnauskas, Pulmonary intravascular and extravascular fluid volumes in exercising cardiac patients, *Circulation*, **44**:620–637 (1971).

99. R. Tancredi, P. Caldini, M. Shanoff, S. Permutt, and K. Zierler, The pulmonary microcirculation evaluated by tracer dilution techniques, In *Cardiovascular Nuclear Medicine.* Edited by H. W. Strauss, B. Pitt, A. E. James, Jr. St. Louis, C. V. Mosby Company, 1974, pp. 255–260.

100. K. L. Zierler, Circulation times and the theory of indicator dilution methods for determining blood flow and volume. In *Handbook of Physiology, Circulation.* Vol. 1. Washington, D.C., American Physiological Society, 1965, pp. 585–615.

101. A. Maseri, P. Caldini, S. Permutt, and K. L. Zierler, Frequency function in transit times through dog circulation, *Circ. Res.*, **5**:527–543 (1970).

102. J. Gamel, W. F. Rousseau, C. B. Kalholi, and E. Meel, Pitfalls in digital computation of the impulse response of vascular beds from indicator-dilution curves, *Circ. Res.*, **32**:516–523 (1973).

103. C. Guintini, Theoretical considerations on the measure of pulmonary blood volume and extravascular lung water in man, *Bull. Physiopath. Respir.* (Nancy), **7**:1125–1160 (1971).

104. F. P. Chinard, G. H. Vosburgh, and T. Enns, Transcapillary exchange of water and of other substances in certain organs of the dog, *Amer. J. Physiol.*, **183**:221–234 (1955).

105. K. L. Brigham, L. H. Ramsey, J. D. Snell, and M. Cullen, III., On defining the pulmonary extravascular water volume, *Circ. Res.*, **29**:385–397 (1971).

106. M. G. Weidner, Jr., A. O. Burford, R. A. Daniel, Jr., and R. L. Light, Autonomic control of the pulmonary vascular bed. II. Detection of pulmonary edema with sodium[22], *Surg. Forum*, **6**:275–278 (1956).

107. J. D. Cooper, N. L. McCullogh, and E. Lowenstein, Determination of pulmonary extravascular water using oxygen 15-labeled water, *J. Appl. Physiol.*, **33**:842–845 (1972).

108. N. A. Lassen, Capillary diffusion capacity of sodium studied by the clearances of Na^{24} and Xe^{133} from hyperemic skeletal muscle in man, *Scand. J. Clin. Lab. Invest.*, **19** (Suppl 99):24–26 (1967).

109.   N. A. Lassen and D. H. Ingvar, Radioisotope assessment of regional cere-
       bral blood flow. In *Progress in Nuclear Medicine*. Vol. 1. Edited by E. J.
       Polchen and V. R. McCready. Basel Karger, New York, 1971, p. 376–
       409.
110.   K. L. Zierler, Equations for measuring blood flow by external monitoring
       of radioisotopes, *Circ. Res.*, 16:309–321 (1965).
111.   J. E. Worsham, Measurement of blood flow by external monitoring of
       isotopes, *J. Appl. Physiol.*, 21:1653–1654 (1966).
112.   B. M. Lewis, L. Sokoloff, R. L. Wechsler, W. B. Wentz, and S. S. Kety, A
       method for the continuous measurement of cerebral blood flow in man
       by means of radioactive krypton (Kr 79), *J. Clin. Invest.*, 39:707–716
       (1960).
113.   P.-E. E. Bergner, Exchangeable mass: Determination without the assump-
       tion of isotopic equilibrium, *Science,* 19:1048–1050 (1965).
114.   W. Perl, R. M. Effros, and F. P. Chinard, The indicator equivalence
       theorem for input rates and regional masses in multi-inlet steady state
       systems, *J. Thoret. Biol.*, 25:297–316 (1969).
115.   W. Perl, Stimulus-response method for flows and volumes in slightly per-
       turbed constant parameter systems, *Bull. Math. Biophysics,* 33:225–233
       (1971).
116.   W. Perl, N. A. Lassen, and R. M. Effros, Matrix proof of flow volume and
       mean transit time theorems for regional and compartmental systems,
       Bull. Math. Biophysics, in press.
117.   A. B. Gorin, J. Weidner, and N. C. Staub, Non-invasive measurement of
       altered protein permeability in lungs of sheep, *Amer. Rev. Resp. Div.,*
       111:941 (1975).
118.   K. Wasserman, S. Kolodny, and D. E. Johnson, Measurement of extra-
       vascular serum albumin in the lung, **in preparation.**
119.   E. D. Robin, C. E. Cross, and R. Zelis, Medical progress, pulmonary
       edema, *N. E. J. Med.,* 288:292–304 (1973).
120.   K. Wasserman and H. S. Mayerson, Dynamics of lymph and plasma pro-
       tein exchange, *Cardiologia,* 21:296–307 (1952).
121.   A. Krogh and J. Lindhard, Measurements of the blood flow through the
       lungs of man, *Scand. Arch. Physiol.,* 27:100–125 (1912).
122.   S. Kety, The theory and applications of the exchange of inert gas at the
       lungs and tissues, *Pharmacol. Rev.,* 3:1–41 (1951).
123.   L. Cander and R. E. Forster, Determination of pulmonary parenchymal
       tissue volume and pulmonary capillary blood flow in man, *J. Appl. Phys-
       iol.,* 14:541–551 (1959).
124.   K. Wasserman and J. H. Comroe, A method for estimating instantaneous
       pulmonary capillary blood flow in man, *J. Clin. Invest.,* 41:401–410
       (1962).
125.   L. Cander, Solubility of inert gases in human lung tissue, *J. Appl. Phys-
       iol.,* 14:538–540 (1959).
126.   M. A. Sackner, K. A. Feisal, and A. B. DuBois, Determination of tissue

volume and carbon dioxide dissociation slope of the lungs in man, *J. Appl. Physiol.*, **19**:374–380 (1964).

127. C. E. Vreim and N. C. Staub, Indirect and direct pulmonary capillary blood volume in anesthetized open-thorax cats, *J. Appl. Physiol.*, **34**: 452–459 (1973).

128. F. J. W. Roughton and R. E. Forster, Relative importance of diffusion and chemical reaction rates in determining rate of exchange of gases in the human lung, with special reference to true diffusing capacity of pulmonary membrane and volume of blood in the lung capillary, *J. Appl. Physiol.*, **11**:290–302 (1957).

129. J. Butler, Measurement of cardiac output using soluble gases. In *Handbook of Physiology*. Section 3, Respiration. Vol. 2. Washington, D.C., American Physiological Society, 1965, pp. 1489–1503.

130. A. A. Affifi and S. P. Azen. *Statistical Analysis: A Computer-Oriented Approach.* New York, Academic Press, 1972.

131. D. V. Huntsberger. *Elements of Statistical Inference.* Boston, Allyn and Bacon, 1961.

132. A. P. Fishman, Dynamics of the pulmonary circulation. In *Handbook of Physiology*. Circulation. Vol. 3. Washington, D.C., American Physiological Society, 1965, pp. 1667–1731.

133. E. P. Sharpey-Shafer, Effect of respiratory acts on the circulation. In *Handbook of Physiology*. Circulation. Vol. 3. Washington, D.C., American Physiological Society, 1965, pp. 1875–1886.

134. A. C. Guyton. *Circulatory Physiology: Cardiac Output and Its Regulation.* Philadelphia, W. B. Saunders, 1963, pp. 427–435.

135. A. Naimark and K. Wasserman, The effect of posture on pulmonary capillary blood flow in man, *J. Clin. Invest.*, **41**:949–954 (1962).

136. J. B. West, Ventilation/Blood Flow and Gas Exchange. Oxford, Blackwell, 1970.

137. K. A. Feisal, J. Soni, and A. B. DuBois, Pulmonary arterial circulation time, pulmonary arterial blood volume and the ratio of gas to tissue volume in the lungs of dogs, *J. Clin. Invest.*, **41**:390–400 (1962).

138. M. A. Sackner, N. Atkins, J. Goldberg, N. Segal, S. Zarzecki, and A. Warner, Pulmonary arterial blood volume and tissue volume in man and dog, *Circ. Res.*, **34**:761–769 (1974).

139. M. A. Sackner, D. Greeneltch, M. S. Neiman, S. Epstein, and N. Atkins, Diffusing capacity, membrane diffusing capacity, capillary blood volume, pulmonary tissue volume and cardiac output measured by rebreathing technique, *Amer. Rev. Resp. Dis.*, **111**:157–165 (1975).

140. B. M. Lewis, T. H. Lin, E. Noe, and E. J. Hayford-Welsing, The measurement of pulmonary diffusing capacity for carbon monoxide by a rebreathing technique, *J. Clin. Invest.*, **38**:2073–2086 (1959).

141. C. E. Cross, H. Gong, C. J. Kurpershoek, J. E. Gillepsie, and R. W. Hyde, Alterations in distribution of blood flow to the lung's diffusion surfaces during exercise, *J. Clin. Invest.*, **52**:414–421 (1973).

142. R. L. Johnson, W. S. Spicer, J. M. Bishop, and R. E. Forster, Pulmonary capillary blood volume, flow and diffusing capacity during exercise, *J. Appl. Physiol.*, **15**:893–902 (1960).

143. F. I. Glauser, A. F. Wilson, M. Hoshiko, M. Watanabe, and J. Davis, Pulmonary parenchymal tissue (V_t) changes in pulmonary edema, *J. Appl. Physiol.*, **36**:648–652 (1974).

144. L. A. Geddes, H. E. Hoff, D. M. Hickman, and A. G. Moore, The impedance pneumograph, *Aerospace Med.*, **33**:28–33 (1962).

145. E. Pasquali, Problems in impedance pneumography: Electrical characteristics of skin and lung tissue, *Med. Biol. Eng.*, **5**:249–258 (1967).

146. J. W. Severinghaus, C. Catron, and W. Noble, A focusing electrode bridge for unilateral lung resistance, *J. Appl. Physiol.*, **32**:526–530 (1972).

147. J. Nyboer. *Electrical Impedance Plethysmography.* 2nd ed. Springfield, Ill., Charles C Thomas, 1970.

148. D. A. Witsoe and E. Kinnen, Electrical resistivity of lung at 100 kHz, *Med. Biol. Eng.*, **5**:239–248 (1967).

149. T. Olsson, W. Daily, and L. Victorin, Transthoracic impedance. I. Theoretical considerations and technical approach, *Acta Pediat. Scand.*, **207**: 15–27 (1970).

150. S. Rush, J. A. Abildskov, and R. McFee, Resistivity of body tissue at low frequencies, *Circ. Res.*, **12**:40–50 (1963).

151. L. A. Geddes and L. E. Baker, The specific resistance of biological material—a compendium of data for the biomedical engineer and physiologist, *Med. Biol. Eng.*, **5**:271–293 (1967).

152. W. L. Cooley, The parameters of transthoracic electrical conduction, *Ann. N.Y. Acad. Sci.*, **170**:702–713 (1970).

153. W. L. Cooley and R. L. Longini, A new design for an impedance pneumograph, *J. Appl. Physiol.*, **25**:429–432 (1968).

154. L. E. Baker and L. A. Geddes, Transthoracic current paths in impedance spirometry, *Proceedings of the Symposium on Biomedical Engineering,* **1**:181–186 (1966).

155. L. Victorin, W. Daily, and T. Olsson, Transthoracic impedance. III. Methodological studies in newborn infants, *Acta Pediat. Scand.*, **207**:37–47 (1970).

156. M. Pomerantz, F. Delgado, and B. Eiseman, Clinical evaluation of transthoracic electrical impedance as a guide to intrathoracic fluid volumes, *Ann. Surg.*, **171**:686–694 (1970).

157. J. M. Van de Water, B. E. Mount, J. R. Barela, R. Schuster, and F. S. Leacock, Monitoring the chest with impedance, *Chest,* **64**:597–603 (1973).

158. R. V. Leupker, J. R. Michael, and J. R. Warbasse, Transthoracic electrical impedance: Quantitative evaluation of a non-invasive measure of thoracic fluid volume, *Amer. Heart J.*, **85**:83–93 (1973).

159. W. G. Kubicek, J. N. Karnegis, R. P. Patterson, D. A. Witsoe, and R. H. Mattson, Development and evaluation of an impedance cardiac output system, *Aerospace Med.*, **37**:1208–1212 (1966).

160. M. Graham, Guard ring use in physiological measurements, *IEEE Trans. Biomed. Eng.*, **12**:197–198 (1965).

161. M. Pomerantz, R. Baumgartner, J. Lauridson, and B. Eiseman, Transthoracic electrical impedance for the early detection of pulmonary edema, *Surgery*, **66**:260–268 (1969).

162. I. Kjellmer, T. Olsson, and L. Victorin, Transthoracic impedance. II. Experimental evaluation of the method in the cat, *Acta Pediat. Scand.*, **207**: 29–35 (1970).

163. L. Victorin and T. Olsson, Transthoracic impedance. IV. Studies of the infant during the first two hours of life, *Acta Pediat. Scand.*, **207**:49–56 (1970).

164. W. Daily, T. Olsson, and L. Victorin, Transthoracic impedance: V. Effects of early and late clamping of the umbilical cord with special reference to the ratio air-to-blood during respiration, *Acta Pediat. Scand.*, **207**:57–72 (1970).

165. W. B. Cannon. *The Way of an Investigator.* New York, Hafner, 1968, p. 35.

12

Heart Failure and Hemodynamic Pulmonary Edema

ALDO A. LUISADA

The Chicago Medical School, University of Health Sciences
and
Oak Forest Hospital
Oak Forest, Illinois

I. Introduction

A. Forms of Edema

Pulmonary edema can be either acute or chronic. Acute pulmonary edema is a paroxysmal phenomenon that starts in the perihilar regions, expands in a butterflylike fashion, and may threaten life because of its severe effects on the circulatory system and the mechanical blocking of the small airways caused by the foam. The "butterfly" type of acute pulmonary edema, revealed in man by x-ray studies, represents the early stage of perivascular edema. Chronic pulmonary edema is a long-standing phenomenon of mild or medium severity; it usually predominates at the bases of the lungs, being influenced by gravity, as revealed by both physical examination and x rays.

B. Heart Failure and Hemodynamic Imbalance

Heart failure is absolute if the heart has actually reduced its work; it is relative if the heart maintains or increases its work but is inadequate for the high requirements of the tissues. Acute heart failure is due to sudden, primary or secondary, disturbance of the heart. The resulting clinical picture resembles that of shock, characterized by signs of arterial depletion. It often ends in "cardiogenic shock." Subacute or chronic heart failure, on the contrary, is mostly revealed by signs and symptoms of congestion of the venous side of the cardiovascular system.

Circulatory failure occurs when the blood flow in the systemic capillaries is not adequate for the needs of the tissues. It may be absolute (when there is actual inadequacy) or relative (when the inadequacy exists only because the needs are increased). Circulatory failure may occur either because there is a reduction of the circulating blood volume or because the capacity of the circulatory system is increased (vasodilation). In both cases, reduced venous return is responsible for the failure.

A third type of reduction of the effective circulating blood volume is caused by one or the other of:

1. Valve stenosis. Not sufficiently compensated for by increased effort of one of the cardiac chambers (the most typical are aortic or mitral stenosis).
2. Inadequacy of left ventricular filling. Caused by constriction or restriction of the ventricular wall (constrictive pericarditis, endocardial fibroelastosis, myocardial fibrosis).

Left ventricular failure has been defined as a decrease in the ratio between venous return and cardiac output. This discrepancy is, of course, only temporary. After a brief stage, two different possibilities exist:

1. The left ventricle increases in size due to a rise of its end-diastolic pressure, which also increases the pressure in the left atrium and the pulmonary vessels. Increase of pulmonary capillary pressure leads to distension of the (usually) closed vessels and to an increase in pulmonary blood volume. This type of failure is accompanied by dyspnea and may be followed by pulmonary edema. Cardiac output usually decreases but may remain adequate.
2. The left ventricle is normal in size and left atrial pressure is not increased. In this eventuality (most commonly found after strong digitalization) there is no tendency to pulmonary congestion. On the other hand, cardiac output is decreased.

It should be emphasized that so far no satisfactory, all-encompassing definition of heart failure has been developed. A few examples will explain this. If we accept that every time the left ventricle is enlarged there is left ventricular failure, then some cases with aortic insufficiency or patent ductus would automatically qualify in spite of an efficient myocardium and an adequate cardiac output. If we accept that every time the left ventricular diastolic pressure is elevated there is heart failure, then we should include cases of constrictive pericarditis, myocardial fibrosis or amyloidosis, or endocardial fibroelastosis, even if the left ventricular contraction is still adequate for the needs of the tissues. If we extend this concept to left atrial pressure, then we additionally should consider many patients with mitral stenosis as having left heart failure, a fact that is only occasionally true and for a different reason. One might claim that in all such cases there is *circulatory failure,* but a better term would be *circulatory imbalance.*

Among the possible causes of an increased left ventricular diastolic pressure is a functional mechanism that will be discussed later. It is due to extreme sympathetic stimulation plus action of large amounts of catecholamines. These seem to decrease the compliance of the left ventricular wall and cause an acute elevation of the left ventricular end-diastolic pressure.

C. Effects of Elevated Left Ventricular Pressure on the Lung Capillaries

High left ventricular diastolic pressure is immediately followed by increased left atrial pressure, a fact that will maintain the circulation in spite of a different pressure level. High left atrial pressure will cause an increased pressure in the pulmonary veins and capillaries. Of course, this can occur only if the right ventricle automatically increases its work, i.e. increases its systolic pressure, and as a result augments the mean pulmonary arterial pressure. Again, this will be possible only if there is an adequate venous return. Thus, an elevated pulmonary capillary pressure may be the result of any increase in the resistance on the left side of the circulation, whether this is in the pulmonary veins (diffuse contraction or compression), in the left atrium (mitral stenosis, left atrial myxoma, etc.), or in the left ventricle (elevation of left ventricular diastolic pressure through any mechanism including ventricular compression, restriction, or failure).

II. The Pulmonary Circulation

A. General Characteristics

The characteristics of the pulmonary circulation have been gradually outlined through the studies of the last fifty years, especially by Starling [1],

Cameron [2], and Spector [3]. The lungs can be considered as consisting of a gigantic, though thin, membrane that permits diffusion of respiratory gases. In close contact with this membrane is an extensive capillary network of 100 to 140 m^2, in which blood and air are separated by only an average of 1.4 μm. When the subject is at rest or is engaged in mild exercise, many capillaries are closed. They open only in severe exertion or emergency situations so that the enlarged pulmonary vascular bed becomes available as a "blood depot."

In man at rest, one-twentieth of the total lung surface is sufficient to maintain normal oxygenation of the blood. This ensures a great margin of safety for emergency or stressful situations. At rest, contraction of the heart expels an average output of 6 to 8 liters/min or 2 to 4 liters/(min × m^2 of body surface). This blood flows through the pulmonary artery at a pressure of 18 to 25 mmHg in systole with a mean pressure of 10 to 12 mmHg. Passage through the lungs takes about 3 sec, less than a third of which is spent in the capillaries. The velocity of flow varies according, not only to the vascular surface area of the lungs, but also to the position of the patient. It is slower at the bases in the sitting and standing positions; there is also an increase in pressure in the capillaries of the dependent areas.

The normal pulmonary capillary pressure is intermediate between the mean pulmonary arterial pressure (10 to 12 mmHg) and the mean pulmonary venous pressure (7 to 8 mmHg). Probably an average of 9 to 10 mmHg is the correct estimate, but it should be noted that there is a difference in both pressure and flow between systole and diastole.*

Any increase of the mean diastolic pressure of the left ventricle (4 to 6 mmHg in normal subjects) would cause an increase of the left atrial, pulmonary venous, pulmonary capillary, and pulmonary arterial pressures, so that flow would continue unimpeded as a result of the increased pumping action of the right ventricle. The resistance of the pulmonary arterioles and of the pulmonary venules is normally very low.

The colloid osmotic pressure of the pulmonary capillary blood is similar to the colloid osmotic pressure of the blood in general, and has been considered to be between 18 and 25 mmHg.

As transudation through the capillary membranes is regulated by the balance between the colloid osmotic and the hydrostatic capillary pressures, retention of fluid within the capillaries is assured, in spite of the subatmospheric (or "negative") intrapleural pressure that varies around a mean of 5 cm H$_2$O and that would favor transudation from the capillaries.

---

*This pressure is measured in all experimental and clinical laboratories in reference to a zero level represented by the level of the right atrium.

An increase of venous return to the right heart does not markedly affect the pressure of the pulmonary capillaries since there is opening of "reserve" capillaries and also reflex increase of heart rate and cardiac output. This is true, however, only if the structure and function of the heart are normal. If there is any structural narrowing (mitral valve stenosis), if the left ventricular wall is constricted or restricted, if this wall is either weakened (left ventricular failure) or less compliant (to be described)—then an increased return will cause an increase of pulmonary capillary pressure as soon as the reserve capillaries are filled.

It has been stated that the lungs can accommodate about twice their normal blood volume without an increase in capillary pressure. Increased venous return usually would cause a pressure rise only if it is more than doubled. On the other hand, if there is any resistance on the left side (inadequate increase in function of the left ventricle, decreased compliance of left ventricular wall, mitral block), then even a moderate increase in venous return can effectively raise the pulmonary capillary pressure.

The functional significance of the pulmonary veins is still debated. The pulmonary venous resistance is 20 to 30% of the total pulmonary vascular resistance, and is probably similar to the pulmonary arterial resistance, thus giving stability to the pulmonary circulation. The resistance of the pulmonary veins increases more than resistance of the pulmonary arteries under the action of histamine [4,5]. Eliakim and Aviado [6] observed an increase of pulmonary venous resistance following the administration of acetylcholine, angiotensin, histamine, and ATP. However, if constriction was first induced by serotonin, these drugs caused venous dilatation.

Diffuse pulmonary venoconstriction has been reported in the pulmonary edema caused by high altitude, alloxan, and inhalation of toxic gases or respiratory burns, as well as in pulmonary embolism, and is also accepted as one of the possible consequences of mitral stenosis by Braun and Stern [7].

B. Capillary Dilatation as a Cause of Increased Transudation

Severe dilatation of the capillaries of the lungs occurs only when the reserve capillaries are already open through increase of flow or pressure. The most significant dilatation is that caused by an increase in capillary pressure because two factors will then operate: (1) a distension of the capillary wall with thinning of the structures; (2) a pressure level that will become higher than that of the colloid osmotic pressure of the blood. When this happens, "permeability" may increase and more protein molecules may escape from the bloodstream. Increased permeability is a phenomenon that takes place in the capillary wall. It causes increased fluid filtration in the interstitial spaces. Then, increase of lymphatic flow and increased tissue pressure will both take place. If the lymphatic flow is unable to drain all or most of the fluid, this will exert a pressure on the alveolar membranes that will be sufficient for causing transudation into the airspaces. The penetration of these molecules was attributed in the past to "dilatation of the pores." More recent studies with the electron microscope, however, have suggested an active process, similar to secretion [8]. Whenever blood cells pass into the alveoli, it is likely that actual rupture of some point of the capillary wall has occurred.

C.   Compensatory Mechanisms Decreasing Pulmonary Capillary Pressure

Several mechanisms have been described that tend to decrease the elevation of pulmonary capillary pressure or its effects. The first is the increased activity of the lymphatic circulation that may be able to drain large amounts of fluid; the second is a dilatation of the existing anastomoses between pulmonary and bronchial veins;* the third (operating only in chronic conditions) is a thickening of the capillary wall.†

D.   Collateral Factors Favoring or Decreasing Pulmonary Edema

Several factors may favor, aggravate, decrease, or complicate pulmonary edema.

Hypoproteinemia

When the blood has a colloid osmotic pressure lower than normal, fluid may escape from the capillaries in the presence of a slightly raised, or even normal, capillary pressure. This factor is so important that a decrease in serum protein

---

*The main bronchial veins are tributaries of the azygos vein and therefore their blood should be drained into the superior cava. There has been speculation that in normal conditions only about one-half of this blood follows such a course while the rest goes into the pulmonary veins. However, whenever the pulmonary venous pressure reaches levels of 50 to 80 mmHg, it is likely that a reversal of flow will occur so that a certain amount of pulmonary venous blood will enter the systemic venous circulation where the pressure is only 3 to 4 mmHg.

†Electron microscopy has revealed definite changes of the basal membrane of the pulmonary capillaries in cases of severe mitral stenosis. In addition, thickening and alteration of the interstitial spaces were also noted.

concentration to 50% of normal would allow pulmonary edema to occur with a capillary pressure of 11 mmHg instead of 25. If this edema occurs only in the lungs, local factors, not occurring in other organs, must be present. Hypoproteinemia can be found in clinical states of malnutrition, chronic lipoid nephrosis, and certain hepatic diseases. More acute hemodilution can occur in postoperative states if a too abundant infusion of physiologic glucose solution is given in order to prevent shock.

Membrane Damage

Inhalation of toxic gases has been thought to cause a direct lesion of the alveolar membranes, and through close proximity, possibly also of capillary membranes. This would greatly favor exudation of plasma from the capillaries into the airspaces.

Hypoxia

It has been stated in the past that hypoxia increases the permeability of the pulmonary capillaries. More recent studies have demonstrated the occurrence of pulmonary arteriolar constriction. If this occurs in selected areas, flow would increase in other areas, thus favoring edema in these other areas. Constriction of the pulmonary venules would, more than constriction of the arterioles, increase the pressure in the capillaries and thus favor pulmonary edema. This has been considered one of the possible causes of high altitude pulmonary edema. In addition, one should always keep in mind that cerebral hypoxia would stimulate the sympathoadrenal system, causing severe vascular and cardiac alterations.

Effect of Edemogenic Substances on Permeability

It has been postulated that liberation of histamine or serotonin in the lungs might cause or favor pulmonary edema. This fact has not been conclusively demonstrated, even though indirect evidence has been found, including a useful preventive or therapeutic effect of "antihistamines." While such a chemical action should still be discussed in several experimental and clinical situations, it is obvious that its most likely action would occur in anaphylactic shock and possibly in certain inflammatory states of the lungs.

Infectious or Infected Pulmonary Edema

Infectious pulmonary edema is a chronic state that is often found in the areas that surround zones of pneumonitis, bronchopneumonia, small pulmonary abscesses, or active tubercular lesions. Infected pulmonary edema is a sub-acute or chronic state that results from the localization of bacteria in areas of the lungs that experience either subacute or chronic edema. In both cases, it is likely that the inflammatory process causes liberation of histamine and thus leads to an increase of permeability and a greater severity of edema.

A different type of edema has been experimentally caused with intra-venous injection of *E. coli*. Apparently the bacterial toxins themselves alter the capillary permeability in such experiments.

Unilateral Edema

Edema of only one lung is a rare occurrence. It may be favored by either the patient's position, as in cases of hemiplegia with the patient lying on the para-lytic side, or an inflammatory process. Unilateral edema is also favored by ex-tensive fibrosis of the contralateral lung.

Adrenocortical Steroids

Adrenocortical steroids appear to be beneficial in preventing experimental pul-monary edema. Their effect in clinical conditions has not been ascertained. One condition that is definitely helped by these substances is acute rheumatic fever. However, adrenocortical steroids indirectly favor pulmonary edema by causing fluid retention.

Thickening of Membranes

Membrane thickening is a pathological process that has been demonstrated in severe mitral stenosis.* Not only is the capillary wall thicker than normal but the interstitial spaces and the alveolar membrane participate, with the process of "brown induration." It has been suggested that passage of proteins through the capillary walls would require a higher hydrostatic pressure.

Chronic Lung Diseases

Pulmonary emphysema consists of the destruction of some of the interalveolar septa with their capillaries resulting in the formation of blebs. As a result, the

*A similar process is likely to occur in (1) left atrial myxoma, (2) endo-cardial fibroelastosis (restrictive type), and (3) constrictive pericarditis of the left heart.

remaining capillaries may be dilated due to the increased blood flow they must accommodate. This is an element favoring pulmonary edema. However, other cardiovascular repercussions have greater importance.

Left Ventricular Damage

Moderate coronary heart disease resulting in myocardial fibrosis is a common process occurring in the hearts of the aged. If these subjects are submitted to stress, like that occurring during anesthesia and surgery, the left ventricle is more likely to fail in the postoperative stage. Whenever hemodilution is an additional factor, even mild left ventricular failure may easily induce pulmonary edema.

Dyspnea

Deep respiration tends to increase the negative pressure of the chest during inspiration. It has been postulated that a "suction effect" would occur and that the degree of transudation would be increased. This view cannot be supported from a dynamic standpoint, however.

III. Clinical Conditions Often Associated with Hemodynamic Forms of Pulmonary Edema

A great variety of clinical conditions may be associated with acute pulmonary edema. While a more complete list has been compiled by the author [9], a partial list (Table 1) shows those conditions in which a hemodynamic sequence causing pulmonary edema is most common and most likely. Some of them often have a preexisting increase of the left ventricular diastolic pressure (aortic insufficiency or stenosis, coarctation, hypertensive heart disease). Others have a preexisting increase in left atrial pressure (mitral insufficiency, left atrial myxoma, mitral stenosis). In others, edema is the result of an acute event, like a myocardial infarct or a cerobrovascular attack.

Pulmonary edema as an autopsy finding was studied by Cameron [2]. In 500 autopsies, he found 94 cases of hypertensive heart disease with edema in 86%; in 66 cases of "coronary occlusion," edema was present in 68%; in 66 cases of cerebral hemorrhage, 67%; in 38 cases of fractured skull, 63%; and in 84 cases of mitral stenosis, 65% had evidence of edema. Of all the cases of pulmonary edema in his series, 68% were related to either cardiac or neurologic conditions.

TABLE 1   Clinical Conditions Most Often Associated
with Hemodynamic Forms of Pulmonary Edema

Cardiovascular Diseases

Aortic insufficiency (rheumatic; syphilitic)

Aortic stenosis (rheumatic; calcific)

Mitral insufficiency (rheumatic; caused by papillary muscle lesion or dysfunction)

Mitral stenosis (rheumatic; caused by or associated with left atrial myxoma)

Coarctation of aorta (congenital)

Hypertensive heart disease (pheochromocytoma; hypertensive nephropaties; toxemia of pregnancy; essential hypertension)

Coronary heart disease (myocardial infarct; prolonged coronary insufficiency)

Diseases or Lesions of the Central Nervous System

Trauma to the skull

Cerebrovascular attack (cerebral or subarachnoid hemorrhage; cerebral thrombosis or embolism)

Cerebral abscess or tumor

Encephalitis; meningitis; poliomyelitis; tetanus; epilepsy; strychnine poisoning

---

The mechanism of the acute pulmonary edema has been clarified by the experimental studies of the last 100 years, and particularly of the last 20 years.

IV.   Experimental Pulmonary Edema

The great variety of clinical conditions causing pulmonary edema is paralleled by a similarly great number of experimental methods for inducing it. In most cases, the investigator tried to reproduce a particular situation existing in a clinical condition. Some methods had no definite clinical parallel, however, even though their results cast some light on clinically encountered disorders.

A.   Heart-Lung Preparations

Fuehner and Starling, working on heart-lung preparations, noted the spontaneous appearance of pulmonary edema. Either an increase in the aortic resistance [10,11], or an obstruction of the pulmonary veins [12], has been shown to favor the occurrence of edema in this preparation.

B. Interference with Left Ventricular Function

The demonstration by Friedlaender [13] that compression or ligation of the rabbit's ascending aorta between the heart and the innominate trunk is often followed by massive pulmonary edema led to the theory of "dissociation between the outputs of the two ventricles." Welch [14], working in Cohnheim's laboratory, obtained similar results both in dogs and rabbits but more often in the latter. He obtained the best results by ligating the aortic arch between the innominate trunk and the left subclavian artery. Of course ligature of the arch is followed by increased pressure in the brain, because in the rabbit or dog, both carotids and the right subclavian artery arise proximally to the ligation as in most animal species. He reported that the right carotid pressure increased, whereas pulmonary arterial pressure showed little change. Crushing of most of the left ventricular wall caused pulmonary edema while crushing of the right did not. This led Welch to develop the theory that "pulmonary edema occurs because the left ventricle is unable to expel all the blood supplied by a normally functioning right ventricle." Several authors were unable to reproduce Welch's experiments, and Cameron [2] criticized the experiments on several grounds. Antoniazzi [15] repeated Welch's experiments in rabbits without opening the thorax (by using a curved needle, introduced into the mediastinum from the suprasternal notch). He succeeded in preventing this type of pulmonary edema by either injecting morphine sulfate or removing the stellate ganglia.

More recently, Sarnoff [16] repeated Welch's experiments and showed that a dramatic reflex constriction of the capacitance vessels of the systemic circulation follows aortic ligation. He considered this the result of reflexes elicited by the low pressure in the aorta below the ligation. This caused the shifting of a large mass of blood from the periphery to the right heart and the lungs while the left ventricle was severely overloaded. Sympatholytics or deep anesthesia prevented the pulmonary edema caused by aortic ligation because they prevented venoconstriction.

C. Volume Overloading

Overloading of the circulation with massive infusions of fluid or blood may cause pulmonary edema in the experimental animals. Large amounts can be injected intravenously, however, without causing pulmonary edema if the heart is normal and the central nervous system is intact [17–20]. Wiggers [21] estimated that physiologic saline solution amounting to three times the blood volume can be infused in anesthetized dogs without causing pulmonary edema.

The author injected either saline solution or blood under high pressure
in the "isolated" head of dogs or rabbits and caused pulmonary edema that,
at the time [1929], was considered to be reflex in nature. Further studies
showed, however, that venous connections at the surface of the spinal cord
still permitted overloading of the circulation. The method has been subsequently refined by Kovách and coworkers (to be described later).

Due to the difficulty of completely excluding the head from the circulation, Luisada and Sarnoff [22] compared the result of infusions injected
either in the common carotids toward the brain (Fig. 1) or into a peripheral
vein or artery. Intracarotid infusion caused pulmonary edema with a smaller
volume and in a more constant fashion. Both central sedation (by phenobarbital or chloral hydrate) and ganglionic block prevented this type of pulmonary edema, and a similar preventive effect was obtained by denervating the
carotid bifurcations.

At first this experimental type of pulmonary edema was thought to be
caused by a carotid sinus reflex, but later studies by Luisada and Contro [23]

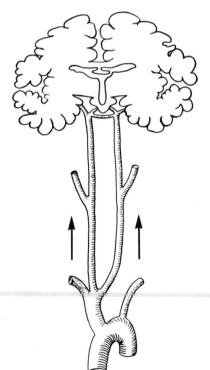

FIGURE 1   Scheme of carotid infusion
toward the brain. Reprinted from A. A.
Luisada and S. J. Sarnoff, *Am. Heart J.*,
31:270–307 (1946), by courtesy of the
publisher.

suggested that a carotid body reflex, elicited by the unoxygenated fluid, was involved. The final interpretation was that a complex cardiovascular reaction took place, including a reflex systemic vasoconstriction.

Pulmonary edema is frequently observed in surgical wards from over-zealous fluid loading after operations. The heart, following anesthesia and possible blood loss or because of the patient's age, may be unable to increase its work adequately to accommodate the extra fluid. Moreover, the hypotonic solutions frequently used add a further element (hypoproteinemia) that favors transudation.

D. Intravenous Catecholamines

Pulmonary edema rapidly develops in rabbits when adrenalin is injected into the marginal vein of the ear. But other routes of injection (subcutaneous, intratracheal) cause a similar response. Within a few minutes after the injection, the animals become depressed and dyspneic, then cyanotic. Convulsions occur, then bloody foam exudes from the nostrils, and a large percentage of the animals die. The lungs show severe hemorrhagic edema [24].

The author, in order to study the effect of drugs in preventing the edema, established the minimal dose that caused death in about 40% of the animals (0.3 mg/kg). He also noted that larger doses were required in summer, and that male albino rabbits should be used in order to obtain consistent results. Tamura [25] found the opposite seasonal influence in ANTU-induced pulmonary edema. Using adrenalin, the author found that the best protection against pulmonary edema was given by chloral hydrate, and that other central sedatives (morphine, clorobutanol, chloretone, phenobarbital) provided slightly less protection. Boggian [26] showed the protective effect of bilateral stellate ganglion removal, and Bariety and Kohler obtained prevention of pulmonary edema by means of sympatholytic agents.

The author [24] had shown that adrenalin caused a marked, sustained rise of left atrial pressure when injected intravenously in the cat. However, this important element of pulmonary edema was not explained at the time. More recently, Siwadlowski et al. [27] restudied adrenalin pulmonary edema. They observed that, while epinephrine was unable to produce pulmonary edema in rabbits, adrenalin (epinephrine plus norepinephrine) induced it systematically. Following injection of adrenalin, the left ventricular end-diastolic pressure rose to levels of 40 to 50 mmHg. This could have been interpreted as evidence of left ventricular failure but that was excluded by the observation that the first derivative (dp/dt) of the left ventricular pressure also markedly increased indicating an increase in left ventricular contractility. They also studied the effects of beta blockers and ganglionic blockers on the prevention of pulmonary edema.

Following previous studies by the author, Kovách et al. [28,29] re-opened the controversy with a new series of experiments. They performed complete vascular isolation of the head of a recipient dog and perfused it from the trunk of a donor dog. A large dose of adrenalin injected into the trunk of the donor caused pulmonary edema in the lungs of both donor and recipient, even though the heart and lungs of the latter were not reached by the drug. Measurements of left atrial pressure in the recipient dog showed an increase up to 20 mmHg. This rise, caused by neurogenic impulses, was attributed to "left ventricular failure."

Subsequent studies on dogs in the author's laboratory (Worthen et al. [30]) were done with epinephrine in blood in order to clarify some unexplained points of Kovách's study. In one group of experiments, epinephrine (Suprarenin, Winthrop) in blood was directly infused headward, where it had the highest concentration; it then reached the other body tissues in lesser concentration, being diluted by the animals' venous blood. In another group of experiments, epinephrine in blood was infused into a vein and presumably entered the vascular beds of the head and trunk at similar concentrations. The most striking result noted was a tremendous rise of left ventricular end-diastolic pressures to levels of 50 to 80 mmHg (Fig. 2). This rise was significantly less in the intravenously infused animals than in those receiving intra-carotid infusions. When such experimental procedures were performed in open-chest, open-pericardium animals, the left ventricular end-diastolic pressure rise also occurred, and marked dilatation of the heart was noted. This rise of diastolic pressure might be considered related to "left ventricular failure." However, the following facts do support such contention, at least in the accepted meaning of such term:

1. In the first period of these experiments, the rise was reversible in spite of the continuing presence of epinephrine in the blood.

2. The first derivative (dp/dt) of left ventricular pressure showed a sharp increase in the early-systolic wave, which persisted higher than control values almost to the end (Fig. 3); it is known that this derivative is an index of myocardial contractility.*

3. Cardiac output decreased less in these experiments than in the controls, where intravenous epinephrine without blood did not result in pulmonary edema.

*It is unfortunate that this increase is favored by an increase in the LV end-diastolic pressure.

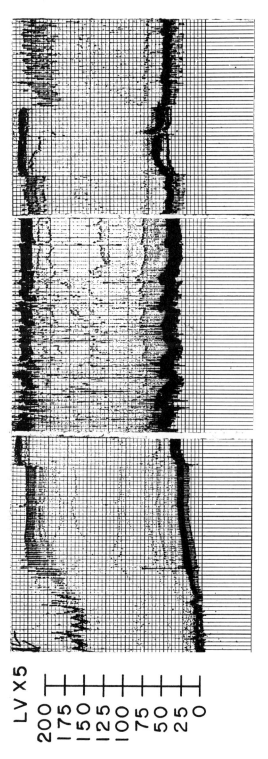

FIGURE 2 Carotid infusion of epinephrine in blood in a dog. Record of left ventricular pressure. LV pressure rose to 240 mmHg while the end-diastolic pressure rose to 77 mmHg. Five minutes elapsed between first and second section, 10 min between second and third. Pulmonary edema resulted with a lungs/body index = 3.2 (normal < 0.9). Pressures in mmHg.

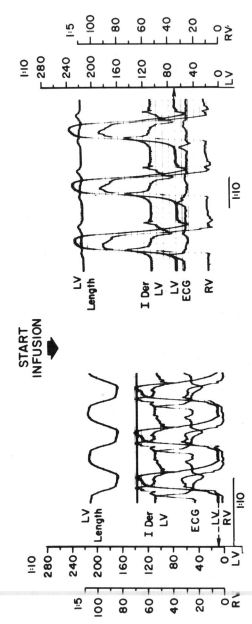

FIGURE 3 High-speed photographic tracing in a standard dog experiment with infusion of epinephrine and blood towards the brain. The two sections of the tracings were taken at a 10-min interval. LV and RV pressures in mmHg. LV length recorded with a mercury gauge sutured to the surface of the left ventricle. Dp/dt of LV pressure (I Der) is also recorded.

LV diastolic pressure rose to 80 mmHg. The I derivative of LV pressure had a remarkable increase throughout the experiment. Pulmonary edema resulted with a lungs/body weight index = 2.7 (normal = <0.9). Reprinted from M. Worthen et al, *Jap. Heart J.*, **10**:133–158 (1969), by courtesy of authors and publisher.

Both the injected volume of blood and the presence of circulating epinephrine were undoubtedly contributing factors. The former caused an augmentation in the amount of blood contained in the pulmonary vessels, overcoming direct constriction of the pulmonary vessels; the latter, because it caused a more powerful systemic arteriolar and venular constriction and a shift of blood from the systemic to the pulmonary circulation. The additional blood alone had little or no effect, however, and the epinephrine alone caused only moderate changes of left ventricular end-diastolic pressure when injected into the carotid artery. The left ventricular systolic pressure rise was significantly higher in the intravenously infused animals than in those receiving the headward infusions. This could be due to either the effect of the higher epinephrine concentration on the carotid body receptors in the headward infused dogs or direct central nervous system stimulation. On the other hand, the greater left ventricular diastolic pressure rise in the headwardly infused dogs might result from the same mechanism, being caused by increased cardiac sympathetic stimulation combined with the increased blood volume. Length-volume measurements were made, comparing the effect of infusion of blood alone with the effect of infusion of blood plus epinephrine. Epinephrine seemed to decrease the compliance of the left ventricle. Decreased distensibility of the left ventricular wall as a result of epinephrine had been noticed by others. Therefore, the tremendous increases in left diastolic pressures observed in our experiments can be explained, at least partly, by this effect of epinephrine.

Experiments with cardiac denervation were then done, in spite of the knowledge that cardiac denervation is often incomplete. In four of eight "cardiac-denervated dogs," both left ventricular end-diastolic pressure rise and pulmonary edema were prevented or decreased. This seemed to confirm an important function of the cardiac nerves in the mechanism of pulmonary edema.

In a subsequent study, Worthen et al. [31] attempted to differentiate between the centrally mediated and the systemic effect of an infusion of blood with epinephrine in the pathogenesis of pulmonary edema. Experiments in cross-circulated dogs showed that the infusion of blood with epinephrine caused an elevation of the left ventricular diastolic pressure, an increase of the left ventricular dp/dt, and pulmonary edema both when it acts only on the heart and systemic vessels (trunk dog) and when it acts only on the cerebral vessels (head dog). In the "head dog," even though epinephrine acted only on the brain centers, a sympathetic discharge, which was probably reinforced by adrenal secretion, may well have caused peripheral vasoconstriction, systolic overloading of the left ventricle, and increased venous return to the right heart. A decrease of left ventricular wall compliance could also occur through stimulation of the sympathetic fibers of the heart without a direct effect of circulating epinephrine.

Subsequent experiments compared cross-circulated dogs in which the epinephrine did or did not act on the cerebral vessels. Even though elevation of left ventricular end-diastolic pressure (or left atrial mean pressure) was higher in the dogs receiving epinephrine throughout the whole circulation (three out of four experiments), the severity of pulmonary edema varied unpredictably in the various experiments between the two dogs of each series (a third dog acted merely as a donor).

Adrenalin has multiple actions, and all of them should be considered in the final evaluation of the results of its administration. By its action on the heart, it increases cardiac output; by its action on the arteries of the splanchnic system, it mobilizes blood, which increases venous pressure; by its action on the veins, it increases right heart and pulmonary vascular pressures. Thus, the pressure effect is a direct result and the volume effect is an indirect one. In addition, adrenalin constricts the large lymphatic vessels. This may decrease the lymphatic flow from the lungs in a situation in which an increase would be beneficial.

The series of experiments described confirms the elevation of left atrial pressure in both animals of a series submitted to cross-circulation and injected with blood and epinephrine; it shows that this elevation is caused by elevation of left ventricular end-diastolic pressure; it also suggests that such an increase, occurring at a time of maximal increase of contractility (as evidenced by an increase of the dp/dt), is related not to left ventricular failure, as Kovách had stated [28,29] but to a particular modification of left ventricular compliance in conjunction with an increased venous return. The latter seems to be caused by either circulating catecholamines, nerve impulses, or both.

E.   Central Nervous System Irritation

Pulmonary edema can be induced by increased intracranial pressure, bilateral lesion of the vagal nuclei, discrete bilateral lesions of the preoptic areas of rats, or bilateral injection of minute amounts of aconitine or veratrine into the preoptic areas of rats or dogs. The edema caused by increased intracranial pressure is preceded by systemic hypertension that is accompanied by bradycardia.

Jarisch et al. [32] demonstrated that injection of veratrine in the cisterna magna of the rat or rabbit is rapidly followed by pulmonary edema. A similar method, based on the injection of thrombin and fibrinogen, was used by Cameron and De [33] in the same two species and with the same results. Sarnoff and coworkers [34–37] used the latter method and documented severe systemic hypertension and a massive increase of venous return taking place in these experiments. They explained the pulmonary edema as resulting from overloading of the left ventricle followed by "relative left ventricular failure." They called this sequence of events "neuro-hemodynamic pulmonary edema."

This concept was inadequate because a simple increase in the blood volume of the lungs would not be followed by edema. But such an increase would become crucial for the mechanism of edema if it were accompanied by severe increase of left atrial pressure.

Applying the method of Jarisch to the dog (Fig. 4) we have been able to confirm the severe systemic hypertension that follows the injection [38], and, by left atrial and ventricular catheterizations, we have documented the occurrence of a "relative" mitral insufficiency, which caused an increase of left atrial mean pressure and thus contributed to the increase of pulmonary capillary pressure [39]. We systematically investigated left ventricular function, peripheral vasoconstriction, and the effect of neurogenic stimuli on the heart in the production of pulmonary edema [38]. Experiments performed with a standard procedure revealed that the behavior of both the systolic and diastolic pressures and the dp/dt of the left ventricle was similar to that observed in experiments with a previously described method, in which massive doses of epinephrine and blood were injected. In other words, central nervous system stimulation was followed by peripheral arterial and venous constriction, systemic hypertension, increased venous return, decreased compliance of the left ventricular wall, and increased contractility of the ventricular myocardium (Table 2). All these actions, caused by central stimuli, are probably potentiated by centrally induced adrenal secretion (Fig. 5).

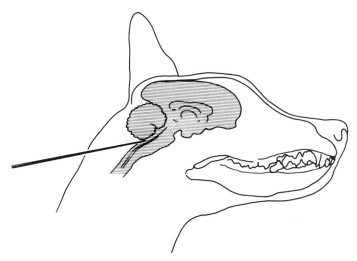

FIGURE 4   Scheme of injection of veratrine in the cisterna magna of a dog.

TABLE 2 Modification of Responses to Intracisternal Veratrine in Dogs

Procedure	No.	Left Ventricle Indices						Lung weight[a]
		Systolic pressure		End-diastolic pressure		dp/dt		Body weight
		C	M	C	M	C	M	
Standard	10	155	300	4	79	10	27	2.00
After high spinal transection	5	139	196	5	17	12	36	1.17
After bilateral removal of stellate ganglia and vagotomy	10	146	263	3	35	7	16	1.08
After vagotomy alone	2	187	231	4	28	12	20	1.66

Note: C = control; M = maximum.
[a] Normal for the dog <0.98.

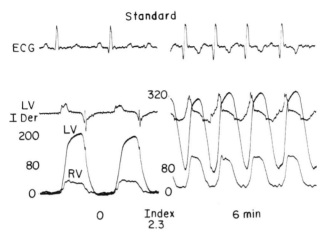

FIGURE 5 Effect of a standard injection of veratrine in the cisterna magna of a dog. At left = control; at right = after 6 min. Left ventricular (LV) and right ventricular (RV) pressures: first derivative (dp/dt) of LV pressure (I Der). Elevation of LV systolic pressure from 200 to 320 mmHg. Elevation of LV diastolic pressure from 0 to 80 mmHg. Increase of LV dp/dt from 12 to 24 mm. Pulmonary edema resulted. The lungs/body index was 2.3 (normal <0.9). Reprinted from M. Worthen et al., *Jap. Heart J.*, **10**:133–158 (1969), by courtesy of the authors and publisher.

    In animals receiving veratrine after high spinal transection (Table 2) the left ventricular systolic pressure rose less, and the left ventricular diastolic pressure was only moderately increased, but a remarkable increase of dp/dt of the left ventricular pressure still occurred (Fig. 6). Central nervous system stimulation did not lead to either peripheral vasoconstriction or adrenal secretion in these animals. In spite of this, adrenergic stimuli reaching the heart increased cardiac contractility. The occurrence of only a moderate increase of left ventricular diastolic pressure suggested that the modification of left ventricular compliance observed in the standard type of experiments requires several factors: (1) *direct*: stimuli affecting the heart; (2) *indirect*: peripheral venous constriction resulting in increased venous return and right and left ventricular diastolic overload; (3) *indirect*: peripheral arterial constriction causing a left ventricular systolic overload; (4) *direct and indirect*: increased adrenal catecholamine secretion. All elements were prevented by spinal transection except the stimuli affecting the heart. In spite of the lesser increase in left ventricular end-diastolic pressure and of lesser venous return, a minimal degree of pulmonary edema was still observed.

    Experiments were then done in animals after bilateral stellectomy and vagotomy (Table 2). These revealed a marked increase in left ventricular

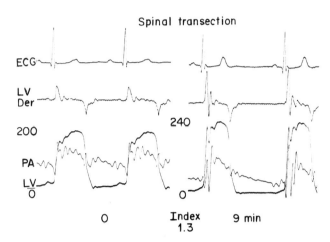

FIGURE 6 Effect of a standard injection of veratrine in the cisterna magna
of a dog after high spinal transection. At left = control; at right = after 9 min.
LV and PA pressures, as well as LV dp/dt, were recorded. LV systolic pressure
rose from 200 to 240 mmHg. LV diastolic pressure remained at 20 mmHg (this
level had been reached by giving a blood transfusion to compensate for expansion of the volume of the capacitance vessels). LV dp/dt increased from 12 to
26 min. The lungs/body index was 1.3 (normal < 0.9) and there was only minimal foam from the trachea. Reprinted from M. Worthen et al., *Dis. Chest.*
(1969), by courtesy of the authors and publisher.

systolic pressure, a moderate increase in left ventricular end-diastolic pressure,
and a less dramatic increase of the dp/dt of the left ventricular pressure. As
the augmented venous return still occurred (spinal cord intact), the less
marked increase of left ventricular end-diastolic pressure and the less marked
increase of left ventricular dp/dt suggested a decrease in adrenergic stimuli
reaching the left ventricle (Fig. 7). It is important to note that pulmonary
edema was minimal or absent in these experiments in spite of the augmented
venous return and the severe overloading of the left ventricle. Vagotomy was
done because, in the dog, the vagus nerve contains numerous sympathetic
fibers. However, vagotomy alone did not prevent the occurrence of pulmonary
edema. These results suggested that stellectomy prevented stimuli that would
be directly responsible for the increase of left ventricular end-diastolic pressure
from reaching the heart. The sympathetic nervous system's action in the
development of pulmonary edema is not limited to the left ventricle but possibly
extends to the pulmonary vessels.

In summary, these experiments suggest that pulmonary edema caused by
central nervous system irritation is the result of two different but interacting

Stellectomy

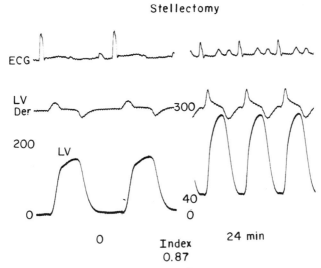

FIGURE 7 Effect of a standard injection of veratrine in the cisterna magna of a dog after bilateral stellectomy. At left = control; at right = after 24 min. LV pressures (in mmHg) and LV dp/dt. Elevation of LV systolic pressure from 160 to 270 mmHg. Elevation of LV diastolic pressure from 0 to 44 mmHg. Increase of LV dp/dt from 6 to 13 mm. The lung/body index was 0.87 (normal <0.9) and there was no foam from the trachea. Reprinted from M. Worthen et al., *Jap. Heart J.*, **10**:133–158 (1969), by courtesy of the authors and publisher.

chains of events: (1) a temporary increase of venous return, which overloads the right heart and favors the congestion of the lungs (this peripheral factor had been already emphasized by Sarnoff); and (2) a lasting increase in the level of left ventricular end-diastolic pressure due to decreased compliance of the wall in combination with central congestion; this is caused by adrenergic stimuli and by circulating catecholamines but is favored by the increased after-load (systemic vasoconstriction) as well as by the tachycardia.

The increase of resistance at the left ventricular level, transmitted to the pulmonary vessels in terms of increased pressure, transforms the results of increased venous return into a maximal increase of capillary pressure. If either the increase of venous return is less marked or the decreased compliance of the left ventricular wall is absent, then the dramatic increase of pulmonary capillary pressure will not occur.

Left ventricular end-diastolic pressure rise in the presence of increased contractility should not be considered evidence of "left ventricular failure" in the conventional sense.

Systematic studies of Coleman et al. [40] have subsequently confirmed the effect of sympathetic stimuli on the compliance of the left ventricular wall.

V. Mechanism of the Most Common Forms of Pulmonary Edema Caused by Heart Failure and Hemodynamic Mechanisms

A.   Myocardial Infarction and Angina Pectoris

Pulmonary edema is most often observed in the acute stage of a myocardial infarction (first to third day). It may occur later, however [41]. One is tempted to explain this type of pulmonary edema as due simply to left ventricular failure. However, myocardial infarction can result in cardiogenic shock without pulmonary edema, pulmonary edema without shock, both, or neither. Experimental studies by Tamura [42] are against the blind acceptance of left ventricular failure per se. When pulmonary and cardiogenic shock occur together, the usual sequence is that pulmonary edema occurs first. Then, as expression of the terminal stage, shock occurs, complicating the picture.

It is obvious that while left ventricular failure would raise the pressure of the pulmonary capillaries, this rise cannot take place without an increased (or at least a normal) output of the right ventricle, which depends on venous return. Thus, unless systemic venous constriction causes a temporary increase of venous return and causes a blood shift in the presence of left ventricular failure, only a moderate rise of pulmonary capillary pressure would take place.

A "stress reaction" causing secretion of catecholamines and sympathetic stimulation has been postulated as a result of myocardial infarction. Increased catecholamine excretion has been documented in myocardial infarction and found highest in the first 48 to 72 hr, but still elevated for several days [43–46]. The mean catecholamine level has been found higher whenever acute pulmonary edema is present [46]. If the "stress reaction" is severe, we should accept that pulmonary edema in these cases results from both left ventricular failure and sympathoadrenal reaction.

Acute pulmonary edema has been observed during severe episodes of precordial pain (angina pectoris, coronary insufficiency). In this respect, it is interesting to note that precordial pain caused by rapid atrial pacing is accompanied by "diastolic stiffening" of the left ventricular wall, resulting in a marked increase of diastolic pressure [47]. In those experiments, the average LV end-diastolic pressure rose 140% (from 12 to 29 mmHg). Since catecholamine secretion and sympathetic stimulation are markedly increased by atrial pacing, one can correlate the mechanisms of pulmonary edema of angina pectoris and of central neurologic conditions.

Another possible result of coronary atherosclerosis has been described by Dodek et al. [48]. In their cases, diffuse coronary artery disease was associated with recurrent pulmonary edema and radiographically normal heart size. The authors accept a reduced left ventricular compliance so that even a minor increase in diastolic volume would result in a significant increase of end-diastolic pressure. The authors attribute this abnormal behavior of the left ventricular wall to myocardial scarring and fibrosis.

B. Central Nervous System Disorders

The appearance of pulmonary edema following cerebrovascular attacks, trauma to the skull, or other neurologic conditions is based on the simultaneous interplay of three elements: (a) left ventricular systolic overload caused by constriction of the systemic resistance vessels; (b) right ventricular (and then left ventricular) diastolic overload caused by blood shift from the periphery to the lungs (due to constriction of the systemic capacitance vessels); and (c) decreased compliance of the left ventricular wall preventing optimal diastolic distension; this will further increase the left ventricular end-diastolic pressure. These changes are caused by a sympathoadrenal storm but, if the cerebrovascular accident takes place in patients with weak myocardium on account of coronary heart disease, left ventricular failure may also be involved.

C. Hypertensive Cardiovascular Disease

Hypertensive cardiovascular disease shows a mechanism of pulmonary edema similar to that of the group of central nervous disorders, except that long-lasting hypertension may have weakened the myocardium by causing an inadequate blood supply of the hypertrophied left ventricle and by favoring coronary lesions. Then, an element of left ventricular failure may be involved, especially if the attack is long-lasting. This type has been reproduced in the experimental laboratory by the i.v. injection of Adrenalin.

D. Mitral Stenosis

In mitral stenosis, there is a fixed obstruction to flow at the mitral level. As previously discussed, any temporary increase of venous return to the right heart will create an imbalance between inflow to the lungs and outflow therefrom, followed by an increase of pulmonary capillary pressure. The most common cause of this hemodynamic imbalance is exertion. This has been clearly shown by catheterization studies of mitral patients exercised on a bicycle. The left atrial pressure of these patients, usually between 20 and 30 mmHg, may rise to 50 or 60 mmHg at the end of exertion. Central stimulation related to anger or excitement, or reflex stimulation brought about by exposure to cold, would cause: (1) a massive shift of blood from the periphery to the lungs; (2) tachycardia, which increases the pressure in the pulmonary capillaries by decreasing the duration of diastoles; and (3) probably a decrease of left ventricular compliance; this would increase the level of left ventricular diastolic pressure and thus the level of left atrial and pulmonary capillary pressures.

Thus, while pulmonary edema of mitral stenosis is basically due to a structural lesion, its actual determinant is connected to either exertion or a sympathoadrenal storm, and may even be favored by chronic left ventricular failure.

Pulmonary arterial vasoconstriction, pulmonary arterial sclerosis, or tricuspid defects would decrease the severity of pulmonary edema by preventing a sudden increase of pulmonary capillary flow. Pulmonary venous sclerosis, on the contrary, would increase the frequency of pulmonary edema.

E. Restriction of the Left Ventricle

Several conditions (constrictive pericarditis predominating over the left ventricle, restrictive type of fibroelastosis, amyloidosis, myocardial fibrosis) may limit the distensibility of the left ventricle. These processes cause a permanent increase of left ventricular end-diastolic pressure. The determinants of the acute attack, however, will be the same as those acting in mitral stenosis.

F. Mitral Insufficiency

The regurgitant jet that enters the left atrium in systole in mitral insufficiency causes an increase of the mean left atrial pressure and of the pulmonary capillary pressure that would favor pulmonary edema. All the various acute changes that may precipitate pulmonary edema in mitral stenosis also are important in mitral insufficiency. The same is true for myocarditis with subsequent left ventricular failure. Moreover, left ventricular failure of these patients is favored by the chronic left ventricular diastolic overload that is typical of this condition.

G. Aortic Insufficiency

The regurgitant jet entering the left ventricle in diastole tends to increase the left ventricular end-diastolic pressure and hence the left atrial and pulmonary capillary pressures. Reflex elements, probably caused by temporary drops in aortic pressure, may favor a sympathoadrenal storm that will then precipitate pulmonary edema by increasing venous return to the right heart and decreasing left ventricular compliance.

Syphilitic aortitis seems to favor the occurrence of reflex sympathetic storms through irritation of aortic receptors. Acute left ventricular failure may also occur, favored by the chronic diastolic overload of the left ventricle.

H. Aortic Stenosis

The decreased compliance and the persistent strain of the left ventricle cause a lasting, compensatory increase of left ventricular end-diastolic pressure in severe aortic stenosis. Whenever either a sympathoadrenal storm or a left ventricular failure occur, pulmonary edema will be precipitated.

I. Coarctation of the Aorta

Coarctation of the aorta causes left ventricular strain similar to that of aortic stenosis. On the other hand, reflexes arising in the various pressoreceptor areas may cause a sudden and massive shift of blood towards the lungs, as experimental studies have demonstrated. It is likely that the same sympathetic stimulation will also decrease the compliance of the left ventricle and add to the severity of the episode.

J. Chronic Congestive Failure

Chronic congestive failure is usually associated with chronic edema of the lungs. In this condition, the failing left ventricle is dilated and has an increase in its end-diastolic pressure, probably related to the lesser compliance that is inherent in the marked stretching of the wall. This factor easily augments left atrial and pulmonary pressures in association with the generally increased blood volume. It is known that catecholamine levels are elevated in congestive failure without infarction [49], and more elevated if there is significant pulmonary edema. It is still undetermined whether this is or not a significant contributory element.

K. Other Conditions

Several other conditions may cause pulmonary edema. Before accepting a mechanism that excludes a hemodynamic element, care should be taken to exclude systemic vasoconstriction, central nervous system stimulation, and catecholamine secretion. This will be particularly necessary in evaluating pulmonary edema caused by hypoxia, uremia, or the effect of several poisons or drugs.

References

1. E. H. Starling, On the absorption of fluids from the connective tissue spaces, *J. Physiol.* (London), **19**:312–326 (1896).
2. G. R. Cameron, Pulmonary oedema, *Brit. Med. J.*, **1**:965–976 (1948).
3. W. G. Spector, Substances which affect capillary permeability, *Pharm. Rev.*, **10**:475–505 (1958).
4. H. Mautner and E. P. Pick, Ueber die durch "Schockgifte" erzeugten Zirkulationstoerungen, *Muench. Med. Wochenschr.*, **62**:1141–1156 (1915).
5. R. P. Gilbert, L. B. Hinshaw, H. Kuida and M. D. Visscher, Effects of histamine, 5-hydroxytryptamine and epinephrine on pulmonary hemodynamics, etc., *Amer. J. Phys.*, **194**:165–170 (1958).
6. M. Eliakim and D. M. Aviado, Effects of nerve stimulation and drugs on the extra-pulmonary portion of the pulmonary vein, *J. Pharm. Exp. Ther.*, **133**:304–312 (1961).
7. K. Braun and S. Stern, Functional significance of the pulmonary venous system, *Amer. J. Card.*, **20**:56–65 (1967).
8. B. Kisch, Electron microscopy of the lungs in acute pulmonary edema, *Exp. Med. Surg.*, **16**:17–33 (1958).
9. A. A. Luisada. *Pulmonary Edema in Man and Animals.* St. Louis, W. Green, 1970, p. 9.
10. Y. Matsuoka, A contribution to the pathology of obstructive oedema of the lung, etc., *J. Path. Bact.*, **20**:53–76 (1915).
11. D. T. Barry, Pulmonary edema and congestion in the heart-lung preparation, *J. Physiol.* (London), **57**:368–378 (1923).
12. W. H. Newton, Pulmonary oedema in the cat heart-lung preparation, *J. Physiol.* (London), **75**:288–304 (1932).
13. K. Friedlaender. *Untersuchungen ueber Lungentzuendung*, etc. Berlin, Hirschwald, 1873.
14. W. H. Welch, Zur Pathologie des Lungenoedems, *Virchows Arch. Path. Anat.*, **72**:375–412 (1878).
15. E. Antoniazzi, Contributo allo studio dell 'edema polmonare acuto, *Arch. Sci. Med.*, **54**:818–846 (1930).
16. S. J. Sarnoff, Some physiological considerations on the genesis of acute pulmonary edema. In *Pulmonary Circulation*. New York, Grune and Stratton, 1959, p. 273.

17. J. Cohnheim and L. Lichtheim, Ueber Hydraemie und hydraemisch Oedem, *Virchows Arch. Path. Anat.*, **69**:106–143 (1877).
18. M. Loewit, Zur Entstehung des Lungenoedems, *Zbl. Allg. Path. Anat.*, **6**: 97–104 (1895).
19. H. Sahli, Zur Pathologie und Therapie des Lungenoedems, *Arch. Exp. Path. Pharm.*, **19**:433–482 (1895).
20. F. Kraus, Ueber Lungenoedem, *Z. Exp. Path. Ther.*, **14**:402–412 (1913).
21. W. J. Wiggers, *Physiology in Health and Disease.* 4th ed. Philadelphia, Lea and Febiger, 1944.
22. A. A. Luisada and S. J. Sarnoff, Paroxysmal pulmonary edema consequent to stimulation of cardiovascular receptors. I. Effect of intra-arterial and intravenous infusions, *Amer. Heart J.*, **31**:270–281 (1946). II. Mechanical and neurogenic elements, *Amer. Heart J.*, **31**:282–292 (1946). III. Pharmacologic experiments, *Amer. Heart J.*, **31**:293–307 (1946).
23. A. A. Luisada and S. Contro, Experimental pulmonary edema following rapid carotid infusion: Mechanism and therapy, *Circ. Res.*, **1**:179–183 (1953).
24. A. A. Luisada, Beitrag zur Pathogenese und Therapie des Lungenoedem und des Asthma cardiale, *Arch. Exp. Path. Pharm.*, **132**:313–329 (1928).
25. H. Tamura, Experimental studies on pulmonary edema. II. Seasonal influence on the production of pulmonary edema, *Jap. Circul. J.*, **26**:188–201 (1962).
26. B. Boggian, Contributo allo studio dell'edema polmonare acute. Turin, Minerva Medica, **2**:967–975 (1929).
27. W. Siwadlowski, C. Aravanis, M. Worthen, and A. A. Luisada, Mechanism of adrenalin pulmonary edema and its prevention by narcotics and autonomic blockers, *Chest*, **57**:554–557 (1970).
28. A. G. B. Kovách, Neurohaemodynamische Zusammenhaenge bei der Entstehung des Lungenoedems, *Allergie Asthma*, **10**:338–343 (1964).
29. A. G. B. Kovách, P. S. Roheim, M. Iranyi, S. Kiss, and J. Antal, Effect of the isolated perfusion of the head on the development of ischaemic and hemorrhagic shock, *Acta Physiol. Acad. Sci. Hung.*, **14**:231–238 (1958).
30. M. Worthen, B. Placik, B. Argano, D. M. Mac Canon, and A. A. Luisada, On the mechanism of epinephrine-induced pulmonary edema, *Jap. Heart J.*, **10**:133–141 (1969).
31. M. Worthen, B. Argano, W. Siwadlowski, D. W. Bruce, D. M. Mac Canon, and A. A. Luisada, Epinephrine-induced pulmonary edema in cross-circulated animals, *Jap. Heart J.*, **10**:142–158 (1969).
32. A. Jarisch, H. Richter, and H. Thoma, Zentrogenes Lungenoedem, *Klin. Wochenschr.*, **18**:1440–1443 (1939).
33. G. R. Cameron and S. N. De, Experimental pulmonary oedema of nervous origin, *J. Path. Bact.*, **61**:375–387 (1949).
34. S. J. Sarnoff and L. C. Sarnoff, Neurohemodynamics of pulmonary edema. I. Autonomic influence on pulmonary vascular pressures and the acute pulmonary edema state. A preliminary report, *Dis. Chest*, **22**:685–698 (1952).

35.   S. J. Sarnoff and L. C. Sarnoff, Neurohemodynamics of pulmonary edema. The role of sympathetic pathways in the elevation of pulmonary and systemic vascular pressures following the intracisternal injection of fibrin, *Circulation*, 6:51–62 (1952).

36.   S. J. Sarnoff, E. Berglund, and L. C. Sarnoff, Neurohemodynamics of pulmonary edema. III. Estimated changes in pulmonary blood volume accompanying systemic vasoconstriction and vasodilatation, *J. Appl. Phys.*, 5:367–374 (1953).

37.   S. J. Sarnoff and E. Berglund, Neurohemodynamics of acute pulmonary edema. IV. Effect of systemic vasoconstriction and subsequent vasodilatation on flow and pressures in systemic and vascular beds, *Amer. J. Phys.*, 170:588–600 (1952).

38.   M. Worthen, B. Argano, W. Siwadlowski, D. W. Bruce, D. M. Mac Canon, and A. A. Luisada, Mechanism of intracisternal veratrine pulmonary edema, *Dis. Chest*, 55:45–48 (1969).

39.   A. Jacono, M. Kaplan, and A. A. Luisada, Relative mitral insufficiency as a factor of paroxysmal pulmonary edema, *Cardiol.* (Basel), 39:1–11 (1961).

40.   B. Coleman, M. C. Worthen, D. M. MacCanon, J. E. Kalal, and A. A. Luisada. Sympathetic influence on ventricular compliance, *Jap. Heart J.*, 17:222–232 (1976).

41.   R. Tricot, P. Nogrette, and B. Ziskind, L'oedème du poumon dans l'infarctus du myocarde, *Arch. Mal. Coeur*, 61:1439–1449 (1968).

42.   H. Tamura, Experimental studies on pulmonary edema. I. Influence of experimentally produced myocardial infarct on the production of pulmonary edema, *Jap. Circ. J.*, 26174–187 (1962).

43.   R. F. Klein, W. G. Troyer, H. K. Thompson, M. D. Bogdonoff, and A. G. Wallace, Catecholamine excretion in myocardial infarction, *Arch. Int. Med.*, 122:476–482 (1968).

44.   C. Valori, M. Thomas, and J. Shillingford, Free noradrenaline and adrenaline excretion in relation to clinical syndromes following myocardial infarction, *Lancet*, 1:127–130 (1967).

45.   D. E. Jewitt, C. J. Mercer, D. Reid, C. Valori, M. Thomas, and J. Shillingford, Free noradrenaline and adrenaline excretion in relation to the development of cardiac arrhythmias and heart failure in patients with acute myocardial infarction, *Lancet*, 1:635–641 (1969).

46.   D. C. Siggers, C. Salter, and D. C. Fluck, Serial plasma adrenaline and noradrenaline levels in myocardial infarction using a new double isotope technique, *Brit. Heart J.*, 33:878–883 (1971).

47.   W. H. Barry, J. Z. Brooker, E. L. Alderman, and D. C. Harrison, Changes in diastolic stiffness and tone of the left ventricle during angina pectoris, *Circulation*, 49:255–263 (1974).

48.   A. Dodek, D. G. Kassebaum, and J. D. Bristow, Pulmonary edema without cardiomegaly: Ischemic cardiomyopathy and the small stiff heart, *Amer. Heart J.*, 85:281–284 (1973).

49.   C. A. Chidsey, E. Braunwald, and A. G. Morrow, Catecholamine excretion and cardiac stores of norepinephrine in congestive heart failure, *Amer. J. Med.*, 39:442–451 (1965).

13

Bronchial Edema

GIUSEPPE G. PIETRA AND ALFRED P. FISHMAN

University of Pennsylvania
Philadelphia, Pennsylvania

I. Bronchial Vascular Anatomy

A pertinent preamble to considering bronchial edema is a brief review of certain features of bronchial anatomy that may pertain to the accumulation of excess water in and around the airways. Comprehensive descriptions of the gross and microscopic anatomy of the bronchial circulation exist elsewhere in excellent monographs and books [1-7].

A. Bronchial Arteries

That the lung has a dual blood supply was recognized more than 500 years ago by Leonardo da Vinci:

> You could say that the trachea and the lung had to be nourished,
> and if you had to do this with a single large venarteria [pulmonary
> artery] this could not remain attached to the trachea without great

The original research on which this report is based was supported, in part, by a grant from the National Heart and Lung Institute, HL-8805.

hindrance to the motion which occurs with the expansion and contraction of the trachea in length as well as in width. Consequently, for this reason, she [nature] gave such veins and arteries to the trachea as were needed for its life and nourishment, and separated a little from trachea the other large branches to nourish the substance of the lung with great convenience [8].

Since the time of Leonardo, progress in understanding the bronchial circulation has been slow, sporadic, and unspectacular. Nonetheless, it is now clear that blood reaching the lungs by the bronchial arteries is only a small fraction of the blood delivered by the pulmonary arterial tree, that it originates from systemic arteries, that it is importantly involved in sustaining the conducting airways, large pulmonary vessels, lymph nodes, and nerve trunks and ganglia, and that its influence on the bronchi extends the entire length of the airways to the respiratory bronchioles [9, 10]. In the region of the respiratory bronchioles, overlap exists with blood supply from the pulmonary artery. Also, in certain species, including man and horse, bronchial arterial blood has access to the alveolar capillary bed [5].

The origin of the bronchial arteries from the thoracic aorta varies among species but the intrapulmonary course of the arteries is very constant [1,3]. Within the lung, a branch of the bronchial artery accompanies each main bronchus; each subsequent subdivision of the bronchial tree is accompanied by a corresponding subdivision of the bronchial artery. The vessels lie in the peribronchial connective tissue sheath and branch to form a sparse, wide-meshed arterial plexus around the bronchus. In animals with a thick pleura, including man, horse, cow, sheep, and pig, the visceral pleura is supplied with blood by the bornchial artery; in animals with a thin pleura, such as the dog, cat, monkey, and rat, blood for the visceral pleura comes from the pulmonary circulation. This anatomical distinction may be important for the rates of removal of fluid from the pleural space in different species. The bronchial arteries can be followed as distinct vessels as far as the distal portions of the terminal bronchioles, where they generally terminate in a capillary network in common with the pulmonary circulation. These connecting vessels are capable of considerable proliferation when exposed to appropriate stimuli. Among the most effective stimuli are sustained and severe curtailment of pulmonary blood flow, as in congenital pulmonary stenosis or atresia [11], chronic fibrosing pulmonary disease [12], chronic suppuration [13], and bronchogenic carcinoma [14].

B. Bronchial Capillaries and Veins

From the bronchial arteries in the peribronchial connective tissue space, fine radicles perforate the muscular layer of the bronchus and reach the submucosa.

Here they give rise to capillaries that branch extensively, forming a rectangular, meshed plexus whose long axis is parallel to the bronchus. The capillaries gradually merge into venules, which in turn give rise to bronchial veins [1, 15].

Quite remarkable is the spatial arrangement of the bronchial veins along the length of the airways, where they are so disposed as to form a communicating network that consists of a plexus on either side of the bronchial muscle linked by transmuscular venous channels (Fig. 1). The submucosal venular plexus parallels another venular plexus that is formed by somewhat larger vessels and located in the peribronchial connective tissue, outside the cartilage plates [1, 15]. As the bronchi subdivide in the lung periphery, their walls become thinner, eventually the cartillage disappears and the muscle layer becomes attenuated. In these distal portions of the airways, the two plexuses approximate each other and fuse, merging in radicles of the pulmonary veins.

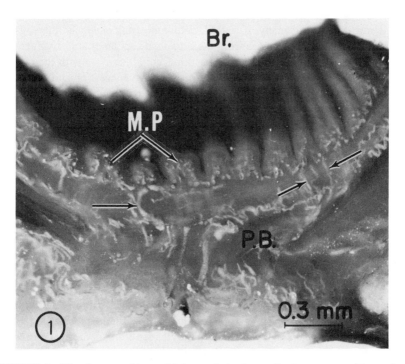

FIGURE 1 Silastic cast of bronchial vessels in the wall of a segmental bronchus of a dog lung. The cast reveals the tortuous vessels of the peribronchial plexus (P.B.); the perforating vessels (arrows) and the mucosal plexus (M.P) composed of fine vessels that follow the mucosal folds. Br. = bronchial lumen. Reprinted from G. G. Pietra et al., *Circ. Res.,* **29**:323-337 (1971), enlargement of section of Figure 6, by courtesy of the publisher.

Three groups of veins drain the tracheobronchial tree and lungs: (1) bronchial veins from the first one or two divisions of the bronchi; these veins empty predominantly into the right atrium via the azygos and hemiazygos veins; (2) bronchial veins from the subsequent bronchi and broncioles; these empty into the pulmonary veins; and (3) the pulmonary veins, which drain blood from the respiratory surface of the lungs into the left atrium. (The last group will not be considered further in this article.)

The bronchial venous flow to the left atrium affords the prospect of venous admixture. Under ordinary conditions, the bulk of the bronchopulmonary flow does not traverse alveolar capillaries [16]. However, the degree of shunting to the alveolar capillaries—or diversion from them—may vary with the physiologic state, the experimental preparation, and the relative performances of the two ventricles.

Particularly intriguing are the implications of the spatial arrangement of this peri- and transmuscular venous network. Contraction of bronchial smooth muscle might interrupt many, if not all, communicating channels, thereby interfering with venous drainage from the bronchial capillaries and submucosal veins. Overactivity of this muscle, as in asthma, could interfere with the circulation through the bronchial walls while predisposing to congestion and mucosal edema. Another untoward prospect is that this hemodynamic disorder could compromise the self-cleansing activities of the airways, thereby predisposing to infection. Another function the submucosal plexus might have is modulating the quantity of blood that reaches the submucosa, since the transmuscular veins that can direct venous blood to or away from connections provide a potential sluicing mechanism. The submucosal plexus, by adjusting the quantity of blood near the surface, may help to control the temperature and humidity of air traversing the bronchi [15, 17].

Ultrastructurally, the small blood vessels of the bronchial capillary-venular plexus are lined by continuous endothelium 0.1 to 0.3 μm thick—except for the perinuclear regions, where it may be 3 to 4 μm thick (Fig. 2). The endothelial cells contain the usual complement of intracellular organelles: a moderate number of mitochondria, a few profiles of smooth and rough endoplasmic reticulum, numerous plasmalemmal vesicles, and abundant irregular bundles of fine fibrils 5 to 10 nm thick. The basal lamina is quite thick and arranged in multiple concentric layers, in which the pericytes are contained. In comparison with small pulmonary blood vessels, bronchial capillaries and venules have a thicker endothelium, a large number of cytofibrils, and prominent pericytes. The number of cytofibrils seems to be higher as one goes from true capillaries (5 μm in diameter) to postcapillary venules.

Much less is known about the stimuli for proliferation of the bronchial *venous* circulation than about the bronchial *arterial* circulation. Large expan-

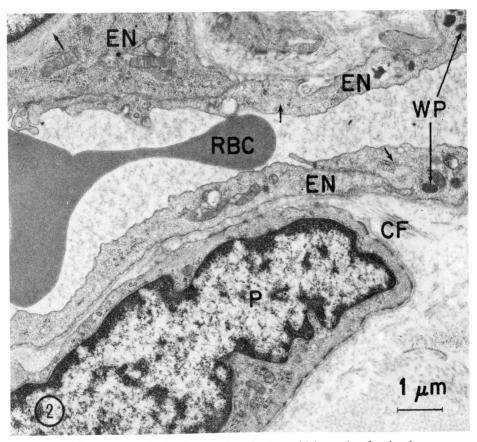

FIGURE 2 Electron photomicrographs of a bronchial venule of a dog lung sectioned longitudinally. This vessel differs from microvessels of the pulmonary circulation in having a relatively thicker endothelial cytoplasm, well-developed pericyte (P), and numerous cytoplasmic filaments (arrows), particularly in the perinuclear region. WP = Weibel-Palade bodies. EN = endothelium. RBC = erythrocye. CF = collagen fibers.

sions of the bronchial veins have been produced experimentally by ligating lobar pulmonary veins [18]. Corresponding enlargement also occurs spontaneously in chronic obstructive lung disease [19, 20]. The functional significance of these changes is obscure. In mitral stenosis, however, the submucosal venules become exceedingly dilated and congested and prone to rupture [21].

C. Bronchial Interstitial Space

It is difficult to picture a substantial three-dimensional complex structure of the
terminal airways and alveolar walls from two-dimensional electron micrographs.
Figure 3 represents our understanding of the interstitial space of a terminal
bronchiole. Towards the lumen there is a monostratified epithelium composed
of ciliated and Clara cells. Neuroepithelial cells [22] are interposed between
ciliated and Clara cells. The submucosa is richly vascularized, as it contains the
the submucosal capillary-venular plexus and small lymphatic vessels. The muscle
layer is not continuous but perforated by arterial and venous radicles to and
from the peribronchial plexuses. Abundant connective tissue surrounds the
muscle layer and is continuous with the adventitia of the pulmonary artery and
with the pericapillary spaces of the lung. No distinct partitions exist to interrupt
the flow of fluid from the most peripheral interstitial spaces of the lungs to the
mediastinum via the peribronchial interstitium. This anatomical continuity is
occasionally shown clinically by the route taken by air that escapes from the
distal interstitial spaces into the peribronchial space and progresses centrally, to
cause mediastinal emphysema. The peribronchial connective tissue consists of
thick collagenous and elastic fibers arranged in a spiral around the bronchus [23,
24] and immersed in a pool of polysaccharides, which has an inconsistent
electron-lucency, probably reflecting various degrees of hydration. In this connective tissue are numerous venules and lymphatic vessels forming a fine-meshed
plexus.

 More distally [25], only a few micrometers may separate the lymphatic
vessels from alveolar lumens. Thus, fluid or inhaled material may easily reach
these "juxtalymphatic capillaries" from the alveolar spaces [25]. Drainage of
fluids from the alveolar interstitium is favored by the architecture of the lungs
in the vicinity of the terminal brochioles, so that pressure gradients favorable to
movement of fluid towards lymphatic capillaries are generated. Additional
propulsive force in this neighborhood is probably provided by contraction of
bronchial muscle, since when this muscle contracts, the veins and lymphatics
in the peribronchial space open wide [26]. The contribution of lymphatic
contraction towards movement of fluid toward the larger ducts (e.g., by creating
a sucking force) is unknown.

D. Mast Cells

Mast cells in the lung are located predominantly in the peribronchial and perivascular connective tissue, although the number and distribution of mast cells
within the lungs vary greatly among species [27]. They also very in histologic
appearance and biochemical structure. The metachromasia of the mast cells is

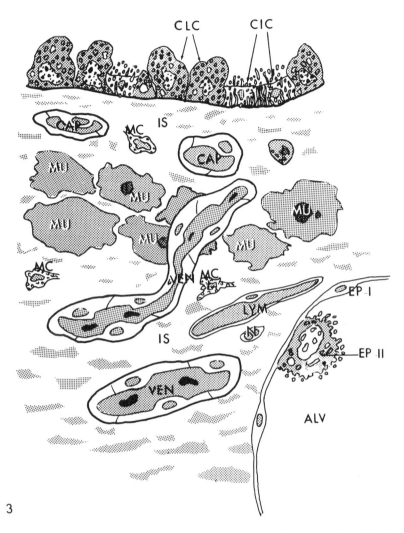

3

FIGURE 3 Diagram of the bronchial interstitial space. Between the epithelium and the muscle layer are capillaries and venules of the submucosal plexus embedded in a connective tissue containing mast cells and other cells. In the more abundant peribronchial interstitium are larger venules of the peribronchial plexus, lymphatic vessels, nerve trunks, and fixed and wandering cells (not shown). Perforating branches connect the submucosal and peribronchial plexuses. The peribronchial interstitium is in direct continuity with the interstitium of the interalveolar septa. CLC = Clara cell. CIC = ciliated cell. CAP = capillary. MC = mast cell. VEN = bronchial venule. MU = muscle. LYM = lymphatic vessel. IS = interstitial space. N = nerve trunk. ALV = alveolus. EpI = type I alveolar cell. EpII = type II alveolar cell.

due to their content of heparin. To the heparin are bound amines (histamine in man and dog; serotonin in the rat), polypeptides (bradykinin, eosinophil chemo-tactic factor of anaphylaxis, or ECF-A), the slow-reacting substance of anaphy-lasis (SRS-A), and so on [28, 29]. These powerful agents may be released from mast cells by a variety of diverse stimuli, including hypoxia, chemical agents, or antigens, after mast cells have been sensitized with IgE immunoglobulins [30, 33]. Histamine, bradykinin, and SRS-A are known to contract smooth muscle and to increase systemic venular and capillary permeability. Therefore, the loca-tion of cells containing these substances in the vicinity of the smaller bronchi and venules may have practical significance. Administration of exogenous histamine or release of endogenous histamine causes interstitial edema limited to the peribronchial connective tissue [15].

II. Leaky Bronchial Vessels

Excess water may accumulate in the interstitial or the alveolar compartments of the lungs, or both. We have described elsewhere the ultra-structural organization of the alveolar-capillary interstitial pressure gradients that favor removal of water from the gas-exchanging surfaces [34]. Pulmonary edema is generally considered in terms of this ultrastructural and hydrodynamic arrangement and explained in terms of a change in the hydrostatic of osmotic forces across the walls of the pulmonary microcirculation and of lymphatic flow. Although this approach has been rewarding relative to hemodynamic pulmonary edema, it has left unanswered questions about certain types of edema that are generally attributed to "increased permeability" of the pulmonary circulation. Among these is pul-monary edema evoked by histamine.

Reexamination of this problem in our laboratory [15], using dogs, has dis-closed that no matter what the route of administration to the lungs—intraven-ously, by nebulization, or by direct injection into the lung—histamine selectively caused the bronchial venules to leak. The effect was consistently independent of dose: pleural injections elicited this selective response, with as little as 0.1 mg of histamine base; larger doses, administered intravenously (up to 30 mg kg^{-1} min^{-1} for 90 min), or by nebulization (2.75 mg/ml for 90 min to one lobe) in the attempt to cause pulmonary capillaries to leak elicited the same qualitative bronchial venular response (Fig. 4) while leaving the pulmonary microcirculation unaffected (Fig. 5). Within 10 min after the agent was administered, leakage stopped, leaving trapped tracer in the bronchial venular adventitia—evidence of antecedent transudation of fluid across the bronchial venular wall (Fig. 4).

The anatomical basis for this transient effect of histamine appears to be "stretching" of interendothelial junctions so that gaps appear between cells, allowing plasma to enter the interstitial space (Fig. 6). The endothelial lining of

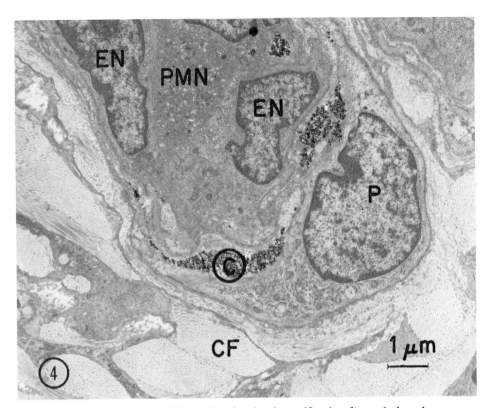

FIGURE 4 Leaky bronchial venule of a dog lung 60 min after subpleural injection of histamine. Colloidal carbon was injected intravenously shortly before histamine administration. The presence of carbon (C) in the adventitia, between endothelium (EN) and pericyte (P) indicates that the vessel had become leaky. A leukocyte (PMN) now fills the lumen of the partially collapsed blood vessel. No evidence of edema is detected at this time; the interstitium contains compact bundles of collagen fibers (CF).

the bronchial venules and capillaries are richly endowed with contractile fibrils, which when they are stimulated to contract seem to be responsible for widening the junctions between adjacent endothelial cells. This behavior on the systematic venules of the lungs is reminiscent of the comparable responses of systemic venules in the cremaster muscle of the rat to the administration of histamine.

Similar responses were elicited by bradykinin injected intrapleurally or intravenously. Biopsy samples of the lung disclosed leakage of carbon from bronchial venules that was apparent within 1.5 min after intrapleural injection; at comparable dosages, bradykinin appeared to exert more leakage of carbon tracer and more widespread involvement of bronchial venules. Subpleural or

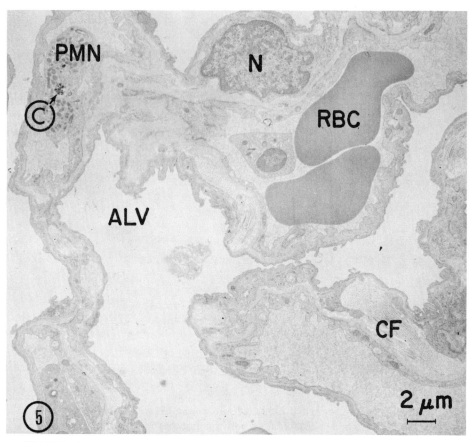

FIGURE 5 An electron photomicrograph of the alveolar capillaries from the same animal as in the previous figure. No leakage of carbon nor any interstitial edema is seen. Carbon is seen within the cytoplasm of leukocyte (PMN). N = nucleus.

intravenous injections of 48/80, a mast cell degranular, evoked the same response without affecting pulmonary microvessels. In contrast, serotonin failed to cause bronchial venular leakage even after huge doses (up to 10 mg intrapleurally).

    Considered together, these obervations seem to allow certain conclusions. (1) Certain agents, traditionally believed to cause pulmonary leakage elicit bronchial venular leakage instead. (2) These agents seem to exert this sterotyped effect independent of the route of administration. (3) In the lungs, as elsewhere in the body, the affected vessels are systemic venules. (4) The discrepant effects

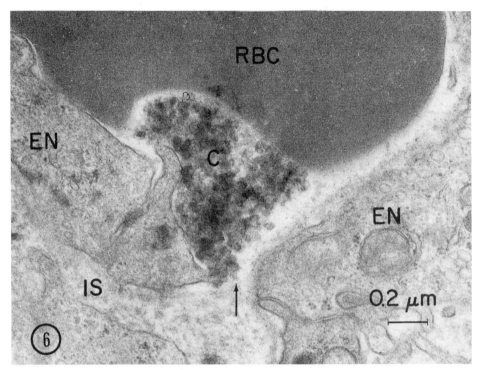

FIGURE 6 Electron photomicrograph of a bronchial venule of a dog lung 60 sec after administration of histamine. Carbon is apparently escaping through a large gap in the vessel's wall.

of histamine on the one hand and serotonin on the other suggest that contraction of the bronchial venular smooth muscle—which occurred in both instances— was not the common denominator responsible for the leakage. Instead, the leakage appears to reflect stimulation of inherent endothelial contractility by one agent (e.g. histamine or bradykinin) and lack of stimulation by another (e.g. serotonin).

These observations focus on the bronchial circulation as a possible source of interstitial edema. Because of the submucosal location of one bronchial venular plexus, local injury, such as bronchitis, should readily evoke peribronchiolar edema as part of the exudative process. Also, that the bronchial circulation is a source of interstitial edema during anaphylaxis was shown many years ago by Schultz and Jordan [35] in chronic studies on anaphylaxis, and by Warren and Dixon [36, 37], who sensitized guinea pigs to albumin and triggered anaphylaxis using $[^{131}I]$albumin, localizing the site of $[^{131}I]$albumin leakage by radioautography.

More mysterious have been the changes produced by increased quantities of circulating bioactive substances, such as endotoxin. By producing endotoxin shock in dogs using *Escherichia coli* lipopolysaccharide that was injected intravenously, with colloidal carbon as a tracer, we could reproduce the bronchial venular leakage that we observed after histamine and bradykinin, again leaving unaffected the pulmonary microcirculation [38]. Only after an hour of persistent hypotension were alveolar-capillary interfaces affected; the alveolar septum then showed focal interstitial edema, the alveolar epithelium showed focal degenerative changes, and damaged leukocytes appeared to be sequestered in the alveolar capillaries. But by then, it was difficult to unravel the relative importance of sustained hypotension from the direct vascular consequences of the endotoxin. Indeed, the demonstration that sustained hemorrhagic hypotension could reproduce the alveolar capillary lexions indicates that hypotension

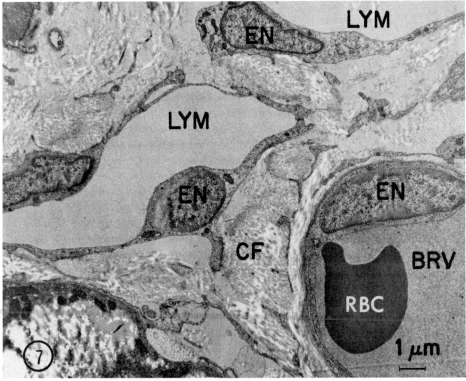

FIGURE 7 Low-power electron photomicrograph of the peribronchial space of a dog lung, showing the close proximity of bronchial venules (BRV) and lymphatic vessels (LYM).

from any cause if allowed to persist will promote secondary damage in the gas-exchanging portions of the lung.

Once interstitial edema exists in the vicinity of the bronchioles, secondary effects may supervene, depending on the compliance of the interstitial space in the affected region and the proximity of other structures involved in water removal from the lungs, e.g. lymphatics. It is now generally accepted that no matter where in the lungs excess fluid begins to accumulate, interstitial forces direct it away from the gas-exchanging surfaces towards lymphatics that will transport it towards exits from the lungs [35, 39, 40]. Whether perilymphatic edema interferes with lymphatic drainage remains to be determined.

Clearly, the demonstration that bronchial venules can suffer an increase in permeability raises questions about using the lymph collected at main exits from the lungs to gain insight into the composition of interstitial fluid in the more remote alveolar interstitial spaces. This uncertainty is heightened by the proximity of bronchial venules and capillaries to lymphatics in the peribronchial lymphatic space (Fig. 7), and the consequent opportunity for physical inter-dependence as well as for the exchange of plasma constituents across the thin endothelial barriers in accord with differences in concentration. Finally, it seems unlikely that the present experience with histamine, bradykinin, histamine releasers, and endotoxin will prove to be unique. Indeed, it seems reasonable that other physiologic processes and bioactive materials also operate to increase selectively the permeability of the bronchial venules. Accordingly, not only do the systemic venules to the lungs provide a potential site, per se, for the patho-geneis of pulmonary edema, but this potential for leakage may also aggravate more conventional types of pulmonary edema by interfering with the interstitial machinery for removing water from the lungs [15, 34].

References

1. W. S. Miller. *The Lung*. 2nd ed. Springfield, Ill., Charles C Thomas, 1947, pp. 74-88.
2. G. Töndury and E. Weibel. Anatomie der Lungengefässe, *Ergebn. ges. Tuberk-Forsch.*, 14:61-100 (1958).
3. W. Florange, Anatomie und Pathologie der Arteria bronchialis, *Ergebn. Path. u. Path. Anatomie*, 39:153-213 (1960).
4. R. F. McLaughlin, Jr., W. S. Tyler, and R. O. Canada. A study of the subgross pulmonary anatomy in various mammals. *Amer. J. Anat.*, 108: 149-165 (1961).
5. R. F. McLaughlin, Jr., W. S. Tyler, and R. O. Canada. Subgross pulmonary anatomy of the rabbit, rat, and guinea pig with additional notes on the human lung, *Amer. Rev. Resp. Dis.*, 94:380-387 (1966).

6. L. Cudkowicz. *Human Bronchial Circulation in Health and Disease.* Baltimore, Williams and Wilkins (1968).

7. H. Von Hayek, *Die menschliche Lunge.* 2nd ed. Berlin, Heidelberg, New York, Springer-Verlag, 1970, pp. 113-158.

8. Leonardo DaVinci. *Quaderni D'Anatomia.* Vol. 2. *Cuòre, Anatomia & Fisiologia.* Ventiquattro Fogli della Royal Library di Windsor. Christiana, Dybwad, 1912.

9. M. D. Daly and C. Hebb. *Pulmonary and Bronchial Vascular Systems.* Baltimore, Williams and Wilkins, 1966.

10. A. P. Fishman, The clinical significance of the pulmonary collateral circulation, *Circulation,* 24:677-690 (1961).

11. A. P. Fishman, G. M. Turino, M. Brandfonbrener, and A. Himmelstein. The "effective" pulmonary collateral blood flow in man, *J. Clin. Invest.,* 37:1071-1086 (1958).

12. A. A. Liebow, M. R. Hales, and W. E. Bloomer. Relation of bronchial to pulmonary vascular tree. In *Pulmonary Circulation.* Edited by W.R. Adams amd I. Veith. New York, Grune and Stratton, 1959, pp. 79-98.

13. P. Marchand, J. C. Gilroy, and V. H. Wilson. An anatomical study of the bronchial vascular system and its variations in disease, *Thorax,* 5:207-221 (1950).

14. L. Cudkowitz, and J. B. Armstrong. Blood supply of malignant pulmonary neoplasm, *Thorax,* 8:152-156 (1953).

15. G. G. Pietra, J. P. Szidon, M.M. Leventhal, and A. P. Fishman. Histamine and interstitial pulmonary edema in the dog, *Circ. Res.,* 29:323-337 (1971).

16. D. M. Aviado, M. D. Daly, C. Y. Lee, and C. F. Schmidt. The contribution of the bronchial circulation to the venous admixture in pulmonary venous blood, *J. Physiol.,* 155:602-622 (1961).

17. T. Hughes. Microcirculation of the tracheobronchial tree, *Nature,* 206: 425-426 (1965).

18. A. Hurwitz, M. Calabresi, R. W. Cooke, and A. A. Liebow. An experimental study of the venous collateral circulation of the lung. 1. Anatomical observations, *Amer. J. Path.,* 30:1085-1116 (1954).

19. E. Zuckerklandl. Über die Anastomosen der Venae pulmonales mit den bronchial Venen und mit dem mediastinalen Venennetze, *S. B. Akad. Wiss. Wien. math. nat. Kl.,* 84:110-152 (1882).

20. A. A. Liebow. The bronchopulmonary venous collateral circulation with special reference to emphysema, *Amer. J. Path.,* 29:251-276 (1953).

21. F. C. Ferguson, R. E. Kobilak and J. E. Dietrick. Varices of the bronchial veins as a source of hemoptysis in mitral stenosis, *Amer. Heart J.,* 28:1-12 (1944).

22. J. M. Lauweryns, M. Cokelaere, P. Theunynck. Neuro-epithelial bodies in the respiratory mucosa of various mammals, *Z. Zellforsch.,* 135:569-592 (1972).

23. F. Orsos. Die Gerüstsysteme der Lunge deren physiologische und pathologische Bedeutung. 1. Normal-anatomische Verhältnisse, *Beitr. Z. Klin. Tuberk. Forsch.,* 87:568-609 (1936).

24. T. H. Rosenquist, S. Bernick, S. S. Sobin, and Y. C. Fung. The structure of the pulmonary interalveolar microvascular sheet, *Microvasc. Res.*, 5:199-212 (1973).

25. J. M. Lauweryns. The blood and lymphatic microcirculation of the lung. In *Pathology Annual*. Edited by S. C. Sommers. New York, Appleton-Century-Crofts, 1971, pp. 365-415.

26. V. E. Krahl. Anatomy of the mammalian lung. In *Handbook of Physiology Respiration*. Section 3, Vol. 1. Washington, D.C., American Physiological Society, 1964, pp. 213-284.

27. C. Hebb. Motor innervation of the pulmonary blood vessels of mammals. In *The Pulmonary Circulation and Interstitial Space*. Edited by A. P. Fishman and H. H. Hecht. Chicago, University of Chicago Press, 1969, pp. 195-222.

28. H. Chiu, and D. Lagunoff. Histochemical comparison of vertebrate mast cells, *Histochem. J.*, 4:135-144 (1972).

29. K. F. Austen. A review of immunological, biochemical and pharmacological factors in the release of chemical mediators from human lung. In *Asthma: Physiology, Immunopharmacology and Treatment*. Edited by K. F. Austen and L. M. Lichtenstein. New York, Academic Press, 1973, pp. 109-122.

30. F. Haas and E. H. Bergofsky. Role of the mast cell in the pulmonary pressor response to hypoxia, *J. Clin. Invest.*, 51:3154-3162 1972.

31. J. M. Kay, J. C. Waymire, and R. F. Grover. Lung mast cell hyperplasia and pulmonary histamine-forming capacity in hypoxic rats, *Amer. J. Physiol.*, 226:178-184 (1974).

32. T. Ishizaka, K. Ishizaka, R. P. Orange, and K. F. Austen. Pharmacologic inhibition of the antigen-induced release of histamine and slow-reacting substance of anaphylaxi s (SRS-A) from monkey lung tissues mediated by human IgE, *J. Immunol.*, 106:1267-1273 (1971).

33. D. Lagunoff. The mechamism of histamine release from mast cells, *Biochem. Pharmacol.*, 21:1889-1896 (1972).

34. A. P. Fishman. Pulmonary edema. The water-exchanging function of the lung, *Circulation*, 46:390-408 (1972).

35. W. H. Schultz and H. E. Jordan. Physiological studies in anaphylaxis. III. A microscopic study of the anaphylactic lung of the guinea pig and mouse, *J. Pharm.*, 2:375-389 (1911).

36. S. Warren, and F. J. Dixon. Antigen tracer studies and histologic observations in anaphylactic shock in the guinea pig, *Amer. J. Med. Sci.*, 216:136-145 (1948).

37. F. J. Dixon and S. Warren. Antigen tracer studies and histologic observations in anaphylactic shick in the guinea pig, *Amer. J. Med. Sci.*, 217:414-421 (1949).

38. G. G. Pietra, J.P. Szidon, H. A. Carpenter and A. P. Fishman. Bronchial venular leakage during endotoxin shock, *Amer. J. Path.*, 77:387-406 (1974).

39. N. C. Staub, H. Nagano, and M. L. Pearce. Pulmonary edema in dogs, especially the sequence of fluid accumulation in lungs, *J. Appl. Physiol.*, 22:227-240 (1967).

40. N. C. Staub. Pulmonary edema, *Physiol. Rev.*, 54:679-811 (1974).

14

Role of Lymphatics in the Genesis of "Shock Lung"
A Hypothesis

DENIS F. J. HALMAGYI

College of Physicians and Surgeons
Columbia University
New York, New York

I. Introduction

The subject index of the *Proceedings* of a comprehensive and authoritative symposium on shock, published in 1961, failed to include the word *lung* [1], whereas in 1968 the National Academy of Sciences convened a special conference on the pulmonary effects of nonthoracic trauma [2]. In 1973 various forms of acute respiratory failure accounted for 50% of all patient-days in the Surgery-Anesthesiology Intensive Care Unit of the Columbia-Presbyterian Medical Center.

The emergence of this new syndrome is considered by some as a sign of improved efficiency in the management of the critically ill, who are now assured of progress towards hitherto uncharted expanses of their illness. More critical observers maintain, however, that this syndrome is largely iatrogenic, caused by overambitious resuscitation with oxygen and fluids; and the potential role of overhydration justifies its inclusion in this monograph.

Ashbough, Bigelow, Petty, and Levine [3] were first to notice the frequent association of critical illness and acute hypoxic (as distinct from hypercapnic) respiratory failure and having found that it failed to respond to "usual methods of treatment," they considered this a separate entity and coined the term *adult respiratory distress syndrome*, alluding to its resemblance to a similar condition seen in the newborn. It appears reasonable to assume that "not responding to the usual methods of treatment" was meant to indicate that these patients could be controlled only by assisted ventilation.

Others used the term *shock lung*, which is commendable for its brevity but wrongly implies that hypotension is a mandatory preamble. The many names under which this illness has become known are summarized in Table 1 [4].

TABLE 1 Synonyms for Acute Hypoxic Respiratory Failure

Adult hyaline membrane disease
Adult respiratory insufficiency syndrome
Bronchopulmonary dysplasia
Congestive atelectasis
DaNang lung
Fat embolism
Hemorrhagic atelectasis
Hemorrhagic lung syndrome
Hypoxic hyperventilation
Oxygen toxicity
Postperfusion lung
Posttransfusion lung
Posttraumatic atelectasis
Posttraumatic pulmonary insufficiency
Progressive pulmonary consolidation
Progressive respiratory distress
Pulmonary edema
Pulmonary hyaline membrane disease
Pulmonary microembolism
Pump lung
Respirator lung
Shock lung
Stiff lung syndrome
Transplant lung
Traumatic wet lung
Wet lung
White lung syndrome

II. Acute Hypoxic Respiratory Failure

A. Definition

Hypoxic respiratory failure is a stereotyped response to various pulmonary insults ranging from lung contusion to severe viral pneumonia, from fluid inhalation to heroin poisoning, and the etiology can be identified only by special tests. Here I propose to discuss only that form of acute hypoxic respiratory failure that is associated with severe trauma or sepsis.

It usually appears 6 to 24 hr following trauma or massive infection and this may be the reason why it has been missed both by clinicians (whose patients may not have lived long enough) and by laboratory investigators (who have concentrated their attention on the immediate response). The characteristically severe dyspnea is the combined result of hypoxemia, which causes hyperventilation, and of the fall in lung compliance, which increases the work of breathing. At this stage the chest roentgenogram reveals widespread opacities [5] indistinguishable from left ventricular failure [6] or from fluid inhalation [7]. The course is variable; many patients continue to deteriorate and require assisted ventilation with various concentrations of inspired oxygen for days or weeks. A small minority cannot be controlled and become candidates for extracorporeal oxygenation, or they die. For a full and lucid description of the physiologic and clinical details and for bibliography the reader is referred to the excellent review by Pontoppidan et al. [8]. Only some aspects of the condition will be discussed here.

Acute hypoxic respiratory failure is frequently preceded by aggressive fluid resuscitation; extracellular lung water is increased [9, 10] and postmortem, the lung weight is about 1 to 2 kg higher than normal [9]. These findings can be interpreted as suggesting that the syndrome represents acute pulmonary edema secondary to fluid overload. On closer scrutiny, however, some important differences are revealed, as summarized in Table 2.

B. Comparison with Hemodynamic Edema

No quantitative correlation could be established between the water content of the lung and the previous fluid balance [9]; peripheral edema is not, as a rule, observed and pleural effusion is absent. More important, even the most severe forms of this condition may develop without any measurable elevation in pulmonary arterial wedge pressure.

It could be argued that hemodynamic alterations do not represent the only pathogenetic mechanism causing lung edema. Many of the patients are septic, and increased pulmonary vascular permeability in bacteremia has not convincingly shown experimentally [11].

TABLE 2   Comparison between Acute Hypoxic Respiratory Failure and Acute
Hemodynamic Lung Edema

	Lung edema	Acute respiratory failure
Total body fluid volume	++	+/=
Right atrial pressure	++	+/=
Pulmonary arterial wedge pressure	++	+/=
Plasma protein concentration	All reduced	Albumin reduced
Pleural effusion	+	−
Physical signs over chest	Typical	Absent/multiform
Radiology of lung	Typical	Variable
Foam in airways	++	−
Effects of diuretics	Curative	Slight/temporary
Effect of digitalis	+	−
Histology	Alveolar edema	Interstitial edema
Increase in compliance following hyperinflation	+	−

Irrespective of etiology, the earliest detectable stage of fluid accumulation in the lung is an expansion of the peribronchial and perivascular spaces and this is followed by a similar expansion of the alveolar interstitium [12]. Accumulation of fluid in the interstitium, more than alveolar edema, is likely to be related to the higher compliance of the interstitial tissue. Cells of the normal alveolar epithelium are joined by continuous, tight intercellular junctions, which prevent the flow of proteinaceous fluid into the alveoli until it overflows the respiratory bronchioles, floods the alveoli, and procudes intra-alveolar lung edema. In contrast, the site of fluid in acute hypoxic respiratory failure is predominantly interstitial with only a few scattered foci of fluid-filled alveoli [13–15], as if in this condition the normal sequence of fluid accumulation in the lung has been arrested. Results of pulmonary mechanics measurements in these patients have been consistent with a predominantly extracellular type of lung edema.

In acute hemodynamic edema, fall in lung compliance is secondary to the presence of bubbles in the alveolar orifices resulting in the reduction of the number of alveoli participating in volume changes [16, 17]. In these patients hyperinflation of the lung with pressures over 50 to 60 cm H_2O opens up previously nonpatent groups of alveoli, resulting in a sharp increase in the slope of the pressure-volume curve.

This does not happen in acute hypoxic respiratory failure. We measured lung volume by N_2 washout and total thoracic compliance (airway pressure plus integrated flow) in patients receiving assisted ventilation for nonpulmonary causes (myasthenia gravis, tetanus, etc.), for exacerbations of chronic obstructive lung disease, for minor acute respiratory distress following surgery, and for acute hypoxic respiratory failure. Details of this work will be published elsewhere [18] but some of the findings are shown in Figure 1. An inflating pressure of about 25 cm H_2O expands the healthy lung to near-total lung capacity, as shown by the interrupted line. The patient with chronic obstructive lung disease (as shown by the increased FRC (curve D) and the patient with minor postoperative respiratory distress (curve C) could be well inflated. These patients were not severely ill and were extubated a few hours later. Lines A and B were obtained on two consecutive days in a patient suffering from severe acute hypoxic respiratory failure. We found that in this condition the pressure-volume curve is not restored towards normal by using high inflating pressure, and the increment in lung volume is likely to be secondary to overdistension of patent alveoli rather than to recruitment of new airspaces. A similar behavior (increased recoil pressure on inflation) was described for mitral stenosis and was interpreted as

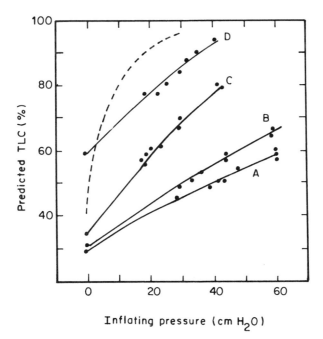

FIGURE 1 The relation between total lung capacity and airway pressure. Dotted line is predicted normal curve. Lines A and B obtained on successive days in a patient with acute hypoxic respiratory failure. Line C represents a patient with minor postoperative respiratory distress; and line D, a patient with chronic obstructive lung disease.

suggesting the presence of interstitial fibrosis and lymphatic engorgement [19]. This is consistent with the predominantly interstitial location of water in the lung of our patients.

The interstitial compartment of the lung, as Hayek described [20], consists of the peribronchial, perivascular, and subpleural spaces, is filled with fibrous connective tissue, and contains the nerves, bronchial vessels, and lymphatics. Its fluid is largely entrapped within a fine meshwork of polymerized chondroitin sulfate and hyaluronic acid, and there is free fluid containing the protein [21]. Early measurements of subcutaneous interstitial fluid pressure with needles inserted into the interstitial space yielded values ranging from 0.4 to 4.9 torr [22], and with a more refined technique in the bat wing it was found to be 1.25 torr [23]. Using a completely different method of measurement, Guyton [24] asserted that interstitial fluid pressures were normally negative, i.e. subatmospheric, and subsequent investigators, with their own techniques, confirmed these surprising findings [25]. Because of the low capillary pressure and the negative intrapleural pressure, the concept of subatmospheric interstitial pressure has been more readily accepted for the lung [26] than for other organs. For a clear and comprehensive summary of this topic, the reader is referred to the very informative review by Hughes [21].

C. Lymphatic Function

Fluid from the interstitial compartment is cleared into the bloodstream by the lymphatics, which form an extensive plexus in the interlobular, perivascular, and peribronchial connective tissue [20, 27, 28]. Since the pulmonary interstitial pressure is subatmospheric and the right atrial pressure is higher than atmospheric, lymph flow is against the pressure gradient and can not be passive. The active propulsion involves extrinsic (i.e., respiratory movements, arterial pulsations) and intrinsic (i.e., lymphatic contractility) forces [29], and it is the latter that is less well known and less widely appreciated, and requires closer scrutiny.

In the cannulated thoracic duct of animals [30, 31] and of man [32] pulsations varying from 1 to 25 torr were recorded at frequencies of 1 to 30 per min, with respiratory fluctuations superimposed. Rate and amplitude of the contractions are influenced by the amount of fluid entering the lymphatics, suggesting that an important intrinsic mechanism regulates the removal of fluid from the tissues [30, 33]. This is consistent with the assumption that lung lymphatics operate as skimming pumps, maintaining a constant level of interstitial fluid [12]. Effectiveness of the contractions are facilitated by the firm anchorage of the vessels to the collagenous fibers of the surrounding tissue [34].

Since fluid accumulation in the interstitium increases the distance between individual collagenous fibers, this mechanism also provides for maximum patency of the vessel during edema formation.

The functional unit of the lymphatics is considered by some [35, 36] to be the segment between two valves, with the distal valve belonging to the segment and the proximal valve forming part of the next, as shown in Figure 2. Lymph is propelled by a coordinated process of contractions and dilatations involving simultaneously several segments and valves. Occlusion of the lymph vessels results in a gradual rise in intraluminal pressure to as high as 50 torr [29]. Since the maximum increment in the pressure of a single segment is only 1 to 2 torr, the high values obtained in the whole vessel must be the result of active coordinated contractions of several segments [37].

Contractions generating such high intraluminal pressures require musculature and this is abundantly present in the wall of the lymphatics, forming mainly longitudinal layers [38], as shown in Figure 3. Musculature first appears in the wall of the medium-sized lymph vessels and gradually increases in thickness proximally. The functionality of this musculature is further underlined by the presence of an extensive network of nutritive blood vessels [39]. Anatomically, physiologically, and pharmacologically, the musculature of the lymphatics is in between the skeletal and cardiac muscles [40], as summarized in Table 3. Comparative histologic studies have shown species differences in the extent of muscle supply; it is richest in ruminants and poorest in dogs and cats, with pigs and humans in the middle [41].

The close topographic relation between nerve fibers and smooth muscles in the lymphatic wall provides morphologic data implicating possible nervous regulation [34], with some nerve endings tentatively identified as receptors [42]. In addition, the lymphatics were shown to respond to various humoral agents, as summarized in Table 4.

In the normal (i.e., negative) tissue pressure range, small increments in interstitial fluid volume produce a disproportionately large increase in tissue pressure [43], as shown in Figure 4. If for any reason fluid commences to accumulate in the lung, the increment in tissue pressure will diminish or abolish the gradient against which the lymph has to be propelled into the veins. Thus the force needed for maintaining lymph transport will be reduced and the increased inflow of tissue fluid into the terminal lymphatics will stimulate lymphatic contractility. These two factors would then increase lymph flow (Fig. 4b) and would tend to create a new dynamic equilibrium between fluid formation and fluid transport, at a higher level of interstitial fluid volume and tissue pressure. This situation would then become reminiscent of heart failure, when cardiac output is maintained at the cost of increased blood volume and rising filling pressure.

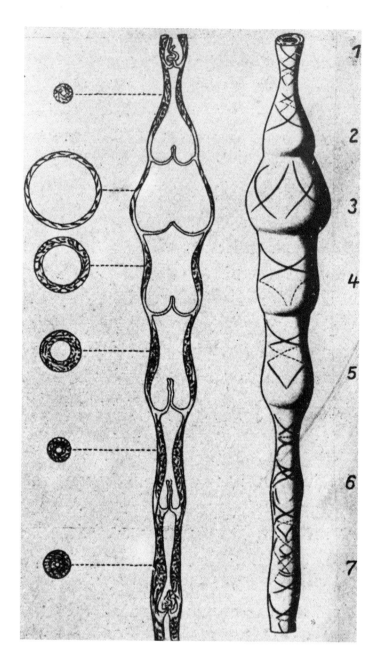

FIGURE 2 Schematic representation of lymph vessel contraction. Numbers at top represent different stages of contraction. Most relaxed segment, no. 3; most contracted, no. 7. Center and right-hand drawings are external and sagittal sections through length of the lymphatic. At the left are representative cross sections. Reprinted from E. Horstmann, *Gegenbaur's Morphol. Jb.*, **91**:483-510 (1952), by courtesy of the publisher.

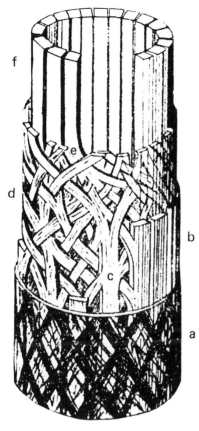

FIGURE 3 Schematic representation of a medium-sized lymph vessel. a = connective tissue. b = external longitudinal muscle. c and d = invasion and ramification of b into media. e = transition of b into intima. f = musculature of intima. Reprinted from G. D. Mall, *Z. Anat. Entwickl.*, **100**:521-558 (1933), by courtesy of the publisher.

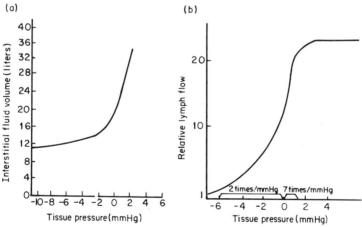

FIGURE 4 Theoretical relation between interstitial tissue fluid pressure and extracellular fluid volume (A) and relative lymph flow (B). Reprinted from A. E. Taylor, et al., *Lymphology*, **6**:192-208 (1973), by courtesy of the publisher.

TABLE 3 Musculature of Lymphatic Vessels: Anatomical and Physiological Characteristics

Features similar to skeletal muscle	Features similar to cardiac muscle
Anatomic	
1. Number and peripheral position of nuclei	1. Abundance of sarcoplasmic reticulum
2. Distribution of mitochondria	2. High number of mitochondria
3. Absence of intercalated discs	3. Length and structure of fibers and myofibrils
4. Endplate-like neuromuscular junctions	4. Surface contacts of the sarcoplasmic reticulum
	5. Intraplasmic granular vesicles
Physiologic	
1. Exhibits tetanic contractions	1. Duration of contractions
2. Paralyzed by curare	2. Paralyzed by acetylcholine
3. Short refractory period	3. Activation of automatism following chronic denervation
4. No compensatory pause	
5. Contractions may sum	
6. Electrophysiology	
7. Neuromuscular transmission	

TABLE 4 Response to Lymphatics to various Humoral Agents

Agent	Frequency response	Amplitude response	Reference
Serotonin	+	+	40
Norepinephrine	+	+	40
Procaine	–	–	45
Histamine	+	=	31
Ornithin	–	–	31
1-Arginin	+	+	31
1-Tyrosin	+	+	44
Bradykinin	+	+	44

NOTE: +, increase; –, decrease; = unchanged.

III. Hypothesis of Lymph Failure

Many potential causes of reduced lymphatic contractility exist in sepsis and trauma. Excessive activation of the autonomous nervous system and release of various humoral agents are known to be associated with these conditions: the lymphatics are known to respond with constriction to many of these secretions [44–46]. In addition, lymph flow may also be impaired by increased intra-luminal resistance [47]. Lymph has the capacity to clot [29], and thrombi have been observed in the lumen of lymph vessels [48]. Severe trauma and sepsis have a profound effect on the clotting mechanism and this has been implicated as a contributor to the pathogenesis of pulmonary changes [4]. It is conceivable that under certain conditions, clots may also form in the lymphatic vessels of the lung, but owing to the time-consuming techniques needed for the postmortem examination of the lung lymphatics, this problem has not yet been studied.

The present hypothesis is offered not as a substitute but as a complement to the many interesting theories on the hitherto unknown pathogenesis of the adult respiratory distress syndrome.

References

1. *Proceedings of a Conference on Recent Progress and Present Problems in the Field of Shock.* Edited by S. F. Seeley and J. R. Wiesiger. *Fed. Proc.,* **20**, suppl. 9 (1961).

2. B. Eiseman and D. G. Ashbaugh, editors, Pulmonary effects of non-thoracic trauma, *J. Trauma,* 8:625-747 (1968).

3. D. G. Ashbaugh, D. B. Bigelow, T. L. Petty, and B. E. Levine, Acute respiratory distress in adults, *Lancet,* 2:319-323 (1967).

4. W. Blaisdell and R. M. Schlobohm, The respiratory distress syndrome, a review, *Surgery,* **74**:252-262 (1973).

5. N. Joffe, Roentgenologic findings in post-shock and postoperative pulmonary insufficiency, *Radiology,* **94**:369-375 (1970).

6. W. T. Meszaros, Lung changes in left heart failure, *Circulation,* **47**:859-871 (1973).

7. D. F. J. Halmagyi and H. J. H. Colebatch, The drowned lung: A physiological approach to its mechanism and management, *Australasian Ann. Med.,* **10**:68-77 (1961).

8. H. Pontoppidan, B. Geffin, and E. Lowenstein, Acute respiratory failure in the adult, *N. E. J. Med.,* **287**:690-698, 743-752, 799-806 (1972).

9. F. E. Gump, Y. Mashima, A. Ferenczy, and J. M. Kinney, Pre- and post-mortem studies of lung fluids and electrolytes, *J. Trauma,* 11:474-482 (1971).

10. F. E. Gump, Y. Mashima, S. Jørgensen, and J. M. Kinney, Simultaneous use of three indicators to evaluate pulmonary capillary damage in man, *Surgery,* **70**:262-270 (1971).

11. K. L. Brigham, W. C. Woolverton, L. H. Blake, and N. C. Staub, Increased sheep lung vascular permeability caused by pseudomonas bacteremia, *J. Clin. Invest.,* **54**:792-804 (1974).

12. N. Staub, The pathophysiology of pulmonary edema, *Physiol. Rev.,* **54**: 678-811 (1974).

13. W. Remmele and U. Goebel, Zur pathologischen Anatomie des Kreislaufschocks beim Menschen. V. Pathomorphologie der Schocklunge, *Klin. Wochenschr.,* **51**:25-31 (1973).

14. G. Nash, F. D. Foley, and P. C. Langlinais, Pulmonary interstitial edema and hyaline membrane in adult burn patients; electron-microscopic observations, *Human Pathol.,* **5**:149-160 (1974).

15. M. Bachofen and F. Roth, Zur Behandlung der akuten Ateminsuffizienz beim chirurgischen Patienten, *Schw. Med. Wochenschr.,* **104**:757-763 (1974).

16. C. D. Cook, J. Mead, G. L. Schreiner, N. R. Frank, and J. M. Craig, Pulmonary mechanics during induced pulmonary edema in anesthetized dogs, *J. Appl. Physiol.,* **14**:177-182 (1959).

17. J. T. Sharp, G. T. Griffith, I. L. Bunnell, and D. G. Green, Ventilatory mechanics in pulmonary edema in man, *J. Clin. Invest.,* **37**:111-117 (1959).

18. D. F. J. Halmagyi, J. Israel, and Z. Eckstein, unpublished data.

19. T. E. Wood, P. McLeod, N. R. Anthonisen, and P. J. Macklem, Mechanics of breathing in mitral stenosis, *Amer. Rev. Resp. Dis.,* **104**:52-60 (1971).

20. H. Hayek, *Die Menschliche Lunge.* Berlin, Springer, 1953.

21. J. M. B. Hughes, Pulmonary interstitial pressure, *Bull. Physio-Pathol. Resp.,* **7**:1095-1123 (1971).

22. P. D. McMaster, The pressure and interstitial resistance prevailing in the normal and edematous skin of animals and man, *J. Exp. Med.,* **84**:473-509 (1946).

23. C. A. Wiederhelm. In *The Pulmonary Circulation and Interstitial Space.* Edited by A. P. Fishman and H. H. Hecht. Chicago, University of Chicago Press, 1969, pp. 29-41.

24. A. C. Guyton, A concept of negative interstitial pressure based on pressures in implanted perforated capsules, *Circ. Res.,* **12**:399-414 (1963).

25. P. F. Scholander, A. R. Hargens, and S. L. Miller, Negative pressure in the interstitial fluid of animals, *Science,* **161**:321-328 (1968).

26. B. J. Meyer, A. Meyer, and A. C. Guyton, Interstitial fluid pressure. V. Negative pressure in the lungs. *Circ. Res.,* **22**:263-271 (1968).

27. W. S. Miller, Das Lungenläppchen, seine Blut- und Lymphgefässe, *Arch. Anat. Entwickl.,* **179**:197-228 (1900).

28. J. M. Lauweryns. In *Pathology Annual.* Edited by S. C. Sommers. New York, Appleton-Century-Crofts, 1971, pp. 365-415.

29. J. M. Yoffey and F. C. Courtice. *Lymphatics, Lymph and the Lymphomyeloid Complex.* London, Academic Press, 1970.

30. J. G. Hall, B. Morris, and G. Wooley, Intrinsic rhythmic propulsion of lymph in the unanesthetized sheep, *J. Physiol.* (London), **180**:336-349 (1965).

31. T. Campbell and T. Heath, Intrinsic contractility of lymphatics in sheep and in dogs, *Quart. J. Exp. Physiol.,* **58**:207-217 (1973).
32. J. B. Kinmonth and G. W. Taylor, Spontaneous rhythmic contractility in human lymphatics, *J. Physiol* (London), **133**:3P (1956).
33. M. Mislin, Die Motorik der Lymphgefässe und die Regulation der Lymphherzen. In *Das Lymphgefässystem, Hb. allg. Pathol.* Vol. 3, Part 6. Edited by H. Meessen. Berlin, Springer, 1972, pp. 219-238.
34. L. V. Leak, The fine structure and function of the lymphatic vascular system. In *Das Lymphgefässystem, Hb. allg. Pathol.* Vol. 3. Part 6. Edited by H. Meessen. Berlin, Springer, 1972, pp. 149-196.
35. E. Horstmann. Über die funktionelle Struktur der mesenterialien Lymphgefässe, *Gegenbaur's Morphol. Jb.,* **91**:483-510 (1952).
36. E. Horstmann, Beobachtungen zur Motorik der Lymphgefässe, *Pflüg. Arch.,* **269**:511-519 (1959).
37. F. Waldeck, Zur Motorik der Lymphgefässe bei der Ratte, *Pflüg. Arch.,* **283**:285-293, 294-300 (1965).
38. G. D. Mall, Über den Wandbau der mittleren und kleineren Lymphefässe des Menschen, *Z. Anat. Entwickl.,* **100**:521-558 (1933).
39. H. M. Evans, The blood supply of lymphatic vessels in man. *Amer. J. Anat.,* **7**:195-208 (1907).
40. R. Schipp and R. Flindt, Zur Feinstruktur und Innervation der Lymphherzmuskulatur der Amphibien *(Rana temporaria), Z. Anat. Entwickl.,* **127**:232-253 (1968).
41. M. Poberai, A. Gellért, I. Nagy, J. Lippai, M. Kozma, and S. Nagy, Comparative histology of the structure of the wall of lymphatic vessels. III. Histological structure of the wall of peripheral lymphatic vessels, *Acta Morphol. Acad. Sci. Hung.,* **11**:229-238 (1962).
42. R. Schipp. In *New Trends in Basic Lymphology.* Edited by J. M. Collette et al. Basel, Birkhäuser, 1967, pp. 50-57.
43. A. E. Taylor, W. H. Gibson, H. J. Granger, and A. C. Guyton, The interaction between intracapillary and tissue forces in the overall regulation of interstitial fluid volume, *Lymphology,* **6**:192-208 (1973).
44. C. Vogel, The pharmacology of the lymph and the lymphatic system. In *Das Lymphgefässystem, Hb. allg. Pathol.* Vol. 3. Part 6. Edited by H. Meessen. Berlin, Sprigner, 1972, pp. 363-404.
45. R. O. Smith, Lymphatic contractility, *J. Exp. Med.,* **90**:497-509 (1949).
46. T. K. C. King, B. Weber, A. Okinaka, S. A. Friedman, J. P. Smith, and W. E. Briscoe, Oxygen transfer in catastrophic respiratory failure, *Chest,* **75**:763-767 (1974).
47. M. Földi, Physiologie und Pathophysiologie des Lymphgefässystems. In *Das Lymphgefässystem, Hb. Allg. Pathol.* Vol. 3. Part 6. Edited by H. Meessen. Berlin, Springer, 1972, pp. 239-310.
48. L. Pfleger, F. Kaindl, E. Mannerhaim, and B. Thurner. In *New Trends in Basic Lymphology.* Edited by J. M. Collette et al. Basel, Birkhäuser, 1967, pp. 138-145.

15

High Altitude Pulmonary Edema

HERBERT N. HULTGREN

Stanford University School of Medicine
Stanford, California
and
Veterans Administration Hospital
Palo Alto, California

I. Introduction

High altitude pulmonary edema (HAPE) occurs in unacclimatized individuals who are rapidly exposed to altitudes in excess of 8000 feet. It is most frequently seen in climbers who ascend to high altitude without prior acclimatization and who engage in heavy physical exertion on arrival. Initial symptoms of dyspnea, cough, fatigue, and occasionally hemoptysis appear, usually within 2 to 7 days after arrival. Common physical signs are tachypnea, tachycardia, rales, cyanosis, and hypotension. In severe episodes, disturbances of consciousness or coma may be observed. Descent to a lower altitude, bed rest, and oxygen administration result in rapid clinical improvement. Fatal episodes continue to occur in many parts of the world as access to high altitudes by unacclimatized visitors is facilitated by modern means of travel. Most deaths occur when a prompt diagnosis is not made, when the victim is not moved to a lower altitude, or when oxygen is unavailable. Subjects who develop HAPE do not have demonstrable preexisting cardiac or pulmonary disease. Physiologic studies during the acute stage have revealed a normal pulmonary artery wedge pressure, marked elevation of pulmonary artery pressure, severe arterial unsaturation and usually a low cardiac output. Pulmonary arteriolar (precapillary) resistance is elevated. The incidence is higher in young males but may occur at any age. HAPE represents one of several varieties of acute pulmonary edema where left ventricular filling pressure is normal.

II. Historical Aspects

Mosso [1] in his monograph entitled "Life of Man in the High Alps" described a fatal episode of HAPE involving a physician climber on Mont Blanc in 1891. An autopsy revealed acute edema of the lungs but pneumonitis was thought to be a contributing cause of death. Ravenhill [2] in 1913 described three patients with probable HAPE sustained in the Bolivian Andes between 15,400 ft and 16,200 ft. Two of the patients died and one recovered after descending to 7000 ft. Ravenhill classified these cases as "a cardiac type of Puña" or mountain sickness, and believed that cardiac failure was the mechanism involved.

Hurtado in 1937 described a native of Casapalca, Peru (altitude 13,665 feet), who traveled frequently to sea level (Lima). On one occasion, on returning to the mountains he developed acute pulmonary edema, which subsided rapidly after return to Lima. Hurtado attributed the pulmonary edema to altitude exposure and suggested that neither pneumonia nor cardiac failure could explain the occurrence [3]. Subsequently several studies appearing in the Peruvian medical literature described the essential clinical features of the syndrome [4-6].

In 1957, Houston published the first report of an episode of HAPE in North America and suggested that deaths in mountaineers previously ascribed to pneumonia were probably instances of HAPE [7]. An analysis of the clinical aspects of 18 patients with HAPE observed in Peru and 13 afflicted mountaineers, with a review of the literature, was reported in 1961 [8]. Singh [9] and Menon [10] published subsequent additional clinical descriptions, concerning cases in India. Fred and his workers [11] reported the first hemodynamic studies in a patient with HAPE. A physician skier developed pulmonary edema at Alta, Utah, and was admitted to the Salt Lake City General Hospital. Cardiac catheterization revealed an elevated pulmonary artery pressure and marked arterial unsaturation. Fortuitously the catheter entered the left atrium via a patent foramen ovale and a normal left atrial pressure was recorded. The pulmonary artery wedge pressure was also normal. There was no evidence of cardiac disease or pneumonia. After two days of bed rest and oxygen therapy the patient recovered. The same patient experienced a recurrence of HAPE two years later while hiking in the Sierras. Further hemodynamic studies done at high altitude on patients with HAPE have confirmed the data Fred reported and clearly excluded left heart failure as a causative mechanism [12-14].

Autopsy studies reported by several workers supported the view that not pneumonia, nor cardiac disease, nor left ventricular failure were the etiologic factors [15-17].

III. Epidemiology and Incidence

A. Altitude of Occurrence and Acclimatization

High altitude pulmonary edema rarely occurs below 8000 ft and the incidence increases with altitude. Episodes occurring between 8000 and 10,000 ft are usually related to heavy physical exertion, but at higher altitudes pulmonary edema may occur with only light activity or even at rest. Individuals who are acclimatized over 1 to 2 weeks rarely develop HAPE except at very high altitudes. At the Mount Everest Base Camp in 1963, several thoroughly acclimatized members of the party had clinical signs of mild pulmonary edema after strenuous climbing during the day. These signs disappeared after bed rest and low-flow oxygen administration during the night [18]. HAPE is rare in fully acclimatized residents of high altitude regions unless there is rapid ascent to a higher altitude.

B. HAPE during Reascent

Full acclimatized individuals who descend to sea level and then return to high altitude may develop HAPE on reascent. HAPE during reascent is rare when the sea-level sojourn is less than 10 to 14 days [8-10]. Reascent pulmonary edema may occur more frequently than pulmonary edema during initial ascent to high altitude [9], but further data are needed to settle this point.

C. Susceptible Individuals

Some individuals appear to be susceptible to HAPE and may experience recurrent episodes when again ascending to high altitude [8, 19, 20]. In Peru, 20% of patients with HAPE had experienced at least one prior episode [20]. Physiologic studies have indicated that subjects with a previous history of HAPE show an abnormal rise in pulmonary arteriolar resistance and an impaired pulmonary oxygen exchange during acute altitude exposure that is not observed in normal subjects [21]. Susceptible subjects also show a more marked rise in pulmonary artery pressure and arteriolar resistance than normal subjects during low oxygen breathing [13, 21-23].

D. Incidence and Age

A study of the incidence of HAPE has been carried out in the mining town of La Oroya (altitude 12,300 ft) in the central Peruvian Andes [19, 20]. Many permanent residents live in this community and make frequent trips to sea level for vacations or business purposes. A survey questionnaire was sent to families living in the area asking for details about altitude exposure, trips to sea level, and occurrence of HAPE in their families during the preceding year. A total of 860 exposures to high altitude in 95 persons was reported. An exposure was defined as a rapid ascent to 12,300 ft or higher from sea level either for the first time or after a sea level visit of greater than two weeks. The overall incidence during 860 exposures to high altitude in 95 persons was reported. An exposure was defined as a rapid ascent to 12,300 ft or higher from sea level either for the first time or after a sea level visit of greater than two weeks. The overall incidence during 860 exposures to high altitude was 3.4%. Only 2 out of 50 adults (4%) experienced HAPE and 17 out of 45 subjects under 21 (38%) experienced HAPE. No cases affecting children under 2 years occurred. Three of the younger group had a total of 9 repeat episodes of HAPE. For a single ascent, the estimated chance of HAPE is 60/1000 for subjects under 21 and 4/1000 for subjects over 21 (Table 1). The incidence in Indian troops transported by air to over 11,500 feet was 5.7%. If travel was by auto, the incidence was 0.3%. About half the patients were 20 to 29 years old [10]. Singh has reported an incidence of 13 to 15% in troops moved rapidly to 11,000 to 18,000 feet [9]. The incidence was similar for men going to high altitude for the first time and those who were returning from a furlough at lower altitude.

Previous studies from Peru have also shown a high incidence of HAPE in children and adolescents compared with adults [8]. The characteristics of HAPE occurring in children have been described [15]. The incidence of HAPE in women is low, but for children there is no sex dominance [8, 20].

E. Subclinical HAPE

The data described refer only to obvious HAPE severe enough to require medical attention. If one includes subclinical HAPE, the true incidence will be substantially higher than indicated. Houston has made observations of climbers before and after an ascent of Mount Rainier, Washington (14,408 ft). Fifteen percent of 140 subjects had pulmonary rales after descent, suggesting the presence of mild pulmonary edema [24]. Singh noted that about one-third of patients with severe acute mountain sickness had pulmonary rales [9]. Thus, subclinical pulmonary edema can be estimated to occur at least three times as frequently as the more severe form.

TABLE 1 Incidence of HAPE during Acute Altitude Exposure

Sex	2 to 21 yr					> 21 yr				
	Number of subjects	Number of ascents	Ascents per subject (mean)	Number episodes HAPE	Incidence HAPE (%)[a]	Number of subjects	Number of ascents	Ascents per subject (mean)	Number episodes HAPE	Incidence HAPE (%)[a]
Males	16	151	9.4	9	6.0	24	228	9.5	1	0.44
Females	29	251	8.7	17	6.8	26	230	8.8	1	0.44
Totals	45	402	.0	26	6.5	50	458	9.2	2	0.44

NOTE: Data obtained from 95 subjects who made a total of 860 ascents from sea level to an altitude between 12,000 and 14,000 feet in Peru. Ascents were either initial ascents or ascent after a sea level stay of longer than two weeks. Incidence is expressed as the percentage of ascents where pulmonary edema occurred.

[a]Expected incidence per each ascent for one subject: under 21, 0.6%; over 21, 0.04%.

IV. Clinical Features

A. Clinical Presentation

The initial symptoms of HAPE usually begin 24 to 96 hr after arrival at high altitude and are commonly preceded by heavy physical exertion such as climbing, skiing, or carrying heavy loads. Dyspnea, a persistent nonproductive cough and marked weakness and fatigue are the most common early symptoms. Headache, nausea, vomiting, or somnolence is often seen in children. As the severity of the pulmonary edema increases, usually during the night, dyspnea at rest becomes severe and the cough becomes productive of clear, copious watery sputum. Audible rhonchi and gurgling sounds can be heard without a stethoscope. Hemoptysis, sometimes involving fairly large quantities of blood, can be seen in about 20% of severe episodes. The patient becomes apprehensive, fears death, and may become incoherent or irrational or experience hallucinations. Coma may follow and precedes death by 1 to 6 hr if oxygen is not administered or the patient is not carried to a lower altitude. In rare instances, stupor progressing to coma may occur, with minimal symptoms or signs of respiratory distress, and the clinical picture may resemble encephalitis or intracranial disease [24-26]. Central nervous system dysfunction and altered consciousness are probably related to hypoxia or cerebral edema, which may be profound in severe HAPE [24].

Common clinical signs include cyanosis, hyperpnea, crepitant rales, and rhonchi. The blood pressure is low. In 21 patients observed in Peru, the mean arterial pressure was 106/69. Tachycardia due to severe hypoxia is present, with heart rates up to 160/min in severe episodes. The mean heart rate in 34 Peruvian episodes was 122/min. The respiratory rate is increased and a mean value of 32/min was observed in Peruvian studies [8].

B. Laboratory Studies

Laboratory studies reveal an elevated hematocrit and an acid urine with a high specific gravity compatible with hemoconcentration. Signs of infection are absent, with only minor temperature elevations, a normal white blood cell count, and a normal sedimentation rate.

Electrocardiograms during acute HAPE reveal tachycardia and signs of acute right ventricular overload, including right axis deviation, P-wave abnormalities compatible with right atrial strain, prominent R waves in the right precordial leads, and S waves in leads V_5-V_6. In one instance transient atrial flutter has occurred. The changes are similar to those occurring during pulmonary embolism and acute cardiac pulmonary edema and subside during treatment. The ECG abnormalities are probably due to acute pulmonary hypertension.

C. Radiologic Features

Radiologic studies have been done in many instances of HAPE and the extent of the edema present on the chest film roughly parallels the clinical severity. In mild episodes, single or several small patchy exudates are present. In severe forms the exudates may nearly fill both lung fields. The exudates are rarely confluent and clear spaces of aerated lung are usually present especially at the lung bases. The edema is more severe and common in the right midlung field. The usual symmetrical, "bat-wing," distribution of edema commonly seen in cardiac pulmonary edema or uremia is rare. The central branches of the pulmonary artery are prominent but the overall heart size is not increased. Left atrial enlargement and pulmonary venous congestion are absent. Kerley lines of pulmonary venous hypertension are absent. Pleural effusion is rare.

Serial chest films during recovery from HAPE reveal clearing of exudates and decrease in prominence of the pulmonary arteries, but no consistent change in heart size [8]. Radiologic features of HAPE are illustrated in Figure 1.

For subjects with severe HAPE, especially when treatment has been delayed or recovery is slow, chest films may reveal exudates persisting for many days or even up to two weeks after clinical recovery [27, 28]. For this reason it is advisable that chest films be obtained on any individual who may have had an episode of HAPE, even though clinical recovery has occurred. The demonstration of a slowly clearing residual pulmonary exudate may thus confirm the diagnosis of suspected HAPE even after return to sea level.

D. Severity

In evaluating treatment and prognosis, objective assessment of the severity of HAPE is important. In an evaluating therapy of HAPE in Peru [28], a simple method of grading severity has been used based on the clinical picture, the ECG, and the chest film (Table 2). General experience indicates that patients with Grade 4 severity usually die unless prompt therapy can be instituted.

The mortality of HAPE is variable and depends on many factors. Studies of large population groups at risk indicate a mortality of 0.5% to 12.7% [9, 10, 20].

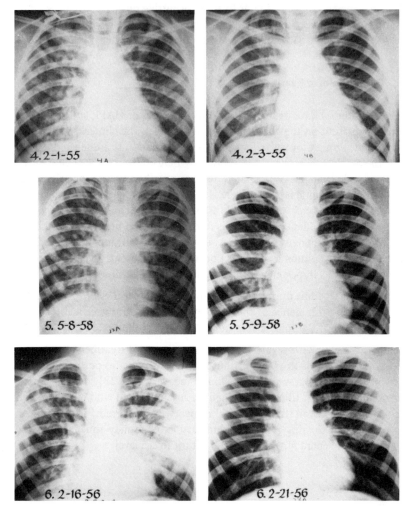

FIGURE 1 Pulmonary edema occurring in 3 subjects following rapid ascent from sea level to an altitude between 12,200 and 14,200 ft. Initial chest films on hospital entry shown on left. Films on right were taken after bed rest and oxygen therapy.

V. Treatment

Prompt recognition of the syndrome, bed rest, descent to a lower altitude, and oxygen are the most effective methods of therapy in HAPE [29, 30].

TABLE 2 Severity Classification of HAPE

Grade[a]	Clinical	ECG	Chest film
1 Mild	Minor symptoms with dyspnea only on heavy exertion.	Tachycardia only. Heart rate at rest < 110.	Minor exudate involving less than one-fourth of one lung field.
2 Moderate	Symptoms of dyspnea, weakness, fatigue on ordinary effort. Headache, dry cough.	Tachycardia with resting heart rate 110–120. P wave changes only.	Exudate involving at least half of one lung field.
3 Serious	Symptoms of dyspnea, headache, weakness, nausea at rest. Loose recurrent productive cough.	Tachycardia with heart rate 120–140. P wave and minor QRS-T wave changes.	Bilateral exudates involving at least half of each lung field.
4 Severe	Stupor or coma, unable to stand or walk. Severe cyanosis. Bubbling rales present with copious sputum, usually bloody.	Tachycardia with heart rate >140. Right axis deviation, QRS, T wave and P wave changes.	Bilateral exudates involving more than half of each lung field.

[a]Grades 1 and 2 can usually be treated with bed rest alone without descent. Grade 4 cases are usually fatal unless immediate descent and oxygen treatment can be instituted.

445

A. Recognition

Severe HAPE and many fatalities among mountain climbers have occurred because the initial symptoms have been ignored or concealed or because an erroneous diagnosis of pneumonia has been made. Recognizing early symptoms permits the prompt institution of therapy and may prevent progression to a more serious stage.

B. Bed Rest

Absolute bed rest is important in therapy since physical exercise will further aggravate existing HAPE by increasing pulmonary artery pressure and reducing arterial oxygen saturation. Studies in Peru have shown that HAPE can be treated by bed rest alone at high altitude without oxygen or descent [20, 28 29]. In severe cases, recovery is slower with bed-rest treatment than when oxygen is used. Mild cases of HAPE can be treated at high altitude without descent by one to two days of bed rest. Serial examinations of the chest and measurement of heart rate and respiratory rate, as well as evaluation of symptoms, are necessary, since if deterioration occurs, prompt assistance to a lower altitude should be carried out.

C. Descent to a Lower Altitude

There are many reports of subjects with HAPE who have improved on descent to a lower altitude [3, 8]. A descent of even 2000 or 3000 ft may result in improvement, since at high altitude one's oxygen saturation lies on the steep part of the O_2 dissociation curve and small changes in altitude and resultant PI_{O_2} will be accompanied by significant changes in arterial oxygen saturation. For climbing parties at high altitude, descent to a lower altitude may be the only method of treatment available. Early recognition of mild symptoms will permit the victim to be helped down to a lower altitude before serious HAPE occurs and the victim is unable to walk. If symptoms are severe evacuation by a litter will be necessary, since the effort of climbing down may increase the severity of the HAPE.

D. Oxygen

The administration of 100% oxygen is the most effective and rapid method of treating HAPE. Studies in Peru have shown that oxygen administration will rapidly increase arterial oxygen saturation, lower pulmonary artery pressure, reduce the heart rate and respiratory rate, and relieve symptoms (Fig. 2). In

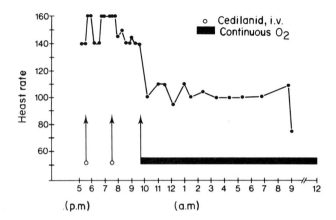

FIGURE 2 Comparison of the effect of intravenous Cedilanid-D (deslanoside) and oxygen in acute high altitude pulmonary edema. Each intravenous injection contained 0.8 mg Cedilanid. No effect on heart rate, cardiac rhythm, respiratory rate, or symptoms was noted. Prompt improvement in all the above features was noted immediately after the administration of 100% oxygen at 6 liters/min by a plastic face mask.

field conditions oxygen can be effectively administered via a plastic face mask [30]. High flow rates of 6 to 8 liters/min should be used for the first 15 to 30 min because of the rapid respiratory rate. To conserve oxygen, rates of 2 to 4 liters/min can be used for 12 to 48 hr until recovery or evacuation to a lower altitude. Rescue teams or helicopters should carry oxygen to the victim so that therapy can be initiated immediately. Treatment by descent and oxygen has been described vividly in a severe case of HAPE occurring on the 1969 American Dhaulagiri expedition [31].

E. Drug Therapy

Evalutating the effect of drug interventions in HAPE is difficult for several reasons: (1) HAPE usually occurs in the mountains, where facilities for systematic studies are not available. (2) Treatment by bed rest, removal to a lower altitude, or oxygen may be instituted at the same time so the effect of a drug intervention alone cannot be evaluated. (3) No animal model of HAPE is available that would permit proper investigation of drug interventions. (4) Anecdotal reports of alleged successful use of drugs are common and tend to be repeated in the literature, whereas failures of drug therapy are rarely reported.

Diuretics such as furosemide have been used in patients with HAPE, and workers in India have recommended furosemide for prevention and treatment of

HAPE has several physiologic features that suggest that a diuretic would be of limited value in treatment: (1) The blood volume is low due to fluid loss into the lungs, fluid loss by the respiratory tract, and inadequate fluid intake. (2) The cardiac output and systemic blood pressure are low. (3) Left ventricular failure is not present. In these circumstances, a further decrease in plasma volume by diuresis may further lower blood pressure, cardiac output, and perfusion of vital organs. In the mountains this may cause an ambulatory patient to become a litter case, with consequent difficulty in evacuation [26]. Furosemide has been shown to be of no value in preventing acute mountain sickness, and it results in a high incidence of postural hypotension and syncope [33, 34]. The degree of body hydration has shown no relation to the incidence of severity of acute mountain sickenss [35]. Proponents of diuretic therapy argue that furosemide has a venous dilating effect and may also reduce cerebral edema. These effects have not been demonstrated in patients with HAPE. With no clear evidence of benefit and with the potential of harmful side effects, it is prudent not to use diuretics for preventing or treating HAPE until further data are available.

Morphine has also been used in treating HAPE, probably because of its traditional use in cardiac pulmonary edema [9, 10, 32]. Morphine use in HAPE has not been subjected to adequately controlled studies, and until beneficial effects have clearly been shown, its use should be avoided. Unfavorable effects have been reported [36]. The depressant effect of morphine on ventilation could further increase the severity of hypoxia, which is an important cause of HAPE.

Other drugs such as digoxin, isoproterenol, and steroids have no proven value (Fig. 2).

VI. Prevention

Since the occurrence of HAPE is related to the speed of ascent, the altitude reached, and the amount of physical exertion done at high altitude, the most effective means of prevention is acclimatization, either by a slow ascent or a sojourn for several days at an intermediate altitude. High altitude pulmonary edema is being reported with increasing frequency in places where unacclimatized individuals are rapidly brought to high altitudes. These places include Colorado ski areas, Mounts Kenya and Kilimanjaro in Africa, the Everest base camp in India, Mount Aconcagua in Chile, and the Peruvian Andes. Houston recommends one day per 500 ft of ascent from 9000 ft upwards, interrupted by a day of partial rest at 14,000 and 18,000 ft [24]. This may be too slow a pace. Experienced Himalayan trekkers advise 2 rest days during ascent at 11,000 and 15,000 ft [24]. It has been shown that acute mountain sickness at 14,110 ft on Pikes Peak is greatly reduced by a 4-day sojourn at an intermediate altitude of

5400 or 11,000 ft [37]. Administration of Diamox during this period provides added protection [38].

Heavy physical activity on arrival at high altitude should be avoided during the first 2 to 5 days after arrival especially if ascent has been rapid. Mild cases of HAPE may be treated at high altitude by 1 to 2 days of bed rest provided that deterioration does not occur.

In well-controlled studies [39], it has been shown that Diamox reduces the incidence and severity of acute mountain sickness. Side effects are minimal and disappear when the drug is stopped. Preliminary studies have suggested that Diamox may be of value in preventing recurrent HAPE is susceptible subjects [40], but other workers have noted failures with this medication [34]. Diamox in a dosage of 250 mg is usually administered once or twice daily beginning the day of ascent and continued for 3 to 5 days after arrival at high altitude. Diamox should not be continued for longer than 7 days.

Furosemide and other diuretics have no demonstrated value in preventing HAPE.

VII. Physiologic Features

A. Hemodynamics

Pulmonary hypertension due to an increased pulmonary vascular resistance is a consistent finding in patients with HAPE. Pulmonary artery wedge and left atrial pressures are normal or low [11-14]. The cardiac output is decreased and the systemic blood pressure is low. Right atrial pressure is normal or occasionally raised. The blood pressure response to the Valsalva maneuver is normal [12]. Hemodynamic features of HAPE are summarized in Table 3.

Hemodynamic studies of subjects who have recoved from HAPE have revealed essentially normal values and normal responses to exercise. Data from a few patients suggest that the rise in pulmonary artery pressure during exercise and during acute hypoxia may be greater than in normal subjects [12, 21-23].

B. Blood Gases

Arterial oxygen saturation is decreased with HAPE, often to very low levels (Table 3). The P_{CO_2} is decreased or normal and the pH is increased [11, 14]. Exercise or induced hypoxia results in a further increase in pulmonary artery pressure and a fall in arterial oxygen saturation.

The administration of 100% oxygen is accompanied by a prompt rise in arterial oxygen saturation but normal values are usually not attained, suggesting

TABLE 3 Hemodynamic Features of HAPE

Case no.	Altitude (ft)	Sex	Age (yr)	PCV (%)	Sa O$_2$ (%)	PA pressure, mean (mmHg)	PA wedge pressure, mean (mmHg)	Cardiac index (liter/min^{-1}/m^2)	Pulmonary vascular resistance (dyn sec^{-1}/cm^{-5})	BA pressure (mmHg)	Heart rate/ min	PCO$_2$ (mm)	pH
1[a]	12,200	M	8	45	76	117	4	2.6	2900	84	129		
2[a]	12,200	M	27	58	64	46	2	2.7	640	85	107		
3[a]	12,200	F	17	49		37	5			94	115		
4[a]	12,200	M	8			33	3			85	110		
5[b]	4,800	M	48	46	76	46	6	2.9	1104	100	100	32	7.38
6[c]	14,200	M	17	64	55	62	1	2.3	1301	80	138		
7[c]	14,200	M	21	54	60	63	2	2.7	1118	86	135		
8[d]	11,000	M	22		87	30	2	2.4	940	95	125	24	7.46
9[d]	11,000	M	23		78		5[g]	4.5		92	75	29	7.45
10[d]	11,000	M	38		78	22	4[g]	3.2	400	80	75	26	7.49
11[d]	11,000	M	28		85	24	9	3.4	350	80	96	34	7.45
12[d]	11,000	M	20		54	24	3	3.0	560	80	110	35	7.43
13[d]	11,000	M	26		66	24	1[g]	3.5		80	140	27	7.52
Mean Values			23	52.5	71	46	3.6	3.0	1035	79	110	28	7.45
Normal values 12,200 ft, n = 36[ef]			30	54	85	22	8	3.4	224	100	77	32	7.43

NOTE: All data were obtained during the acute state at high altitude and following minimal treatment. The altitude at which the study was done is indicated. Cases 8–13 may have had their hemodynamic status changed by descent to a lower altitude (11,000 ft) from the altitude where HAPE occurred (15,000 ft).

[a]Hultgren[12]; [b]Fred [11]; [c]Peñaloza [13]; [d]Roy [14]; [e]Hultgren [62]; [f]Sevringhaus [89]; [g]LA pressure.

450

the presence of intrapulmonary shunting. Oxygen administration will rapidly lower pulmonary artery pressure, but normal levels are not usually attained.

VIII. Pathology

Autopsy studies of fatal cases of HAPE have been reported by several workers [15-17]. Severe, confluent pulmonary edema is present, with a protein-rich exudate filling the alveoli. In some cases fibrinous intra-alveolar exudates or hyaline membranes are present that are like those seen in influenzal pneumonia in patients with mitral stenosis, or in the respiratory distress syndrome of infants. Such deposits are usually found when very high capillary pressures occur or when capillary injury is present with increased permeability to protein. Hemorrhage into alveoli may be present. Marked capillary congestion and distension of capillaries by erythrocytes is commonly found. Obstruction of capillaries and arterioles by thrombi consisting of platelet aggregates, leucocytes red cells, and fibrin strands or clumps have been described. Numerous megakaryocytes may be present in such aggregates [15]. Marked dilatation of preterminal arterioles, capillaries, and small pulmonary veins has also been observed [16].

Pneumonitis is rare. In one patient in whom pneumonitis was present the clinical history suggested that a viral respiratory infection existed before the HAPE occurred [15]. The pneumonitis may have encouraged the HAPE, since pneumonia in experimental animals increases capillary permeability and susceptibility to pulmonary edema.

The right atrium, right ventricle, and large pulmonary arteries are usually distended and hepatic congestion may be present. Signs of left heart failure are absent. The left ventricle, left atrium, and pulmonary veins are not distended. Underlying cardiac or pulmonary disease is absent.

Cerebral edema probably related to severe hypoxia may occur [9, 24, 26].

IX. Etiology

Several concepts of the mechanism of HAPE have been proposed.

A. Antidiuresis and Fluid Retention

Many normal subjects respond to acute high altitude exposure by a diuresis. It has been proposed by investigators in India that a failure of diuresis and consequent water retention is an important causative mechanism of HAPE [9, 10, 32]. This has been the reason for recommending that diuretics such as furosemide be used to prevent and treat HAPE. Critical data to support this concept are lacking. An increase in plasma volume and a decrease in hematocrit would be expected to be present in subjects before HAPE occurred. This has not been shown. Subjects who have had a prior history of HAPE do not have a decrease in hematocrit on exposure to high altitude [41, 42]. Antidiuresis and water retention with the occurrence of edema of the face and extremities are occasionally seen in normal subjects when they are exposed to high altitude, particularly women, but such subjects do not develop pulmonary edema and HAPE is rare in women [43]. It is clearly possible that antidiuresis and fluid retention may facilitate the occurrence of HAPE in some subjects, but it seems unlikely as a primary causative agent.

B. Increased Capillary Permeability

The hemodynamics of HAPE are somewhat similar to the hemodynamics of pulmonary edema that occurs from agents such as alloxan, which increase pulmonary capillary permeability, since left atrial and pulmonary arterial wedge pressures are normal under these circumstances. Pulmonary hypertension, however, is mild or absent. Many studies of the isolated and intact pulmonary circulation have failed to demonstrate any significant increase in pulmonary capillary permeability due to even profound degrees of hypoxia [44, 45]. Besides, if an increase in capillary permeability were a primary cause of HAPE, one would not expect a significant elevation of pulmonary arterial pressure to be a constant finding in the early stage of the disease.

C. Transarterial Leakage

Whayne produced pulmonary edema in rats exercised by swimming and subjected to hypoxia [46]. Histologic studies revealed cuffing of edema fluid around arterioles. These workers suggested that the high pulmonary arterial pressure resulted in the leakage of fluid across the walls of arterioles and precapillary vessels, and they proposed this process as an important factor in the etiology of HAPE. Hemodynamic data were not obtained during these studies, and therefore left ventricular failure cannot be excluded. Histologic studies of lungs from fatal cases of HAPE have not revealed similar lesions, and capillaries are usually markedly congested, which suggests that a high capillary pressure and not only a high arterial pressure was present.

D. Centrogenic Origin Due to Cerebral Edema

It has long been recognized that head injury and cerebral edema may be accompanied by severe pulmonary edema even in the absence of pulmonary or cardiac disease [47, 48]. This type of centrogenic pulmonary edema has been investigated experimentally. Usually left ventricular filling pressures are raised as a consequence of central shifts in blood volume. Some observations indicate that left atrial pressure elevation may not always precede the onset of this type of pulmonary edema and reflex construction of small pulmonary veins may be an additional causative factor. Acute exposure to high altitude may result in severe headache, neurologic signs, retinal hemorrhages, and symptoms compatible with cerebral edema [24-26]. Cerebral edema has been demonstrated in monkeys exposed to a hypoxic atmosphere [49]. Hypoxia is a cause of cerebral edema [50]. Although this is an attractive hypothesis, clinical observations of HAPE do not support the etiologic role of cerebral edema in HAPE. Only rarely is HAPE preceded by any signs or symptoms suggesting cerebral edema. When disturbances of consciousness or neurologic signs occur in HAPE, their appearance follows the clinical picture of HAPE. Cerebral edema thus appears more likely to be a complication of HAPE rather than a primary initiating factor.

E. Fluid Shift from Periphery to the Lungs

During the first few days after rapid ascent to high altitude, cardiac output is increased [51] and peripheral vasoconstriction occurs [52]. It has been shown that hypoxia in normal subjects increases intrathoracic and pulmonary blood volume [53, 54]. Calves placed in a high altitude chamber have exhibited an increase in pulmonary extravascular water [55].

Such fluid shifts may facilitate the occurrence of HAPE but cannot be regarded as essential etiologic mechanisms.

F. Heart Failure

Hemodynamic and autopsy studies have securely eliminated the possibility that HAPE is due to left ventricular failure [11-17].

G. Overperfusion Concept

General

The etiologic mechanisms of HAPE must be considered within the framework of the following well-established features of this unusual form of pulmonary edema.

　1.　Presence of a rapid rise in pulmonary artery pressure due to high altitude ascent, with a low pulmonary artery wedge and left atrial pressure.

2. Presence of acute hypoxic pulmonary arteriolar vasoconstriction, which is reversed by breathing oxygen.

3. Absence of left ventricular failure or pneumonia.

4. Marked pulmonary capillary congestion and presence of capillary and arterial thromboses in many fatal cases.

5. Harmful effect of heavy exercise, but improvement on bed rest.

In 1966, the author proposed the following concept of the etiology of HAPE, which deserves review and comment at this time [56,57]. It was proposed that the primary cause of HAPE was nonhomogeneous obstruction of the pulmonary vascular bed by hypoxic vasoconstriction and possibly intravascular thromboses. During periods of exercise and increased pulmonary blood flow, unobstructed areas of the pulmonary circulation would be subjected to high pressure and flow; the precapillary arterioles would thereupon be dilated, permitting the high pulmonary artery pressure to be transmitted directly to the capillary bed, with resulting interstitial and alveolar edema. With dilation of arterioles and capillaries, the pulmonary veins may then become the site of resistance to flow, which would also result in a high capillary pressure. Thus, an important mechanism of HAPE is a failure of hypoxic vasoconstriction and dilatation of nonconstricted vessels in local areas of the lung (Fig. 3). A similar concept has been proposed for the mechanism of hypertensive encephalopathy in systemic hypertension. It is proposed that in this condition cerebral edema is due to failure of cerebral vasoconstriction, permitting a high arterial pressure to be transmitted to the capillary bed with resultant edema. Failure of vasoconstriction seems to occur when a very high arterial pressure is present. The degree of pressure elevation is thought to be the etiologic factor. Clinical and experimental evidence is available to support this concept [58-60].

Indirect Evidence

The proposed etiology for HAPE can be supported by the following general lines of evidence.

1. A rise in pulmonary arterial pressure due to hypoxic pulmonary arteriolar constriction occurs in normal subjects acutely exposed to high altitude [61-65]. Under conditions of exercise in such individuals, the pulmonary arterial pressure may rise to mean values of 32 mmHg [64].

2. Subjects who have experienced prior episodes of HAPE respond to high altitude exposure by a greater rise in pulmonary pressure than normal subjects experience (Table 4). This rise in pressure occurs in

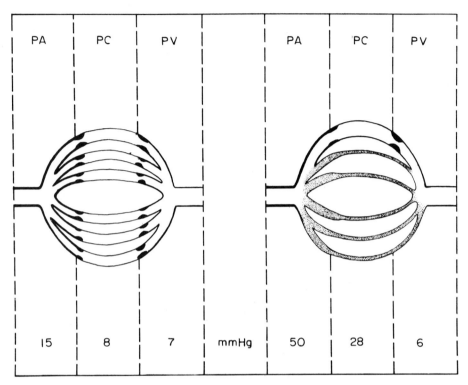

FIGURE 3 The normal pulmonary circulation with normal pressure values are indicated on the left. Resistances at pulmonary arterioles and pulmonary veins are indicated. On the right, 80% of the pulmonary circulation has been occluded and increased blood flow is present in the remaining protion of the pulmonary vascular bed. Pressure measurements correspond to those obtained in canine experiments. PA = pulmonary artery. PC = pulmonary capillary. PV = pulmonary vein.

the absence of clinical evidence of pulmonary edema, and thus probably represents the initial abnormality in patients who later develop HAPE [12, 22, 23]. Normal subjects acutely exposed to high altitude have similar changes in pulmonary arterial pressure, A-a gradients, and ventilation-perfusion relation to those observed in subjects with a prior history of HAPE, but the responses in normals are of a lesser magnitude [21, 64-66].

3. Further obstruction of the pulmonary vascular bed may occur as the result of arterial and capillary thromboses, such as those that have been observed in fatal cases at autopsy [15-17]. Indirect evidence

TABLE 4 Hemodynamic Feature of Acute Altitude Exposure in Subjects with a Prior History of HAPE

Case no.	Altitude (ft)	Sex	Age (yr)	PCV (%)	Sa O$_2$ (%)	P$_{CO_2}$ (mm)	pH	PA pressure, mean (mmHg)	PA wedge pressure, mean (mmHg)	Cardiac index (liter min^{-1}/m^2)	Pulmonary vascular resistance	BA pressure, mean (mmHg)	Heart rate/ min
1	11,200	M	22	43	87.8	32	7.45	22	8	3.2	265	100	89
2	11,200	M	36	42	84.8	33	7.46	41	12	4.1	420	98	95
3	11,200	M	37	40	91.3	33	7.50	47		3.1	450	78	82
4	11,200	M	38	40	91.0	26	7.54	37	11	2.9	540	103	96
5	11,200	M	54	40	83.1	28	7.50	47	11	3.4	555	128	107
Mean values			37.4	41	87.6	30.4	7.49	38.8	10.5	3.36	446	101	94
Mean values, sea level				43	96.9	40.4	7.40	13.8	7.4	3.40	171	98	65

NOTE: Mean values on the same subjects at sea level are shown at the bottom of the chart. Upper values were obtained after ascent to 10,200 ft and following several hours of strenuous physical activity at 12,500 ft [21]. Note increase in pulmonary artery pressure despite drop in P$_{CO_2}$ and rise in pH with arterial unsaturation and increase in heart rate.

has been presented that is compatible with intrapulmonary thromboses, platelet count decreases, shortening of the whole-blood coagulation time, and platelet accumulation in the lungs during high altitude exposure [67-71].

4. Experimental studies of perfused intact dog lungs have demonstrated that when blood flow to a pulmonary lobe is increased more than fourfold, the pressure drop in the precapillary vessels is diminished, capillary pressure rises, and the site of resistance to flow is shifted to pulmonary veins, with an increase in small vein pressure [72] (Fig. 4).

5. Constriction of pulmonary veins is a possible mechanism. It is difficult to evaluate the possible role of pulmonary venous constriction in generating HAPE. A *primary* etiologic role seems unlikely but venous constriction may be secondarily important in increasing pulmonary capillary pressure. Intravascular pulmonary thrombosis may bring about pulmonary venous constriction. It has been shown that this happens in pulmonary embolism either from massive vascular obstruc-

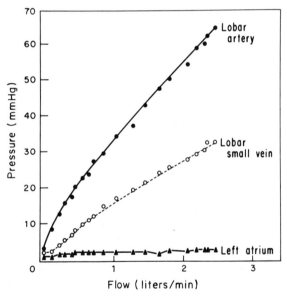

FIGURE 4 Lobar vascular pressures during pump perfusion of three-fourths of left lower lobe in six intact dogs. The maximum flow of 2.5 liters/min is approximately 5.4 times normal basal flow to this portion of the lung. Note progressive increase in lobar small vein pressure with increasing flow. Reprinted from A. Hyman, *J. Appl. Physiol.*, **27**:179-185 (1961), by courtesy of the publisher.

tion or from particulate embolism [73-75]. Another possible mechanism is release of serotonin from platelets [74].

6. Sea-level hemodynamic analogs of HAPE are rare but have been seen. A simple analog is massive pulmonary embolism. In most clinical instances, right ventricular failure and a low cardiac output are present, so that pulmonary arterial pressure is not markedly elevated. However, Alexander and his workers have described patients with severe pulmonary embolism who had pulmonary edema in areas of the lung where blood flow was not blocked [76]. Pulmonary edema has also been described in other instances of pulmonary embolism [77, 78]. Case reports have been published describing surgical removal of large pulmonary emboli and pulmonary arterial thromboses, followed by severe pulmonary edema [79-82].

7. Recently three cases of HAPE have been observed in Colorado in association with congenital absence of one pulmonary artery [83]. One patient died and the diagnosis of congenital absence of the left pulmonary artery was confirmed at autopsy. The diagnosis was established in two surviving patients by typical roentgenographic findings and lung scans. Unilateral absence of a pulmonary artery not associated with other congenital cardiac lesions is rare and only 32 cases had been reported up to 1962. Pulmonary hypertension was observed in 19% of the cases [84]. The rarity of this congenital lesion and its presence in three patients with HAPE suggest that this is not a fortuitous occurrence.

Clearly the increased pulmonary blood flow to the normal lung and the elevated pulmonary artery pressure would facilitate the occurrence of HAPE in such patients if the overperfusion concept is an acceptable explanation of the syndrome.

8. The proposed concept would explain the radiologic features of HAPE. Even in severe instances of HAPE, the distribution of the exudate is patchy, and clear areas are usually found adjacent to areas of exudate. Clear areas of lung are commonly seen at the base of the lungs. It is quite likely that such clear areas are zones of vasoconstriction of vascular obstruction that are not perfused, and that areas of exudate represent areas of overperfusion and resulting edema. The lung bases are usually clear because hypoxic vasoconstriction is more severe in these areas [85].

9. Hypoxia and exercise will increase pulmonary arterial pressure at high altitude. If a high pulmonary arterial pressure is a necessary factor in the genesis of HAPE, the beneficial effect of bed rest, descent, and oxygen, all of which lower pulmonary arterial pressure, is compatible with the proposed mechanism.

10. Inhomogeneity of the pulmonary vasoconstrictive response to hypoxia has been demonstrated. Lehr subjected rabbits to hypoxia and perfused the lungs with India ink particles before sacrifice. Patchy distribution of the particles suggested that the vasoconstrictive response to hypoxia was not homogeneous [86]. Ventilation-perfusion studies of normal subjects have also suggested that disturbances of perfusion occur following ascent to high altitude [21, 65, 66].

Experimental Evidence

A hemodynamic analog of HAPE has been examined and it supports the concept already described. A brief summary of these studies follows.

Methods

Large mongrel dogs (mean weight 16 kg) were anesthetized with nembutal anesthesia and the chest was opened via a left thoractomy. Ventilation was controlled by a Bennett apparatus, which supplied room air. The pericardium was opened and the following measurements were made: (1) Arterial and right atrial oxygen contents, blood gas tensions, and pH. (2) Pressures from the femoral artery, right atrium, left atrium, and pulmonary artery, and pulmonary artery wedge pressure. Right and left atrial pressures were recorded via plastic cannulas tied into the atrial appendages. Pulmonary artery pressure and wedge pressure were recorded via a double-lumen catheter inserted into the left-upper-lobe pulmonary artery. After control measurements had been made, the right pulmonary artery was ligated and after a 10-min stabilization period, blood gas values and pressures were again determined. The right atrium was then cannulated via catheters from the femoral and jugular vein. A roller pump inflow cannula was inserted via a stab wound into the main pulmonary artery and secured by ligatures. A roller pump withdrew blood from the right atrium and delivered a constant flow to the main pulmonary artery, thus bypassing the right ventricle. Bypass of the right ventricle is necessary to prevent right ventricular failure and to maintain and vary the pulmonary flow. Initial bypass flow was started at 500 ml/min. Blood samples and pressures were again recorded. Ligatures were then placed around the isolated branches of the pulmonary artery to the left lower lobe and the left middle lobe. The ligatures were then slowly tightened so that total pulmonary flow was diverted through the left upper lobe (Fig. 5). After 10 min, blood gas and pressure values were determined; this was repeated at 10-min intervals. Similar measurements were made with bypass flows of 1.0 and 1.5 liters/min. Cardiac output was determined by the Fick principle. Expired air was collected in a meteorological balloon and analyzed. All pressures were referred to the midchest.

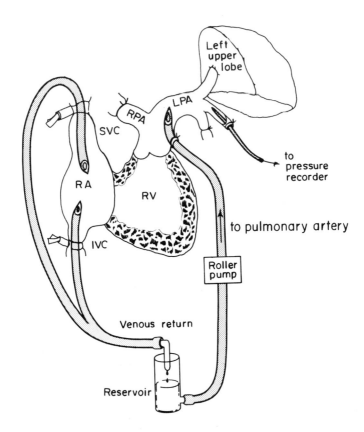

FIGURE 5   Diagram of experimental method of producing pulmonary edema by increased blood flow through a single lobe of a canine lung. RA = right atrium, RV = right pulmonary artery, IVC = inferior vena cava, SVC = superior vena cava.

At the termination of each experiment, the arteries, veins, and bronchi to each lobe were tied. The lobes were removed and weighed in air. The volume was determined by water displacement. Sections were taken for histologic study.

Results

Ligation of the right pulmonary artery resulted in a moderate increase in pulmonary arterial pressure from a control value of 16.2 to 30.5 mmHg (mean). Femoral arterial pressure, left atrial pressure, and cardiac output did not change significantly.

Ligation of pulmonary arterial branches to left lower and left middle lobe was then performed. When perfusion of the left upper lobe along began, the lobe became engorged and a continuous thrill and murmur appeared over the upper lobe artery and surface of the lung. After 10 to 20 min of perfusion the lobe became stiff and cyanotic, blood-tinged fluid filled the bronchus, and arterial oxygen saturation fell rapidly. Examination of the lobe after removal from the animal revealed diffuse pulmonary edema, and fluid oozed from the cut surface. The means specific grativy of 8 edematous lobes was 0.93, and the uninvolved, ligated lobes had a mean specific gravity of 0.56. The mean specific gravity of normal lobes of the lung removed immediately after ligation from 3 anesthetized dogs was 0.36. The protein content of the edema fluid removed from the bronchi was 4.3 to 5.3%. Histologic studies revealed marked capillary dilatation and engorgement with red cells and diffuse hemorrhagic pulmonary edema.

The hemodynamic data from 8 dogs are summarized in Table 5. The left atrial and pulmonary arterial wedge pressures remained normal throughout each study and showed no significant changes from the control pressures. The mean pulmonary arterial pressure was 48 mmHg (range 31-68 mean) just before gross pulmonary edema appeared. The cardiac output, i.e., total pulmonary flow, was not significantly different from control values. The calculated pulmomary vascular resistance rose from 9.6 units (following ligation of the right pulmonary artery) to 20 units. From measurements of the weight of normal lung lobes, it was found that the left upper lobe is approximately 25% of the weight of the total lung. Assuming that the capacity of the vascular bed is uniformly distributed in the dog lung, one can estimate that in these studies the blood flow through the left upper lobe was increased by 600%.

Conclusions

These data demonstrate that a sixfold increase in blood flow to a portion of a normal dog lung will result in severe pulmonary edema. Under the experimental conditions leading to pulmonary edema, the mean pulmonary artery pressure was 48 mmHg and the pulmonary arterial and pulmonary artery wedge pressures were normal. Hemodynamic studies of HAPE have revealed similar values, i.e., pulmonary arterial mean pressure of 46 mmHg with normal pulmonary artery wedge and left atrial pressures (Table 3).

In summary, the overperfusion concept of the etiology of HAPE is supported by numerous physiologic observations in man and experimental animals. Sea-level analogs are numerous and include pulmonary edema occuring during pulmonary embolism and following the surgical correction of obstruction of the pulmonary artery. The concept is similar to current views on the genesis of cerebral edema during hypertensive encephalopathy.

TABLE 5   Hemodynamic Features of Overperfusion Pulmonary Edema

	Control[a]	Pulmonary edema
PA mean, mmHg	26[b]	48
LA mean, mmHg	5	4
PA wedge, mmHg	5	6
Cardiac output, liter/min	2.3	2.0[c]
A-V difference, ml/100 ml	4.9	6.1
FA mean, mmHg	131	73
Heart rate, beats/min	157	135

[a]Control values were obtained after ligation of the right pulmonary artery but before right ventricular bypass was established. Values on the right were obtained just before the onset of pulmonary edema.
[b]RPA ligated.
[c]On bypass.

X. Future Areas of Research

Continued investigations of HAPE are essential for practical reasons and for understanding the basic mechanisms of pulmonary edema that occurs in the absence of left ventricular failure.

In the past few years, backpacking and mountaineering have increased enormously. Package tours are bringing many people to high altitude regions of the world, including the South American Andes, the Himalayas, and Mounts Kenya and Kilimanjaro. Annually, over 900 tourists reached the top of Mount Kenya (15,860 ft), and 9000 individuals ascended the lower slopes (13,500 ft). In a 30-month period, 33 episodes of severe pulmonary edema were observed among climbers on Mount Kenya. During 1975, over 4000 individuals ascended Mount Rainier in Washington (14,410 ft), and several times that number climbed Mount Whitney in California (14,495 ft). It is estimated that approximately 100 fatalities per year in climbers are due to HAPE and about 1000 to 2000 nonfatal episodes occur annually in various parts of the world. Differences of opinion still exist about appropriate methods of treatment and prevention. Continued research will minimize fatalities and prevent many nonfatal episodes.

It is evident that pulmonary edema in several different clinical conditions at sea level has hemodynamic features similar to those of HAPE. Pulmonary edema in heroin addicts and in patients with acute myocardial infarction are familiar examples. Other associated clinical conditions include pulmonary embolism, head injury, and open-heart surgery. Continued research on HAPE may very likely provide important information about the genesis of these familiar kinds of pulmonary edema.

Future lines of research should include the following.

1. Development of an animal model of HAPE. A small-animal model is desirable, one that would permit large numbers to be studied at sea-level altitude chambers. The animal should be large enough to permit simple hemodynamic studies and exercise methods. Viswanathan and his associates have produced pulmonary edema in guinea pigs, rats, and mice under such conditions [87]. The incidence of pulmonary edema was 30 to 66%. Animals that respond to hypoxia by a large rise in pulmonary artery pressure would be most suitable. At the present time, calves appear to be the most sensitive for this, but right ventricular failure and not pulmonary edema is the usual clinical feature seen on altitude exposure. An animal model may require interventions other than hypoxia and exercise to produce pulmonary edema consistently. Such interventions should include: (1) Ligation of one pulmonary artery in young and adult animals. (2) Exposure to high altitude for 1 to 3 months, with a return to sea-level atmosphere for 2 to 4 weeks then reexposure to high altitude. (3) Salt and water loading during initial exposure to high altitude. (4) Use of immature animals.

2. Noninvasive studies of the pulmonary circulation during acute altitude exposure in normal man and subjects with a prior history of HAPE. Such studies should examine, by isotope or radiologic methods, the homogeneity of pulmonary perfusion. Changes in plasma volume and water balance should be measured, to evaluate more completely the antidiuresis concept [35]. Measurements of lung water content and evaluation of lung compliance should be made to detect early pulmonary edema. The respiratory center and carotid body response to hypoxia should be examined in susceptible subjects, since it is possible that HAPE may be partly due to a decreased response of respiratory control mechanisms to hypoxia. Echocardiography may be useful in evaluating the changes in pulmonary arterial pressure during ascent and following interventions [88].

3. Invasive studies of the pulmonary circulation in subjects with a prior history of HAPE should be performed to examine more thoroughly the response of the pulmonary circulation to acute hypoxia. Preliminary studies have suggested that susceptible subjects show an abnormal elevation of pulmonary arterial pressure during hypoxia [21–23]. Further studies of this phenomenon are needed.

4. Field studies during acute exposure to high altitude should be carried out to evaluate simple methods of early diagnosis of HAPE. These studies should include ventilatory studies (vital capacity and airflow

velocity), basal heart rate and respiratory rate, ventilatory response to exercise, and measurement of arterial P_{O_2} at rest and during sleep. Simple field methods of detecting early HAPE would permit early preventive measures such as oxygen administration, bed rest, and removal to a lower altitude.

5. The reason for the higher incidence of HAPE in subjects under 20 years of age should be investigated. Younger individuals may respond to hypoxia by more vigorous pulmonary vasoconstriction. Younger individuals may maintain a higher cardiac output during hypoxic pulmonary hypertension with a resultant higher pulmonary arterial pressure.

6. Systematic studies of pharmacologic methods of prevention and treatment should be performed in animal models and under field conditions in human subjects. Controversy still exists over the value of diuretics, Diamox, morphine, digitalis, and other drugs in prevention and therapy. Diamox appears to be the most promising preventive drug for study.

7. To provide systematic data on severe or fatal episodes of HAPE, a central registry of all available cases should be developed. This registry should contain accurate clinical data and also results of any special studies like ECG's, blood gases, chest films, and autopsy data.

8. Support of studies in high altitude areas in other countries should be facilitated. The decrease in research support for high altitude studies in Peru, for example, resulted in a sharp decrease in the productive high altitude studies carried out in the Andes.

References

1. A. Mosso, *Life of Man in the High Alps.* London, T. F. Unwin, 1898.
2. T. Ravenhill, Some experiences of mountain sickness in the Andes, *J. Trop. Med. Hyg.,* **16**:313-320 (1913).
3. A. Hurtado, *Aspectos Fisiologicos y Patologicos de la Vida en la Altura.* S. A. Lima, Imp. Edit. Rimac, 1937.
4. E. Lundberg, Edema agudo del pulmon en el soroche, *Conferencia sustenada en la Asociacion Medica de Yauli, Oroya,* 1952.
5. L. Lizarraga, Edema agudo del pulmon, *Anal. Fac. Med., Lima,* 38:244 274 (1955).
6. A. Bardales, Edema pulmonar agudo por soroche grave, *Revista Peruana de Cardiologia,* **6**(2):115-136 (1957).
7. C. Houston, Acute pulmonary edema of high altitude, *N. E. J. Med.,* **263**: 478-480 (1960).

8. H. Hultgren, W. Spickard, K. Hellriegel, and C. Houston, High altitude pulmonary edema, *Medicine,* **40**:289-313 (1961).
9. I. Singh et al., High altitude pulmonary edema, *Lancet,* pp. 229-234, Jan. 30, 1965.
10. N. Menon, High altitude pulmonary edema, *N. E. J. Med.,* **273**:66-73 (1965).
11. H. Fred, A. Schmidt, T. Bates, and H. Hecht, Acute pulmonary edema of altitude. Clinical and physiologic observations, *Circulation,* **25**:929-937 (1962).
12. H. Hultgren, C. Lopez, E. Lundberg, and H. Miller, Physiologic studies of pulmonary edema at high altitude, *Circulation,* **29**:393-408 (1964).
13. D. Penaloza and F. Sime, Circulatory dynamics during high altitude pulmonary edema, *Amer. J. Cardiol.,* **23**:369-378 (1969).
14. S. Roy et al., Hemodynamic studies in high altitude pulmonary edema, *Brit. Heart J.,* **31**:52-58 (1969).
15. H. Hultgren, W. Spickard, and C. Lppez, Further studies of high altitude pulmonary edema, *Brit. Heart J.* **24**:95-102 (1962).
16. J. Arias-Stella and H. Kruger, Pathology of high altitude pulmonary edema, *Arch. Pathol.,* **76**:147-157 (1963).
17. N. Nayak, S. Roy, and D. Narayanan, Pathologic features of altitude sickness, *Amer. J. Pathol.,* **45**:381-391 (1964).
18. G. Roberts, In *Americans on Everest.* Philadelphia and New York, J. B. Lippincott, 1964.
19. H. Hultgren and E. Marticorena, Epidemiological observations in high altitude pulmonary edema, *Clin. Res.,* **16**:142 (1968). Abstract.
20. E. Marticorena, Edema agudo pulmonar de altura. Epedemeologica, estandardization de su severidad y evaluation de su terapia, Ph.D. Thesis, Lima, Emelio A. Marticorena Pimentel, 1971.
21. H. Hultgren, R. Gover, and L. Hartley, Abnormal circulatory responses to high altitude in subjects with a previous history of high altitude pulmonary edema, *Circulation,* **44**:759-770 (1971).
22. J. Kleiner and W. Nelson, High altitude pulmonary edema. A rare disease? *JAMA,* **234**:491-495 (1975).
23. R. Viswanathan et al., Pulmonary edema of high altitude, *Amer. Rev. Resp. Dis.,* **100**:334-349 (1969).
24. C. Houston and J. Dickinson, Cerebral form of high altitude illness; *Lancet,* pp. 758-761, Oct. 18, 1975.
25. P. Radford, High altitude oedema presenting as coma, *Brit. Med. J.,* **3**: 294-295 (1973).
26. R. Wilson, Acute high altitude illness in mountaineers and problems of rescue, *Ann. Intern. Med.,* **78**:421-428 (1973).
27. H. Hultgren, High altitude pulmonary edema. In *Hypoxia, High Altitude and the Heart.* First conference on Cardiovascular Disease. Vol. 5. Aspen, Colo. 1970. Basel, Munich, Paris, New York, Karger, 1970, pp. 24-31.
28. E. Marticorena and J. Severino, Remision espontanea del edema agudo pulmonary de aitura, *Arch. Inst. Biol. Andina,* **1**:157-178 (1966).

29. E. Marticorena and H. Hultgren, Treatment of high altitude pulmonary edema by bed rest alone, *Circulation*, **33, 34**(2): 163 (1966). Abstract.

30. H. Hultgren, Treatment and prevention of high altitude pulmonary edema, *American Alpine Club J.*, 1965, pp. 363-372.

31. W. Read, J. Morrissey, and L. Reichardt, American Dhaulagiri Expedition 1969, *American Alpine J.*, **17**:19-26 (1970).

32. I. Singh et al., Acute mountain sickness, *N. E. J. Med.*, **280**:175-184 (1969).

33. H. Hultgren, J. Bilisoly, H. Fails, M. Stone, J. Pfeifer, and E. Marticorena, Plasma volume changes during acute exposure to high altitude, *Clin. Res.*, **21**:224 (1973).

34. G. Gray et al., Control of acute mountain sickness, *Aerospace Med.*, **48**: 81-84 (1971).

35. V. Aoki and S. Robinson, Body hydration and the incidence and severity of acute mountain sickness, *J. Appl. Physiol.*, **31**:363-366 (1971).

36. T. Bates, Pulmonary oedema of mountains, *Brit. Med. J.*, **3**:829 (1972).

37. S. Robinson, W. Evans, R. Sterner and D. Stamper, Effect of intermediate altitude staging upon acute mountain sickness, *Fed. Proc.*, **33**:307 (1974). Abstract No. 581.

38. S. Robinson et al., The amelioration of the symptoms of acute mountain sickness (AMS) by staging and acetazolamide, *Fed. Proc.*, **34**:409 (1975). Abstract.

39. S. Forwand et al., Effect of acetazolamide on acute mountain sickness, *N. E. J. Med.*, **279**:839-845 (1968).

40. R. Grover, personal communication.

41. M. Malhotra et al., Electrolyte changes at 3500 m in males with and without high altitude pulmonary edema, *Aviation Space and Environ. Med.*, **46**:409-412 (1975).

42. M. Surks, K. Shinn, and L. Matovsh, Alterations in body composition in man after acute exposure to high altitude, *J. Appl. Physiol.*, **21**:1741-1746 (1966).

43. K. Sumiyoshi et al., Changes of blood elements and the circulatory system in climbing, *Jap. Circ. J.*, **26**:535-457 (1962).

44. M. Visscher, Basic factors in the genesis of pulmonary edema and a direct study of the effects of hypoxia upon edemogenesis. In *Biomedicine Problems of High Terrestrial Elevations.* Edited by A. H. Hegnauer. Natick, Mas., U.S. Army Research Institute of Environmental Medicine, 1969, p. 90.

45. R. Courtice and P. Korner, The effect of anoxia on pulmonary edema produced by massive intravenous infusions, *Aust. J. Exp. Biol. Med. Sci.*, 30:511-526 (1952).

46. T. Whayne, Jr., and J. Sevringhaus, Experimental hypoxic pulmonary edema in the rat, *J. Appl. Physiol.*, **25**:729-732 (1968).

47. J. Theodore and E. Robin, Pathogenesis of neurogenic pulmonary edema, *Lancet*, pp. 749-751, Oct. 18, 1975.

48. T. Drucker, Increased intracranial pressure and pulmonary edema, *J. Neurosurg.*, **28**:112-117 (1968).

49. G. Kennedy, T. Bucci, R. Myers, C. Alden, R. Demaree, and I. Plaugh, Effects of altitude on the Cebus monkey with emphasis on the central nervous system, *Fed. Proc.,* **29**:591 (1970). Abstract No. 1927.

50. J. White et al., Changes in brain volume during anesthesia: The effects of anoxia and hypercapnia, *Arch. Surg.,* **44**:1-21 (1942).

51. R. Grover, Influence of high altitude on cardiac output response to exercise. In *Biomedical Problems of High Terrestrial Elevation.* Edited by A. H. Hegnauer. Natick, Mass., U.S. Army Research Institute of Environmental Medicine, 1969, p. 223.

52. J. Weil, D. Battock, R. Grover, and C. Chidsey, Venoconstriction in man upon ascent to high altitude: Studies on potential mechanisms, *Fed. Proc.,* **28**:1160 (1969).

53. H. Fritts, Jr., J. Odell, P. Harris, E. Braunwald, and A. Fishman, Effects of acute hypoxia on the volume of blood in the thorax, *Circulation,* **22**: 216-219 (1960).

54. S. Roy et al., Immediate circulatory response to high altitude hypoxia in man, *Nature,* **217**:1177-1178 (1968).

55. R. Smith and L. Ramsey, The measurement of pulmonary extravascular water volume during exposure to simulated high altitude. Naval Aerospace Medical Research Laboratory. Bureau of Medicine and Survery. 3 Jan. 1973.

56. H. Hultgren, M. Robinson, and R. Wuerflein, Overperfusion pulmonary edema, *Circulation,* **33,** 34(3):132 (1956). Abstract.

57. H. Hultgren, High altitude pulmonary edema. In *Biomedicine of High Terrestrial Elevations.* Edited by A. Hegnauer. Nattick, Mass., U.S. Army Research Institute of Environmental Medicine, 1969.

58. N. Lassen, Control of cerebral circulation in health and disease, *Circ. Res.,* **34**:749-760 (1974).

59. B. Johansson, S. Strandgaard, and N. Lassen, On the pathogenesis of hypertensive encephalopathy, *Circ. Res.,* **34,** 35:167-171 (1974).

60. E. Skinhoj and S. Strandgaard, Pathogenesis of hypertensive encephalopathy, *Lancet,* **1**:461-462 (1973).

61. D. Penaloza, F. Sime, N. Banchero, and R. Gamboa, Pulmonary hypertension in healthy men born and living at high altitudes. In *Normal and Abnormal Pulmonary Circulation.* Edited by R. Grover, Basel, Karger, 1963, p. 25.

62. H. Hultgren, J. Kelly, and H. Miller, Pulmonary circulation in acclimatized man at high altitude, *J. Appl. Physiol.,* **20**:233-238 (1965).

63. R. Grover, J. Vogel, G. Voight, and S. Blount, Jr., Reversal of high altitude pulmonary hypertension, *Amer. J. Cardiol.,* **18**:928-932 (1966).

64. J. Vogel, J. Goss, M. Mori, and H. Brammell, PA pressure rise with high altitude and exercise, *Clin. Res.,***15**:95 (1967). Abstract.

65. R. Kronenberg et al., Pulmonary artery pressure and alveolar gas exchange in man during acclimatization to 12,470 feet, *J. Clin. Invest.,* **50**:827-837 (1971).

66. P. Haab, R. Held, E. Ernst, and L. Farhi, Ventilation-perfusion relationships during high altitude adaptation, *J. Appl. Physiol.,* **26**:77-81 (1969).

67. I. Singh, I. Chohan, and N. Mathew, Fibrinolytic activity in high altitude pulmonary oedema, *Indian J. Med. Res.*, **57**:210-217 (1969).
68. I. Singh and I. Chohan, Blood coagulation changes at high atltitude predisposing to pulmonary hypertension, *Brit. Med. J.*, **34**:611-617 (1972).
69. J. Torres, Tiempo de coagulation, tiempo de sangria y prueba de Rumpel Leeds en la hypoxia aguda por ascension a les grandes altures. Ph.D. Thesis, University of Peru, "Cayetano Heredia," Lima, Peru, 1968.
70. E. Genton and J. Vogel, Altitude and blood coagulation factors, *Clin. Res.*, **17**:133 (1961).
71. G. Gray, A. Bryan, M. Freedman, C. Houston, W. Lewis, D. McFadden, and G. Newell, Effect of altitude exposure on platelets, *J. Appl. Physiol.*, **39**:648-651 (1975).
72. A. Hyman, Effects of large increases in pulmonary blood flow on pulmonary venous pressure, *J. Appl. Physiol.*, **27**:179-185 (1961).
73. H. Weisberg, J. Lopez, M. Juria, and L. Katz, Persistence of lung edema and arterial pressure rise in dogs after lung emobli, *Amer. J. Physiol.*, **207**: 641-646 (1964).
74. G. Daicoff, F. Chavez, A. Anton, and E. Swenson, Serotonin-induced pulmonary venous hypertension in pulmonary embolism, *J. Thorac. Cardiovasc. Surg.*, **56**:810-815 (1968).
75. D. Singer, C. Hesser, R. Pick, and L. Katz, Diffuse bilateral pulmonary edema associated with unilobar miliary pulmonary embolism in the dog, *Circ. Res.*, **6**:4-9 (1958).
76. J. Alexander, personal communication.
77. S. Kovacs, J. Hill, T. Aberg, A. Blesousky, and F. Gerbode, Pathogenesis of arterial hypoxemia in pulmonary embolism, *Arch. Surg.*, **93**:813-823 (1966).
78. L. Parmley, Jr., R. North, and B. Ott, Hemodynamic alterations of acute pulmonary embolism, *Circ. Res.*, **11**:450-465 (1962).
79. S. Brown et al., Massive pulmonary hemorrhagic infarction following revascularization of ischemic lungs, *Arch. Surg.*, **108**:795-797 (1974).
80. A. Makey et al., Fatal intra-alveolar pulmonary bleeding complicating pulmonary embolectomy, *Thorax*, **26**:466-471 (1971).
81. C. Couves et al., Hemorrhagic lung syndrome, *Ann. Thorac. Surg.*, **15**: 187-195 (1973).
82. Case records of the Massachusetts General Hospital. Edited by B. Custleman. *N. E. J. Med.*, **271**:40-50 (1964).
83. C. Houston, personal communication.
84. P. Pool, J. Vogel, and G. Blount, Congenital unilateral absence of a pulmonary artery. The importance of flow in pulmonary hypertension, *Amer. J. Cardiol.*, **10**:706-732 (1962).
85. C. Hales, B. Amluwalia, and H. Kazemi, Strength of pulmonary vascular response to regional alveolar hypoxia, *J. Appl. Physiol.*, **38**:1083-1087 (1975).
86. D. Lehr, M. Triller, L. Fisher, K. Ellis, and A. Fishman, Induced changes in the pattern of pulmonary blood flow in the rabbit, *Circ. Res.*, **13**:119-131 (1963).

87. R. Viswanathan, S. Jain, S. Subramanian, and B. Puri, Pulmonary edema of high altitude. I. Production of pulmonary edema in animals under conditions of simulated high altitude, *Amer. Rev. Resp. Dis.*, **100**:327-333 (1969).

88. P. Mills, G. Leech, A. Leatham, and W. Ginks, Non-invasive estimation of pulmonary artery end-diastolic pressure. *Circulation,* **52**(2):50 (1975).

89. J. W. Severinghaus and A. Carcelen, Cerebrospinal fluid in man native to high altitude, *J. Appl. Physiol.,* **19**:319-321 (1964).

16

Treatment of Pulmonary Edema

CARROLL E. CROSS

University of California at Davis
Davis, California

RICHARD W. HYDE

University of Rochester School of Medicine and Dentistry
Rochester, New York

I. Introduction

Pulmonary edema is generally defined as an increase in the volume of water in the interstitium and alveoli of the lung. Its presence reflects a disturbance in the mechanisms that control movements of liquid in the pulmonary microcirculation and can usually be ascribed to (1) increased hydrostatic pressure secondary to cardiac abnormalities or (2) increased permeability to liquid and solutes secondary to injury to lung cells [1,2]. Hemodynamic forms of pulmonary edema are fairly well understood and usually respond to cardiotonic regimens [3]. In contrast, pathologic processes leading to increased permeability of alveolar epithelium and pulmonary capillary endothelium [2,4] or possibly bronchial endothelium [5] are poorly understood and specific therapeutic agents are lacking. Therapeutic approaches will likely develop from a better understanding about injury to the lungs.

This work partly supported by National Institutes of Health grants, HL 70820-02, HL 17853, and AP 00628.

This account focuses on mechanisms of noncardiogenic forms of pulmonary edema and strategies that could lead to newer therapeutic agents for its treatment. Current techniques for clinical detection, evaluation, and treatment of pulmonary edema are discussed, with emphasis on general measures of treatment useful in all forms of pulmonary edema and on speculations concerning future approaches.

II. Pulmonary Capillary Permeability

Three main pathways for increased passage of liquid from the pulmonary microvasculature have been identified: (1) an intracellular cell membrane pathway permeable to water and lipid-soluble solutes but impermeable to lipid-insoluble solutes; (2) a "pore" pathway via the relatively "tight" intercellular junctions, where permeability is a function of a poorly characterized operational "pore" size, possibly transcapillary hydrostatic pressures, and forces of cell membranes and associated junction complexes; and (3) a second intracellular pathway consisting of cytoplasmic vesicles. Little is known about the contributions of each of the three transcapillary transport pathways to net transcapillary liquid transport in normal and diseased states. A fourth pathway, via relatively "leaky" fenestrations in the bronchial microvasculature, has been demonstrated to exist under certain experimental circumstances but has yet to be evaluated [5,6].

Recent studies of capillary permeability in general have focused on the metabolic and transport functions of endothelial cells [7]. These functions may include active contraction of endothelial cells, possibly in response to vasoactive mediators such as histamine, serotonin, and bradykinin [8,9]. It is clear that interendothelial junctional sealing elements, which have marked anatomical and functional variabilities [10,11], can undergo rapid configurational change in response to various pathophysiologic conditions such as local osmotic forces, adjacent endothelial cell wall tensions, and endothelial cell glutathione concentrations [12–14]. The factors involved in the assembly and modulation of junctions are of special interest because their temporary opening or irreversible injury may take place in some forms of pulmonary edema. Advances in understanding normal and abnormal capillary permeability states will likely require detailed knowledge of the molecular architecture, permeability properties, breakdown and mode of assembly, growth, and repair of lung endothelial junctions.

Permeability of the lung microcirculation can be altered by numerous agents known to damage capillary endothelium [15]. Pulmonary edema may result from interactions between pulmonary endothelial cells and the main hemostatic systems of contained blood, such as the coagulation-fibrinolytic system and platelets; from permeability factors related to type I allergic reactions (such as histamine), phagocytes, the kinin-generating system, complement and other immunological phenomena, arachidonic acid, and prostaglandins; and from the substructure of the endothelial cells themselves.

The nature of these interactions at the cellular and subcellular levels, particularly those relating to endothelial cell functions, is poorly understood. Potentially fruitful areas for further research include: (1) delineation of the molecular organization of the membrane in endothelial cells; (2) expanded knowledge of how the membrane responds to a wide variety of agents known to alter membrane functions; (3) explanation of phenomena leading to endothelial membrane disruptions and also endothelial cell immune and osmotic lysis; (4) investigation of the role of the endothelial microskeleton, such as the actinlike contractile microfilaments and the microtubules, in endothelial permeability; (5) studies of the interrelations among this endothelial microskeleton, endothelial plasma membranes, and endothelial junctional assemblies in modulating transmural permeabilities [8,14,16]; (6) a better definition of the organization and role of the endothelial microskeleton and intercellular junctions when pulmonary capillary permeability is increased; (7) studies of the functions of the basal lamina and other components of the extravascular interstitial space of the lung (such as connective tissue fibers, ground substance, pericytes, and interstitial cells) in lung liquid transport; (8) investigation of interrelations among endothelial injury, cellular and organelle edema, changes in cell metabolism, and changes in capillary permeability [17,18]; and (9) explanations of the regulation of phagocyte adherence and diapedesis by normal and by injured endothelium. As endothelial cell swelling itself has potentially serious consequences to both capillary permeability and to cell viability, the ability of hyperosmotic agents such as mannitol to enhance cellular functions or survival or both in injured endothelial cells deserves further evaluation.

Current sketchy knowledge of the function of the endothelial cell in health and disease severely limits development of rational methods of controlling and modulating capillary permeability. Especially needed are investigations of endothelial cellular responses to injury, particularly to determine their mode of interaction with inflammatory mediators and phagocytes and to determine whether they are primary immunologic targets in life. Studies of isolated endothelial cells and their junctional apparatus, and of the effects of perturbators such as platelet components [19], should lead to new techniques for detailed analysis of their cellular functions and provide a way of obtaining useful clues about the pathophysiology of pulmonary endothelial cells.

III. Lung Inflammatory Responses

Physical and chemical agents damage lung cells. Such agents include trans-thoracic insults such as irradiation, airway toxins (inhaled oxidants), microbes and aspirated acid, and bloodborne toxins (paraquat, a herbicide; and phthal-ate esters, plasticizers). These agents presumably cause pulmonary edema by direct cellular injury.

Treatment strategies are complicated because cellular injuries coexist with variable inflammatory reactions (defined as local reactions to injury) capable of amplifying and propagating the initial injury mechanism, thereby worsening the cellular injury. In addition, necessary treatments such as high inspired O_2 tensions or high intravascular volume (which may be required to maintain tissue O_2 delivery) have further deleterious effects. In some situa-tions, the stimulus provoking the reaction would be innocuous to the lung were it not for its ability to induce an inflammatory reaction via activation of mediator and phagocyte amplification systems. Possible examples of this mechanism are anaphylaxis, the Arthus reaction, endotoxemia, some viral in-fections, and even severe nonthoracic trauma.

Since one of the cardinal features of inflammation is increased micro-vascular permeability, the inflammatory response to primary lung injury will either initiate or worsen existing permeability disorders. It is possible that suppression of immune responses would be helpful in some forms of lung in-jury where inflammatory defenses are excessive. Pharmacologic modulations of putative inflammatory responses by drugs that affect microtubular function, intracellular esterase, or cyclic nucleotide activities might be particularly help-ful in this regard. Appreciating the role of mediators in inflammatory re-sponses instead of focusing only on inflammation itself will likely enhance the outlook for treatment through inhibitors and antagonists of these mediators.

The pattern of inflammation-related increased vascular permeabilities in injury is often biphasic, with an early phase that is mild and often brief, and a later phase that is more severe and often prolonged. The time course of in-flammatory events is distinctive and suggests involvement of different chem-ical substances responsible for each inflammatory event. Considerable varia-tion in inflammatory response may occur, according to the nature, severity, and mechanisms of the primary cell injury and according to the autoregulatory factors that control the intensity, extent, and duration of the host inflamma-tory reactions.

The activity of mediators of inflammation in causing either "early" or "delayed" types of increased vascular permeability may be important in in-dicating what mechanisms are responsible for the increased permeability re-sponse and in determining susceptibilities to inhibitors of inflammatory permeability factors such as antihistaminics [20–23]. Treatment or prevention of the delayed pulmonary edema secondary to such lung insults as smoke inhalation and near drowning may develop from such studies.

Knowledge of the inflammatory process has increased immeasurably in recent years. Special attention has been focused on inflammatory mediators derived from plasma proteins, phagocytes, and platelets. Much has been learned about how complement, coagulation, and kinin cascades and how vasoactive peptides, prostaglandins, and lymphokines affect inflammatory processes. Unfortunately, the interrelations of important primary injury mechanisms and the secondary inflammatory responses in the lung are poorly understood. Information gathered from studies of inflammatory responses has not often been directly applied to inflammations in the lung [24]. Inflammatory mediators undoubtedly are important in the range of noncardiogenic pulmonary edema. Indeed, sequential interactions between injured pulmonary endothelium and vascular and perivascular constituents presumably contribute in varying degrees to the increased vascular permeability that characterizes these disorders.

Primary injury to lung endothelial and epithelial cells can be accompanied by a variety of potential mediator-amplification systems [20–26], some of which are listed in Figure 1. A big problem in lung biology today is the lack of basic knowledge concerning these potential mediator-amplification systems in noncardiogenic forms of pulmonary edema.

With suitable mild primary injury or with exposure to low concentrations of mediators of increased permeability, the permeability effects are entirely and rapidly reversible. With more severe primary injury secondary to large concentrations of mediator infusion or release, irreversible endothelial injuries associated with big increases in permeability occur. Following some forms of lung injury such as smoke inhalation and near drowning, there is often a delay (6–24 hr) in the maximal permeability response, suggesting activation of complex time-dependent inflammatory cascades. Alternatively, if the damage in these conditions is less than catastrophic, the delay in the appearance of pulmonary edema might be due merely to a slow leakage of intravascular liquid. Until more information is obtained, treatments of both early and late (or delayed) secondary inflammatory states occurring subsequent to primary injuries will be both supportive and empirical.

Polymorphonuclear leukocytes and macrophages are likely important contributors of reactants found in the lung and pulmonary circulation in pulmonary edema that is accompanied by increased permeability [27,28]. Margination of phagocytes and platelets in the pulmonary capillaries accompanies many forms of pulmonary injury manifested by increased permeability and occurs in some clinical circumstances in which the lung damage is secondary

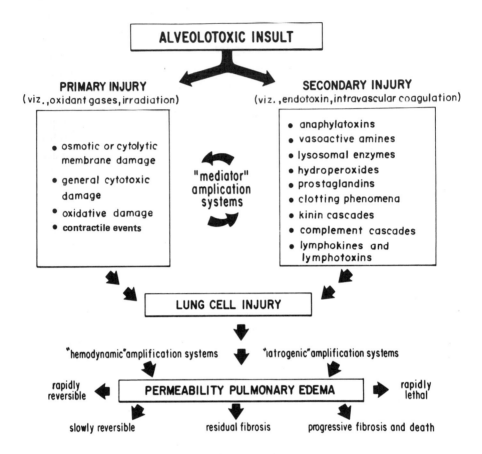

FIGURE 1   Theoretical diagram of mechanisms of lung cell injury, depicting the potential secondary inflammatory amplification systems that could initiate, amplify, or propagate primary lung damage mechanisms. The modifying aspect of cardiogenic and iatrogenic factors (overinfusion, hypotonicity) are shown, and also the possible outcome of the induced "permeability" pulmonary edema.

to nonpulmonary tissue insults such as nonthoracic trauma, shock, and hemodialysis [27–31].

Sequestered, recruited, or activated phagocytes may be toxic to lung cells. Accumulated phagocytes may cause increased permeability by direct lysosomal enzyme injury or oxidative injury, or may possibly cause indirect injury via activation of cascade reactants on the critical endothelial membranes. These consequences of lung phagocyte sequestration, activation, and degranulation raise important questions for therapeutic consideration. For example, it is not clear whether or not phagocyte sequestration and degranulation initiates, causes (wholly or partially), or results from lung endothelial injury. If sequestration is important as a causative mechanism of lung injury, then administration of anti-inflammatory agents such as steroids and aspirin, which diminish phagocyte adherence [32], would be useful.

IV. Phagocytes

Circulating phagocytes (predominantly leukocytes) normally are in dynamic equilibrium with marginated phagocytes that are stuck to endothelium. Under conditions of tissue injury or inflammation, however, phagocytes undergo increased adherence [32], and this equilibrium is shifted so that an increasing proportion of bloodborne phagocytes are attracted to vessel walls. Phagocyte adherence to pulmonary capillary endothelium characterizes pulmonary responses to most forms of sublethal lung injury [27].

Chemattractant and receptor mechanisms responsible for phagocyte adherence to injured pulmonary endothelium are not known [32]. They presumably involve intermembrane charges, membrane receptors, changes in plasmalemmal phospholipid or protein composition, or changes in membrane fluidity or membrane surface sulfhydryl groups, or they may depend on mediator activations such as those that thrombogenic or immunologic stimuli provide. It is probable that phagocyte attachment to endothelium represents a stimulus for "activation" of phagocytes, leading to local release of lysosomal enzymes and oxidants that may affect phagocyte diapedesis through endothelium, similar to the process whereby chemotactic factors "activate" release of lysosomal enzymes [32–34].

That phagocyte margination can be injurious to the lung is suggested by evidence in other tissues, where phagocyte accumulation induced by local injury causes endothelial basement membrane and tissue injury, presumably by releasing or secreting lysosomal proteases, lipases, or oxidants [35–39]. In experimental models, the state of existing immunity can influence the character and severity of antigen-mediated lung inflammatory responses characterized by immunoglobulin and complement deposition, phagocyte activation, and tissue injury [40]. In such cases phagocytes undoubtedly are very important in causing the increased vascular permeability. In the majority of instances, however, it is uncertain whether phagocytic accumulations and activations, which characterize the inflammatory response to injury, amplify or perpetuate the existing injury or are merely the result of the injury itself [41]. Cell damage by lysosomes and oxidants have potential therapeutic significance.

A. Lysosomal Mechanisms

The overall importance of lysosomal enzyme release by sequestered phagocytes in mediating the increased permeability seen in noncardiogenic pulmonary edema is not known. A variety of phagocytic and nonphagocytic stimuli,
including small peptide fragments of C3 and C5 and a number of other chemo-
tactic factors, cause phagocytes to liberate their lysosomal enzymes [33,34,42–
44]. Endothelial adherence may itself stimulate phagocytes to increase their
synthesis and release of potentially damaging lysosomal enzymes. A wide
variety of substances in perfusate blood, including intravascular microaggregates
of platelets and red cells (seen in shock), antigen-antibody complexes, and
activated complement components, are able to induce phagocytic release of
lysosomal enzymes into the immediate microenvironment [42–46]. Presumably sequestration and activation of phagocytes could account for the leukoag-
glutin-induced pulmonary edemas that multiple leukocyte transfusions precipitate [47].

Phagocytic lysosomal enzyme systems include phospholipases, nonspecific proteases, and specific neutral proteases such as plasminogen activators, col-
lagenases, and elastases. Although we know that these enzyme systems can
injure interstitium, including basement membranes [48], we do not know
whether they are directly detrimental to endothelial cell membranes and their
junctional complexes. Nor do we know whether the release of lysosomal enzymes activates potential mediator amplification systems in blood and lung
tissue and whether the serum antiproteases and antilipases can neutralize these
potentially harmful systems. The gradual accumulation of lysosomal proteolytic enzymes from phagocytes following lung injury may account for the delayed injury and inflammation seen in the lung following smoke inhalation,
near drowning, and nonthoracic trauma. Although more evidence is needed,
it seems probable that lysosomal enzymes released from sequestered platelets
and megakaryocytes damage the lung in several types of noncardiogenic pulmonary edema [27,42–46,48–51].

If the sequestration of phagocytes and platelets is important in initiating
some forms of noncardiogenic pulmonary edema, then suppressing the activities of the enzymes they release would be fundamentally important in atten-
uating the harmful aspects of the inflammatory process. For example, it may
be possible to modify phagocyte adhesiveness to lung capillaries [32,52].
Agents that might have therapeutic value are immunosuppressive drugs, agents
that effect the release of lysosomal enzymes and functions of microtubules
and microfilaments, autonomic neurohormones, and protease and prostaglandin
synthetase inhibitors [49,53–57].

B. Oxidative Mechanisms

Recent studies of lung damage by oxygen, ozone, or paraquat have focused on the biochemical and physiologic features of lung oxidant stress, and may lead to therapeutic approaches to noncardiogenic forms of pulmonary edema [58–61]. Of special interest are recent demonstrations that phagocytes can generate superoxide anion radicals (O_2^-), hydrogen peroxide (H_2O_2), and perhaps hydroxyl radical and singlet O_2 at the level of the plasma membrane [62–64], thereby providing a chemical insult to surrounding healthy tissue. This finding may explain why the products of peroxidation are found at sites of inflammation [25,62,65]. Numerous nonphagocytic and phagocytic stimuli cause phagocytes to elaborate toxic oxygen metabolites that could mediate lung damage at sites of their sequestration [66–68]. A somewhat similar injury mechanism has been shown with erythrocytes that have been exposed to either phagocytosing leukocytes [69] or cultured macrophages [70]. These findings suggest that lung oxidative damage may be more common than previously thought. Since the lung parenchyma must cope with much higher oxygen tensions than those found in other organs and since therapeutic administration of O_2-enriched gas is common for critically ill patients, oxidant damage may be significant in noncardiogenic pulmonary edema.

Mechanisms of oxidant-induced lung cell injury have been discussed in several reviews [58,60,61,71]. Most theories involve generation of activated unstable O_2 derivatives such as O_2^-, H_2O_2, hydroxyl radical, singlet O_2, or other free radicals. Further information about these substances is needed. These reactive and unstable O_2 metabolites are thought to be able to damage tissue directly by oxidative and peroxidative decomposition of thiol groups and essential membrane-associated fatty acids [60]. Peroxide decomposition may result in free-radical production that can initiate further oxidation and peroxidation—of other sulfhydryl groups, amino acids, pyridine-nucleotide systems, and polyunsaturated fatty acids. These mechanisms of molecular damage presumably could alter the permeability of critical endothelial cell membranes, producing endothelial cell damage, intracellular edema, organelle swelling, and finally pulmonary edema. Operationally important amplification systems include changes in permeability to lysosomal enzymes with subsequent labilization of hydrolytic enzyme systems. One such enzyme, phospholipase A, by hydrolyzing arachidonic acid from membrane phospholipids, stimulates prostaglandin synthesis, whereas labilized proteases can activate clotting, kinin, and immune cascades as well as cause direct cellular proteolytic damage.

Many agents may help to protect the oxidant-sensitive components of the cell from damage by the above mechanisms. These agents include enzyme

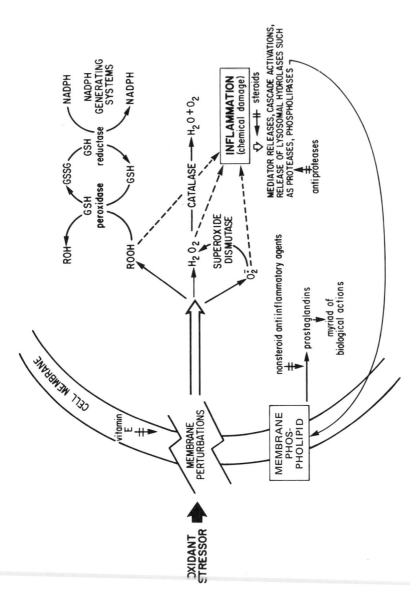

FIGURE 2 Oxidant-induced membrane damage subsequent to generation of lipid peroxides (ROOH), H_2O_2, and O_2^-, which are believed to represent an important primary mechanism of oxidative lung damage. The protective effect of endogenous antioxidant substances and the potential intracellular mechanisms for amplifying damage via lysosomal enzyme activations and stimulated prostaglandin biosynthesis are shown.

systems such as the selenium-containing glutathione peroxidase pathways, catalase, superoxide dismutase, sulfhydryl reductases, antioxidant factors such as α-tocopherols, and factors capable of modifying prostaglandin metabolism (see Fig. 2).

The possibility of oxidant-induced endothelial damage and resultant pulmonary edema raises several specific questions concerning possible directions for future research and therapy. Do substances known to have a protective effect in vitro on the viability and integrity of phagocytosing phagocytes (such as superoxide dismutase, catalase, and mannitol) have a part in anti-inflammatory pulmonary treatment [64]? Are antioxidant substances such as α-tocopherols, selenium, and superoxide dismutase important in treating oxidant-induced pulmonary edema? Recent unconfirmed experiments have shown, for example, that superoxide dismutase administration modified cell injury induced by paraquat and irradiation [59,72]. Since the protective effect of administered superoxide dismutase appeared to last well beyond the lifetime of the short-lived, radiation-produced O_2^- radical, superoxide dismutase may cause stabilization of cell membranes or influence secondary inflammatory responses such as prostaglandin biosynthesis [73].

The development of a small-molecule analog of superoxide dismutase that could cross cell membranes would be of potential therapeutic importance so far as oxidant-induced and phagocyte-induced lung damages are concerned. Can injured cells with moderately severe oxidant-induced membrane injuries be rescued by treatment? What do mediator systems do in cells injured by oxidants? Do amplification systems permit other therapeutic approaches? Lastly, since some forms of oxidant damage appear to have radiomimetic properties, could radioprotective compounds be effective in treating acute lung injury states [74]?

V. Hemostatic Systems

Components of the blood-clotting mechanisms significantly affect tissue responses to inflammation and may influence the inflammatory response, as seen in noncardiogenic pulmonary edema. Following endothelial injury, platelets become more "sticky," and they agglutinate and adhere to subendothelial tissue. Stimuli such as basement membrane collagen, thrombin, prostaglandins, catecholamines, and infection with microorganisms that can trigger the production of circulating immune complexes probably spur this phenomenon. Adherence is followed by release of vasoactive amines (5-hydroxytryptamine, which may increase endothelial permeability; adenosine diphosphate, which initiates further platelet activation; and thromboxanes, prostaglandin intermediates which are extremely potent inducers of platelet aggregation and which are involved in the lipid peroxide production associated with platelet release reactions [75]). In some forms of pulmonary edema, like those seen with intravascular coagulation [2], platelets appear to affect complement activation [76].

Platelet entrapment in pulmonary capillaries is histologically apparent in a variety of lung injuries, including traumatic shock induced by soft tissue injury, endotoxemia, and anaphylaxis [27,51,77,78]. Platelets have also been shown to contain proteolytic enzymes, including collagenase, elastase, and mediators of increased vascular permeability [4,79,80]. It is probable that platelet adherence and release of biologically active agents such as prostaglandin intermediates and proteolytic enzymes [81,82] either limit or amplify endothelial injury mechanisms.

Pharmacologic inhibition of platelet reactivity is a form of antithrombotic therapy that has gained considerable favor [83]. Areas needing further study are the experimental assessment of the effect in noncardiogenic pulmonary edema of platelet antiaggregating agents, including those that inhibit platelet release (agents, for instance, that modulate platelet cyclic nucleotide levels; and also nonsteroidal anti-inflammatory drugs and α-tocopherols) [75,83,84].

Extravascular pulmonary fibrinogen and fibrin deposition accompanies many forms of noncardiogenic pulmonary edema. With lysis, their degradation products cause a further increase in capillary permeability and attract granulocytes; a complex interrelation is thereby suggested for inflammatory reactions and proteolytic clotting and anticlotting cascades in the lung [85–89]. Endothelial and tissue injury, by exposing negatively charged surfaces (basement membranes), can activate Hagemen factor [89,90]. Hageman factor activation triggers clotting, kinin generation, and fibrinolysis, and via plasmin generation, activates complement. Microparticulate substances and bacteria also can activate Hageman factor. The blood coagulation systems thus can be seen to be closely involved with inflammatory responses.

VI. Complement

The activation of the complement system (C_1–C_9) by classic or alternative pathways may represent a general inflammatory trigger to injury [91–93]. Since lysosomal proteases, thrombin, and plasmin activate complement, activated complement components must interact with inflammatory processes [94]. Complement activations have two distinct biological consequences: (1) irreversible damages to the phospholipid moieties of biological membranes (resulting in lysis of certain cells); and (2) initiation of phagocyte migration. The effect of complement is thus achieved both directly and via secondary effects of phagocytes.

Because of the complex interaction with inflammatory processes, it has been difficult to delineate what complement does in noncardiogenic pulmonary edema. It is not known, for example, whether lung endothelial or epithelial cells possess receptors for activated complement components nor whether activation of the complement cascade occurs in noncardiogenic forms of pulmonary edema. The degree to which activation of complement causes injury to pulmonary endothelium has not been explored. Complement activation has been incriminated in some forms of noncardiac pulmonary edema, such as those associated with endotoxin or circulating immune complexes [92,95]. Recently, complement activation by the equipment used during hemodialysis or cardiopulmonary bypass has been suspected as a contributor to the pulmonary edema seen in some patients receiving this therapy [96,97].

Interventions that influence serum complement activities may represent a potential mechanism for combating undesirable inflammatory processes in the lung. Related fields needing further investigation include the interactions among complement, other blood constituents, endothelial cell membranes, and lung complement receptors, and complement's effect on lung phagocyte activation processes. Such studies may lead to new therapeutic approaches for controlling noncardiogenic pulmonary edema.

VII. Vasoactive Amines

Although the activity of potent vasoactive amines such as histamine, serotonin, kinins, and catecholamines in various pathologic phenomena has been fairly well characterized, the importance of these substances in noncardiogenic forms of pulmonary edema has not been precisely defined. These substances increase permeability of blood vessels by briefly affecting endothelial cell contractile structures [9]. Studies on other regions of the body show that the vasoactive amines are significant in the increased permeability present in immediate hypersensitivity reactions, trauma, burns, and infections.

What histamine does in the immediate hypersensitivity component of the biphasic Arthus reaction is well defined. Local antihistamines can inhibit this early phase [98]. Histamine may even act in increasing permeabilities elicited by the releases of proteases from phagocytes [49], although other pharmacologically active peptides such as kinins may also be activated by proteases and affect inflammatory reactions [99]. Histamine itself can increase pulmonary vascular permeability to protein and liquid [22], but the effects on lung microvascular porosity are more modest than on systemic vessels [100].

Studies on the release of vasoactive amines in noncardiac forms of pulmonary edema deserve further study. For example, their activation or release can be prevented by hormones or drugs capable of changing intracellular cyclic nucleotide levels [54,98,101]. In human lung models, prostaglandin E_2 and β-adrenergic agents inhibit immune-mediated histamine release whereas α-adrenergic agents and cholinergic agents potentiate histamine releases [102]. Histamine H_2-receptor activity itself may modulate histamine release induced by immune reactants from mast cells and also influence certain phagocytes and lymphcyte-mediated cytotoxicity mechanisms [102].

Stimulation of H_1 and H_2 receptors appears to have opposing effects on pulmonary vasculature [103]. Activation of both H_1 and H_2 receptors, along with activation of kinin cascades, may seriously affect many kinds of noncardiogenic pulmonary edema. The therapeutic application of inhibitors of biogenic vasoactive amines and activators of kinins will require a more precise definition of their pathophysiologic activities. Moreover, because histamine itself inhibits antigen-induced release of endogenous histamine [98], vasoactive amines may partly self-regulate the extent of inflammatory processes.

Experimentally, catecholamine infusions can produce a florid pulmonary edema [104]. It remains to be documented whether or not the localized release of catecholamines in or near the pulmonary circulation contributes, at least partly, to the pulmonary edema associated with acute critical illness, such as sepsis, shock from various causes and cerebral injury.

VIII. Prostaglandins

Prostaglandins, and their precursors and related compounds, are believed to be significant potentiators and mediators of the increased vascular permeability seen in inflammatory reactions [105-108]. Their biosynthetic mechanisms are activated by a wide variety of cell injuries, possibly via activations of cellular microsomal and lysosomal phospholipases [108,109]. Activated phospholipases presumably free prostaglandin precursors such as arachidonic acid from membrane phospholipids. Recently, very potent short-lived intermediates such as cyclic endoperoxides and thromboxanes have been described. These prostaglandin precursors may be involved in the increased vascular permeability associated with ischemia, shock, anaphylaxis, cell injury, inflammation, and related phenomena [82,110,111].

It will be difficult to study how these compounds affect noncardiogenic pulmonary edema. Problems in defining their action in modulating capillary permeabilities include (1) their rapid synthesis and degradation; (2) the opposing effects of prostaglandins of the E and the F series in some models of capillary permeability; (3) their complex interrelations with other cell types such as endothelial cells, phagocytes, and platelets; (4) their interactions with intermediary mediators and effectors such as steroids, catecholamines, vasoactive peptides, and cyclic nucleotides; (5) their ubiquitousness; and (6) the lack of specificity of inhibitor compounds that are frequently used to define their relation to inflammation.

The lungs have a very high prostaglandin content and an active enzyme mechanism for the production, transport, and metabolism of prostaglandins and their intermediate compounds [112-118]. Prostaglandins and their precursors may therefore cause increased permeability in the lung. The presence of active phagocytic lysosomal enzyme systems in the lung is a potentially strong stimulus to prostaglandin formation. Also, both the high O_2 tensions available to lung tissue and the numerous phagocytes and platelets that can produce endoperoxides suggest the possible activity of prostaglandin in noncardiogenic forms of pulmonary edema [27,111,113]. Such mild maneuvers as hyperinflation and hyperventilation stimulate lung prostaglandin release [116].

No evaluations of the contribution of prostaglandins to the increased permeability seen clinically in noncardiogenic forms of pulmonary edema have been reported. It is likely, however, that prostaglandins are important in lung injury and inflammation [116]. For example, in experimental models of pulmonary embolism, microembolization, anaphylaxis, and hemorrhagic shock, the lung releases prostaglandins capable of increasing vascular permeability [117-121]. The recent demonstration of active prostaglandin synthesis in cultured endothelial cells [122] further suggests that these compounds may seriously affect endothelial permeability.

The most rewarding investigations will probably include (a) evaluating nonsteroidal anti-inflammatory compounds such as the antisynthetases aspirin, indomethacin, aminopyrine, antipyrine, and quinoline antimalarials [123,124]; (b) studying antiphospholipases and antilipases, which may be expected to decrease availability of the prostaglandin precursor arachidonic acid; and (c) examining antioxidant compounds such as phenolic antioxidants, which may inhibit formation of endoperoxides [125,126].

IX. Immune Complexes

Immune complexes composed of immunoglobin and antigen can propagate inflammatory responses [39,95,127]. Inflammatory processes induced by immune complexes are typified by the phagocyte infiltrations and degranulations that characterize the Arthus reaction, for which selective release of lysosomal enzymes from phagocytes and platelets has been well documented [128].

Many of these immune complexes can directly activate the complement, clotting, and kinin-forming systems, thereby generating mediators that increase vascular permeability and cause tissue injury. Although the pulmonary edema associated with anaphylaxis due to IgE-mediated immediate-hypersensitivity phenomena is fairly well understood, the activity of circulating or intrapulmonary immune complexes in the pathogenesis of noncardiogenic forms of pulmonary edema, including those forms due to severe septic shock and viral infections, is not well defined.

X. Lymphokines and Lymphotoxins

Soluble lymphocyte factors, or lymphokines, affect the activities of phagocytes and may be important in delayed types of inflammatory responses [129–130]. These factors exert influences on surface adherence, cell recruitment, phagocytosis, and lysosomal enzyme synthesis and release. Under some circumstances activated lymphoid cells can themselves mediate cytolysis of host tissues by elaborating a material called lymphotoxin [131]. However, it is currently not known whether lymphokines, lymphotoxin-elaborating lymphocytes, or other products of lymphocyte-mediated immunologic activations act in noncardiogenic forms of pulmonary edema.

XI. Clinical Assessments

Understanding pathogenesis is essential for treating pulmonary edema rationally. Diagnosing pulmonary edema due to left ventricular failure is usually simple and treatment is straightforward, whereas there is no specific treatment for pulmonary edema due to lung injury with increased permeability. Although a few studies indicate that mediators act in the inflammatory response and the various associated proteolytic cascades, no studies indicate that pharmacologic agents can modify the mechanisms responsible for the increased permeability. Treating such cases is complicated because multiple etiologic factors that need complex treatment strategies are often present. In some of these patients, lung biopsy seems indicated [132].

An early diagnosis of pulmonary edema is extremely important. In many instances anticipating the problem and instituting vigorous prophylactic and monitoring measures represent the most efficient strategy in treatment. In other instances differentiating hemodynamic and permeability forms of pulmonary edema may be difficult, or both mechanisms may be involved. Although there are well-accepted methods for assessing pulmonary capillary hemodynamics, there is no reliable clinical test for detecting abnormal pulmonary capillary permeability.

A. Assessing Lung Water Content

Pulmonary edema is generally assessed clinically through physical and laboratory findings, including rapid and shallow respirations, auscultation of the chest, roentgenographic findings of pulmonary venous and later pulmonary lymphatic congestion with varying degrees of interstitial edema, and pulmonary function tests. Abnormalities are more easily detectable when extravascular liquid accumulation has progressed to the point that liquid begins to leak into alveolar spaces, setting the stage for rapid alveolar filling. In the earlier phases, the pulmonary edema is confined to the loose interstitial space and peribronchial and pervascular tissues, and is not easily identified clinically. At this point one may have few clinical signs. The four classical clinical manifestations of pulmonary edema to be seen sequentially include (1) dyspnea, tachypnea, decreased lung compliance, and decreased arterial O_2 tensions; (2) increased opacification through roentgenographic stages until lung "whiteout" is observable; (3) rales; and (4) frothy sputum.

In the past few years, techniques have been developed for more accurate measurement of lung liquid [1,133,134]. Techniques include delivery of indicator via airways or blood, measurements of transthoracic electrical impedance, video-densitometric techniques, sequential measurements of regional redistribution of pulmonary blood flow, and measurement of peripheral airway resistance. If these techniques were developed into practical clinical tools, early diagnosis of pulmonary edema would be helped; treatment could then be started promptly and causative factors removed.

B. Recognition of Hemodynamic Factors

When the flow-directed Swan-Ganz catheter was introduced in 1970 [135], sequential measurement of pulmonary artery pressure became practical. When the balloon is inflated, pulmonary wedge pressure can be determined. Under most circumstances, wedge pressure is a reasonable approximation of left atrial pressure and left ventricular filling pressures. The catheter is easily introduced from a peripheral vein into the pulmonary artery under fluoroscopic control or by pressure monitoring alone [136]. Placing a thermistor at the catheter tip permits repetitive measurement of cardiac output by the thermodilution technique. Also, measuring O_2 tensions in mixed venous blood samples drawn through the catheter provides an indirect monitoring of overall tissue oxygenation. Complications from the Swan-Ganz catheter are not common but do exist; they are arrhythmias, pulmonary infarction, pulmonary artery rupture, and catheter knotting and infections [137].

Indications for hemodynamic monitoring with the catheter are still being clarified but the procedure has proved helpful in several circumstances. First, the most important use of the catheter is to confirm the diagnosis of cardiogenic pulmonary edema in cases in which the clinical findings are not diagnostic. Although the presence of a normal wedge pressure does not completely exclude the possibility that a previously elevated wedge pressure initiated the pulmonary edema, it strongly suggests that the edema is noncardiogenic. Second, patients who have mild left ventricular failure without frank pulmonary edema have a high risk of developing progressive refractory pulmonary edema from diseases such as acute myocardial infarction with hypotension. Pulmonary wedge pressure monitoring makes it feasible to administer fluid to produce the reported optimal left ventricular filling pressures of 16 to 18 mmHg, while minimizing the danger of pulmonary edema from overinfusion [138].

Hemodynamic monitoring is also an important aid in managing patients with permeability edema. For example, the patient with a permeability abnormality will have greater capillary filtration than the patient with normal permeability at any comparable pulmonary capillary pressure (Fig. 3). With the Swan-Ganz catheter, fluid and diuretic therapy can be adjusted to maintain a minimal wedge pressure while avoiding low cardiac output, hypotension, and renal failure.

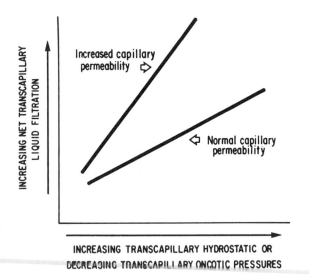

FIGURE 3   Hypothetical relation between increasing *net* transcapillary pulmonary liquid filtration and increasing Starling forces (increasing transcapillary hydrostatic pressures or decreasing oncotic pressures) using two different theoretical values for capillary permeability.

TABLE 1   Methods for Assessing Pulmonary Capillary Permeability

1. Analysis of pulmonary edema fluid
2. Single-pass indicator dilution with "marker" molecular species
3. Analysis of pulmonary lymphatic flow
4. Analysis of pulmonary lymphatic protein concentration
5. Radioisotope injection techniques
6. Lung tracer isotope equilibration

Some cases of pulmonary edema associated with shock may have been initiated by the rapid administration of fluids during resuscitation. In addition, some forms of noncardiogenic pulmonary edema such as those precipitated by hemorrhagic shock, pancreatitis, or endotoxemia may be accompanied by significant myocardial depression. Patients may also have coexisting subclinical congestive heart failure. Since pulmonary edema can result from minimal fluid overload in such patients, ventricular filling pressure should be monitored. Such monitoring has the additional advantage of detecting sudden and transient depressions of left ventricular function, a not unusual occurrence in seriously ill patients.

Concomitant measurements of both colloid osmotic pressure and wedge pressure may provide a more reliable basis for guiding infusion therapy in patients with risks of developing pulmonary edema than determinations of wedge pressure alone [139].

C. Monitoring Permeability Factors

Table 1 lists some of the methods that have been used in assessing pulmonary capillary permeability in experimental models. The various experimental techniques have been recently reviewed [1]. A big challenge lies in developing practical and reliable techniques for measuring abnormal permeability in clinical settings. Such determinations would allow prompt treatment for these disorders and thereby avoid in some instances the development of more extensive lung injury and accompanying pulmonary edema.

XII.   Life Support Measures

Since hypoxemia is the most life-threatening consequence of pulmonary edema, initial therapy in any form of pulmonary edema should be directed towards improving tissue O_2 delivery. This is achieved by increasing the transfer of O_2 into the pulmonary capillaries, by optimizing cardiac output, and by maintaining an adequate blood O_2-carrying capacity and a satisfactory hemoglobin O_2 affinity.

A. Oxygenation

The goal of each sequential therapeutic oxygenation maneuver is undertaken to optimize tissue O_2 delivery. Oxygenation is most easily improved by increasing the O_2 in inspired gas. Oxygen should initially be given at high flow rates (up to 12 liters/min) by face mask or nasal catheter, with arterial blood gas measurements to monitor its effectiveness. If administration of 100% O_2 by a rebreathing mask does not achieve an arterial O_2 tension greater than 50 mmHg, tracheal intubation and intermittent positive pressure ventilation (IPPV) is indicated.

Patients with severe pulmonary edema may fail to maintain arterial O_2 tensions above 50 mmHg even when intubated and mechanically ventilated with high oxygen concentrations. In these patients more aggressive forms of oxygenation are indicated.

B. Continuous Positive Pressure Ventilation (CPPV)

In severe pulmonary edema, increased inspired O_2 tensions may fail to maintain arterial O_2 tensions at acceptable levels (approximately 50 mmHg or greater). The application of CPPV has gained widespread recognition as an effective therapy for increasing arterial O_2 tensions above this critical level [140–142]. Although it has frequently been used in infants with pulmonary edema secondary to the infant respiratory distress syndrome and lately in patients with cardiogenic pulmonary edema [143], in adults it generally requires intubation and mechanical ventilation for effectiveness. Its use often allows inspired O_2 tensions to be reduced, sparing the lung from potential damage caused by O_2 toxicity.

The ability of CPPV to increase arterial O_2 tension is apparently due to the increase in lung volume rather than to the increased alveolar pressure that it produces. The increased lung volume is believed to have the following effects: (1) a more uniform ratio of ventilation to perfusion throughout the lung, (2) a decreased thickness of the alveolar blood diffusion barrier; (3) ventilation of damaged alveoli that would collapse without the positive distending pressure (in effect, CPPV reduces the size of the right to left shunt through collapsed alveoli); (4) a decreased pulmonary capillary blood volume; and (5) an increased pulmonary interstitial liquid hydrostatic pressure. The two last-mentioned mechanisms could reduce the Starling transcapillary hydrostatic pressure gradient and the capillary surface area available for liquid exchange, thus decreasing net transcapillary liquid transfer from capillaries into lung interstitium. Since CPPV appears to decrease lung lymph flow [1,144], it neither reduces the amount of lung edema present nor facilitates its removal. High levels of CPPV (above 25 cm H_2O) may even favor liquid accumulation in lung extravascular spaces [145].

Institution of CPPV in patients with pulmonary edema usually raises arterial blood O_2 tensions [137-141]. Patients with the greatest degree of hypoxemia and the largest loss of lung volume appear to receive the most benefit [142,146]. There is not necessarily a concomitant increase, however, in O_2 transport to the tissues because applying CPPV may cause a fall in cardiac output, especially in patients with hypovolemia or normal lung compliance, or when very high levels of CPPV are used [146]. Its use in critically ill patients therefore requires careful monitoring of cardiac output or mixed venous blood by direct or indirect methods.

Continuous positive pressure ventilation is frequently effective in opening collapsed lung units, preventing closure of unstable alveoli, and increasing both lung compliance and arterial oxygenation without seriously compromising venous return or cardiac output. Tissue O_2 delivery is therefore increased. With greater increases in transpulmonary pressures (end-expiratory pressures of 15 to 60 cm H_2O), alveolar overdistension will eventually predominate, with a resultant decrease in lung compliance, venous return, and cardiac output [147]. If this fall in cardiac output is sufficiently severe, there may be an overall decrease in O_2 transport to the tissues despite an increased oxygenation of arterial blood. Therefore, CPPV in patients with reduced cardiac outputs is potentially dangerous, especially if lung compliance is not markedly reduced or if any degree of hypovolemia is present [146]. Volume replacement, however, may permit using CPPV in patients who previously could not tolerate it due to the development of hypotension.

Numerous techniques are recommended for identifying the CPPV providing optimal tissue O_2 delivery (see Table 3). The optimal level depends on a complex interrelation of airway resistance, transpulmonary and intrathoracic pressures, lung compliance, venous return, myocardial contractility and afterload, and O_2 saturation. Probably most important is the level of CPPV above which cardiac output may drop significantly, thus negating any value of the increased arterial O_2 tension.

In most hospitals it is not feasible to base ventilation adjustments on an assessment of all or most of the items listed in Table 3. In this circumstance, monitoring total thoracic compliance, arterial P_{O_2}, intrapulmonary shunt, and mixed venous O_2 tensions has indicated the most practical physiologic variables to follow [147,148]. In cases in which pulmonary capillary wedge pressures are being monitored, a correlation between increased wedge pressures and decreased cardiac outputs following institution of CPPV has been noted [149]. Particularly striking is the increase in wedge pressures observed at the level of CPPV where big falls in cardiac output occur [146]. Under these conditions, the wedged catheter is probably sensing alveolar pressure rather than left atrial pressure and is no longer a reliable indication of left atrial or left ventricular end-diastolic pressures [149].

Mixed venous O_2 tension or saturation may provide the most practical indicator of overall tissue oxygenation. Monitoring arterial blood gases, cardiac output, and lung-inflating pressures allows identifying patients with pulmonary edema unresponsive to conventional levels of CPPV (5 to 15 cm H_2O). In such refractory cases, CPPV levels over 40 cm H_2O have been claimed to improve oxygenation [148]. In this circumstance spontaneous voluntary inspiratory activity, called intermittent mandatory ventilation, may partially prevent the marked reduction in venous return and cardiac output that these extraordinarily high mean intrathoracic pressures may cause [150]. The use of intermittent spontaneous inspiratory efforts provides a brief reduction in mean intrathoracic pressures, and therefore cardiac output can be augmented at any level of CPPV.

Other adverse effects from CPPV include the complications from endotracheal tubes, pneumothorax, possibly diffuse lung damage due to overdistension, and also depression of cardiac output. In the presence of hypovolemia or hypotension or both, CPPV tends to cause a more marked fall in cardiac output. Purposefully induced hypervolemia, however, can offset the adverse effects of CPPV on cardiac output, even at CPPV levels of 25 cm H_2O or higher [150,151]. When blood volume is augmented to overcome the hemodynamic deterioration caused by CPPV, care must be exercised when CPPV is discontinued because the sudden increase in filling pressures may produce hypervolemic pulmonary edema.

Two innovative approaches that theoretically avoid some of the undesirable features of intubation CPPV are controlled or spontaneous ventilation while negative pressure is applied to the chest wall [152] and introduction of spontaneous breathing with increased end-expiratory pressure simply with a tightly fitted plastic mask [153]. These techniques provide an effective way of increasing lung volume and improving arterial oxygenation without significant decreases in venous return and without endotracheal intubation. These techniques show promise in becoming a helpful adjunct to ventilatory support in selected cases in which CPPV is not required or in cases in which CPPV causes unacceptable decreases in cardiac output.

C. Membrane Oxygenation

When CPPV techniques have failed to maintain tissue oxygenation, selected patients have survived for 1 to 2 weeks with the use of extracorporeal circulation and oxygenators that maintain separation of blood and O_2 with silicon rubber membranes [154-156]. Experience to date suggests that these extracorporeal membrane oxygenators (ECMO) can delay death from hypoxemia [157]. There has only been limited clinical and experimental experience with this therapy for progressive hypoxemia due to noncardiac pulmonary edema refractory to other forms of therapy. Recently investigators have performed pulmonary lavage while maintaining cardiopulmonary function with ECMO in order to clear the lung of undesirable materials [158]. This therapy may develop into a technique that could shorten the ECMO treatment or permit introducing therapeutic agents into the lungs. Therapeutic indications for treatment with ECMO are not now clearly established.

D. Fluid, Colloid, and Diuretic Therapy

Pulmonary edema in normal healthy subjects from intravenous infusions means that massive rapid administration precipitated it [159,160]. In patients with increased pulmonary capillary permeabilities, even minimal degrees of overinfusion may precipitate fulminating pulmonary edema.

Early rapid volume replacement to achieve hemodynamic stability is clearly indicated in hypovolemic, hemorrhagic, or traumatic shock because the incidence of pulmonary complications appears related to the duration of the hypoperfusion [161]. Most experts recommend that intravascular oncotic pressures be maintained by administering blood, plasma, salt-poor albumin, or artificial macromolecular colloids to avoid pulmonary edema secondary to decreases in plasma oncotic pressures [162,163]. Such resuscitative therapy, however, can precipitate "hypervolemic" pulmonary edema.

In the presence of increased pulmonary capillary permeability, as it typically occurs in late stages of traumatic and septic shock, the combination of moderately increased hydrostatic pressures, hypervolemia, and reduced plasma oncotic pressure may initiate pulmonary edema. It has been suggested, with some experimental validation, that peripheral vasoconstriction caused either by stress-induced adrenergic activity or by infusion of vasoconstrictor drugs contributes to the development of pulmonary edema by causing hypervolemia in the pulmonary circulation [164,165]. In critically ill patients, poor correlation exists between blood volume, hematocrit, central venous pressures, and wedge pressure determinations [166]. Estimating left ventricular filling pressures with the wedged pulmonary artery catheter during fluid administration should theoretically permit early detection of ventricular overload and avoidance of this form of pulmonary edema.

Studies of the effectiveness of osmotic agents for removing liquid from edematous lungs have not been encouraging [167]. The difficulty in promoting reabsorption of pulmonary edema liquid results from rapid equilibration of the administered osmotic agents, such as albumin, urea, mannitol, or dextran, between the lung extravascular and vascular compartments. This equilibration will unfortunately take place even more rapidly in patients with increased capillary permeability, negating the therapeutic value of the infused colloid. Mannitol and dextran have the added liability of precipitating allergic reactions and interfering with clotting phenomena. Therapeutic successes have been reported from combining osmotic agents and diuretics, hemodialysis, and ultrafiltration, but the clinical value of extracting pulmonary edema liquid by

TABLE 2   General Measures Available for Treating Pulmonary Edema

I.   Supportive measures useful in most forms of pulmonary edema
      A.   Supportive measures to improve respiratory gas exchange
            1.   Oxygen enrichment of inspired air
            2.   Aminophylline
            3.   Nasotracheal suction
            4.   Mechanical ventilation (IPPB or CPPB)
            5.   Membrane oxygenators
      B.   Measures to counteract Starling forces
            1.   Combat hypervolemia – diuretics
            2.   Treat "subclinical" heart failure
            3.   Correct decreased plasma oncotic pressure
      C.   Measures to improve acid-base derangements

II.   General measures directed primarily against hemodynamic factors
      A.   Enhancement of myocardial contractility
            1.   Cardiac glycosides
            2.   β-Adrenergic stimulation
            3.   Aminophylline
            4.   Oxygen
      B.   Reduction of left ventricular "preload" and "afterload"

III. General measures directed against permeability factors
      A.   Hypovolemia
      B.   Empirical use of anti-inflammatory drugs, viz. steroids
      C.   Increase plasma oncotic pressure

TABLE 3   Modalities for Assessing Optimal
CPPV Therapy

1.   Alveolar-arterial O_2 gradient
2.   Arterial O_2 tension and O_2 content
3.   Cardiac output
4.   Mixed venous O_2 tension or O_2 content or both
5.   Venous admixture (intrapulmonary shunt)
6.   Function residual capacity
7.   Alveolar dead space
8.   Thoracic pressure/volume relations
9.   Pulmonary capillary wedge pressure

these means has not been extensively studied [168–170]. The potential of hyperosmotic agents for restoring normal cell functions by reducing intracellular endothelial swelling has received little attention. Mannitol has an additional free-radical scavenger activity that may have therapeutic benefit [64].

When overexpansion of the intravascular volume has contributed to the development of noncardiac pulmonary edema, diuretics are accepted as effective therapeutic agents [162]. Reduced plasma osmotic pressures during the initial volume loading may contribute to this fluid overload syndrome. In these patients, diuretic administration has the dual effect of reducing the hypervolemia and increasing osmotic pressures [162].

Patients on ventilators frequently go into positive water balance because the humidified gas supplied by the ventilator markedly diminishes the insensible water loss and because starvation in these severely ill patients leads to conversion of fat stores into water. Diuretic administration frequently produces a significant improvement in lung function by diminishing intrathoracic blood volume or intrapulmonary liquid retention or both in these patients [162,169].

XIII.   Measures Directed Primarily Against Hemodynamic Factors

In managing hemodynamic forms of pulmonary edema, the aim of therapeutic intervention is to reduce the increased transmural pulmonary capillary hydrostatic pressure. As outlined in Table 2, this is achieved by reducing the left atrial transmural pressure. More extensive discussions of treatments of cardiogenic pulmonary edema are available elsewhere [3,171].

A.   Enhancement of Myocardial Contractility

Cardiac glycosides increase myocardial contractility, increasing stroke volume at a lower left atrial pressure, and thereby reduce pulmonary capillary pressure. When the digitalis glycosides are used, the enhanced myocardial contractility takes hours to appear, depending on the form and route of administration. Because of this delay, the initial treatment of severe pulmonary edema should also include measures to decrease central blood volume, venous return, and afterload. The gradual onset of digitalis action can help prevent recurrence of pulmonary edema. Beta-adrenergic receptor stimulation by isoproterenol and dopamine rapidly produce increased contractility. However, the usefulness of these drugs is limited by the tachycardia and ventricular arrhythmias they produce. Because isoproterenol also increases myocardial oxygen consumption and reduces coronary blood flow, it is considered less helpful than dopamine or low doses of norepinephrine in acute myocardial infarction complicated by pulmonary edema and hypotension.

Aminophylline increases myocardial contractility and potentiates endogenous and exogenous beta-receptor stimulation by hormones and drugs. It has the additional beneficial effect of dilating airways and improving gas exchange. However, in the presence of significant hypoxia-induced pulmonary vasoconstriction, it may decrease arterial O_2 tensions by increasing regional blood flow through areas of the lung that are hypoventilated. Fortunately this hypoxia is usually readily reversed by modest increases in inspired O_2 tension.

Newer inotropic agents, such as synthetic sympathomimetics, have selective myocardial inotropic beta-receptor stimulating activity with little peripheral or chronotropic effects [172,173]. Their therapeutic value remains to be determined.

B.   Measures Designed to Reduce
Left Ventricular "Preload" and "Afterload"

In left ventricular failure, the cardiac work does not have a strong dependency on filling pressure (end-diastolic fiber length), i.e., the left ventricular function curve is flat. Small reductions in filling pressure (venous return) will produce a relatively large drop in left atrial transmural pressure without significantly compromising cardiac work. This can be readily accomplished by having the patient with pulmonary edema sit with the head elevated and legs dependent, thus pooling blood in peripheral capacitance vessels. When rotating tourniquets are used for this purpose cuff pressure should be just below arterial diastolic pressure, thereby facilitating fluid loss into the peripheral extravascular spaces.

Intermittent positive pressure breathing has also been advocated as a means of reducing venous return.

Morphine is administered to many patients with acute cardiogenic pulmonary edema. It should be given intravenously in small, titrated, intermittent doses. Its mechanism of action is not entirely understood. It produces a reduction in arterial resistance and an increase in venous capacitance, presumably through "central sympatholysis" [174]. Its circulatory action is therefore dual, reducing both the preload and the afterload.

When acute pulmonary edema is superimposed on chronic left heart failure, hypervolemia frequently coexists. The potent, rapidly acting diuretics furosemide and ethacrynic acid have traditionally been given in acute pulmonary edema to reduce total blood volume and thus to help prevent the recurrence of pulmonary congestion. It has recently been shown that furosemide has an immediate peripheral vascular effect similar to that of morphine and unrelated to its diuretic properties [175]. Thus, these drugs may share one common mechanism of action. Agents that produce venous pooling or hypovolemia may also unload the heart excessively, producing an undesirable reaction in cardiac output, causing prerenal axotemia, mental confusion, and other undesirable effects. By monitoring the mixed venous oxygen saturation, one can estimate whether the reduction in cardiac output has dangerously decreased tissue oxygenation.

Afterload reduction with the use of phentolamine or nitroprusside is a recent trend in treating myocardial infarction complicated by elevated left ventricular filling pressures [176]. Afterload reduction can sustain cardiac output with a reduced preload and thereby reduce pulmonary capillary pressure. This reduction in capillary pressure should theoretically be useful in treating both the cardiogenic and noncardiogenic forms of pulmonary edema. Nitroglycerin, which reduces arterial resistance and increases systemic vascular capacity, has also been advocated in the treatment of pulmonary edema from acute myocardial infarction [177]. Nitroprusside may prove to be more useful than sublingual nitroglycerin because the afterload reduction can be more precisely controlled, with consequent optimum balance between preload reduction and blood pressure reduction [178].

C. Special Forms of Hemodynamic Edema

Hemodynamic pulmonary edema from isolated aortic stenosis, acute hypertension, and pure mitral stenosis requires specialized treatment and is discussed elsewhere [171]. Hemodynamic pulmonary edema can also result from pulmonary venous hypertension secondary to left atrial myxoma, congenital absence of pulmonary veins, mediastinal fibrosis, and pulmonary veno-occlusive disease. In severe forms of pulmonary arterial hypertension, forward transmission of arterial pressure to capillaries may possibly result in pulmonary capillary hypertension and pulmonary edema [2].

Obstruction limited to large pulmonary veins can conceivably be treated surgically. Glucocorticoids may be useful in some cases of mediastinal fibrosis. In patients with obvious clotting abnormalities, anticoagulant administration has been recommended [179]. If pulmonary capillary hypertension is thought to result from functional constriction of pulmonary venules, such as release of serotonin or histamine might occasion, treatment should be directed towards the underlying disease. For example, heparin would presumably diminish serotonin release in pulmonary embolic disease.

In normal subjects the pulmonary wedge pressure provides an accurate index to pressures in the large pulmonary veins and left atrium. With pulmonary venous disease, however, the wedge pressure does not necessarily reflect pressures in either pulmonary veins or capillaries and may give misleading information [179].

In some cases of severe pulmonary arterial hypertension of relatively rapid onset, one can speculate that the normal structural or autoregulatory arteriolar resistance breaks down, resulting in dilatation of the precapillary arterioles. Then high pressures are transmitted to the pulmonary capillaries. Such mechanisms may be a factor in the pulmonary edema resulting from brain damage or high altitude or from acute pulmonary embolism. Treatment should theoretically be directed at lowering the elevated pulmonary artery pressures.

In certain patients, coexisting permeability disorders may cause pulmonary edema to develop at lower pulmonary capillary pressures than hemodynamic considerations alone would indicate. Diseases in this category may include uremia, disorders with reduced serum oncotic pressure such as cirrhosis and nephrosis, and pulmonary lymphatic obstruction such as seen in silicosis or pulmonary lymphangitic carcinomatosis. These patients should show a response to a "cardiogenic" regimen even though the etiology of the pulmonary edema is not purely cardiogenic.

Excessive fluid administration or severe congestive failure may so markedly increase intrapulmonary blood volumes that the capillaries become overdistended; leakage into the interstitium is thereby caused. This mechanism may account for pulmonary edema following brain damage. Treatment in such cases is directed towards decreasing total blood volume and redistributing central blood volume to the periphery.

XIV. Adult Respiratory Distress Syndrome

The adult respiratory distress syndrome embraces a diverse group of disorders that are probably noncardiogenic forms of pulmonary edema stemming from abnormalities of vascular permeability brought about by many different mechanisms [2]. Similarities in clinical presentation, pathophysiologic findings and treatment are striking even though the initiating pathophysiologic processes are multiple. While it now seems likely that lung phagocyte and platelet sequestration and degranulation contribute to the increased capillary permeability that characterize the clinical presentation, other mechanisms are undoubtedly significant.

Table 4 lists some of the conditions causing this syndrome. It is clear that a wide variety of different etiological factors can result in alveolotoxic forms of cell injury and accompanying pulmonary edema. Since this disorder has been extensively discussed elsewhere [161,180–183], we shall focus only on certain forms that have the potential for unique types of treatment.

A. Influenza

Inflammatory pulmonary edema associated with influenzal viral pneumonia appears to be related to direct bronchial and alveolar epithelial injury produced by the virus under suitable circumstances [184], leading to intense

TABLE 4   Causes of the Adult Respiratory Distress Syndrome

Overinfusion	Drug overdose (especially opiates)
Shock or trauma	Paraquat
Viral infection	Radiation
Microembolism (including fat embolism)	Systemic lupus erythematosis
Oxidant gases	Leukoagglutins
Aspiration and near drowning	Uremia
Sepsis endotoxemia, other toxic products from bacterial infections	Burn lung
Intravascular coagulation	Prolonged cardiopulmonary bypass
Cerebral injury	Pancreatitis
Toxemia of pregnancy	Pulmonary oxygen toxicity

intracellular and extracellular edema throughout the lung parenchyma with swelling of capillary endothelial cells and disruption of capillary integrity [185]. This disorder is often found in patients with prior abnormalities of the pulmonary circulation, most notably preexisting heart and lung disease. Potential strategies for handling involve prevention with immunization, development of methods for more rapid recognization, use of newer antiviral agents such as interferon, amantadine, and similar drugs, and further delineation of how inflammatory mediators like the platelets [186] modify the clinical severity of the infection. Steroids have been advocated for the most severe form of this disorder [187,188]. As with other forms of increased intra-alveolar lung liquid, secondary bacterial infection is a frequent accompanying factor contributing to the morbidity.

B.   Hemorrhagic Shock

Resuscitation from hypotensive, hemorrhagic shock may be followed by respiratory insufficiency from acute pulmonary edema [189]. Electron-microscopic studies show destructive lesions of the pulmonary endothelial ultrastructure [190]. Suspected initiating factors include prolonged stasis of blood in peripheral and splanchnic circulations, release of toxic humoral or enzymatic substances from the splanchnic bed [191-193], intravascular cellular aggregation from platelets and leukocytes [190], severe acidosis, vasoconstriction, and microembolism [194]. Current treatment stresses the early reestablishment of an effective circulating blood volume with normalization of microcirculatory flow and avoidance of prolonged splanchnic ischemia and correction of the severe acidosis. Unfortunately, aggressive fluid replacement can lead to overperfusion and significant decreases in plasma oncotic pressures. These factors may initiate or accelerate the development of pulmonary edema in these patients with increased pulmonary vascular permeability [195]. Although a comprehensive controlled study of the relative usefulness of steroids and heparin in this condition is not available, steroids are frequently used empirically [177].

Other therapeutic modalities have been advocated to prevent intravascular cellular aggregation and the accompanying increased blood viscosity such as administration of dextran 40 to prevent cellular microaggregates [183,184,196] and protection of the pulmonary microvasculature by filtering all transfused blood through fine screens [180].

C.   Gram-Negative Sepsis

Pulmonary edema frequently accompanies gram-negative sepsis. Studies in sheep infused with *Pseudomonas* bacteria clearly show that alterations in the permeability of lung capillaries initiate the sequence leading to pulmonary edema [1]. Bronchial venular leakage also occurs in endotoxin shock [5]. Endotoxin may directly injure endothelial cells [197] or induce phagocyte sequestration, degranulation, and fragmentation [27,78] with release of lysosomal proteases, activating kinin, complement, and clotting cascades and thereby causing further damage to pulmonary endothelium. As endotoxin can induce pulmonary capillary damage in animals that are severely leukopenic from radiation, gram-negative sepsis may produce pulmonary edema via mechanisms independent of phagocytes [198]. Gram-negative bacteremia also causes platelet aggregation with release of vasoactive amines (such as serotonin), which are capable of causing pulmonary edema. Release of the phospholipid procoagulant platelet factor 3 from the membrane of degraded platelets may further activate both coagulation and fibrinolysis [199,200]. Phagocyte activations appear to be important in triggering the frequently associated intravascular coagulation seen in endotoxemia [201].

Endotoxin activations of complement generate chemotactic factors that could contribute to the lung granulocyte sequestrations. Since septic shock is accompanied by the liberation of many potent humoral agents such as catecholamines, histamine, kinins, and prostaglandins, it is difficult to ascribe the increase in capillary permeability to any one mediator system.

Future development of more specific therapeutic maneuvers will include further evaluations of the activity of both steroidal and nonsteroidal antiinflammatory agents, evaluation of blocking agents effective against a variety of mediators of inflammation, and possible use of specific antitoxins [202,203].

D.   Fat Embolism

The fat embolism syndrome, in which hemorrhagic pulmonary edema is a prominant feature, is a rare but definite clinical entity commonly recognized in patients one to four days after extensive long-bone fractures. It also occurs in patients with sickle-cell crisis, extensive burns, or diabetic acidosis, and also follows cardiopulmonary bypass and renal transplantation [204]. Both mechanical and chemical agents seem to be involved. In experimental animals, intravenous administration of oleic acid or arachidonic acid produces a diffuse toxic vasculitis and a hemorrhagic pulmonary edema that closely resembles the syndrome in humans [2]. Infusions of neutral fat or of homogenized homologous or autologous fat produce a milder form of pulmonary edema [205]. The delay in onset of symptoms may result from the time required for the conversion of neutral fats by the action of lipoprotein lipase to the more toxic fatty acids. The mainstay of therapy of human subjects includes all the usual measures for treating the adult respiratory distress syndrome. Investigators have also advocated therapy with heparin, intravenous alcohol, and adrenal corticosteroids, but the efficacy of these therapeutic agents is not well established [206–208].

E.   Neurogenic Pulmonary Edema

Acute pulmonary edema may develop after injuries to the central nervous system [209,210]. Brain injury by hemorrhage, infection, neoplasm, or compression and trauma can experimentally or clinically lead to this syndrome. Many investigators believe that the initiating event is a massive hypothalamus-mediated central sympathetic discharge from the acutely injured brain [210,211] that causes a reduced left ventricular compliance and a generalized peripheral vasoconstriction; the result is transient left atrial hypertension and a shift in blood from the systemic to the pulmonary circulation. This shift of blood may contribute to the pulmonary edema by causing pulmonary hypervolemia, pulmonary capillary hypertension, pulmonary capillary rupture, and finally pulmonary edema and hemorrhage [164]. Pulmonary venous constriction may have some effect [212]. This form of pulmonary edema thus appears to have components of both increased capillary hydrostatic pressure and increased permeability [210]. A variety of sympatholytic and general anesthetic agents protect against the development of experimental neurogenic pulmonary edema [213,214]. These findings support the hypothesis that the pulmonary edema is due to sympathetic overactivation produced by hypothalamic discharge. Elevations of cerebrospinal fluid pressures may be responsible in some forms of this syndrome [214].

The pulmonary edema following experimental hypoglycemia is also prevented by adrenergic blockage [215], suggesting that similar mechanisms are responsible for this form of pulmonary edema. Neurogenic pulmonary edema also closely resembles the pulmonary edema observed after bilateral cervical vagotomy, after massive injections of epinephrine into the pulmonary circulation, and after overdoses of opiates [104,209,210].

Intense cerebral hypoxia in animals can induce acute pulmonary edema that is prevented by prior denervation of the lung [216]. These provocative experiments suggest that severe cerebral hypoxemia also triggers a massive sympathetic discharge that results in a neurogenic type of pulmonary edema. If this is so, severe cerebral hypoxemia may also contribute to the pulmonary edema seen following opiate overdoses [210].

These exotic forms of pulmonary edema usually respond to the therapy used for cardiogenic pulmonary edema. Occasional patients have a protracted course and therapeutic maneuvers to manage the adult respiratory distress syndrome are needed. If indeed these disease entities are due to transient left ventricular failure following sympathetic overactivity, careful monitoring of pulmonary vascular pressures in patients at risk should permit prompt detection of the onset of the disease process and administration of preventive therapy with α-adrenergic blocking agents.

F. Pancreatitis

Pulmonary edema and respiratory failure may occur in patients with acute pancreatitis [217–219]. The mechanism may be related to coexistent fluid overload, excessive crystalloids, left ventricular failure, impaired respiratory excursions, hemorrhagic shock, or sepsis. Acute pancreatitis leads to the release of pancreatic phospholipases and proteolytic enzymes into the circulation. These substances may damage the pulmonary capillary endothelium or deactivate pulmonary surfactant and cause pulmonary edema due to altered pulmonary permeability. As both hemodynamic and permeability factors may be involved in the genesis of this disorder [220], carefully monitored replacements of blood, plasma, and crystalloid solution in conjunction with the traditional therapy for pancreatitis are indicated. In some cases CPPV and diuretics are required. Some investigators have advocated corticosteroids [218]. Newer experimental treatments include the use of peritoneal dialysis and the administration of proteolytic enzyme inhibitors such as antitrypsin and the bovine protease inhibitor Trasylol [221]. Perfection of methods to administer pulmonary surfactant by inhalation would presumably be effective therapy if indeed the circulating phospholipases deactivate pulmonary surfactant [222,223].

XV. Treatments Directed Towards Cellular Damage Mechanisms

Many useful therapeutic interventions designed to save jeopardized lung cellular functions are potentially available. As damage to cell membranes may represent a central theme of irreversible injury, the efficacy of interventions is likely to be related to the degree of primary membrane injury, the persistence of secondary amplification mechanisms, and temporal constraints. For example, such nonspecific measures as treatment with agents to reduce cell swelling and inflammation appear to decrease injury in some models of myocardial damage [224] and may apply to treatments of injured lung cells. Before such treatments have clinical application based on scientific principles, however, much more information than what is currently available is needed about lung cellular metabolisms, the mechanisms of cytotoxic damage in noncardiogenic pulmonary edema, and the factors that determine the irreversibility of cellular repair processes in the lung.

A. Steroids

Adrenal glucocorticoids in high doses are used in the management of many
diseases, with the goal of suppressing inflammation or modifying undesirable
immunologic processes [225,226]. High pharmacologic doses have been used
for noncardiogenic forms of pulmonary edema from acute aspiration
pneumonia (peptic pneumonitis), smoke inhalation, near drowning, hydrocar-
bon aspiration, severe viral pneumonia, endotoxemia, hemorrhagic shock, and
radiation pneumonitis [187,188,206,227–233]. Controlled clinical trials to
evaluate the benefit of glucocorticoids in these diseases are meager. Results in
animal studies are controversial. For example, recent studies on experimental
animals with pneumonia from hydrochloric acid aspiration or freshwater near-
drowning, and treated with continuous positive pressure ventilation and oxygen, have failed to indicate that steroid administration altered the clinical
course [234,235]. Other investigators claim, however, that glucocorticoids
can modify aspiration pneumonia caused by tracheal installation of hydrochloric acid [236].

The effects of steroid administration on the course of noncardiac forms
of pulmonary edema may depend on the specific time at which steroid therapy is initiated and on the dose. In most of the uncontrolled clinical studies,
patients received large doses of glucocorticoids, such as 60 to 100 mg dexa-
methasone or 1 to 2 g methylprednisone per day, in the early stages of the
disease [229]. There exists surprisingly little understanding of how these
compounds might modify noncardiac pulmonary edema and lung inflammation. Anti-inflammatory effects at supraphysiologic doses cannot be explained
by interaction with cytoplasmic and nuclear steroid receptors [237]. Their
anti-inflammatory potencies may be related to their abilities to permeate hydrophobic regions of cell membranes [238]. They also appear to counteract
the increase in capillary permeability produced by compounds such as histamine and kinins [239]. In addition, corticosteroids appear to interfere with
margination and migration of phagocytes into inflamed areas [53]. This
activity would inhibit adherence of phagocytes to endothelium and subsequent
diapedesis through capillary walls [53,239,240], decreasing the recruitment of
potentially damaging phagocytes into the lung.

Glucocorticoids also interfere with phagocytosis and presumably with
phagocytosis-associated exocytosis of proteolytic lysosomal enzymes. In some
systems, high doses interact with lipid moieties of biomembranes. Steroids
thus seem capable of influencing the abilities of lysosomal enzymes to provoke
tissue injury by modifying intra- and extracellular lysosomal release of hydrolytic enzymes [240,241]. There is suggestive evidence that steroids may
modify myocardial damage in experimental myocardial infarction by this

mechanism [242]. However, the high concentrations of glucocorticosteroids required to demonstrate lysosomal membrane "stabilization" in most inflammatory models are unachievable clinically, and the balance of evidence indicates that phagocyte lysosomes are not "stabilized" by clinical doses of steroids [41,243,244]. Massive doses cause many perturbations in metabolic activities of phagocytes, including inhibition of guanylate cyclase activity and calcium influx [245]. It has lately been shown that concentrations of hydrocortisone in the range 10^{-9} to 10^{-10} M inhibit release in vitro of arachidonic acid from cellular lipids, thus inhibiting endogenous prostaglandin production [246]. It seems probable that their anti-inflammatory effects are best explained by the combined influence on phagocyte kinetics and cellular metabolism, like modulating cyclic nucleotide levels, rather than by direct interaction with lysosomal membranes.

Other potentially important actions of glucocorticoids on the lung include their possible effects on phagocyte, lymphocyte, and endothelial cell surfaces, their possible effects on T-lymphocyte functions, their inhibitory effects on protein synthesis, their inhibition of overall prostaglandin metabolism and release, and their influence on prolyl hydroxylase activity and collagen biosynthesis [225,239,247–249]. Whether or not steroid therapy is a helpful adjuvant in forestalling the fibrogenic reactions that follow some cases of lung injury [250] warrants further study.

Glucocorticoids may in fact inhibit nearly all aspects of inflammation. The inflammatory response is a highly integrated process including various cell types, mediators, enzymes, and vascular responses—sufficiently complex that it is difficult to develop a unitary hypothesis that would satisfactorily encompass all aspects of anti-inflammatory actions of steroids. Because of this multiplicity of complex effects and the imprecise methods of documenting lung inflammatory responses in humans, current understanding of the anti-inflammatory properties of glucocorticoids is rudimentary. No definitive recommendation can be made for their use in the varying forms of noncardiogenic pulmonary edema. Proponents favor their use where processes mediated by inflammatory and immunologic causes are themselves presumably causing further damage to alveolar-capillary membranes.

B.   Nonsteroidal Anti-inflammatory Substances

Efforts to develop nonsteroidal drugs that could reduce inflammation or increased capillary permeability without the general systemic action of glucocorticoids have had limited success. Nonsteroidal anti-inflammatory drugs like aspirin and indomethacin may inhibit prostaglandin biosynthesis or have

membrane- and protein-stabilizing actions [124,251,252]. The naphthoquin-
ones and eriodictyol [253] and numerous antioxidant compounds have had
limited therapeutic success in selected instances of noncardiac pulmonary
edema. It can be predicted that as the mechanism of lung injury becomes better understood, these compounds will have an increasing applicability in the
treatment of pulmonary edema of the noncardiogenic type.

C. Anticoagulants

Fulminating forms of disseminated intravascular coagulation may precipitate
noncardiogenic pulmonary edema [254]. More subtle forms of clotting are
frequently associated with lung injury. Since increased intravascular coagu-
lability of mild degree accompanies the normal postoperative recovery [255],
it should not be surprising that organ injuries accompanied by tissue damage
with or without pulmonary edema are etiologically related to mild clotting abnormalities. The recommended rule is to treat the underlying cause, such as
infection, hemolysis, or shock. If the underlying cause is not readily correct-
able and if bleeding is life-threatening, heparin is a possibility; it has been rec-
commended by some experts but not by others. Besides directly affecting
blood coagulation, heparin may also reduce platelet and fibrinogen interaction
with immune complexes [256] and with some viruses [186], presumably by
interfering with deposition of microthrombi and injury of adjacent endothelium.

In many forms of severe hypotensive shock, including that due to endotoxin, fibrin thrombi and platelet-phagocyte plugs may be influential in initiating endothelial damage. A fraction of snake venom has lately been shown
to induce blood incoagulability by rapid defibrination. Its use is currently
undergoing clinical testing in severe shock states; and antiplatelet serum is also
being tested in these conditions.

The use of anticoagulants in noncardiogenic pulmonary edema is potentially disadvantageous, since fibrin generation may prevent spreading of
edema liquid. For example, in experimental alloxan-induced pulmonary
edema, heparin administration has been shown to increase the edema liquid
volume and to decrease survival [88].

D. Sympatholytic Compounds

Marked stimulation of the sympathetic nervous system, causing activation of
α-adrenergic receptors in small arteries and veins, may affect some forms of
noncardiogenic pulmonary edema, such as cerebrogenic pulmonary edema
[211,257,258]. This form of pulmonary edema can be antagonized by an
α-receptor blocking agent [257,258]. A recent study has shown an increase in

pressure in small intrapulmonary veins in response to sympathetic nerve stimulation [212]. Treatment with α-adrenergic blocking agents in clinical conditions in which sympathetic activity may be contributing to noncardiac forms of pulmonary edema deserves further study.

E. Antiproteases

The capacity of serum and body fluids to inhibit kinin, plasmin, thrombin and several phagocytic lysosomal proteases is well established [4]. In particular, several potentially injurious phagocytic lysosomal proteases are inhibited by the plasma protease inhibitors, α_1-antitrypsin and α_2-macroglobulin, which neutralize the enzymes rapidly, thereby preventing the injurious effects of free proteolytic enzymes. The finding of complexes of proteases and α_1-antitrypsin and α_2-macroglobulin in the peritoneal cavity in diffuse peritonitis, and the observation that experimental irreversible pancreatic shock does not occur until the antiproteases in the ascitic fluid from around the pancreas become fully saturated with enzyme and free active protease activity becomes demonstrable [259], strongly suggest that protease inhibitors are important in local defenses against proteases.

Although plasma antiprotease activity in pulmonary diseases has been intensively investigated, it is not known whether proteolytic events initiate noncardiogenic pulmonary edema. However, intratracheal and intravenous instillations of proteolytic enzymes cause lung damage and pulmonary edema [4,260] and macrophages and phagocytes in the injured lung are known to contain abundant lysosomal proteases. In addition, antiproteases are consumed in inflamed lungs [261]. On the other hand, circulating endogenous plasma antiproteases may not be accessible to proteases released from phagocytes and in direct contact with endothelial cells, or to lung tissue proteases released in inflamed lung tissue. Further assessment of the role of endogenous antiproteases such as α_1-antitrypsin and α_2-macroglobulin in pulmonary inflammation is needed. In this regard, small protease inhibitors of microbial origin, such as elastatinal and chymostatin, which inhibit numerous phagocytic proteases and which are able to penetrate tissue, may prove to have therapeutic value in combating selected instances of pulmonary edema in which lung inflammation is an important cause [262].

XVI. Prospects

In the past decade, respiratory intensive-care teams have applied physiologic principles at the bedside and significantly lowered the mortality of patients with noncardiac pulmonary edema. During this time, new information has accumulated concerning membrane biology, capillary permeability, and inflammatory processes. Considerable attention has been focused on inflammatory mediators, coagulation, and immune cascades derived from tissues, plasma proteins, and blood cells. The proteolytic cascades relating complement, clotting, vasoactive peptides, and cellular inflammation have been defined more clearly. Sequential proteolysis of peptides characterizes the complement, clotting, and kinin cascades. Disorders of these sequences should become susceptible to manipulation as our knowledge increases, but therapeutic maneuvers still are gross and nonspecific. Examples of such attempts include giving antiproteases and enzyme-inhibiting agents like indomethacin to inhibit prostaglandin synthesis.

Unfortunately, this new information has not been extended to the inflammatory processes in noncardiogenic forms of pulmonary edema. It is highly probable that future therapeutic advances managing these diverse disorders will come from advances in basic knowledge of inflammatory reactions in the lung [263]. In particular, how do these processes increase lung capillary permeability? How can they be modified by experimentally administered agents? Additional questions seem especially relevant.

Many different agents presumably cause noncardiogenic pulmonary edema—by direct damage to either alveolar epithelial or bronchial and pulmonary endothelial cells (Table 4). What mechanisms damage these cells? Do mediators of inflammation and coagulation amplify or cancel primary lung cytotoxic processes? Are there certain aspects of inflammation or coagulation that are unique for the lung besides the deleterious effects of lung edema on gas exchange? If inflammation, coagulation, and immune mediators influence processes that are accompanied by increased pulmonary capillary permeability, can new strategies based on increased understanding of lung inflammatory processes be developed?

Other therapeutic approaches for improved management of pulmonary edema are expected to evolve from continued research on (1) noninvasive tests for the early diagnosis of increased lung water; (2) methods of objective assessing increased capillary permeability; (3) further refinements in techniques of artificial ventilation and membrane oxygenators; and (4) better understanding of lung damage and repair mechanisms, including diagnostic approaches for assessing degrees of reversibility of severe lung damage and the development of methods for modifying life-threatening fibrogenic reparative processes.

Acknowledgments

The authors thank Drs. G. A. Lillington, K. Kilburn, G. M. Turino, and J. Shan for helpful editorial suggestions.

References

1. N. C. Staub, Pulmonary edema, *Physiol. Rev.*, **54**:678–811 (1974).
2. E. D. Robin, C. E. Cross, R. Zelis, Medical progress: Pulmonary edema, *N. E. J. Med.*, **288**:239–246, 292–304 (1974).
3. *Congestive Heart Failure.* Edited by D. T. Mason. New York, York Medical Books, 1976.
4. G. M. Turino, J. R. Rodriguez, L. M. Greenbaum, and I. Mandl, Mechanisms of pulmonary injury, *Amer. J. Med.*, **57**:493–505 (1974).
5. D. G. Pietra, J. P. Szidon, H. A. Carpenter, and A. P. Fishman, Bronchial venular leakage during endotoxin shock, *Amer. J. Pathol.*, **77**:387–401 (1974).
6. E. M. Renkin and F. E. Curry, Transport of water and solutes across capillary endothelium. In *Transport across Biological Membranes.* Vol. 4. Edited by G. Geibish, D. C. Tosteson, and H. H. Ussing. New York, Springer-Verlag, in press, 1976. Chap. 1.
7. A. F. Junod, The metabolic activity of pulmonary endothelial cells, *Pneumol.*, **153**:169–175 (1975).
8. G. Majno, G. B. Ryan, G. Gabbiani, B. J. Hirshel, C. Irle, and I. Joris, Contractile events in inflammation and repair. In *Inflammation Mechanisms and Control.* Edited by I. Lepow and P. Ward. New York, Academic Press, 1972, pp. 13–27.
9. I. A. Oyvin, P. Y. Gaponyuk, V. M. Volodin, V. I. Oyvin, and O. Y. Tokaryev, Mechanisms of blood vessel permeability derangement under the influence of permeability factors (histamine, serotonin and histamine) and inflammatory agents, *Biochem. Pharmacol.*, **21**:89–95 (1972).
10. L. A. Staehelin, Structure and function of intercellular junctions. *Internat. Rev. Cytol.*, **39**:191–283 (1974).
11. M. Simionescu, N. Simionescu, and G. E. Palade, Segmental differentiations of cell junctions in the vascular endothelium: The microvasculature. *J. Cell Biol.*, **67**:863–885 (1975).
12. S. T. Rapoport, M. Hori, and I. Klatzo, Reversible osmotic opening of the blood-brain barrier, *Science,* **173**:1026–1028 (1971).
13. A. Martinez-Palomo and D. Erlig, Structure of tight junctions in epithelia with different permeability, *Proc. Natl. Acad. Sci. US,* **72**:4487–4491 (1975).
14. H. F. Edelhauser, D. L. Van Horn, P. Miller, and H. J. Pederson, Effect of thiol-oxidation of glutathione with diamide on corneal endothelial function, junctional complexes, and microfilaments, *J. Cell Biol.*, **68**:567–578 (1976).
15. I. Klatzo, Pathophysiological aspects of brain edema. In *Steroid and Brain Edema.* Edited by H. J. Reulen and K. Schurmann. New York, Springer-Verlag, 1972, pp. 1–8.
16. J. M. Lauweryns, J. Baert, and W. Deloecker, Fine filaments in lymphatic endothelial cells, *J. Cell Biol.*, **68**:163–167 (1976).

17.   H. Sugihara, M. Hagedorn, D. Bottcher, H. Neuhof, and C. Mittenmayer,
      Interstitial pulmonary edema following bromocarbamide intoxication,
      Amer. J. Pathol., **75**:457–468 (1974).
18.   E. D. Robin and J. Theodore, Intracellular and subcellular oedema and
      dehydration. In CIBA International Symposium Issue, *Lung Liquids,* Sym-
      posium 38, North-Holland, 1976, pp. 273–289.
19.   S. R. Saba and R. G. Mason, Effects of platelets and certain platelet com-
      ponents on growth of cultured human endothelial cells, *Thrombosis Res.,*
      7:807–812.(1975).
20.   *Mediators of Inflammation.* Edited by G. Weissman. New York, Plenum
      Press, 1974.
21.   C. G. Cochrane, The participation of cells in the inflammatory injury of
      tissue, *J. Invest. Dermatol.,* **64**:301–306 (1975).
22.   K. L. Brigham, R. E. Bowers, and P. J. Owen, Effects of antihistamines on
      the lung vascular response to histamine in unanesthetized sheep, *J. Clin.
      Invest.,* **58**:391–398 (1976).
23.   G. B. Ryan and G. Majno, Acute inflammation. A review, *J. Pathol.,* **86**:
      185–276 (1977).
24.   *NIH Guide for Grants and Contracts,* Vol. 4(9): October 22, 1975.
25.   P. J. Edelson and Z. A. Cohn, Peroxidase-mediated mammalian cell cyto-
      toxicity, *J. Exp. Med.,* **138**:318–323 (1973).
26.   P. A. Ward, Complement-derived inflammatory mediators. The C_5 clearing
      enzyme in biological reactions. In *The Phagocyte in Host Resistance.*
      Edited by J. A. Bellanti and D. H. Dayton. New York, Raven Press, 1975,
      pp. 117–126.
27.   J. W. Wilson, Pulmonary disease and the microcirculation. In *The Micro-
      circulation in Clinical Medicine.* Edited by R. Wells. New York, Academic
      Press, 1973, pp. 169–194.
28.   L. H. Burbaker, Unsticky neutrophils, *N. E. J. Med.,* **291**:674–675 (1974).
29.   J. W. Wilson, Treatment or prevention of pulmonary cellular damage with
      pharmacologic doses of corticosteroid, *Surg. Gynecol. Obstet.,* **134**:675–
      681 (1972).
30.   L. W. Henderson, M. E. Miller, R. W. Hamilton, and M. E. Norman, Hemo-
      dialysis, leukopenia and polymorph random mobility—A possible correla-
      tion, *J. Lab. Clin. Med.,* **85**:191–197 (1975).
31.   J. B. L. Gee, A. S. Khandwala, Motility, transport, and endocytosis in lung
      defense cells. In *Lung Defense Systems.* Vol. 5, Pt. II. Edited by J. D.
      Brain, D. F. Proctor, and L. M. Reid. New York, Marcel Dekker, 1977,
      pp. 927–981.
32.   A. L. Lentnek, A. D. Schreiber, and R. R. MacGregor, The induction of
      augmented granulocyte adherence by inflammation: Mediation by a
      plasma factor, *J. Clin. Invest.,* **57**:1098–1103 (1976).
33.   H. J. Showell, R. J. Freer, S. H. Zigmond, E. Schiffman, S. Aswanikumar,
      B. Corcoran, and E. L. Becker, The structure-activity relations of synthetic
      peptides as chemotactic factors and inducers of lysosomal enzyme secre-
      tion for neutrophils, *J. Exp. Med.,* **143**:1154–1169 (1976).
34.   J. I. Gallin, The role of chemotaxis in the inflammatory-immune response
      of the lung. In *Immunologic and Infectious Reactions in the Lung.* Edited

by C. H. Kirkpatrick and H. Y. Reynolds. New York, Marcel Dekker, 1976, pp. 161–178.

35. H. Z. Movat, D. R. L. Macmorine, and Y. Takeuchi, The role of PMN-leukocyte and lysosome in tissue injury, inflammation and hypersensitivity. VII. Liberation of vascular permeability factors from PMN-leukocytes during "in vitro" phagocytosis, *Int. Arch. Allergy*, **40**:218–235 (1971).

36. M. Dukes, W. C. Chan, and D. A. Willoughby, The effect of various immunosuppressive agents on the vascular response to carrageenan in the rat, *J. Path.*, **109**:151–161 (1973).

37. G. J. Stewart, G. M. Ritchie, and P. R. Lymch, Venous endothelial damage produced by massive stocking and emigration of leukocytes, *Amer. J. Pathol.*, **74**:507–532 (1974).

38. A. Janoff, At least three human neutrophil lysosomal proteases are capable of degrading joint connective tissues. In *Mechanisms of Tissue Injury with Reference to Rheumatoid Arthritis*. Vol. 256. Edited by R. J. Perper. *Ann. N.Y. Acad. Sci.*, 1975, pp. 402–408.

39. I. Goldstein, Polymorphonuclear leukocyte lysosomes and immune tissue injury, *Prog. Allergy* **20**:301–340 (1976).

40. D. O. Slauson and M. A. Dahlstron, The pulmonary inflammatory response, *Amer. J. Pathol.*, **79**:119–126 (1975).

41. R. C. Haynes, Biochemical mechanisms of steroid effects. In *Steroid Therapy*. Edited by D. L. Azarnoff. Philadelphia, W. B. Saunders, 1975, pp. 15–26.

42. P. D. Henson, Pathologic mechanisms in neutrophil-mediated injury, *Amer. J. Pathol.*, **68**:593–606 (1972).

43. I. M. Goldstein, S. T. Hoffstein, and G. Weissman, Mechanisms of lysosomal enzyme release from human polymorphonuclear leukocytes. Effects of phorbol myristate acetate, *J. Cell Biol.*, **66**:647–652 (1975).

44. H.-U. Schorlemmer, P. Davies, and A. C. Allison, Ability of activated complement components to induce lysosomal enzyme release from macrophages, *Nature*, **26**:48–49 (1976).

45. I. Goldstein, S. Hoffstein, J. Gallin, and G. Weissman, Mechanisms of lysosomal enzyme release from human leukocytes: Microtubule assembly and membrane fusion induced by a component of complement. *Proc. Nat. Acad. Sci. U.S.A.*, **70**:2916–2920 (1973).

46. R. B. Zurier, G. Weissman, S. Hoffstein, S. Kammerman, and H. H. Tai, Mechanisms of lysosomal enzyme release from human leukocytes. II. Effects of cAMP and cGMP, autonomic agonists and agents which affect microtubule function, *J. Clin. Invest.*, **53**:297–309 (1974).

47. J. A. Thompson, C. D. Severson, M. J. Parmely, B. J. Mormoestein, and A. Simmons, Pulmonary "hypersensitivity" reactions induced by transfusion of non-HL-A leukoagglutinins, *N. E. J. Med.*, **284**:1120–1125 (1971).

48. C. G. Cochrane and B. S. Aikin, Polymorphonuclear leukocytes in immunologic reactions: The destruction of vascular basement membrane in vivo and in vitro, *J. Exp. Med.*, **124**:733–752 (1966).

49. H. Hayashi, The intracellular neutral SH-dependent protease associated

with inflammatory reactions. In *International Review of Cytology*. Vol. 40. Edited by G. H. Bourne and J. F. Danielli. New York, Academic Press, 1975, pp. 101–151.

50. M. E. Bentfeld and D. F. Bainton, Cytochemical localization of lysosomal enzymes in rat megakaryocytes and platelets, *J. Clin. Invest.*, **56**:1635–1649 (1975).

51. P. M. Henson and R. N. Pinckard, Platelet activating factor (PAF) as a mediator in IgE anaphylaxis, *Fed. Proc.*, **35**:516 (1976).

52. R. E. Bryant and M. C. Sutcliffe, The effect of 3',5'-adenosine monophosphate on gradulocyte adhesion, *J. Clin. Invest.*, **54**:1241–1244 (1974).

53. G. E. Davis and A. Thompson, Effects of corticosteroid treatment in inflammation on the cellular content of blood and exudate in mice, *J. Pathol.*, **115**:17–26 (1975).

54. H. R. Bourne, M. L. Lichtenstein, K. L. Melmon, C. S. Henney, Y. Weinstein, and G. M. Shearer, Modulation of inflammation and immunity by cyclic AMP. Receptors for vasoactive hormones and mediators of inflammation regulate many leukocyte functions, *Science*, **184**:19–28 (1974).

55. L. J. Ignarro, T. F. Lint, and W. J. George, Hormonal control of lysosomal enzyme release from human neutrophils. Effects of autonomic agents on enzyme release, phagocytosis and cyclic nucleotide levels, *J. Exp. Med.*, **139**:1395–1414 (1974).

56. E. L. Pesanti and S. G. Axline, Colchicine effects on lysosomal enzyme induction and intracellular degradation in the cultivated macrophage, *J. Exp. Med.*, **141**:1030–1046 (1975).

57. C. Finaly, P. Davies, and A. C. Allison, Changes in cellular enzyme levels and the inhibition of selective release of lysosomal hydrolases from macrophages by indomethacin, *Agents and Actions*, **5**:345–353 (1975).

58. J. M. Clark and C. J. Lambertson, Pulmonary oxygen toxicity: A review, *Pharmacol. Rev.*, **23**:37–133 (1971).

59. J. S. Bus, S. D. Aust, and J. E. Gibson, Superoxide- and singlet-oxygen-catalyzed lipid peroxidation as a possible mechanisms for paraquat (methyl viologen) toxicity, *Biochem. Biophys. Res. Commun.*, **58**:749–755 (1974).

60. D. B. Menzel, The role of free radicals in toxicity of air pollutants (nitrogen oxides and ozone). In *Free Radicals in Biology*. Vol. 2. Edited by W. A. Pryor. New York, Academic Press, 1976, pp. 181–202.

61. C. E. Cross, A. J. DeLucia, A. K. Reddy, M. A. Hussain, C. K. Chow, and M. G. Mustafa, Ozone interactions with lung tissue: Biochemical approaches, *Amer. J. Med.*, **60**:929–935 (1976).

62. J. T. Curnutte and B. M. Babior, Bacterial defense systems: The effects of bacteria and serum on superoxide production by granulooyton, *J. Clin. Invest.*, **53**:1662–1672 (1974).

63. T. P. Stossel, R. J. Mason, and A. L. Smith, Lipid peroxidation by human blood phagocytes, *J. Clin. Invest.*, **54**:638–645 (1974).

64. M. L. Salin and J. McCord, Free radicals and inflammation. Protection of

phagocytosing leukocytes by superoxide dismutase, *J. Clin. Invest.,* **56**: 1319–1323 (1975).

65. S. C. Sharma, H. Mukhtar, S. K. Sharma, and C. R. Murt, Lipid peroxide formation in experimental inflammation, *Biochem. Pharmacol.,* **21**:1210–1214 (1972).

66. J. M. McCord and M. L. Salin, Free radicals and inflammation: Studies on superoxide-mediated NBT reduction by leukocytes. In *Erythrocyte Structure and Function.* Edited by G. J. Brewer. New York, Alan R. Liss, 1975, pp. 731–746.

67. I. M. Goldstein, D. Roos, H. B. Kaplan, and G. Weissman, Complement and immunoglobulins stimulate superoxide production by human leukocytes independently of phagocytosis, *J. Clin. Invest.,* **56**:1155–1163 (1975).

68. R. B. Johnston and J. E. Lehmeyer, Elaboration of toxic oxygen by-products by neutrophils in a model of immune complex disease, *J. Clin. Invest.,* **57**:836–841 (1976).

69. R. L. Baehner, D. G. Nathan, and W. B. Castle, Oxidant injury of caucasian glucose-6-phosphate dehydrogenase-deficient red blood cells by phagocytosing leukocytes during infection, *J. Clin. Invest.,* **50**:2466–2473 (1971).

70. H. Melsom, T. Sanner, and R. Seljelid, Macrophage cytolytic factor, *Exp. Cell Res.,* **94**:221–226 (1975).

71. G. L. Plaa and H. Witschi, Chemicals, drugs and lipid peroxidation, *Ann. Rev. Pharmacol. Tox.,* **16**:125–141 (1976).

72. A. Patkau, K. Kelly, W. S. Chelack, S. D. Pleskach, C. Barefoot, and B. E. Meeker, Radioprotection of bone marrow stem cells by superoxide dismutase, *Biochem. Biophys. Res. Commun.,* **67**:1167–1173 (1975).

73. Y. Oyanagui, Participation of superoxide anions at the prostaglandin phase of carrageenan foot edema, *Biochem. Pharmacol.,* **25**:1465–1472 (1976).

74. R. Brinkman, H. B. Lamberts, and T. S. Veninga, Radiometric toxicity of ozonised air, *Lancet,* **1**:133–136 (1964).

75. M. Steiner and J. Anastasi, Vitamin E, an inhibitor of the platelet release reaction, *J. Clin. Invest.,* **57**:732–737 (1976).

76. S. Kalowski, E. L. Howes, W. Margertten, and D. G. McKay, Effects of intravascular clotting on the activation of the complement system. The role of the platelet, *Amer. J. Pathol.,* **78**:525–536 (1975).

77. S. E. Bergentz, D. H. Lewis, and V. Ljungquist, Trapping of platelets in the lung after experimental injury. In *Sixth European Conference on Microcirculation.* Edited by J. Ditcel and D. H. Lewis. New York, Basel, Karger, 1971, pp. 35–40.

78. D. G. McKay, Vessel wall and thrombogenesis endotoxin, *Thromb. Diath. Haemorrh.,* **29**:11–26 (1973).

79. C. M. Chesney, E. Harper, and R. Colman, Human platelet collagenase, *J. Clin. Invest.,* **53**:1647–1654 (1974).

80. R. L. Nachman, B. Weksler, and B. Ferris, Increased vascular permeability produced by human platelet granule cationic extract, *J. Clin. Invest.,* **49**: 274–281 (1970).

81. M. K. White, D. Shepro, and H. B. Hechtman, Pulmonary function and platelet-lung interaction, *J. Appl. Physiol.*, **34**:697–703 (1973).

82. J. B. Smith, C. Ingeman, J. J. Kocsis, and M. J. Silver, Formation of an intermediate in prostaglandin biosynthesis and its association with the platelet release phenomena, *J. Clin. Invest.*, **53**:1468–1472 (1974).

83. E. Genton, M. Gent, J. Hirsh, and L. A. Harker, Medical Progress: Platelet-inhibiting drugs in the prevention of clinical thrombotic disease, *N. E. J. Med.*, **293**:1174–1179, 1236–1240, 1296–1300 (1975).

84. J. P. Casenave, M. A. Packham, M. A. Guccione, and J. F. Mustard, Inhibition of platelet adherence to a collagen-coated surface by agents that inhibit platelet shape change and clot retraction, *J. Lab. Clin. Med.*, **84**:483–493 (1974).

85. M. I. Barnhart, L. Sulisz, and G. B. Bluhm, Role for fibrinogen and its derivatives in acute inflammation. In *Immunopathology of Inflammation.* Edited by B. K. Forscher and J. C. Houck. Amsterdam, Excerpta Medica, 1971, pp. 52–58.

86. C. G. Cochrane and K. D. Whepper, The first component of kinin forming system in human and rabbit plasma: Its relationship to clotting factor XII (Hageman factor), *J. Exp. Med.*, **134**:986–1004 (1971).

87. D. G. McKay, Participation of components of the blood coagulation system in the inflammatory response, *Amer. J. Pathol.*, **67**:181–204 (1972).

88. E. C. Meyer and R. Ottavioano, The effect of fibrin on the morphometric distribution of pulmonary exudative edema, *Lab. Invest.*, **29**:320–328 (1973).

89. A. P. Kaplan and K. F. Austen, Activation and control mechanisms of Hageman factor-dependent pathways of coagulation, fibrinolysis, and kinin generation and their contribution to the inflammatory response, *J. Allergy Clin. Immunol.*, **56**:491–506 (1975).

90. S. D. Revak, C. G. Cochrane, A. R. Johnson, and T. E. Hugli, Structural changes accompanying enzymatic activation of human Hageman factor, *J. Clin. Invest.*, **54**:619–627 (1974).

91. J. P. Giroud and D. A. Willoughby, The interrelations of complement and a prostaglandin-like substance in acute inflammation, *J. Pathol.*, **101**:241–249 (1970).

92. E. S. Tucker, The role of complement and other biochemical mediators in immunologic disease. In *Immunopathology: Clinical Laboratory Concepts and Methods.* Edited by R. M. Nakamura. Boston, Little, Brown, 1974, pp. 104–137.

93. J. J. Muller-Eberhard, Chemistry and function of the complement system, *Hosp. Pract.*, **12**:33–43 (1977).

94. D. L. Brown, Annotation: Complement and coagulation, *Brit. J. Hematol.*, **30**:377–382 (1975).

95. J. R. Brentjens, D. W. O'Connell, I. B. Pawlowski, K. C. Hsu, and G. A. Andres, Experimental immune complex disease of the lung: The pathogenesis of a laboratory model resembling certain human interstitial diseases, *J. Exp. Med.*, **140**:105–125 (1974).

96. P. R. Craddock, J. Fehr, K. L. Brigham, R. S. Kronenberg, and H. S. Jacob, Complement and leukocyte-mediated pulmonary dysfunction in hemodialysis, *N. Eng. J. Med.*, **296**:769–774 (1977).

97. D. J. Parker, S. Cook, and M. Turner-Warwick, Serum complement studies during and following cardiopulmonary bypass. In *Lung Metabolism.* Edited by A. F. Junod and R. de Haller. New York, Academic Press, 1975, pp. 581–588.

98. D. A. Levy, Histamine and serotonin. In *Mediators of Inflammation.* Edited by G. Weissman. New York, Plenum Press, 1974, pp. 141–161.

99. L. M. Greenbaum, Leukocyte kininogenases and leukokinins from normal and malignant cells, *Amer. J. Pathol.*, **68**:613–623 (1972).

100. K. L. Brigham and P. J. Owen, Increased sheep lung vascular permeability caused by histamine, *Circ. Res.*, **37**:647–657 (1975).

101. A. P. Kaplan, The pharmacologic modulation of mediator release from human basophils and mast cells. In *Immunologic and Infectious Reactions in the Lung.* Edited by C. H. Kirkpatrick and H. Y. Renolds. New York, Marcel Dekker, 1976, pp. 445–459.

102. M. A. Beaven, Histamine, *N. E. J. Med.*, **294**:320–325 (1976).

103. A. Tucker, E. K. Weir, J. T. Reeves, and R. F. Grover, Histamine H_1 and H_2 receptors in pulmonary and systemic vasculature of the dog, *Am. J. Physiol.*, **229**:1008–1013 (1975).

104. J. L. Berk, J. F. Hagen, R. Koo, W. Beyer, G. R. Dochat, M. Rupright, and S. Nomoto, Pulmonary insufficiency caused by epinephrine, *Ann. Surg.*, **178**:423–435 (1973).

105. S. H. Ferreira, S. Moncada, and J. R. Vane, Prostaglandins and signs and symptoms of inflammation. In *Prostaglandin Synthetase Inhibitors.* Edited by H. J. Robinson and J. R. Vane. New York, Raven Press, 1974, pp. 175–187.

106. T. J. Williams and J. Morley, Prostaglandins as potentiators of increased vascular permeability in inflammation, *Nature*, **246**:215–217 (1973).

107. J. Panagides and E. L. Tolman, Effect of various pharmacological agents on prostaglandin-induced increases in microvascular permeability, *Res. Commun. Chem. Pathol. Pharmacol.*, **12**:609–612 (1975).

108. G. Markelonis and J. Garbus, Alterations of intracellular oxidative metabolism as stimuli evoking prostaglandin biosynthesis. A review of prostaglandins in cell injury and a hypothesis, *Prostaglandins*, **10**:1087–1106 (1975).

109. H. J. Robinson and J. R. Vane, editors. *Prostaglandin Synthetase Inhibitors–Their Effects on Physiological Functions and Pathological States.* New York, Raven Press, 1974.

110. B. Samuelson and M. Hamberg. Role of endoperoxides in the biosynthesis and action of prostaglandins. In *Prostaglandin Synthetase Inhibitors–Their Effects on Physiological Functions and Pathological States.* Edited by H. J. Robinson and J. R. Vane. New York, Raven Press, 1974, pp. 107–119.

111. G. B. Kolata, Thromboxanes: The power behind the prostaglandins? *Science*, **190**:770–771 (1975).

112.   R. B. Zurier, Prostaglandins, inflammation and asthma, *Arch. Intern. Med.*, **133**:101–110 (1974).
113.   Y. S. Bakhle and J. R. Vane, Pharmacokinetic functions of the pulmonary circulation, *Pharmacol. Rev.*, **54**:1007–1043 (1974).
114.   P. T. Russell, A. J. Eberle, and H. C. Cheng, The prostaglandins in clinical medicine. A developing role for the clinical chemist, *Clin. Chem.*, **21**: 653–666 (1975).
115.   L. Z. Bito and R. A. Baroody, Inhibition of pulmonary prostaglandin metabolism by inhibitors of prostaglandin biotransport (probenecid and bromcresol green), *Prostaglandins*, **10**:633–639 (1975).
116.   P. J. Piper, Release and metabolism of prostaglandins in lung tissue, *Pol. J. Pharmacol.*, **26**:61–72 (1974).
117.   H. E. Lindsey and J. H. Wyllie, Release of prostaglandins from embolized lungs, *Brit. J. Surg.*, **57**:738–741 (1970).
118.   A.A. Mathe, P. Hedqvist, K. Strandberg, and C. A. Leslie, Affects of prostaglandins in the lung, *N. Eng. J. Med.*, **296**:850–855 and 910–914 (1977).
119.   K. J. Barrett-Bee and L. R. Green, The relationship between prostaglandin release and lung c-AMP levels during anaphylaxis in the guinea pig, *Prostaglandins*, **10**:589–598 (1975).
120.   B. A. Jakschik, J. L. Kourik, and P. Needleman, Prostaglandin metabolism and release by the lung during hemorrhage, *Pharmacol.*, **18**:197 (1974).
121.   J. Vaage and P. J. Piper, The release of prostaglandin-like substances during platelet aggregation and pulmonary microembolism, *Acta Physiol. Scand.*, **94**:8–13 (1975).
122.   M. A. Gimbrone and R. A. Alexander, Angiotensin II stimulation of prostaglandin production in cultured human vascular endothelium, *Science*, **189**:219–220 (1975).
123.   J. Carr, The effect of anti-inflammatory drugs on increased vascular permeability induced by chemical mediators, *J. Pathol.*, **108**:1–14 (1972).
124.   S. H. Ferreira and J. R. Vane, New aspects of the mode of action of non-steroid anti-inflammatory drugs, *Ann. Rev. Pharmacol.*, **14**:57–73 (1974).
125.   L. Levy and T. L. Kerley, The use of DPPD (N,N'-diphenyl-p-phenylenediamine) as an anti-inflammatory agent, *Life Sci.*, **14**:1917–1925 (1974).
126.   W. C. Hope, C. Dalton, L. J. Machlin, R. J. Filipski, and F. M. Vane, Influence of dietary Vitamin E on prostaglandin biosynthesis in rat blood, *Prostaglandins*, **10**:557–571 (1975).
127.   K. J. Johnson and P. A. Ward, Acute immunologic pulmonary alveolitis, *J. Clin. Invest.*, **54**:349–357 (1974).
128.   P. M. Henson, Interaction of cells with immune complexes: Adherence, release of constituents and tissue injury, *J. Exp. Med.*, **134** (Suppl. 3): 114s–135s (1971).
129.   R. M. Pantalone and R. C. Page, Lymphokine-induced production and release of lysosomal enzymes by macrophage, *Proc. Nat. Acad. Sci. USA*, **72**:2091–2094 (1975).

130. S. Cohen, Cell-mediated immunity and the inflammatory system, *Human Pathol.*, 7:249–264 (1976).

131. W. K. Podleski, Cytodestructive mechanisms provoked by lymphocytes, *Amer. J. Med.*, 61:1–8 (1976).

132. J. D. Hill, J. L. Ratliff, J. C. Parrott, M. Lamy, R. J. Fallat, E. Keoniger, E. M. Yaeger, and G. Whitmer, Pulmonary pathology in acute respiratory insufficiency: Lung biopsy as a diagnostic tool, *J. Thorac. Cardiovasc. Surg.*, 71:64–71 (1976).

133. F. P. Chinard, Estimation of extravascular water by indicator dilution techniques, *Circ. Res.*, 37:137–145 (1975).

134. F. Fazio, T. Jones, H. Jones, C. G. Rhodes, and J. M. B. Hughes, Measurements of extravascular lung water in vivo by external counting, *J. Nucl. Biol. Med.*, 20:81–83 (1976).

135. J. H. C. Swan, W. Ganz, J. Forrester, H. Marcus, G. Diamond, and D. Chonette, Catheterization of the heart in man with use of a flow-directed balloon-tipped catheter, *N. E. J. Med.*, 283:447–456 (1970).

136. A. A. Gilbertson, Pulmonary artery catheterization and wedge pressure measurement in the general intensive therapy unit, *Brit. J. Anaesth.*, 46:97–104 (1974).

137. M. P. Colvin, T. M. Savege, and C. T. Lewis, Pulmonary danage from a Swan-Ganz catheter, *Brit. J. Anaesth.*, 47:1107–1109 (1975).

138. J. A. Forrester, G. Diamond, T. J. McHugh, and H. J. C. Swan, Filling pressures in the right and left sides of the heart in acute myocardial infarction. A reappraisal of central venous pressure monitoring, *N. E. J. Med.*, 285:190–193 (1971).

139. P. L. Luz, H. Shubin, M. H. Weil, E. Jacobson, and L. Stein, Pulmonary edema related to changes in colloid osmotic and pulmonary artery wedge pressure in patients after myocardial infarction, *Circulation*, 51:350–357 (1975).

140. D. G. Ashbaugh, T. L. Petty, D. B. Bigelow, and T. M. Harris, Continuous positive pressure-breathing (CPPB) in adult respiratory distress syndrome, *J. Thorac. Cardiovasc. Surg.*, 57:31–41 (1969).

141. A. Kumar, K. J. Falke, B. Geffin, C. F. Aldridge, M. B. Laver, E. Lowenstein, and H. Pontoppidan, Continuous positive-pressure ventilation in acute respiratory failure, *N. E. J. Med.*, 283:1430–1436 (1970).

142. D. G. Ashbaugh and T. L. Petty, Positive end-expiratory pressure: Physiology, indications and contraindications, *J. Thorac. Cardiovasc. Surg.*, 65:165–170 (1973).

143. F. Kerr, D. J. Ewing, J. B. Irving, M. F. Sudlow, and B. J. Kirby, Positive expiratory pressure plateau breathing in spontaneously breathing patients with myocardial infarction and pulmonary oedema, *Thorax*, 29:690–694 (1974).

144. R. N. Pilon and D. A. Bittar, The effect of positive end-expiratory pressure on thoracic-duct lymph flow during controlled ventilation in anesthetized dogs, *Anesthesiology*, 39:607–612 (1973).

145. P. Caldini, J. D. Leith, and M. J. Brennan, Effect of continuous positive-pressure ventilation (CPPV) on edema formation in dog lung, *J. Appl. Physiol.*, **39**:672–679 (1975).

146. C. F. Hobelmann, D. E. Smith, R. W. Virgilio, A. R. Shapiro, and R. M. Peters, Hemodynamic alterations with positive end-expiratory pressure: The contribution of pulmonary vasculature, *J. Trauma*, **15**:951–959 (1975).

147. P. M. Suter, H. B. Fairley, and M. D. Isenberg, Optimum end-expiratory airway pressure in patients with acute pulmonary failure, *N. E. J. Med.*, **292**:284–289 (1975).

148. R. R. Kirby, J. B. Downs, J. M. Civetta, J. H. Modell, F. J. Dannemiller, E. F. Klein, and M. Hodges, High-level positive end-expiratory pressure (PEEP) in acute respiratory insufficiency, *Chest*, **67**:156–163 (1975).

149. L. Lozman, O. R. Powers, T. Older, R. E. Dutton, R. J. Roy, M. English, D. Marco, and C. Eckert, Correlation of pulmonary wedge and left atrial pressures: A study in the patient receiving positive end-expiratory pressure ventilation, *Arch. Surg.*, **109**:270–277 (1974).

150. R. R. Kirby, J. C. Perry, H. W. Calderwood, B. Ruiz, and D. S. Lederman, Cardiorespiratory effects of high positive end-expiratory pressure, *Anesthesiology*, **43**:533–539 (1975).

151. J. Qvist, H. Pontoppidan, R. S. Wilson, E. Lowenstein, and M. B. Laver, Hemodynamic responses to mechanical ventilation with PEEP: The effect of hypervolemia, *Anesthesiology*, **42**:45–55 (1975).

152. S. K. Sanyal, C. Mitchell, W. T. Hughes, S. Feldman, and J. Caces, Continuous negative chest-wall pressure as therapy for severe respiratory distress in older children, *Chest*, **68**:143–148 (1975).

153. G. J. Taylor, W. Brenner, and W. R. Summer, Severe viral pneumonia in young adults: Therapy with continuous positive airway pressure, *Chest*, **69**:722–728 (1976).

154. E. C. Pierce, A. L. Thebaut, B. B. Kent, J. A. Kirkland, W. E. Goetter, and B. G. Wright, Techniques of extended perfusion using a membrane lung, *Ann. Thorac. Surg.*, **12**:451–470 (1971).

155. J. D. Hill, J. L. Ratliff, R. Fallat, H. J. Tucker, M. Lamy, J. P. Dietrich, and F. Gerbode, Prognostic factors in the treatment of acute respiratory insufficiency with long-term extracorporeal oxygenation, *J. Thorac. Cardiovasc. Surg.*, **68**:905–917 (1974).

156. W. M. Zapol, J. Qvist, H. Pontoppidan, A. Liland, T. McEnany, and M. B. Laver, Extracorporeal perfusion for acute respiratory failure. Recent experience with the spiral coil membrane lung, *J. Thorac. Cardiovasc. Surg.*, **69**:439–449 (1975).

157. Case Records of the Massachusetts General Hospital. Weekly clinopathological exercises. Case 21-1975, *N. E. J. Med.*, **292**:1174–1181 (1975).

158. J. D. Cooper, J. Duffin, M. F. Glynn, D. Phil, J. M. Nelems, S. Teasdale, and A. A. Scott, Combination of membrane oxygenator support and pulmonary lavage for acute respiratory failure, *J. Thorac. Cardiovasc. Surg.*, **70**:304–308 (1976).

159. J. F. Collins, G. M. Cochrane, J. Davis, S. R. Genatar, and T. J. H. Clark, Some aspects of pulmonary function after rapid saline infusion in healthy subjects, *Clin. Sci. Med.,* 45:407–410 (1973).

160. J. D. Cooper, M. Maeda, and E. Lowenstein, Lung water accumulation with acute hemodilution in dogs, *J. Thorac. Cardiovasc. Surg.,* 69:957–965 (1975).

161. F. D. Moore, J. H. Lyone, E. C. Pierce, A. P. Morgan, P. A. Drinker, J. D. MacArthur, and G. J. Dammin, *Post-Traumatic Pulmonary Insufficiency.* Philadelphia, W. B. Saunders, 1969.

162. L. Stein, J. Berand, M. Morissette, P. Luz, M. H. Wel, and H. Shubin, Pulmonary edema during volume infusion, *Circulation,* 52:483–489 (1975).

163. W. C. Shoemaker, Comparison of the relative effectiveness of whole-blood transfusions and various types of fluid therapy in resuscitation, *Crit. Care Med.,* 4:71–78 (1976).

164. H. I. Chen and C. Y. Chai, Pulmonary edema and hemorrhage as a consequence of systemic vasoconstriction, *Amer. J. Physiol.,* 227:144–151 (1974).

165. J. H. Ellis and J. F. Murray, Effect of norepinephrine and fluid administration on pulmonary extravascular water volume in dogs, *Circ. Res.,* 37:80–87 (1975).

166. S. Baek, G. G. Makabali, C. W. Bryan-Brown, J. M. Kusek, and W. C. Shoemaker, Plasma expansion in surgical patients with high central venous pressure (CVP): The relationship of blood volume to hematocrit, CVP, pulmonary wedge pressure, and cardiorespiratory changes, *Surgery,* 78:304–315 (1975).

167. P. W. Brown, J. R. McCurdy, R. C. Elkins, and L. J. Greenfield, Effects of albumin and urea on hydrostatic edema in the perfused lung, *J. Surg. Res.,* 14:440–447 (1970).

168. J. J. Skillman, B. M. Parikh, and B. J. Tanenbaum, Pulmonary arteriovenous admixture: Improvement with albumin and diuresis, *Amer. J. Surg.,* 119:440–447 (1970).

169. A. Sladen, M. B. Laver, and H. Pontoppidan, Pulmonary complications and water retention on prolonged mechanical ventilation, *N. E. J. Med.,* 279:448–453 (1968).

170. M. E. Silverstein, C. A. Ford, M. J. Lysaght, and L. W. Henderson, Treatment of severe fluid overload by ultrafiltration, *N. E. J. Med.,* 291:747, 752 (1974).

171. C. E. Cross and R. Zelis, Pathophysiology of pulmonary edema. In *The Peripheral Circulations.* Edited by R. Zelis. New York, Grune and Stratton, 1975, pp. 315–362.

172. S. F. Vatner, R. J. McRitchie, and E. Braunwald, Effects of dobutamine on left ventricular performance, coronary dynamics and distribution of cardiac output in conscious dogs, *J. Clin. Invest.,* 53:1265–1273 (1974).

173. A. Schwartz, R. M. Lewis, H. G. Hanley, R. G. Junson, F. D. Dial, and M. V. Ray, Hemodynamic and biochemical effects of a new positive inotropic agent, *Circ. Res.,* 34:102–111 (1974).

174.   R. Zelis, E. J. Mansour, R. J. Capone, and D. T. Mason, The cardiovascu-
       lar effects of morphine: Ther peripheral capacitance and resistance ves-
       sels in human subjects, *J. Clin. Invest.*, 54:1247–1258 (1974).
175.   K. Dikshit, J. K. Vyden, J. S. Forrester, K. Chatterjee, R. Prakash, and
       H. J. C. Swan, Renal and extrarenal hemodynamic effects of furosemide
       in congestive heart failure after myocardial infarction, *N. E. J. Med.*, **288**:
       1087–1090 (1973).
176.   R. R. Miller, L. A. Vismara, R. Zelis, E. A. Amsterdam, and D. T. Mason,
       Comparative pharmacologic mechanisms of left ventricular unloading in
       clinical congestive heart failure: Differential effects of nitroprusside,
       phentolamine and nitroglycerin on cardiac function and peripheral cir-
       culation, *Circ. Res.*, **39**:127–133 (1976).
177.   D. O. Williams, E. A. Amsterdam, and D. T. Mason, Hemodynamic ef-
       fects of nitroglycerin in acute myocardial infarction. Decrease in ven-
       tricular preload at the expense of cardiac output, *Circulation*, **51**:421–
       427 (1975).
178.   R. R. Miller, L. A. Vismara, R. Zelis, E. A. Amsterdam, and D. T. Mason,
       Clinical use of sodium nitroprusside in chronic ischemic heart disease.
       Effects on peripheral vascular resistance and venous tone on ventricular
       volume, pump and mechanical performance, *Circulation*, **51**:328–336
       (1975).
179.   U. Thadami, C. Burrow, W. Whitaker, and D. Heath, Pulmonary veno-
       occlusive disease, *Quart. J. Med.*, **44**:133–159 (1975).
180.   F. W. Blaisdell and R. M. Schlobohm, The respiratory distress syndrome:
       A review, *Surgery*, **74**:251 (1973).
181.   A. J. Rosen, Shock lung: Fact or fancy? *Surg. Clin. N. A.*, **55**:613–626
       (1975).
182.   P. C. Hopewell and J. F. Murray, The adult respiratory distress syndrome,
       Ann. Rev. Med., **27**:343–356 (1976).
183.   D. F. J. Halmagyi, Role of lymphatics in the genesis of "shock lung": A
       hypothesis. In *Lung Water and Solute Exchange*, Vol 7. Edited by N. C.
       Staub. New York, Marcel Dekker, 1977, pp. 423–435.
184.   J. F. P. Hers, Disturbances of the ciliated epithelium due to influenza
       virus, *Amer. Rev. Resp. Dis.*, **93**:612–671 (1966).
185.   J. G. Weg, S. D. Greenberg, F. Gyorkey, P. Gyorkey, and D. E. Jenkins,
       Electron microscopic demonstration of disruption of capillary integrity
       in acute diffuse pneumonia, *Clin. Res.*, **19**:56 (1971) (Abstr.).
186.   H. M. Sottneck, W. A. Cassel, and W. G. Campbell, Jr., The pathogenesis
       of vaccinia virus toxicity. I. The role of virus-platelet interaction, *Lab.
       Invest.*, **33**:514–521 (1975).
187.   J. H. Triebwasser, R. E. Harris, R. E. Bryant, and E. R. Rhodes, Varicella
       pneumonia in adults, *Medicine*, **46**:409–423 (1967).
188.   J. E. Ferstenfeld, D. P. Schlueter, M. W. Rytel, and R. P. Molloy, Recog-
       nition and management of adult respiratory distress syndrome second-
       ary to viral interstitial pneumonia, *Amer. J. Med.*, **58**:709–718 (1975).
189.   N. B. Ratliff, J. W. Wilson, D. W. Hackel, and A. M. Martin, The lungs in

hemorrhagic shock: Observations on alveolar and vascular ultrastructure, *Amer. J. Pathol.*, **58**:353–373 (1970).

190. R. S. Connel, R. L. Swank, and M. C. Webb, The development of pulmonary ultrastructural lesions during hemorrhagic shock, *J. Trauma*, **15**: 116–129 (1975).

191. W. W. Feguson, T. M. Glenn, and A. M. Lefer, Mechanisms of production of circulatory shock factors in isolated perfused pancreas, *Amer. J. Physiol.*, **222**:450–457 (1972).

192. A. M. Lefer, Blood-borne humoral factors in the pathophysiology of circulatory shock, *Circ. Res.*, **32**:129–139 (1973).

193. L. R. Soma, G. R. Neufeld, D. C. Codd, and B. E. Marshall, Pulmonary function in hemorrhagic shock: The effect of pancreatic ligation and blood filtration, *Ann. Surg.*, **179**:395–402 (1974).

194. R. Procelli, W. M. Foster, E. H. Bergofsky, A. Bicker, R. Kaur, M. Demeny, and T. Reich, Pulmonary circulatory changes in pathogenesis of shock lung, *Amer. J. Med. Sci.*, **268**:250–261 (1974).

195. I. Dawidson, J. Barrett, E. Miller, and S. L. Martin, Effect of intravascular cellular aggregate dissolution in postoperative patients, *Ann. Surg.*, **182**: 776–781 (1975).

196. M. S. Litwin, Blood viscosity changes after trauma: Use of dextran-40 in correction of microcirculatory insufficiency, *Crit. Care Med.*, **4**:67–70 (1976).

197. R. G. Gerrity, M. Richardson, B. A. Caplan, J. F. Cade, J. Hirsh, and C. J. Schwartz, Endotoxin-induced vascular endothelial injury and repair. II. Focal injury in face morphology, [^{3}H] thymidine uptake and circulating endothelial cells in the dog, *Exp. Molecul. Pathol.*, **24**:59–69 (1976).

198. W. W. Pingleton, J. J. Coalson, and C. A. Guenter, Significance of leukocytes in endotoxic shock, *Exp. Mol. Pathol.*, **22**:183–184 (1975).

199. J. Hawiger, A. Hawiger, and S. Timmon, Endotoxin-sensitive membrane component of human platelets, *Nature*, **256**:125–128 (1975).

200. T. Eckhards and G. Muller-Berghaus, The role of blood platelets in the precipitation of soluble fibrin by endotoxin, *Scand. J. Haematol.*, **14**: 181–189 (1975).

201. G. Müller-Berghaus, E. Bohn, and W. Höbel, Activation of intravascular coagulation by endotoxin: The significance of granulocytes and platelets, *Brit. J. Hematol.*, **33**:213–220 (1976).

202. D. H. Gilbert, J. A. Barnett, and J. P. Stanford, *Escherichia coli* bacteremia in the squirrel monkey, *J. Clin. Invest.*, **52**:406–413 (1973).

203. D. T. Fearon, S. Ruddy, P. H. Schur, and W. R. McCabe, Activation of the properdin pathway of complement in patients with gram-negative bacteremia, *N. E. J. Med.*, **292**:937–940 (1975).

204. D. E. Dines, L. W. Burgher, and H. Okazaki, The clinical and pathologic correlation of fat embolism syndrome, *Mayo Clin. Proc.*, **50**:407–411 (1975).

205   S. Cotev, E. Rosenmann, Z. Eyal, H. Weinberg, E. Shafrir, and J. T.
        Davidson, The role of hypovolemic stress in the production of fat em-
        bolism in rabbits, *Chest,* **69**:523–528 (1976).
206.   J. E. Fischer, R. H. Turner, J. H. Herndon, and E. J. Riseborough, Mas-
        sive steroid therapy in severe fat embolism, *Surg. Gynecol. Obstet.,* **132**:
        667–672 (1971).
207.   A. A. Scott and R. P. Welsh, Fat embolism: A rational approach to treat-
        ment, *Can. Med. Assoc. J.,* **109**:867–871 (1973).
208.   D. G. Murray and G. B. Racz, Fat-embolism syndrome (respiratory insuf-
        ficiency syndrome): A rationale for treatment, *J. Bone Joint Surg.,* **56**-A:
        1338–1349 (1974).
209.   J. S. Callcutt. *Pulmonary Edema.* Baltimore, Williams and Wilkins, 1969.
210.   E. D. Robin and J. Theodore, Speculations on neurogenic pulmonary
        edema, *Amer. Rev. Resp. Dis.,* **113**:405–411 (1976).
211.   R. W. Reynolds, Pulmonary edema as a consequence of hypothalamic
        lesions in rats, *Science,* **141**:930–932 (1963).
212.   P. J. Kaodwitz, P. D. Joiner, and A. L. Hyman, Influence of sympathetic
        stimulation and vasoactive substances on the canine pulmonary veins, *J.
        Clin. Invest.,* **56**:354–365 (1975).
213.   J. W. Bean and D. L. Beckman, Centrogenic pulmonary pathology in
        mechanical head injury, *J. Appl. Physiol.,* **27**:807 (1969).
214.   A. B. Malik, Pulmonary vascular response to increase in intracranial pres-
        sure: Role of sympathetic mechanisms, *J. Appl. Physiol.: Respirat. En-
        viron. Exercise Physiol.,* **42**:335–343 (1977).
215.   E. M. MacKay and E. F. Pecka, Experimental pulmonary edema. III. Hy-
        poglycemia, a cause of pulmonary edema, *Proc. Soc. Exp. Biol. Med.,* **73**:
        568–569 (1950).
216.   G. Moss, The role of the central nervous system in shock: The centro-
        neurogenic etiology of the respiratory distress syndrome, *Crit. Care Med.,*
        2:181–185 (1974).
217.   B. Interiano, D. Stuard, and R. W. Hyde, Acute respiratory distress syn-
        drome in pancreatitis, *Ann. Int. Med.,* **77**:923–926 (1972).
218.   M. F. Hayes, Jr., R. W. Rosenbaum, M. Zibelman, and R. Matsumoto,
        Adult respiratory distress syndrome in association with acute pancreatitis,
        Amer. J. Surg., **127**:314–319 (1974).
219.   J. L. Cameron, Lipid abnormalities and acute pancreatitis, *Hosp. Pract.,*
        12:95–101 (1977).
220.   W. W. Gerguson, T. M. Glenn, and A. M. Lefer, Mechanisms of produc-
        tion of circulatory shock factors in isolated perfused pancreas, *Amer. J.
        Physiol.,* **222**:450–457 (1972).
221.   J. M. Kellum, T. R. DeMeester, R. C. Elklus, and G. D. Zuidoma, Res-
        piratory insufficiency secondary to acute pancreatitis, *Ann. Surg.,* **175**:
        657–662 (1972).
222.   B. Robertson and G. Enhorning, The alveolar lining of the premature
        newborn rabbit after pharyngeal deposition of surfactant, *Lab. Invest.,*
        31:54–59 (1974).

223. D. C. Shannon, H. Kazemi, E. W. Merrill, K. A. Smith, and P. S.-L. Wong, Restoration of volume-pressure curves with a lecithin fog, *J. Appl. Physiol.*, **28**:470–473 (1969).

224. E. Corday, Introduction: Interventions that might influence viability of ischemic jeopardized myocardium, *Amer. J. Cardiol.*, **37**:461–466 (1976).

225. D. L. Azarnoff. *Steroid Therapy*. Philadelphia, W. B. Saunders, 1975.

226. A. S. Fauci, D. C. Dale, and J. E. Baloe, Glucocorticosteroid therapy: Mechanisms of action and clinical considerations, *Ann. Int. Med.*, **315**: 304–315 (1976).

227. T. L. Petty and D. G. Ashbaugh, The adult respiratory distress syndrome: Clinical features, factors influencing prognosis and principles of management, *Chest*, **60**:233–239 (1971).

228. P. M. James and R. T. Myers, Experience with steroids, albumin, and diuretics in progressive pulmonary insufficiency, *South. Med. J.*, **65**: 945–948 (1972).

229. L. J. Kettel and J. O. Morse, Corticosteroids in the treatment of pulmonary disease. In *Steroid Therapy*. Edited by D. L. Azarnoff. Philadelphia, W. B. Saunders, 1975, pp. 287–312.

230. C. A. Ribaudo and W. J. Grace, Pulmonary aspiration, *Amer. J. Med.*, **50**: 77–88 (1971).

231. J. H. Christy, Treatment of gram-negative shock, *Amer. J. Med.*, **50**:77–88 (1971).

231a. J. Schumer, Steroids in the treatment of clinical septic shock, *Ann. Surg.*, **184**:333–341 (1976).

232. T. M. Glenn and A. M. Lefer, Anti-toxic action of methylprednisolone in hemorrhagic shock, *Eur. J. Pharmacol.*, **13**:230–238 (1971).

233. J. A. Moylan, M. Birnbaum, A. Katz, and M. A. Everson, Fat emboli syndrome, *J. Trauma*, **16**:341–347 (1976).

234. H. W. Calderwood, J. H. Modell, and B. C. Ruiz, The ineffectiveness of steroid therapy for treatment of fresh-water near-drowning, *Anesthesiology*, **43**:642–650 (1975).

235. R. L. Chapman, J. B. Downs, J. H. Modell, C. I. Hood, The ineffectiveness of steroid therapy in treating aspiration of hydrochloric acid, *Arch. Surg.*, **108**:858–861 (1974).

236. D. W. Lawson, A. J. DeFalco, J. A. Phelphs, B. E. Bradley, and J. E. McClenathan, Corticosteroids as treatment for aspiration of gastric contents: An experimental study, *Surgery*, **59**:845–852 (1966).

237. I. S. Edleman, Mechanisms of action of steroid hormones, *J. Steroid Biochem.*, **6**:147–159 (1975).

238. P. Ahmad, C. A. Fyfe, and A. Mellors, Anti-inflammatory steroids, lysosomal stabilization and parachor, *Can. J. Biochem.*, **53**:1047–1053 (1975).

239. R. G. Dluhy, S. R. Newmark, D. P. Lauler, and G. W. Thorn, Pharmacology and chemistry of adrenal glucocorticoids. In *Steroid Therapy*. Edited by D. L. Azarnoff. Philadelphia, W. B. Saunders, 1975, pp. 1–14.

240. R. B. Zurier and G. Weissman, Anti-immunologic and anti-inflammatory effects of steroid therapy, *Med. Clin. North Am.*, **57**:1295–1307 (1973).

241. G. Weissman, Corticosteroids and membrane stabilization, *Circulation*, 53 (Suppl. 1):1171–1172 (1976).

242. S. Hoffstein, G. Weissman, and A. C. Fox, Lysosomes in myocardial infarction: Studies by means of cytochemistry and subcellular fractionation with observations on the effects of methylprednisolone, *Circulation*, 53 (Suppl. 1):134–139 (1976).

243. R. H. Persellin and L. C. Ku, Effects of steroid hormones on human polymorphonuclear leukocyte lysosomes, *J. Clin. Invest.*, 54:919–925 (1974).

244. S. L. Wiener, R. Weiner, M. Urivetsky, S. Shafer, H. D. Isenger, C. Janov, and E. Meilman, The mechanism of action of a single dose of methylprednisolone on acute inflammation in vivo, *J. Clin. Invest.*, 56:679-689 (1975).

245. L. J. Ignarro and S. Y. Cech, Lysosomal enzyme secretion from human neutrophils mediated by cyclic GMP: Inhibition of cyclic GMP accumulation and neutrophil function by glucocorticosteroids, *J. Cyc. Nucleotide Res.*, 1:283–292 (1975).

246. S. L. Hong and L. Levine, Inhibition of arachidonic acid release from cells as the biochemical action of anti-inflammatory compounds, *Proc. Nat. Acad. Sci. US*, 73:1730–1734 (1976).

247. G. P. Lewis and P. J. Piper, Inhibition of release of prostaglandins as an explanation of some of the actions of anti-inflammatory corticosteroids, *Nature*, 254:308–311 (1975).

248. K. R. Cutroneo and D. F. Counts, Anti-inflammatory steroids and collagen metabolism: Glucocorticoid-mediated alterations of prolyl hydryxylase activity and collagen synthesis, *Mol. Pharmacol.*, 11:632–639 (1975).

249. S. Murota, Y. Koshihara, and S. Tsurufuji, Effects of cortisol and tetrahydrocortisol on the cloned fibroblast derived from rat carrageenin granuloma, *Biochem. Pharmacol.*, 25:1107–1113 (1976).

250. J. W. Wilson, N. B. Ratliff, D. B. Hackel, E. Mikat, and T. Graham, Inflammatory response in reaction of lung to acute hemodynamic injury. In *Immunopathology of Inflammation*. Edited by B. K. Forsher and J. C. Houch. Amsterdam, Excerpta Medica, 1971, pp. 183-196.

251. J. Carr, The effect of anti-inflammatory drugs on increased vascular permeability induced by chemical mediators, *J. Pathol.*, 108:1–14 (1972).

252. Y. Mizuchina, Y. Ishii, and S. Masumoto, Physico-chemical properties of potent anti-inflammatory drugs, *Biochem. Pharmacol.*, 24:1589–1592 (1975).

253. D. M. Aviado, L. V. Bacalzo, and M. A. Belej, Prevention of acute pulmonary insufficiency by oriodictyol, *J. Pharmacol. Exp. Ther.*, 189:157–166 (1974).

254. D. G. McKay. *Disseminated Intravascular Coagulation: An Intermediate Mechanism of Disease.* New York, Harper & Row, 1965.

255. C. A. Owen, Jr., and E. J. Bowie, Chronic intravascular coagulation syndromes: A summary, *Mayo Clin. Proc.*, 49:673–679 (1974).

256. J. F. Mustard and M. A. Packham, Factors influencing platelet function: Adhesion, release and aggregation, *Pharmacol. Rev.*, **22**:97–187 (1970).

257. N. Doba and D. J. Reis, Acute fulminating neurogenic hypertension produced by brainstem lesions in the rat, *Circ. Res.*, **32**:584–593 (1973).

258. G. Moss, Shock lung: A disorder of the central nervous system? *Hosp. Pract.*, **9**:77–86 (1974).

259. O. Kjell, Collagenase and elastase released during peritonitis are complexed by plasma protease inhibitors, *Surgery*, **79**:652–657 (1976).

260. K. H. Kilburn, A. R. Dowell, and P. C. Pratt, Morphological and biochemical assessment of papain-induced emphysema, *Arch. Intern. Med.*, **127**:884–890 (1971).

261. A. G. Maran and F. Kueppers, Pulmonary arteriovenous differences in serum antiprotease activity during experimental pneumonitis, *Amer. Rev. Resp. Dis.*, **112**:527–534 (1975).

262. G. Feinstein, C. J. Malemud, and A. Janoff, The inhibition of human leukocyte elastase and chymotrypsin-like protease by elastatinal and chymostatin, *Biochim. Biophys. Acta*, **429**:925–932 (1976).

263. J. F. Murray, Conference report: Mechanisms of acute respiratory failure, *Amer. Rev. Respir. Dis.*, **115**:1071–1078 (1977).

AUTHOR INDEX

A

Aarseth, P., 82[33], *94*

Aberg, T., 458[77], *468*

Abildskov, J. A., 361[150], 362 [150], *374*

Abrams, M. E., 311[123], *320*

Acevedo, T. C., 303, *320*

Adams, S., 81[25], *93*

Adamson, I. Y. R., 296[94,95], *319*

Adamson, J. S., 185[25], *223*

Affifi, A. A., 357, *373*

Agostini, E., 135, 138[44], *162*, 170[10,11,12], *181*, 241[35], *271*

Ahmad, P., 505[238], *523*

Ahmed, S. S., 337[84], 340[84], *370*

Aikin, B. S., 478[48], *511*

Alden, C., 453[49], *467*

Alderman, E. L., 400[47], *406*

Aldridge, C. F., 490[141], 491[141], *517*

Alexander, J., 458[76], *468*

Alexander, R. A., 485[122], *516*

Allen, J., 249[70], *273*

Allison, A. C., 478[43,57], *511, 512*

Ames, A., III, 221[141], *230*

Amluwalia, B., 458[85], *468*

Amsterdam, E. A., 497[176,177,178], 500[177], *520*

Anastasi, J., 482[75], *513*

Ancheta, O., 297[102], *319*

Andres, G. A., 483[95], 485[95], *514*

Andreucci, V., 247[64], *273*

Anggard, E., 262[103], *275*

Antal, J., 390[29], 394[29], *405*

Anthonisen, N. R., 428[19], *434*

Anthonisen, P., 335, *370*

Anton, A., 458[74], *468*

Antoniazzi, E., 387, *404*

Aoki, V., 448[35], 463[35], *466*

Aravanis, C., 389[27], *405*

Areskog, N. H., 283[57], *317*

Argano, B., 390[30], 393[31], 395 [38], *405, 406*

Arias-Stella, J., 439[16], 451[16], 453[16], 455[16], *465*

Armstrong, J. B., 408[14], *420*

Aronson, S. B., 280[21], *315*

527

SUBJECT INDEX